VOLUME **2**

DISEASE CONTROL PRIORITIES • THIRD EDITION

Reproductive, Maternal, Newborn, and Child Health

DISEASE CONTROL PRIORITIES • THIRD EDITION

Series Editors

Dean T. Jamison
Rachel Nugent
Hellen Gelband
Susan Horton
Prabhat Jha
Ramanan Laxminarayan
Charles N. Mock

Volumes in the Series

Essential Surgery
Reproductive, Maternal, Newborn, and Child Health
Cancer
Mental, Neurological, and Substance Use Disorders
Cardiovascular, Respiratory, and Related Disorders
HIV/AIDS, STIs, Tuberculosis, and Malaria
Injury Prevention and Environmental Health
Child and Adolescent Development
Disease Control Priorities: Improving Health and Reducing Poverty

DISEASE CONTROL PRIORITIES

Budgets constrain choices. Policy analysis helps decision makers achieve the greatest value from limited available resources. In 1993, the World Bank published *Disease Control Priorities in Developing Countries* (*DCP1*), an attempt to systematically assess the cost-effectiveness (value for money) of interventions that would address the major sources of disease burden in low- and middle-income countries. The World Bank's 1993 *World Development Report* on health drew heavily on *DCP1*'s findings to conclude that specific interventions against noncommunicable diseases were cost-effective, even in environments in which substantial burdens of infection and undernutrition persisted.

DCP2, published in 2006, updated and extended *DCP1* in several aspects, including explicit consideration of the implications for health systems of expanded intervention coverage. One way that health systems expand intervention coverage is through selected platforms that deliver interventions that require similar logistics but deliver interventions from different packages of conceptually related interventions, for example, against cardiovascular disease. Platforms often provide a more natural unit for investment than do individual interventions. Analysis of the costs of packages and platforms—and of the health improvements they can generate in given epidemiological environments—can help to guide health system investments and development.

DCP3 differs importantly from *DCP1* and *DCP2* by extending and consolidating the concepts of platforms and packages and by offering explicit consideration of the financial risk protection objective of health systems. In populations lacking access to health insurance or prepaid care, medical expenses that are high relative to income can be impoverishing. Where incomes are low, seemingly inexpensive medical procedures can have catastrophic financial effects. *DCP3* offers an approach to explicitly include financial protection as well as the distribution across income groups of financial and health outcomes resulting from policies (for example, public finance) to increase intervention uptake. The task in all of the *DCP* volumes has been to combine the available science about interventions implemented in very specific locales and under very specific conditions with informed judgment to reach reasonable conclusions about the impact of intervention mixes in diverse environments. *DCP3*'s broad aim is to delineate essential intervention packages and their related delivery platforms to assist decision makers in allocating often tightly constrained budgets so that health system objectives are maximally achieved.

DCP3's nine volumes are being published in 2015 and 2016 in an environment in which serious discussion continues about quantifying the Sustainable Development Goal (SDG) for health. *DCP3*'s analyses are well-placed to assist in choosing the means to attain the health SDG and assessing the related costs. Only when these volumes, and the analytic efforts on which they are based, are completed will we be able to explore SDG-related and other broad policy conclusions and generalizations. The final *DCP3* volume will report those conclusions. Each individual volume will provide valuable, specific policy analyses on the full range of interventions, packages, and policies relevant to its health topic.

More than 500 individuals and multiple institutions have contributed to *DCP3*. We convey our acknowledgments elsewhere in this volume. Here we express our particular gratitude to the Bill & Melinda Gates Foundation for its sustained financial support, to the InterAcademy Medical Panel (and its U.S. affiliate, the Institute of Medicine of the National Academy of Medicine), and to the External and Corporate Relations Publishing and Knowledge division of the World Bank. Each played a critical role in this effort.

Dean T. Jamison
Rachel Nugent
Hellen Gelband
Susan Horton
Prabhat Jha
Ramanan Laxminarayan
Charles N. Mock

VOLUME **2**

DISEASE CONTROL PRIORITIES • THIRD EDITION

Reproductive, Maternal, Newborn, and Child Health

EDITORS

Robert E. Black
Ramanan Laxminarayan
Marleen Temmerman
Neff Walker

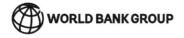 **WORLD BANK GROUP**

ISBNs and DOIs:

Softcover:

ISBN: 978-1-4648-0348-2
ISBN (electronic): 978-1-4648-0368-0
DOI: 10.1596/978-1-4648-0348-2

Hardcover:

ISBN: 978-1-4648-0347-5

DOI: 10.1596/978-1-4648-0347-5

Cover photo: Foune Kouyate waits to vaccinate her baby, Kadidia Goulibaly, at the Centre De Sante Communautaire De Banconi (ASACOBA), a health clinic in Bamako, Mali, on November 4, 2013. © Dominic Chavez/World Bank. Further permission required for reuse.
Cover and interior design: Debra Naylor, Naylor Design, Washington, DC.

Library of Congress Cataloging-in-Publication Data
Names: Black, Robert E., editor. | Laxminarayan, Ramanan, editor. | Temmerman, Marleen, editor. | Walker, Neff, editor.
Title: Reproductive, maternal, newborn, and child health / volume editors, Robert Black, Ramanan Laxminarayan,
   Marleen Temmerman, Neff Walker.
Other titles: Disease control priorities ; v. 2.
Description: Washington, DC : World Bank, 2016. | Series: Disease control priorities ; volume 2 | Includes bibliographical
   references and index.
Identifiers: LCCN 2015038391| ISBN 9781464803475 (hc : alk. paper) | ISBN 9781464803482 (alk. paper) |
   ISBN 9781464803680 (e-book)
Subjects: | MESH: Child Welfare. | Maternal Welfare. | Reproductive Health. | Child Mortality. | Developing Countries. |
   Infant Mortality.
Classification: LCC RG940 | NLM WA 395 | DDC 362.1982--dc23
LC record available at http://lccn.loc.gov/2015038391

Contents

Foreword

When I became the Deputy Director of the Child Survival Partnership in 2004, I knew the task at hand was a challenging one. We were only four years into the Millennium Development Goals (MDGs), but we already knew that moving the needle on maternal and child survival would take more headway and greater advances. Since then, and particularly since 2010, we have accelerated progress in an unprecedented manner, mobilized actors and partners, and improved our way of working.

We have undergone an extraordinary transformation, halving maternal and child mortality under the MDGs. As we transition to the Sustainable Development Goals (SDGs), we are in a much better position to achieve the global and equitable progress we seek for all people. Goal 3 of the 17 SDGs is "to ensure healthy lives and promote well-being for all at all ages." This broad goal embraces the unfinished agenda of the MDGs and goes beyond—to virtually end preventable maternal, newborn, and child deaths and to improve access to sexual and reproductive health, as well as access to medicines and vaccines. By moving toward this goal, we are working to protect the future and well-being of those closest to us: our mothers, children, and communities.

The 2010–15 Global Strategy for Women's and Children's Health brought together hundreds of partners around the Every Woman Every Child movement to jointly achieve the ambitious goals for maternal and child health. Building on this progress, the United Nations (UN) Secretary-General, in September 2015, launched a follow-up roadmap for 2016–30 at the UN General Assembly, The Global Strategy for Women's, Children's, and Adolescents' Health. The new strategy aligns fully with the SDGs, embracing the vision of a future where we reach the highest attainable standard of health for all women, children, and adolescents. A new funding mechanism, The Global Financing Facility in Support of Every Woman, Every Child, aims to bring together existing and new sources of financing for "smart, scaled, and sustainable financing" to accelerate efforts to end preventable maternal, newborn, and child deaths by 2030.

Strategy, financing, and delivery of services need to be guided by the best available scientific knowledge on the efficacy of interventions and the effectiveness of programs. This volume of the *Disease Control Priorities*, third edition (*DCP3*) series, *Reproductive, Maternal, Newborn, and Child Health*, provides this rigorous knowledge base. Readers now have at their fingertips the most relevant technical information on which interventions, programs, service delivery platforms, and policies can best help all to reach the ambitious Global Goal 3 targets—maternal mortality rates lower than 70 maternal deaths per 100,000 live births, neonatal mortality rates of 9 per 1,000 live births, and stillbirth rates of 9 per 1,000 total births. It is a source of great pride to know that my WHO team, led by Professor Dr. Marleen Temmerman, Director of the Department of Reproductive Health and Research, contributed to this work. My team will continue its efforts to end preventable mortality worldwide and to achieve the three broad goals embraced by the new Global Strategy—survive, thrive, and transform.

We all have a role to play as we put this Global Strategy into practice in every corner of the globe. We need everyone's continued engagement, support, and commitments. We have the knowledge, the tools, and the will. A transformation by 2030 is within our reach.

Dr. Flavia Bustreo
Assistant Director-General, Family, Women, and Children's Health, World Health Organization

Preface

Reproductive, maternal, newborn, and child health (RMNCH) encompasses health concerns spanning the life course from adolescent girls to women before and during pregnancy to newborns and older children. In recent years, it has been recognized that appropriately addressing these concerns requires organizing services in a continuum of care that encompasses these stages in the life course. The rationale for the organization of the RMNCH volume is based on the link between interventions at each stage and health effects at that stage and future stages, and consequently the need to deliver integrated, preventive, and therapeutic interventions for mothers and children.

In considering interventions that span the RMNCH continuum, *DCP3* has departed from the disease-specific framing of interventions that was followed in previous editions. *DCP1*, published in 1993, largely focused on individual diseases and conditions with those regarding RNMCH. *DCP1* referred to the "unfinished agenda" that included major diseases, such as acute respiratory infection, diarrhea, malaria, and poliomyelitis, as well as malnutrition, HIV/AIDS and sexually transmitted infections, "excess fertility," and maternal and perinatal health, but it did not include the broader issue of neonatal health. In *DCP2*, published in 2006, nine of the 73 chapters were on RMNCH, reflecting the broader scope of that edition including a greater emphasis on noncommunicable diseases, health system strengthening, and cross-cutting issues.

The "unfinished agenda" of RMNCH continues to be as important today as it was in 1993. This volume contains 19 chapters that range from descriptions of the current levels and causes of reproductive ill health, maternal and child morbidity and mortality, undernutrition, and compromised child development, to consideration of preventive and therapeutic interventions, as well as cost-effectiveness of these interventions and health system considerations for their implementation. The volume gives particular attention to the efficient and effective use of delivery platforms to provide packages of interventions—a framing that supports country decision-making for universal health care. Despite our objective of covering a broad range of RMNCH topics in this volume, some topics of relevance to women and children were found to fit better in other volumes. These include surgical conditions, cancer, mental and developmental disorders, HIV/AIDS and sexually transmitted infections, malaria, injuries, and adolescent health and development.

RMNCH interventions have received significant attention in low- and middle-income countries and among international donors. The reasons for this include the high burden of disease and the evidence that many efficacious and cost-effective interventions are available to dramatically reduce the burden of ill health. The promulgation of the Millennium Development Goals, with their strong focus on RMNCH concerns, gave further impetus to implementation of the proven interventions. It has been important that review of the evidence for new interventions and program approaches has continued through academic journals such as *The Lancet*, *DCP*, and other critical exercises that have identified the needs and opportunities in RMNCH. Substantial success has been achieved with unprecedented declines in maternal and child mortality and fertility; however, problems remain, including large inequities among and within low- and middle-income countries in health services and outcomes.

We intend for this volume to provide an update of the evidence and help to shape what can be implemented in integrated packages of services for reproductive health, maternal and newborn health, and child health to achieve the new Sustainable Development Goals. In addition, we hope that consideration of delivery of interventions with greatest coverage and equity will prioritize strengthening of the three interlinked platforms: communities, primary health centers, and hospitals. We now have the knowledge and means to fully address the unfinished agenda of RMNCH and must not miss the opportunity and the obligation to act.

We thank the following individuals who provided valuable assistance and comments in the development of this volume: Brianne Adderley, Kristen Danforth, Alex Ergo, Victoria Fan, Mary Fisk, Glenda Gray, Rajat Khosla, Nancy Lammers, Rachel Nugent, Rumit Pancholi, Helen Pitchik, Carlos Rossel, Lale Say, Rachel Upton, Kelsey Walters, and Gavin Yamey. We also thank the RMNCH Authors Group for the preparation of the chapters and the reviewers organized by the National Academy of Medicine (formerly the Institute of Medicine).

Robert E. Black
Ramanan Laxminarayan
Marleen Temmerman
Neff Walker

Abbreviations

ACT	artemisinin-based combination therapy
AFHS	Adolescent Friendly Health Services
ANC	antenatal care
ARI	acute respiratory infection
ART	antiretroviral therapy
ASHA	accredited social health activist
BCG	Bacille Calmette-Guérin
BEP	balanced protein energy
BES	balanced energy and protein supplementation
BF	breastfeeding
BMI	body mass index
CBD	community-based distribution
CCM	community case management
CCT	conditional cash transfer
CEA	cost-effectiveness analysis
CF	complementary feeding
CFR	case fatality rate
CHERG	Child Health Epidemiology Reference Group
CHV	community health volunteer
CHW	community health worker
CI	confidence interval
CLTS	Community-Led Total Sanitation
CMAM	community-based management of acute malnutrition
CQI	continuous quality improvement
CRS	congenital rubella syndrome
CS	cesarean section
CSB	corn-soy blend
CYP	couple-years of protection
DALY	disability-adjusted life year
DHS	demographic and health survey
DPT	diphtheria, pertussis, and tetanus
DTP3	third dose of DTP
EBF	exclusive breastfeeding
ECEA	extended cost-effectiveness analysis
ECV	external cephalic version
EED	environmental enteric dysfunction

EPI	Expanded Program on Immunization
FBF	fortified blended flour
FRP	financial risk protection
GAM	global acute malnutrition
Gavi	Global Alliance for Vaccines and Immunization
GBS	Group B streptococcus
GDP	gross domestic product
GNI	gross national income
HAZ	height-for-age Z-score
HBNC	home-based neonatal care
HEP	health extension program
HEW	health extension worker
HiB	*Haemophilus influenzae* B
HICs	high-income countries
HIV	human immunodeficiency virus
HR	hazard ratio
HSV-2	herpes simplex virus-2
IAP	intrapartum antibiotic prophylaxis
iCCM	Integrated Community Case Management
ICD	International Classification of Diseases
ICPD	International Conference on Population and Development
IDA	iron deficiency anemia
IIV	inactivated influenza vaccine
IMCI	Integrated Management of Childhood Illness
IMNCI	Integrated Management of Neonatal and Childhood Illness
IMPAC	Integrated Management in Pregnancy and Childcare
IPT	intermittent preventive treatment
ITN	insecticide-treated bednet
IU	international unit
IUD	intrauterine device
IUGR	intrauterine growth restriction
IYCF	infant and young child feeding
JE	Japanese encephalitis
LBW	low birth weight
LHWs	Lady Health Workers
LICs	low-income countries
LiST	Lives Saved Tool
LMICs	low- and middle-income countries
LNS	lipid-based nutrient supplement
LRI	lower respiratory tract infections
LYS	life-year saved
MAM	moderate acute malnutrition
MD	mean difference
MDG	Millennium Development Goal
MgSO$_4$	magnesium sulphate
MICs	middle-income countries
MMR	maternal mortality ratio
MNP	multiple micronutrient powder
MUAC	mid-upper arm circumference
NIMS	Nutrition Impact Model Study
NMR	newborn mortality rate
NPV	net present value
OHT	One Health Tool

OOP	out-of-pocket
OPV	oral polio vaccine
ORS	oral rehydration solution
PBF	performance-based financing
PCV	pneumococcal conjugate vaccination
PPH	postpartum hemorrhage
PUFA	polyunsaturated fatty acids
QALY	quality-adjusted life year
RCT	randomized controlled trial
RDS	respiratory distress syndrome
RDT	rapid diagnostic test
RMNCH	reproductive, maternal, newborn, and child health
RR	relative risk
RUF	ready-to-use food
RUSF	ready-to-use supplementary food
RUTF	ready-to-use therapeutic food
SAM	severe acute malnutrition
SFP	supplementary feeding program
SGA	small for gestational age
STI	sexually transmitted infection
TFC	therapeutic feeding center
TFR	total fertility rate
UCTs	unconditional cash transfers
UHC	universal health coverage
UMICs	upper-middle-income countries
UN	United Nations
UNICEF	United Nations Children's Fund
UPF	universal public finance
USAID	United States Agency for International Development
VLY	value of a life-year saved
WASH	Water, sanitation, and hygiene
WHO	World Health Organization
WHZ	weight-for-height z-score
YICSSG	Young Infants Clinical Signs Study Group

Chapter 1

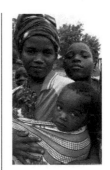

Reproductive, Maternal, Newborn, and Child Health: Key Messages of This Volume

Robert E. Black, Neff Walker, Ramanan Laxminarayan, and Marleen Temmerman

VOLUME SUMMARY

Reproductive, Maternal, Newborn, and Child Health (RMNCH) covers the health concerns and interventions across the life course involving women before and during pregnancy; newborns, that is, the first 28 days of life; and children to their fifth birthday. The volume identifies 61 essential interventions and because of the timing of their delivery in the life course, groups them into three packages: 18 for reproductive health, 30 for maternal and newborn health, and 13 for child health, although some interventions, such as vaccines for immunization, have multiple components. The volume considers the health system needs for implementing these interventions in health service platforms in communities, in primary health centers, and in hospitals and the cost-effectiveness of interventions for which data are available. This chapter summarizes the volume and considers the potential impact and cost of scaling up proven interventions to reduce maternal, newborn, and child deaths and stillbirths.

- The annual number of global maternal and child deaths has dropped markedly in the past 25 years, yet the rate of reduction in many countries has been too slow to achieve Millennium Development Goals 4 and 5 by 2015.

- Progress could be accelerated by scaling up integrated packages of essential interventions across the continuum of care for RMNCH. These interventions are highly cost-effective and result in benefit-cost ratios of 7–11 to 2035 (net present value in U.S. dollars of benefits to costs).
- Scaling up all interventions in the packages of maternal and newborn health, plus folic acid before pregnancy, and child health from the existing rate of coverage to 90 percent would avert 149,000 maternal deaths; 849,000 stillbirths; 1,498,000 neonatal deaths; and 1,515,000 child deaths, representing the impact in 2015 at current rates of pregnancy, birth, and mortality.
- The reproductive health package is particularly important for providing contraceptive services. Addressing 90 percent of unmet need in 2015 would reduce annual births by almost 28 million, which would consequently prevent 67,000 maternal deaths; 440,000 neonatal deaths; 473,000 child deaths; and 564,000 stillbirths from avoided pregnancies.
- Individual interventions that have the highest impact on deaths are provision of contraception; management of labor and delivery; care of preterm births; treatment of severe infectious diseases, including pneumonia, diarrhea, malaria, and neonatal sepsis; and management of severe acute malnutrition.

Corresponding author: Robert E. Black, Johns Hopkins Bloomberg School of Public Health, rblack1@jhu.edu.

- The three packages of reproductive, maternal and new-born, and child health interventions have an annual incremental cost of US$6.2 billion in low-income countries, US$12.4 billion in lower-middle-income countries, and US$8.0 billion in upper-middle-income countries. The average per capita cost of these three packages is US$6.7, US$4.7, and US$3.9 in low-, lower-middle-, and upper-middle-income countries, respectively.
- These packages of interventions are delivered through three key service platforms: community workers and health posts, primary health centers, and hospitals (first level and referral). Community and primary health center platforms could reduce 77 percent of maternal, newborn, and child deaths and stillbirths that are preventable by these essential interventions in the maternal and newborn health and child health packages. Hospitals contribute the remaining averted deaths through more advanced management of complicated pregnancies and deliveries, severe infectious diseases, and malnutrition in these calculations. Contraceptive services are considered to be almost entirely delivered at primary health centers.
- Weaknesses in RMNCH delivery platforms, including limited access to care, poor quality of services, and shortages of health workers or medicines, are a major barrier to improving RMNCH outcomes. To overcome these weaknesses and expand access to RMNCH services, innovative delivery approaches are being deployed, such as task-shifting to other cadres of workers, household visitation, community mobilization and service delivery, financial incentives for households and health workers, and supervision and accreditation.

INTRODUCTION

Reproductive, maternal, newborn, and child health (RMNCH) has been a priority for both governments and civil society in low- and middle-income countries (LMICs). This priority was affirmed by world leaders in the Millennium Development Goals (MDGs) that called for countries to reduce child mortality by 67 percent and maternal mortality by 75 percent between 1990 and 2015. Although substantial progress on these targets has been made, few countries achieved the needed reductions. The United Nations (UN) Secretary-General's Global Strategy for Women's and Children's Health, launched in 2010 and expanded in 2015 to include adolescents, is an indication of the continued global commitment to the survival and well-being of women and children (Ban 2010). Annual official development assistance for maternal, newborn, and

child health has increased from US$2.7 billion in 2003 to US$8.3 billion in 2012, when there was an additional US$4.5 billion for reproductive health (Arregoces and others 2015). A continued focus on RMNCH is needed to address the remaining considerable burden of disease in LMICs from unwanted pregnancies; high maternal, newborn, and child mortality and stillbirths; high rates of undernutrition; frequent communicable and non-communicable diseases; and loss of human capacity. Cost-effective interventions are available and can be implemented at high coverage in LMICs to greatly reduce these problems at an affordable cost.

RMNCH encompasses health problems across the life course from adolescent girls and women before and during pregnancy and delivery, to newborns and children. An important conceptual framework is the continuum-of-care approach in two dimensions. One dimension recognizes the links from mother to child and the need for health services across the stages of the life course. The other is the delivery of integrated preventive and therapeutic health interventions through service platforms ranging from the community to the primary health center and the hospital.

This volume presents the levels and trends of RMNCH indicators, proven interventions for prevention of mortality, costs of these interventions and potential health service delivery platforms, and system innovations. Other volumes in the third edition of *Disease Control Priorities* also cover topics of importance to women and children that are related to the RMNCH health services packages (box 1.1). These topics include the following:

- Trauma care; obstetric surgery; obstetric fistula; surgery for family planning, abortion, and postabortion care; and surgery for congenital anomalies (Volume 1, *Essential Surgery*)
- Breast cancer, cervical cancer and precancer, childhood cancer, and cancer pain relief (Volume 3, *Cancer*)
- Childhood mental and developmental disorders (Volume 4, *Mental, Neurological, and Substance Use Disorders*)
- Cardiovascular and respiratory disorders (Volume 5, *Cardiovascular, Respiratory, and Related Disorders*)
- HIV/AIDS and other sexually transmitted infections, tuberculosis, and malaria (Volume 6, *HIV/AIDS, STIs, Tuberculosis, and Malaria*)
- Road traffic injury and interpersonal violence (Volume 7, *Injury Prevention and Environmental Health*)
- Child (older than five years) and adolescent development (the subject of the entire Volume 8, *Child and Adolescent Development*).

Box 1.1

From the Series Editors of *Disease Control Priorities*, Third Edition

Budgets constrain choices. Policy analysis helps decision makers achieve the greatest value from limited available resources. In 1993, the World Bank published *Disease Control Priorities in Developing Countries* (*DCP1*), an attempt to systematically assess the cost-effectiveness (value for money) of interventions that would address the major sources of disease burden in low- and middle-income countries (Jamison and others 1993). The World Bank's 1993 *World Development Report* on health drew heavily on *DCP1*'s findings to conclude that specific interventions against noncommunicable diseases were cost-effective, even in environments in which substantial burdens of infection and undernutrition persist (World Bank 1993).

DCP2, published in 2006, updated and extended *DCP1* in several respects, including explicit consideration of the implications for health systems of expanded intervention coverage (Jamison and others 2006). One way that health systems expand intervention coverage is through selected platforms that deliver interventions that require similar logistics but address heterogeneous health problems. Platforms often provide a more natural unit for investment than do individual interventions, and conventional health economics has offered little understanding of how to make choices across platforms. Analysis of the costs of packages and platforms—and of the health improvements they can generate in given epidemiological environments—can help guide health system investments and development.

The third edition is being completed. *DCP3* differs substantively from *DCP1* and *DCP2* by extending and consolidating the concepts of platforms and packages and by offering explicit consideration of the financial-risk-protection objective of health systems. In populations lacking access to health insurance or prepaid care, medical expenses that are high relative to income can be impoverishing. Where incomes are low, seemingly inexpensive medical procedures can have catastrophic financial consequences. *DCP3*

offers an approach that explicitly includes financial protection as well as the distribution across income groups of financial and health outcomes resulting from policies (for example, public finance) to increase intervention uptake (Verguet, Laxminarayan, and Jamison 2015). The task in all the volumes has been to combine the available science about interventions implemented in very specific locales and under very specific conditions with informed judgment to reach reasonable conclusions about the impact of intervention mixes in diverse environments. *DCP3*'s broad aim is to delineate essential intervention packages—such as the essential packages in this volume—and their related delivery platforms. This information will assist decision makers in allocating often tightly constrained budgets so that health system objectives are maximally achieved.

DCP3's nine volumes are being published in 2015 and 2016 in an environment in which serious discussion continues about quantifying the sustainable development goal (SDG) for health (United Nations 2015). *DCP3*'s analyses are well placed to assist in choosing the means to attain the health SDG and assessing the related costs. Only when these volumes, and the analytic efforts on which they are based, are completed will we be able to explore SDG-related and other broad policy conclusions and generalizations. The final *DCP3* volume will report those conclusions. Each individual volume will provide valuable specific policy analyses on the full range of interventions, packages, and policies relevant to its health topic.

Dean T. Jamison

Rachel Nugent

Hellen Gelband

Susan Horton

Prabhat Jha

Ramanan Laxminarayan

Charles N. Mock

LEVELS AND TRENDS IN RMNCH INDICATORS

Reproductive Health

Poor reproductive health outcomes for women and their children may result from a broad spectrum of morbid conditions and adverse circumstances and risk factors, such as unsafe sex leading to unwanted pregnancies and sexually transmitted infections, as well as violence against women and girls. Because these are sensitive matters and are often related to gender inequality in a cultural and social context, measuring and quantifying the burden of these conditions and risk factors remains a challenge. This *DCP3* volume focuses on four conditions and risk factors that have significant impacts on reproductive health: unwanted pregnancies, unsafe abortions, infertility, and violence against women.

In 2015, 12 percent of married or in-union women of reproductive age worldwide want to delay or avoid pregnancy but are not using any method of contraception. For example, women in Sub-Saharan Africa are twice as likely to have an unmet need for family planning compared with the rest of the world (UN 2015). The total fertility rate remains very high in many countries in Sub-Saharan Africa (map 1.1, panel a).

An estimated 74 million unintended pregnancies occurred in LMICs in 2012 (Sedgh, Singh, and Hussain 2014). Some of these ended by unsafe abortion, a major cause of maternal morbidity and mortality (Singh, Sedgh, and Hussain 2010). About 8.5 million women worldwide suffer complications from unsafe abortions annually (Singh, Darroch, and Ashford 2014). Regardless of legal status or policies on abortion, it can be fairly stated that preventing unsafe abortion is critical and that effective programming for reproductive health needs should be uncoupled from laws on the legal status of abortion. The large effects of reducing unwanted pregnancies on maternal, neonatal, and child deaths and stillbirths are estimated in a later section of this chapter.

Another hidden burden of reproductive health is infertility. In 2010, an estimated 48.5 million women were involuntarily childless as a result of male or female infertility, or both. This is especially concerning in LMICs, where infertility can lead to severe stigmatization, economic deprivation and denial of inheritance, divorce, and social isolation (Chachamovich and others 2010; Cui 2010).

As an extreme manifestation of social and gender inequality, violence against women and girls is often a hidden problem, with serious health consequences. Women exposed to intimate partner violence are more likely to have poor pregnancy outcomes; acquire HIV

Map 1.1 Total Fertility, Maternal Mortality Ratios, and Under-Five Mortality Rates by Country, 2015

a. Total Fertility (children per woman) 2010–15

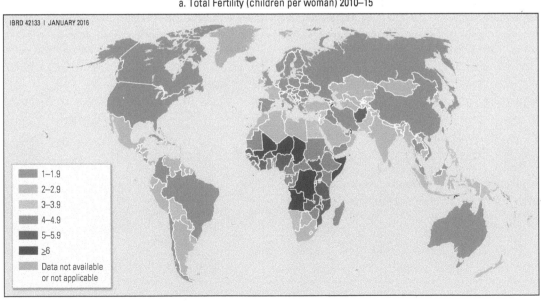

Source: Based on UNPD 2015 (http://esa.un.org/unpd/wpp); map re-created based on WHO 2015.

map continues next page

Map 1.1 Total Fertility, Maternal Mortality Ratios, and Under-Five Mortality Rates by Country, 2015 (continued)

b. Maternal Mortality Ratios, 2015

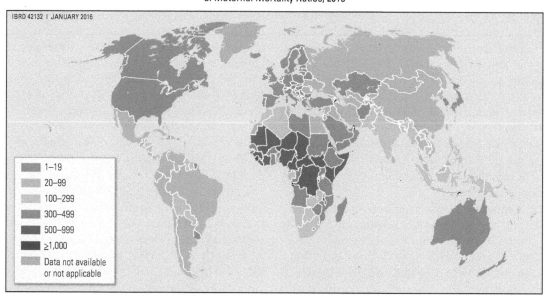

Source: Based on WHO 2015; map re-created based on WHO 2015.

c. Under-Five Mortality per 1,000 Live Births, 2015

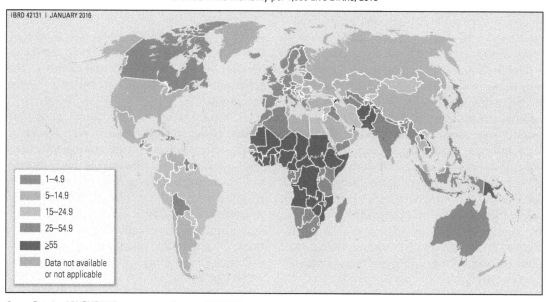

Source: Based on UN IGME 2015; map re-created based on WHO 2015.

(in some regions), syphilis, chlamydia, or gonorrhea; experience depression; or have alcohol abuse disorders (WHO, Department of Reproductive Health and Research, London School of Hygiene and Tropical Medicine, and South African Medical Research Council 2013). Studies have found between 3 percent and 31 percent of women report partner violence during pregnancy (Devries and others 2010). Worldwide, 30 percent of women age 15–49 years in a relationship experience physical or sexual violence by their intimate partner at some point in their lives (WHO, Department of Reproductive Health and Research, London School of Hygiene and Tropical Medicine, and South African Medical Research Council 2013). Tragically, many women do not seek help following these events.

Maternal Mortality and Morbidity

Globally, the total number of maternal deaths decreased by 43 percent, from 532,000 in 1990 to 303,000 in 2015, and the global maternal mortality ratio declined by 44 percent, from 385 maternal deaths per 100,000 live births in 1990 to 216 in 2015 (Alkema and others 2015). LMICs continue to account for 99 percent (302,000 out of 303,000) of global maternal deaths. The highest risks of maternal death are in countries in South Asia and Sub-Saharan Africa (map 1.1, panel b). Thus, while considerable progress has been made, particularly in recent years, the goal of reducing maternal mortality by 75 percent by 2015 was not met.

The risk of maternal death has two components: the risk of getting pregnant, which is a risk related to fertility and its control or lack of control; and the risk of developing a complication and dying while pregnant, in labor, or postpartum. Chapter 3 of this volume, on maternal morbidity and mortality, focuses on the risk during pregnancy, delivery, and postpartum, which is highest at the time of delivery (Filippi and others 2016).

The most important causes of maternal death are obstetric hemorrhage, hypertension, abortion, and sepsis (figure 1.1, panel a). The overall proportion of HIV-related maternal deaths is highest in Sub-Saharan Africa (Say and others 2014). Most maternal deaths do not have well-defined medical causes, and given that many occur in the community rather than health facilities, determining the cause is challenging. Deaths due to abortive outcomes (for example, ectopic pregnancy, induced abortion, and miscarriage), obstructed labor, and indirect causes are of considerable programmatic interest, but are particularly difficult to capture because of poor reporting resulting from lack of knowledge and the sensitive nature of abortion and maternal deaths in facilities. Deaths due to abortion are often not reported to avoid stigma. Despite the availability of proven interventions, the persistence of deaths due to hemorrhage and hypertension are particularly concerning.

The common causes of maternal morbidity in the community vary by region; these causes include anemia, preexisting hypertension or diabetes, depression, and other mental health conditions. Prolonged and obstructed labor is associated with a high burden of morbidity and disability, including that due to obstetric fistula. The true extent of maternal morbidity is not known because of difficulties in definition and measurement. The World Health Organization (WHO) is currently working with partners to develop standard definitions and tools to close this gap.

Perinatal, Neonatal, and Child Mortality

The under-five mortality rate (U5MR), the probability of dying between a live birth and the fifth birthday, is one of the most important measures of the health of a population. Although MDG 4 was not achieved globally, some high-mortality countries in South Asia and Sub-Saharan Africa have achieved this target (Afnan-Holmes and others 2015; Amouzou and others 2012). The U5MR remains very high, especially in many countries in Sub-Saharan Africa (map 1.1, panel c).

The U5MR in 2015 is 42.5 per 1,000 live births, a decline from 90.6 per 1,000 live births in 1990 (You and others 2015). The U5MR fell by half or more from 1990 to 2015 in all world regions. The UN estimates that only 24 of 82 low- or lower-middle-income countries achieved the MDG 4 target (You and others 2015). However, it is important to note that compared with historical trends, the reduction of U5MR has accelerated since 2000, when the MDGs were approved (You and others 2015).

The neonatal mortality rate is now widely followed as an important population health measure because a large proportion (45 percent in 2015) of the deaths in children under age five years occurs in the first month of life. In addition, the rate of stillbirths has received more attention with the recognition of the large number of viable fetuses (2.6 million in 2015) who die after 28 weeks of gestation, often at the time of delivery (Blencowe and others 2016).

Of the 5.9 million deaths occurring after a live birth before age five years, pneumonia, diarrhea, and neonatal sepsis or meningitis are the leading infectious causes (figure 1.1, panel b). The leading single cause of child deaths was complications from preterm birth, followed by pneumonia and intrapartum-related complications, formerly known as birth asphyxia. In the next 15 years, with further implementation of proven health interventions, it is anticipated that the infectious causes of death will decline more quickly than noninfectious causes (Liu and others 2014).

The proportion of global live births in Sub-Saharan Africa is projected to increase from 24.9 percent currently to 32.6 percent by 2030 because of the region's high fertility rate compared with other regions. If the current regional trends in child mortality are continued to 2030, global child deaths will fall to 4.4 million (Liu and others 2014). However, because of both the high number of births and high U5MR, Sub-Saharan Africa's share of global child deaths is expected to increase from 49.6 percent to 59.8 percent by 2030.

Figure 1.1 Causes of Maternal and Child Deaths

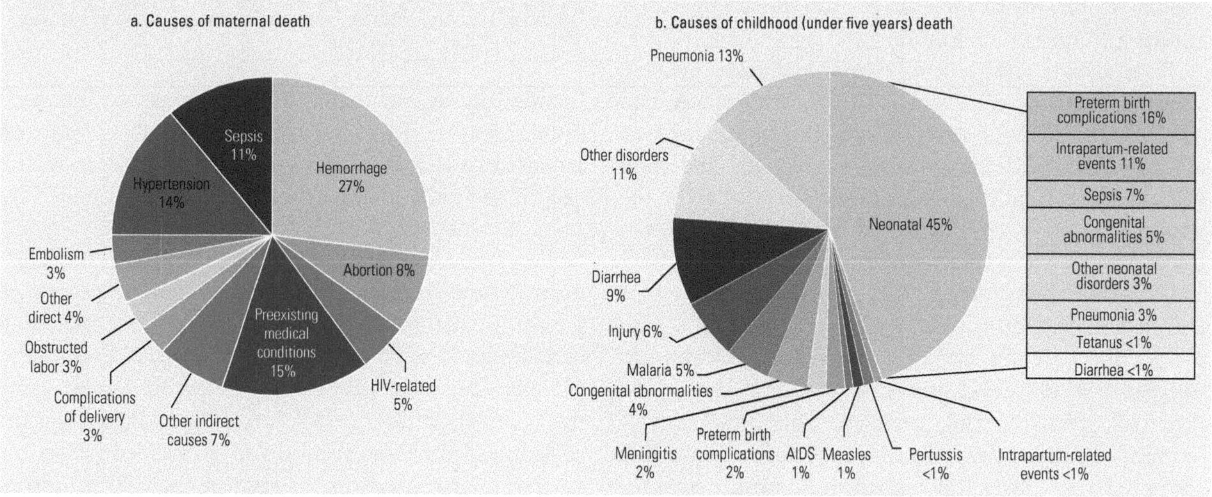

a. Causes of maternal death

- Sepsis 11%
- Hemorrhage 27%
- Hypertension 14%
- Embolism 3%
- Other direct 4%
- Obstructed labor 3%
- Complications of delivery 3%
- Other indirect causes 7%
- Preexisting medical conditions 15%
- Abortion 8%
- HIV-related 5%

Source: Say and others 2014.

b. Causes of childhood (under five years) death

- Pneumonia 13%
- Other disorders 11%
- Neonatal 45%
- Diarrhea 9%
- Injury 6%
- Malaria 5%
- Congenital abnormalities 4%
- Meningitis 2%
- Preterm birth complications 2%
- AIDS 1%
- Measles 1%
- Pertussis <1%
- Intrapartum-related events <1%

- Preterm birth complications 16%
- Intrapartum-related events 11%
- Sepsis 7%
- Congenital abnormalities 5%
- Other neonatal disorders 3%
- Pneumonia 3%
- Tetanus <1%
- Diarrhea <1%

Source: Liu and others 2016.

MATERNAL, FETAL, AND CHILD MALNUTRITION AND EARLY CHILD DEVELOPMENT

Malnutrition includes both undernutrition and the growing problem of overweight, both important problems in women and children under age five years. In women of reproductive age (age 20–49 years), a body mass index (BMI) of less than 18.5 kilograms weight/height in meters squared (kg/m²) is defined as undernutrition or excessive thinness, and a BMI of greater than or equal to 25 kg/m² is considered overweight. The prevalence of maternal undernutrition has fallen from almost 20 percent in Asia and Africa to about 10 percent, which is still too high (Black and others 2013). The prevalence of overweight in women has steadily increased during the same period in all world regions, reaching more than 50 percent in the Americas and in Oceania, 30 percent in Africa, and 20 percent in Asia (Black and others 2013). Deficiencies of iodine, calcium, zinc, iron, and other essential vitamins and minerals are also prevalent and have particular relevance to maternal and fetal health.

Restriction of fetal growth, usually assessed by a low weight for gestational age at birth, is due to poor maternal nutrition and other morbidity, infection, and toxic in-utero exposures (Das and others 2016). Compared to a U.S. birthweight reference, more than a quarter of all live births in LMICs, or 32.4 million babies, were born small-for-gestational age (Black and others 2013). A new international birthweight standard has subsequently been published (Villar and others 2014). Compared with this standard, the estimated global prevalence of small-for-gestational-age births is about one-quarter lower (Kozuki and others 2015). As neonates and infants, these babies have a higher risk of mortality than babies who were appropriate weight for gestational age, and this risk is similar using either the U.S. reference or the new international standard (Kozuki and others 2015). They also have an increased risk of stunted linear growth (Black and others 2013; Christian and others 2013). The risk of mortality with small-for-gestational age birth increases if they are also premature.

Compared with an international growth standard, it was estimated that in 2011 26 percent of children globally had stunted linear growth (height-for-age of less than −2 standard deviations of the growth standard), totaling 165 million children (Black and others 2013). The prevalence of stunting has declined in LMICs since 1990, more in Asia and Latin America than in Africa. Stunting prevalence has declined at similar rates in rural and urban areas but remains higher in rural areas (Stevens, Paciorek, and Finucane 2016). Severe wasting, which was estimated to affect 3 percent, or 19 million, of the world's children in 2011, requires urgent intervention with therapeutic feeding and treatment of concurrent infections (Lenters, Wazny, and Bhutta 2016). Of the micronutrient deficiencies, vitamin A and zinc deficiencies are associated with increased risk of mortality and infectious disease morbidity (Black and others 2013; Das and others 2016). At the same time, overweight (greater than 2 standard deviations of the growth standard weight for height) has steadily increased since 1990 to 7 percent, an increase of more than 50 percent, affecting 43 million children.

Fetal growth restriction, suboptimal breastfeeding, stunting, wasting, and deficiencies of vitamin A and zinc, usually in combination with infectious diseases, are important underlying causes of neonatal and child deaths. These conditions have been estimated to be the underlying causes of 45 percent of deaths in children under age five years (Black and others 2013).

Grantham-McGregor and International Child Development Committee (2007) estimate that a high proportion of the world's surviving children do not reach their developmental potential, based on rates of stunting and poverty. This poor development outcome has numerous causes, including antenatal and postnatal nutrition, exposure to violence, brain injuries or infections, and environments with insufficient stimulation (Aboud and Yousafzai 2016). Critical periods for brain development are during fetal growth and in the first two years of life. Micronutrient deficiencies in pregnancy have important consequences, such as compromised mental development with iodine deficiency and neural tube defects with folic acid deficiency (Black and others 2013). Inadequate diets and high rates of infectious diseases in the first two years of life lead to short stature (stunting) and permanent deficits in cognitive and social development. Additional important determinants of development in children are the amount and quality of household psychosocial stimulation (Singla, Kumbakumba, and Aboud 2015) and the effects of maternal illness, including depression (Walker and others 2007).

INTERVENTIONS TO REDUCE MATERNAL AND CHILD MORBIDITY AND MORTALITY

The RMNCH volume identifies essential interventions, based on their efficacy and appropriateness, to address important health conditions. Tables 1.1–1.3 list these interventions in the least advanced service platform at which their delivery is possible. The three platforms represent services that can be provided by (1) community health workers or health posts; (2) primary health centers; or (3) hospitals, both first-level and referral. The interventions are grouped by the point at which they are needed in the continuum of care. We also consider the nature of their delivery (urgent, continuing care, or routine care), which has important implications for the organization and responsibilities of the health system.

ESSENTIAL INTERVENTIONS ON STILLBIRTHS AND MATERNAL, NEONATAL, AND CHILD DEATHS

In this volume, we define three packages of interventions across the RMNCH continuum with the greatest potential to reduce deaths and disability: reproductive health, maternal and newborn health, and child (age 1–59 months) health.

We report on estimated morbidity and mortality from 75 countries that include more than 95 percent of the world's maternal and child deaths, the countries that had been monitored in the Countdown to 2015 initiative (Requejo and others 2015). Estimates are derived using the Lives Saved Tool (LiST; box 1.2) by increasing the coverage of each intervention to 90 percent from the current level of coverage in each of these 75 countries (Requejo and others 2015).

The deaths averted by individual interventions in the maternal and newborn health and the child health packages are shown in figure 1.2. The immediate (for 2015) impact on deaths of the individual interventions and their combined effects if implemented together was estimated. For these estimates, the effects of folic acid supplementation in the reproductive health package are considered, and these effects are combined with the maternal and newborn package for presentation.

A separate analysis was undertaken for family planning services in the reproductive health package, in which the provision of contraception is scaled up to cover 90 percent of current unmet need (Walker, Tam, and Friberg 2013). Because this reduces the number of pregnancies, we calculated the number of maternal, neonatal, and child deaths and stillbirths that would be prevented if the rates of mortality in 2015 had applied to these pregnancies and births. Estimates of the effects of other interventions such as human papillomavirus vaccination or targeted health care approaches for adolescents are considered in other volumes (for example, volume 3 *Cancer* and volume 8 *Child and Adolescent Development*).

The impact is also considered for interventions provided by each of three platforms for health services (see tables 1.1–1.3). The community platform includes all interventions that can be delivered by a community-based health worker with appropriate training and support or by outreach services, such as child health days, immunizations, vitamin A, and other interventions. For ill children, the integrated community case management (iCCM) approach is assumed to include diagnosis and treatment of pneumonia, diarrhea, and malaria cases without danger signs that indicate the need for referral (Hamer and others 2012; Young and others 2012).

Lives Saved Tool

The Lives Saved Tool (LiST) has been continually developing since 2003. The initial version of the software was developed as part of the work for the Child Survival Series in *The Lancet* in 2003 (Jones and others 2003). The original purpose of the program was to estimate the impact that scaling up community-based interventions would have on under-five mortality (Jones and others 2003). The Bill & Melinda Gates Foundation provided support for the further development and maintenance of the software as part of the work of the Child Health Epidemiology Reference Group (CHERG). At that point, the software was shifted into the free and publicly available Spectrum software package, to take advantage of the demographic capabilities in that software and to provide links to other models for family planning and AIDS (Stover, McKinnon, and Winfrey 2010). Since that time, LiST has expanded its scope to examine the impact of interventions on birth outcomes and stillbirths (Pattinson and others 2011), maternal mortality, and incidence of pneumonia and diarrhea (Bhutta and others 2013), as well as neonatal and child mortality.

LiST has been characterized as a linear, mathematical model that is deterministic (Garnett and others 2011). It describes fixed relationships between inputs and outputs that will produce the same outputs each time one runs the model. The primary inputs in LiST are coverage of interventions with the condition that the quality of that intervention is sufficient to be effective, what is commonly referred to as *effective coverage*. The outputs are changes in population-level risk factors (such as wasting or stunting rates, birth outcomes such as prematurity,

or size at birth) and cause-specific mortality (neonatal, child mortality for those age 1–59 months, maternal mortality, and stillbirths). The relationship between an input (change in intervention coverage) and one or more outputs is specified as a measure of the effectiveness of the intervention in reducing the probability of that outcome. The outcome can be cause-specific mortality or a risk factor. The overarching assumption in LiST is that mortality rates and cause-of-death structure will not change except in response to changes in coverage of interventions.

The roughly 70 separate interventions within LiST (see tables 1.1–1.3) target stillbirths, neonatal mortality, mortality in children age 1–59 months, maternal mortality, or risk factors such as stunting and wasting, within the model. In LiST, interventions can be linked to multiple outcomes, with some interventions linked to multiple causes of death and risk factors. LiST allows the impact of scaling up coverage of multiple interventions to be examined simultaneously.

CHERG, along with its institutional sponsors, the WHO and UNICEF, developed rules of evidence to decide what interventions should be included in the model as well as how to develop the estimates of effectiveness (Walker and others 2010). The assumptions used within LiST are drawn from various sources, but most of the evidence about effectiveness of interventions is presented in three journal supplements (Fox and others 2011; Sachdev, Hall, and Walker 2010; Walker 2013). The set of assumptions and their sources can be found at the LiST website (http://www.livessavedtool.org).

The primary health center (PHC) platform is a facility with a doctor or a nurse midwife (or both), nurses and support staff, as well as basic diagnostic and treatment capabilities. The PHC provides facility-based contraceptive services, including long-acting reversible contraceptives (implants, intrauterine devices); surgical sterilization (vasectomy, tubal ligation); care during pregnancy and delivery for uncomplicated pregnancies; provision of medical care for adults and children, such as injectable antibiotics, that cannot be done in the community; and

training and supervision of community-based workers. For LiST modeling, the effects of meeting the unmet need for contraceptives are considered to be delivered by the PHC platform. For young infants and children, the Integrated Management of Childhood Illness approach is assumed to be used at the PHC level (Bryce and others 2004). The hospital platform, consisting of both first-level and referral hospitals, includes more advanced services for management of labor and delivery in high-risk women or those with complications, including operative

Figure 1.2 Deaths Averted by Individual Interventions in the Maternal and Newborn Health and Child Health Packages

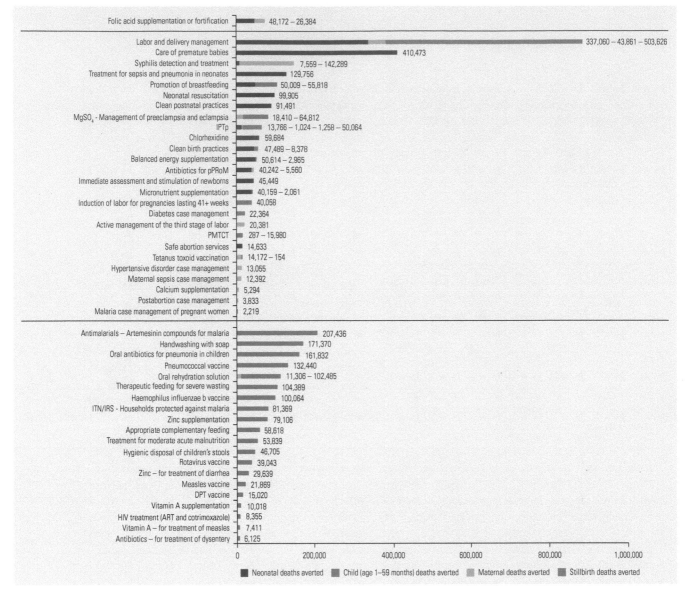

Note: ART = antiretroviral therapy; DPT = diphtheria, pertussis, tetanus; HIV = human immunodeficiency virus; IPTp = intermittent preventive treatment in pregnancy; ITN/IRS = insecticide-treated net/indoor residual spraying; MgSO₄ = magnesium sulfate; PMTCT = prevention of mother-to-child transmission; pPRoM = preterm premature rupture of membranes.

delivery, full supportive care for preterm newborns, and children with severe infection or severe acute malnutrition with infection.

The reproductive health package, other than provision of contraceptive services, consists primarily of educational interventions that are not expected to have a direct impact on deaths, but are important to encourage behaviors to prevent infections, ensure proper nutrition of girls before pregnancy, or to seek care for antenatal or delivery services at other levels. The effects of these practices or treatments are included in LiST and are assigned to the level at which the practice or treatment occurs.

Some deaths are averted through provision of folic acid before conception and in early pregnancy, reducing both stillbirths and neonatal deaths by preventing fetal neural tube defects, resulting in a reduction of stillbirths of 26,000 and neonatal deaths of 48,000 at the current rates of fertility. These deaths are included in the maternal and newborn package for presentation in this chapter.

The largest effect of the reproductive health package is from the contraceptive services that prevent unintended pregnancies. It is estimated that if 90 percent of current unmet need for contraceptives had been met, 28 million births would have been prevented in 2015. This level of

Table 1.1 Essential Interventions for Reproductive Health

	Delivery platform[a]		
	Community workers or health post	**Primary health center**	**First-level and referral hospitals**
Information and education	1. Sexuality education		
	2. Nutritional education and food supplementation		
	3. Promotion of care-seeking for antenatal care and delivery		
	4. Prevention of sexual and reproductive tract infections	1. Detection and treatment of sexual and reproductive tract infections	
	5. Prevention of female genital mutilation (may be for daughters of women of reproductive age)	2. Management of complications following female genital mutilation	
	6. Prevention of gender-based violence	3. Post-gender-based violence care (prevention of sexually transmitted infection and HIV, emergency contraception, support and counseling)	
	7. Information about cervical cancer and screening	4. Screening and treatment of precancerous lesions, referral of cancers	1. Management of cervical cancer
Service delivery	8. Folic acid supplementation[b]		
	9. Immunization (human papillomavirus, hepatitis B)		
	10. Contraception: Provision of condoms and hormonal contraceptives[b]	5. Tubal ligation, vasectomy, and insertion and removal of long-lasting contraceptives[b]	2. Management of complicated contraceptive procedures

Note: Red type denotes urgent care, blue type denotes continuing care, and black type denotes routine care. In this table, the community worker or health post consists of a trained and supported health worker based in or near communities working from home or a fixed health post. A primary health center is a health facility staffed by a physician or clinical officer and often a midwife to provide basic medical care, minor surgery, family planning and pregnancy services, and safe childbirth for uncomplicated deliveries. First-level and referral hospitals provide full supportive care for complicated neonatal and medical conditions, deliveries, and surgeries.
HIV = human immunodeficiency virus.
a. All interventions listed for lower-level platforms can be provided at higher levels. Similarly, each facility level represents a spectrum and diversity of capabilities. The column in which an intervention is listed is the lowest level of the health system in which it would usually be provided.
b. The intervention effect was included in the Lives Saved Tool (LiST).

Table 1.2 Essential Interventions for Maternal and Newborn Health

	Delivery platform[a]		
	Community worker or health post	**Primary health center**	**First-level and referral hospitals**
Pregnancy	1. Preparation for safe birth and newborn care; emergency planning		
	2. Micronutrient supplementation[b]		
	3. Nutrition education[b]		

table continues next page

Table 1.2 Essential Interventions for Maternal and Newborn Health (continued)

	Delivery platform[a]		
	Community worker or health post	**Primary health center**	**First-level and referral hospitals**
	4. IPTp[b]		
	5. Food supplementation[b]		
	6. Education on family planning	1. Management of unwanted pregnancy[b]	
	7. Promotion of HIV testing	2. Screening and treatment for HIV and syphilis[b]	
		3. Management of miscarriage or incomplete abortion and postabortion care[b]	
		4. Antibiotics for pPRoM[b]	
		5. Management of chronic medical conditions (hypertension, diabetes mellitus, and others)	
		6. Tetanus toxoid[b]	
		7. Screening for complications of pregnancy[b]	
		8. Initiate antenatal steroids (as long as clinical criteria and standards are met)[b]	1. Antenatal steroids[b]
		9. Initiate magnesium sulfate (loading dose)[b]	2. Magnesium sulfate[b]
		10. Detection of sepsis[b]	3. Treatment of sepsis[b]
			4. Induction of labor postterm[b]
			5. Ectopic pregnancy case management[b]
			6. Detection and management of fetal growth restriction[b]
Delivery (woman)	8. Management of labor and delivery in low-risk women by skilled attendant[b]	11. Management of labor and delivery in low-risk women (BEmNOC) including initial treatment of obstetric and delivery complications prior to transfer[b]	7. Management of labor and delivery in high-risk women, including operative delivery (CEmNOC)[b]
Postpartum (woman)	9. Promotion of breastfeeding[b]		
Postnatal (newborn)	10. Thermal care for preterm newborns[b]	12. Kangaroo mother care[b]	8. Full supportive care for preterm newborns[b]
	11. Neonatal resuscitation[b]		
	12. Oral antibiotics for pneumonia[b]	13. Injectable and oral antibiotics for sepsis, pneumonia, and meningitis[b]	9. Treatment of newborn complications, meningitis, and other very serious infections[b]
		14. Jaundice management[b]	

Note: Red type denotes urgent care, blue type denotes continuing care, black type denotes routine care. In this table, the community worker or health post consists of a trained and supported health worker based in or near communities working from home or a fixed health post. A primary health center is a health facility staffed by a physician or clinical officer and often a midwife to provide basic medical care, minor surgery, family planning and pregnancy services, and safe childbirth for uncomplicated deliveries. First-level and referral hospitals provide full supportive care for complicated neonatal and medical conditions, deliveries, and surgeries.

BEmNOC = basic emergency newborn and obstetric care; CEmNOC = comprehensive emergency newborn and obstetric care; HIV = human immunodeficiency virus; IPTp = intermittent preventive treatment in pregnancy; pPRoM = preterm premature rupture of membranes.

a. All interventions listed for lower-level platforms can be provided at higher levels. Similarly, each facility level represents a spectrum and diversity of capabilities. The column in which an intervention is listed is the lowest level of the health system in which it would usually be provided.

b. The intervention effect was included in the Lives Saved Tool (LiST).

Table 1.3 Essential Interventions for Child Health

Delivery platform[a]		
Community worker or health post	**Primary health center**	**First-level and referral hospitals**
1. Promote breastfeeding and complementary feeding[b]		
2. Provide vitamin A, zinc, and food supplementation[b]		
3. Immunizations[b,c]		
4. Cotrimoxazole for HIV-positive children[b]	1. Antiretroviral therapy for HIV-positive children[b]	
5. Education on safe disposal of children's stools and handwashing[b]		
6. Distribute and promote use of ITNs or IRS[b]		
7. Detect and refer severe acute malnutrition[b]	2. Treat severe acute malnutrition[b]	1. Treat severe acute malnutrition associated with serious infection[b]
8. Detect and treat serious infections without danger signs (iCCM[d]); refer if danger signs[b]	3. Detect and treat serious infections with danger signs (IMCI[d])[b]	2. Detect and treat serious infections with danger signs with full supportive care[b]

Note: Red type denotes urgent care, blue type denotes continuing care, black type denotes routine care. In this table, the community worker or health post consists of a trained and supported health worker based in or near communities working from home or a fixed health post. A primary health center is a health facility staffed by a physician or clinical officer and often a midwife to provide basic medical care, minor surgery, family planning and pregnancy services, and safe childbirth for uncomplicated deliveries. First-level and referral hospitals provide full supportive care for complicated neonatal and medical conditions, deliveries, and surgeries.

HIV = human immunodeficiency virus; iCCM = integrated community case management; IMCI = integrated management of childhood illness; IRS = indoor residual spraying; ITN = insecticide-treated net.

a. All interventions listed for lower-level platforms can be provided at higher levels. Similarly, each facility level represents a spectrum and diversity of capabilities. The column in which an intervention is listed is the lowest level of the health system in which it would usually be provided.

b. The intervention effect was included in the Lives Saved Tool (LiST).

c. Immunizations included in the standard package are those for diphtheria, pertussis, tetanus, polio, bacillus Calmette-Guerin, measles, hepatitis B, Haemophilus influenzae type b, pneumococcus, rotavirus.

d. Components of iCCM are treatments for diarrhea, pneumonia, and malaria; and of IMCI are treatments of diarrhea, pneumonia, malaria, AIDS (acquired immune deficiency syndrome), other infections, and severe acute malnutrition.

contraception, in turn, would reduce maternal deaths by 67,000, neonatal deaths by 440,000, child deaths by 473,000, and stillbirths by 564,000. Because about half of unwanted pregnancies are ended in abortion, preventing these pregnancies would also reduce millions of abortions, more than half of which would have been unsafe (Singh and others 2009). In addition, delayed age of first pregnancy and avoidance of short interpregnancy intervals would reduce adverse birth outcomes such as preterm delivery. It is important to note that these potential deaths averted by preventing unplanned pregnancies cannot be added to the potential lives saved by the maternal and newborn and child health packages (plus folic acid supplementation), which are estimated at the current rates of fertility and mortality.

The maternal and newborn package provides many interventions resulting in large effects on all of the mortality outcomes in the current year (figure 1.3). We estimate that 2,574,000 deaths would be averted, including 149,000 maternal deaths, 849,000 stillbirths, 1,498,000 neonatal deaths, and 78,000 child deaths (figure 1.2).

For stillbirths, 19 percent could be averted with the community platform, 46 percent with the PHC platform, and an additional 35 percent in hospitals. For maternal deaths, 13 percent could be averted with the community platform, 71 percent with the PHC platform, and the remaining 16 percent with hospital care. For neonatal deaths, the relative effects on level of services are different from maternal deaths, with a possible 48 percent of newborn deaths averted with the community platform, an additional 12 percent with the PHC platform, and a further 40 percent with hospital care. The interventions with the largest effects are labor and delivery management, care of preterm births, and treatment of neonatal sepsis and pneumonia (figure 1.2).

The child health package includes essential interventions across all three service platforms and together these could avert 1,437,000 child deaths. The largest impact (93 percent of avertable child deaths) can be realized by interventions in the community platform (figure 1.3), especially through immunizations and treatment of infectious diseases (figure 1.2). The PHC platform

Figure 1.3 Deaths Averted by Health Care Packages through Three Service Platforms

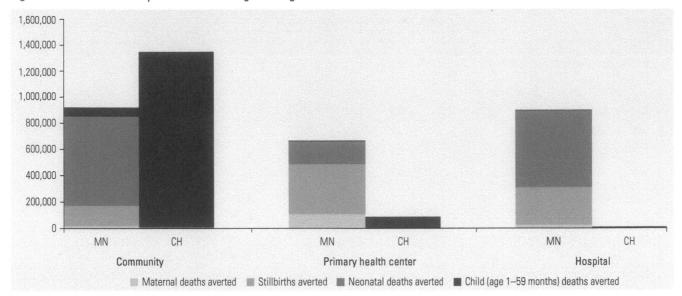

Source: Analyses using the Lives Saved Tool (LiST).
Note: CH = child health package; MN = maternal and newborn package.

results in additional effects on child deaths primarily through treatment of severe infectious diseases and of severe acute malnutrition (SAM). SAM can be managed on an outpatient basis with therapeutic feeding but is placed in the PHC platform because of the need for initial assessment and stabilization. The hospital platform averts some additional deaths with full supportive care for very severe infectious diseases and malnutrition.

Scaling up all interventions in the maternal and newborn health and child health packages in 2015 would avert 149,000 maternal deaths, 849,000 stillbirths, 1,498,000 neonatal deaths, and 1,515,000 child deaths, a total of 4,011,000 deaths averted. Then, interventions would result in a reduction in about half of the estimated global 303,000 maternal deaths in 2015 and also about half of the 5,900,000 global newborn and child deaths (Alkema and others 2015; You and others 2015). However, they would result in a reduction of only about one-third of the 2,600,000 stillbirths (Blencowe and others, forthcoming). Well-functioning community and PHC platforms could avert 77 percent of maternal, newborn, and child deaths and stillbirths that are preventable by these essential interventions, with hospitals contributing the remaining averted deaths through more advanced management of complicated pregnancies and deliveries and newborn and child conditions.

An additional consideration for the organization of health services is whether the interventions can be provided as scheduled routine care (shown in black in

tables 1.1–1.3); provided as continuing care such as for chronic conditions (shown in blue in tables 1.1–1.3); or if the service has to be available at all times and offered as urgent care (shown in red in tables 1.1–1.3). Because of the unpredictable nature of most life-threatening conditions in maternal, newborn, and child health, such as complications of labor and delivery or acute illnesses, most of the essential interventions must be available for urgent care at all times of the day.

COST-EFFECTIVENESS

Individual RMNCH interventions, summarized in figure 1.4, have been shown to be cost-effective (Horton and Levin 2016). This volume explores the cost-effectiveness of packages of interventions that have not yet been scaled up across LMICs. It also reports on new results from extended cost-effectiveness analyses that look at financial-risk-protection outcomes in addition to the health outcomes that are part of traditional cost-effectiveness analyses.

Expansion of coverage of the traditional Expanded Program on Immunization package of bacillus Calmette-Guerin; diphtheria, pertussis, and tetanus; measles; polio; and hepatitis B vaccines remains highly cost-effective, regardless of delivery modality. Introduction of pneumococcal and rotavirus vaccines at Gavi (the Global Vaccine Alliance) prices can avert deaths at a cost of less

Figure 1.4 Cost-Effectiveness Ranges of Selected Interventions for Reproductive, Maternal, Neonatal, and Child Health for Cost per Death Averted (2012 U.S. dollars)

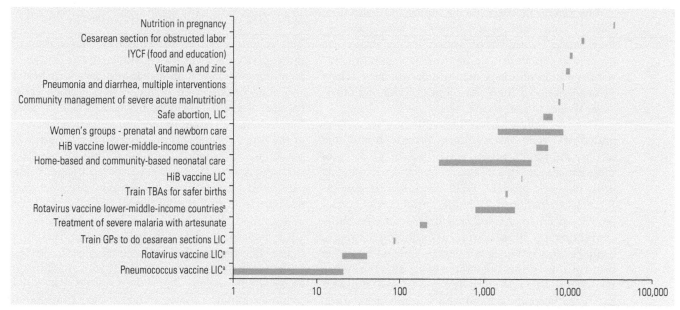

Note: Some vaccine results are for lower-middle-income countries. If country group is not specified, results refer to low and lower-middle-income countries combined.

GP = general practitioner; HiB = Haemophilus influenzae B; IYCF = infant and young child feeding interventions (education combined with food distribution to poorest); LIC = low-income country; TBA = traditional birth attendant.

a. Cost-effectiveness of vaccines is sensitive to vaccine price. Rotavirus and pneumococcus vaccine costs to LICs are a fraction (for example, 5 percent) of the price paid by Gavi, the Vaccine Alliance to procure the vaccines; Gavi, in turn, receives prices that are more favorable than what upper-middle-income countries pay as a result of volume discounts and other factors.

than US$100 per death (Horton and Levin 2016), but these estimates do not include reduced out-of-pocket expenditures, improved financial risk protection for households, or long-term benefits of improved cognition and lifetime productivity (Barnighausen and others 2014). Megiddo and others (2014) find that introduction of a rotavirus vaccine in India was cost-saving and was estimated to avert 34.7 (95 percent uncertainty range [UR], 31.7–37.7) deaths and US$215,569 (95 percent UR, US$207,846–US$223,292) out-of-pocket expenditure per 100,000 children under age five years.

Chapters in this volume have calculated that home-based management of maternal and neonatal care, including interventions to train traditional birth attendants for safer births (Sabin and others 2012), can be cost-effective with lower-end estimates of cost-effectiveness of less than US$1,000 per death averted. Scaling up midwifery services with referral when needed and family planning would cost US$2,200 per death averted (Bartlett and others 2014).

Using extended cost-effectiveness analysis (Verguet and others 2015), it was shown that investing in the provision of universal public finance for pneumonia treatment and for combined treatment with

pneumococcal conjugate vaccine provides substantially higher financial risk protection and saves more lives for the poor in Ethiopia than the current situation. Financial risk protection associated with an intervention is measured using the money-metric-equivalent value of insurance, which is simply what an individual would pay as an insurance premium to ensure that they are fully protected against the disease or adverse health condition.

India alone accounts for 28 percent of neonatal deaths globally. In 2011, India introduced a home-based newborn care (HBNC) package to be delivered by community health workers across rural areas of the country. Nandi and others (2015) estimate the disease and economic burdens averted by scaling up the HBNC among households in rural India. Compared with a baseline of no coverage, providing the care package through the existing network of community health workers could avert 48 (95 percent uncertainty range [UR] 34–63) incident cases of severe neonatal morbidity and 5 (95 percent UR 4–7) related deaths, save US$4,411 (95 percent UR US$3,088–US$5,735) in out-of-pocket treatment expenditure, and provide US$285 (95 percent UR US$200–US$371) in insurance value per 1,000 live births in rural India. Intervention benefits were greater for lower socioeconomic groups.

Investments that increase the supply and demand for RMNCH interventions can have long-lasting effects—for example, the benefits of investments in nutrition can go beyond the immediate improvement in nutritional status by also improving cognitive development, school performance, and future earnings (Victora and others 2008; Walker and others 2007).

The economic and social benefits of a set of integrated RMNCH interventions include health and fertility impacts (Stenberg and others 2014). Some of these benefits are strictly economic, reflected in higher gross domestic product (GDP) from increased workforce participation and higher productivity. Other benefits, denoted as *social benefits*, are not reflected in conventional GDP measures. For example, the value of a child's life saved does not depend only on his or her participation in the labor force when an adult. When taking into consideration the *full-income* approach that goes beyond GDP to also capture these social benefits, including from reducing morbidity and controlling fertility, the benefit-cost ratios indicate high returns on increased investment in RMNCH in most countries, especially when benefits beyond the intervention period are included. For all LMICs considered as a group, the benefit-cost ratio is 8.7 for the intervention period to 2035 at a 3 percent discount rate (Stenberg and others 2014; Stenberg and others 2016).

COST OF SCALING UP ESSENTIAL INTERVENTIONS FOR REPRODUCTIVE, MATERNAL, NEWBORN, AND CHILD HEALTH

This volume estimates the annual cost of scaling up three service packages for reproductive health (family planning costs only), maternal and newborn health, and child health in 74 of the 75 Countdown countries (Sudan is not included because of lack of data). These countries account for more than 95 percent of the world's maternal and child deaths. We estimate the annual incremental costs of scaling up the three packages described in table 1.1, based on per capita cost estimates from a global reproductive, maternal, newborn, and child health investment case (Stenberg and others 2014). Using population estimates for 2015 associated with the health impact shown in figure 1.3, the annual incremental cost is US$6.2 billion in low-income countries, US$12.4 billion in lower-middle-income countries, and US$7.9 billion in upper-middle-countries (table 1.4). Considering a longer time horizon of 2013 to 2035, the annual incremental costs of scaling up the three packages increases slightly depending on the country income groups, reflecting a larger target population, consistent with Stenberg and others (2014) and chapter 16 in this volume (Stenberg and others 2016). These estimates include health system strengthening costs, such as program management, infrastructure needs, improved

Table 1.4 Cost of Essential Reproductive Health (family planning only), Maternal and Newborn Health, and Child Health Packages by Country Income Group for 2015 and 2035 (million 2012 U.S. dollars, except per capita costs)

Package	Low-income countries		Lower-middle-income countries		Upper-middle-income countries		Total cost per package	
	2015	2035	2015	2035	2015	2035	2015	2035
Reproductive health package costs[a]	$562	$603	$520	$630	$151	$164	$1,233	$1,397
Cost per capita	$0.6	$0.5	$0.2	$0.2	$0.1	$0.1	$0.2	$0.2
Maternal and newborn health package costs[a]	$1,183	$1,268	$2,922	$3,542	$1,768	$1,923	$5,872	$6,733
Cost per capita	$1.3	$1.0	$1.1	$1.1	$0.9	$0.9	$1.0	$1.0
Child health package costs[a]	$4,484	$4,810	$8,838	$10,712	$6,060	$6,591	$19,382	$22,113
Cost per capita	$4.8	$3.9	$3.4	$3.3	$2.9	$2.9	$3.5	$3.3
Total costs	$6,229	$6,681	$12,406	$14,884	$7,979	$8,679	$26,614	$30,243
Total per capita costs	$6.7	$5.4	$4.7	$4.6	$3.9	$3.9	$4.7	$4.5

Note: Estimates have been inflated to 2012 U.S. dollars using U.S. consumer price index data (World Bank World Development Indicators).
a. Package costs include commodities, front-line health workers, and additional health system strengthening costs for scaling up services.

governance, and health system information and logistics systems. These costs account for 73 percent of total package costs in low-income countries, 50 percent in lower-middle-income countries, and 41 percent in upper-middle-income countries.[1]

The child health package requires the greatest additional cost to scale up to 2035 with an additional US$22 billion per year. It includes a wide range of commodities and services to prevent and treat childhood illness, including immunization, malaria, and HIV. Scaling up the maternal and newborn package requires an additional US$6.7 billion per year. The reproductive health package is the least costly to scale up and requires an additional US$1.4 billion per year, covering commodities and personnel costs of front-line workers delivering modern family planning methods associated with the greatest reductions in fertility. The estimate does not include the costs of educational interventions in the reproductive health package because these were not available. One reproductive health package service, folic acid, is included in the maternal and newborn health package in this chapter, while human papillomavirus vaccination is included and costed in the package of essential cancer services.

The cost of family planning is low at an average of US$0.20 per capita per year and an annual incremental cost of US$1.4 billion per year. However, because the model only estimates the cost of adding an average 104 million new users for the period, we also estimated the cost of eliminating unmet need for all women who desire to prevent a pregnancy, but do not currently use effective contraceptive methods, by 2035 (Stenberg and others 2014). In this scenario, 208 million additional users are reached during this period at a total cost of US$2.9 billion or US$14.0 per additional user (US$15.8 per additional user for low-, US$10.0 for lower-middle-, and US$24.4 for upper-middle-income countries) (table 1.5).

For comparison, a recent study by the Guttmacher Institute (Singh, Darroch, and Ashford 2014) estimates that meeting all women's needs for modern contraceptives will cost US$5.3 billion per year more than current spending. Although the services included are very similar to those included in our reproductive health package, the Guttmacher estimate covers all LMICs rather than the 74 Countdown countries, includes the costs of improving the quality of care for current family planning users, and includes costs of scaling up services for an estimated 225 million women with unmet need (Singh, Darroch, and Ashford 2014). In sum, differences between this and our estimate reflect differences in scope (all LMICs compared with only Countdown countries), methods, and underlying

Table 1.5 Average Additional Modern Contraceptive Users, Cost per Additional User, and Incremental Costs over the Period 2013–35 (2012 U.S. dollars)

	Low-income countries	Lower-middle-income countries	Upper-middle-income countries	Total
Additional modern contraceptive users (million)	75	106	27	208
Cost per additional user	$15.8	$10.0	$24.4	$14
Incremental costs (US$ million)	$1,188	$1,065	$663	$2,916

assumptions regarding the rate of scaling up and the methods mix of modern family planning among the target population.

Scaling up the three essential packages will require an average additional investment of US$4.7 per person per year in the 74 countries with 95 percent of the global maternal and child mortality burden. It provides rates of return based on economic and social benefit that are up to nine times the investment by 2035 (Stenberg and others 2016). The current (2015) cost of the three packages, inclusive of health system costs, ranges from US$6.70 per capita in low-income settings to US$4.80 and US$3.90 in lower-middle-income and upper-middle-income country settings. These estimates may be higher or lower depending on the country context and current levels of investment and commitment to health system strengthening.

Results from the RMNCH investment case (Stenberg and others 2014) are complemented by new evidence on individual interventions in reproductive, maternal and newborn, and child health interventions also presented in this volume. Although information on empirical costs has grown substantially in the past decade, it remains imperfect and lacks up-to-date data on relatively well-established interventions, such as vitamin A capsule distribution and family planning where modern contraceptive coverage is low in spite of high expressed unmet need. In emerging areas, such as maternal depression and intimate partner violence, few published studies are available. However, the literature does support trends in relative costs across the essential packages and provides a wealth of information especially for child illness and for a variety of platforms. For example, average unit costs (cost per beneficiary) are lower for family planning interventions, antenatal care visits, and normal deliveries at home or health centers with trained birth attendants. Costs per beneficiary tend to increase with the complexity of the service (that is, treatment of obstetric or abortion complications, treatment of severe acute child malnutrition, and a range of community-based nutrition interventions). For example, breastfeeding support and prevention of micronutrient deficiencies are inexpensive compared with facility-based treatment of severe acute malnutrition. Within packages, costs are also likely to vary depending on the context and condition—the prevention and treatment of malaria and diarrheal disease are less expensive per child (US$20 to US$100) than treating pneumonia and meningitis, which more often require inpatient admission (US$150 per visit, or US$800 per child treated for pneumonia; US$300 to US$500 for inpatient care treatment of meningitis and pneumonia).

IMPROVING INTERVENTION UPTAKE AND QUALITY

Supply- and demand-side interventions to improve intervention uptake and quality are increasingly used to ensure that essential RMNCH services are delivered with quality and used appropriately.

Supply-Side Interventions

On the supply side, interest has been growing in the use of pay-for-performance, which rewards providers or health care organizations for achieving coverage or quality targets. One study in Rwanda shows a 23 percent increase in facility delivery and larger increases in preventive care visits by young children in facilities enrolled in a payment plan compared with randomly selected controls (Basinga and others 2011).

A study of performance-based financing in Rwanda in which the government implemented an incentive program in several districts to motivate providers to improve the quality of care and increase service output found no significant differences in the use of maternal health services between intervention and control sites (Priedeman Skiles and others 2013). Only facility birth deliveries (p = 0.014) were 10 percentage points higher for the intervention sites compared with controls. Performance-based financing may be useful if targeted at specific services, such as facility deliveries, but only if service use was consistently low. Peabody and others (2014) considered payment-for-performance incentives and child health outcomes in the Philippines using clinical performance vignettes among randomly

chosen physicians every six months during a three-year period to assess physicians' quality indicators. Bonus payments were awarded if qualifying scores were met. Outcomes of interest—including age-adjusted wasting, C-reactive protein, hemoglobin level, parental self-reported health of children, and children under age five years hospitalized for diarrhea or pneumonia—were not improved in intervention sites. Only two indicators improved. Parental self-reported health of children increased by 7 percentage points and wasting declined by 9 percentage points. A Cochrane review suggests that the quality of evidence is too poor to draw general conclusions about the effectiveness of pay for performance and notes that several studies arrive at contradictory results (Witter and others 2012).

Safe childbirth (intrapartum care) checklists have been proposed as a way of reducing newborn deaths, but there are gaps in the evidence base. The WHO childbirth safety checklist was developed to help reduce the major causes of these deaths (hemorrhage, infection, obstructed labor, and others) (Spector and others 2013; Temmerman, Khosla, Bhutta, and Bustreo 2015; Temmerman, Khosla, Laski, and others 2015). Since most deaths associated with childbirth occur within a 24-hour window and the major causes are well described, checklists have promise for improving healthy delivery. Follow-up studies are currently underway that focus directly on health outcomes attributable to the increase in these practices. The quality of RMNCH services can also be improved using supportive supervision for front-line health workers, which is associated with small benefits for provider practice and knowledge (Bosch-Capblanch, Liaqat, and Garner 2011).

Recent efforts have been made in task-shifting—an innovative approach to increase the delivery of RMNCH services by reassigning certain tasks to community workers. Lay community health workers are increasingly being deployed to classify and treat childhood infectious diseases, such as pneumonia, diarrhea, and malaria, and approaches such as iCCM for their management are expanding widely (Young and others 2012). A recent WHO Guidance Panel on Task Shifting suggested that health workers could carry out many tasks related to maternal and newborn health, provided they received adequate training and support (WHO 2012). These personnel include lay workers (for example, for promotion of appropriate care-seeking behavior and antenatal care during pregnancy, administration of misoprostol to prevent postpartum hemorrhage, and promotion and support of breastfeeding), auxiliary nurses (for example, for administration of injectable contraceptives), auxiliary nurse midwives (for example, for neonatal resuscitation and insertion and removal of intrauterine devices), nurses (for example, for administration of a loading dose of magnesium sulfate to prevent or treat eclampsia), midwives (for example, for vacuum extraction during childbirth), and associate clinicians (for example, for manual removal of the placenta).

Demand-Side Interventions

Countries are increasingly relying on demand-side interventions to expand coverage. Brazil's Bolsa Família, launched in 2003, transfers payments to families on the condition that beneficiaries obtain health services (such as vaccinations and prenatal care for pregnant women) and that children maintain a minimum daily attendance rate at school. The program was associated with a 9.3 percent (p < 0.01) decline in the infant mortality rate and a 24.3 percent (p < 0.01) decrease in the postneonatal mortality rate (Shei 2013).

Lagarde, Haines, and Palmer (2009) conducted a systematic review of conditional cash transfers (CCTs) in low- and middle-income countries to see whether CCTs improve access to and use of health care services as well as health outcomes. Of the 11 CCT studies reviewed, 10 find significant positive effects on the outcome variable being examined. Only the Janani Suraksha Yojana program in India had no significant benefit, but its failure to lower the maternal mortality rate likely stems from beneficiaries' lack of access to quality health care facilities (Lim and others 2010). A 2009 Cochrane review finds that CCTs were associated with higher service use and may be an effective approach to promoting use of frequently undervalued preventive interventions, such as immunization (Lagarde, Haines, and Palmer 2009). Removal of user fees can result in increased use of the targeted RMNCH service, sometimes by a large margin (Lagarde and Palmer 2008; Ponsar and others 2011). Although few rigorous evaluations have been conducted, vouchers have been linked to increases in use of facility delivery and family planning (Bellows and others 2013; Bellows, Bellows, and Warren 2011). A meta-analysis of women's participatory learning and action groups finds that vouchers could potentially reduce maternal mortality by 37 percent and newborn mortality by 23 percent (Prost and others 2013).

CONCLUSIONS

Despite sizable recent reductions in child and maternal deaths, the rate of mortality decline has been too slow to achieve MDGs 4 and 5 globally. Particular regions, especially Sub-Saharan Africa, have high rates of fertility,

maternal mortality, and under-five mortality, providing a compelling case for integrated RMNCH interventions. Most deaths from RMNCH conditions could be greatly reduced by scaling up integrated packages of interventions across the continuum of care. Many of these interventions, especially family planning, labor and delivery management, promotion of breastfeeding, immunizations, improved childhood nutrition, and treatment of severe infectious diseases, are among the most cost-effective of all health interventions. Nevertheless, implementation research is still needed to adapt these interventions to the local health service context and achieve the greatest effects. The benefits of scaling up packages extend beyond health to also include substantial economic and social outcomes. Improved access and quality of care around childbirth can generate a quadruple return on investment by saving maternal and newborn lives and preventing stillbirths and disability. Furthermore, these benefits extend beyond survival—for example, investing in early childhood nutrition and stimulation can reduce losses in cognitive development and adult capacity. Strengthening health systems and improving data for decision making are, among others, key strategies to drive improvement, equity, and accountability.

The 2015 UN Global Strategy for Women's, Children's, and Adolescents' Health builds on evidence presented in this volume, as well as the need to focus on critical population groups such as adolescents and those living in fragile and conflict settings; build the resilience of health systems; improve the quality of health services and equity in their coverage; and work with health-enhancing sectors on issues such as women's empowerment, education, nutrition, water, sanitation, and hygiene (Temmerman, Khosla, Bhutta, and Bustreo 2015). The objectives of universal health coverage, including public health interventions and preventive as well as curative services (Schmidt, Gostin, and Emanuel 2015), and ensuring financial security and health equity are critical if the Sustainable Development Goals are to be achieved. A new vision and commitment to realize good health and human rights for all women, adolescents, and children needs to be articulated.

ACKNOWLEDGMENTS

The Bill & Melinda Gates Foundation provides financial support for the Disease Control Priorities Network project, of which this volume is a part. Carol Levin provided sections of the chapter on cost-effectiveness and cost of interventions. Doris Chou assisted with sections on reproductive health and maternal morbidity and mortality, and Li Liu on child mortality. The following individuals provided valuable assistance and comments on this chapter: Brianne Adderley, Rachel Nugent, Lale Say, and Gavin Yamey. Members of the RMNCH Authors Group wrote chapters on which this initial chapter draws. The group includes Frances Aboud, Fernando Althabe, Ashvin Ashok, Henrik Axelson, Rajiv Bahl, Akinrinola Bankole, Zulfiqar Bhutta, Lori Bollinger, Deborah Hay Burgess, Doris Chou, John Cleland, Daniela Colaci, Simon Cousens, Valérie D'Acremont, Jai Das, Julia Driessen, Alex Ezeh, Daniel Feikin, Veronique Filippi, Mariel Finucane, Christa Fischer Walker, Brendan Flannery, Ingrid Friberg, Bela Ganatra, Claudia García-Moreno, Marijke Gielen, Wendy Graham, Metin Gulmezoglu, Demissie Habte, Mary J. Hamel, Davidson H. Hamer, Peter Hansen, Karen Hardee, Julie M. Herlihy, Natasha Hezelgrave, Justus Hofmeyr, Dan Hogan, Susan Horton, Aamer Imdad, Dean Jamison, Kjell Arne Johansson, Jerry Keusch, Margaret Kruk, Rohail Kumar, Zohra Lassi, Joy Lawn, Theresa Lawrie, Ramanan Laxminarayan, Lindsey Lenters, Colin Mathers, Solomon Tessema Memirie, Arindam Nandi, Olufemi T. Oladapo, Shefali Oza, Clint Pecenka, Carine Ronsmans, Rehana Salam, Lale Say, Peter Sheehan, Joao Paulo Souza, Meghan Stack, Karin Stenberg, Gretchen Stevens, John Stover, Kim Sweeny, Stéphane Verguet, Kerri Wazny, Aisha Yousafzai, and Abdhalah Ziraba.

NOTES

World Bank Income Classifications as of July 2014 are as follows, based on estimates of gross national income (GNI) per capita for 2013:

- Low-income countries (LICs) = US$1,045 or less
  Middle-income countries (MICs) are subdivided:
  - Lower-middle-income = US$1,046 to US$4,125
  - Upper-middle-income (UMICs) = US$4,126 to US$12,745
- High-income countries (HICs) = US$12,746 or more.

1. For the maternal and newborn health package, health system costs are assumed to constitute 19 percent, 23 percent, and 22 percent of the total package for low-, lower-middle, and upper-middle-income groups, respectively. For the child health package, they are 72 percent, 71 percent, and 76 percent of the total for low-, lower-middle, and upper-middle-income groups, respectively.

REFERENCES

Aboud, F. E., and A. Yousafzai. 2016. "Very Early Childhood Development." In *Disease Control Priorities* (third edition): Volume 2, *Reproductive, Maternal, Newborn, and Child Health*, edited by R. E. Black, R. Laxminarayan, N. Walker, and M. Temmerman. Washington, DC: World Bank.

Afnan-Holmes, H., M. Magoma, T. John, F. Levira, G. Msemo, and others. 2015. "Tanzania's Countdown to 2015: An Analysis of Two Decades of Progress and Gaps for Reproductive, Maternal, Newborn, and Child Health, to Inform Priorities for post-2015." *The Lancet Global Health* 3 (7): e396–409. doi:10.1016/S2214-109X(15)00059-5.

Alkema, L., D. Chou, D. Hogan, S. Zhang, A. B. Moller, and others. 2015. "Global, Regional, and National Levels and Trends in Maternal Mortality between 1990 and 2015, with Scenario-Based Projections to 2030: A Systematic Analysis by the UN Maternal Mortality Estimation Inter-Agency Group." *The Lancet*. doi:10.1016/S0140-6736(15)00838-7.

Amouzou, A., O. Habi, K. Bensaid, and Niger Countdown Case Study Working Group. 2012. "Reduction in Child Mortality in Niger: A Countdown to 2015 Country Case Study." *The Lancet* 380 (9848): 1169–78. doi:10.1016/S0140-6736(12)61376-2.

Arregoces, L., F. Daly, C. Pitt, J. Hsu, M. Martinez-Alvarez, and others. 2015. "Countdown to 2015: Changes in Official Development Assistance to Reproductive, Maternal, Newborn, and Child Health, and Assessment of Progress between 2003 and 2012." *The Lancet Global Health* 3 (7): e410–21. doi:10.1016/S2214-109X(15)00057-1.

Ban, K. 2010. "Global Strategy for Women's and Children's Health." Partnership for Maternal, Newborn and Child Health, New York, NY.

Barnighausen, T., S. Berkley, Z. A. Bhutta, D. M. Bishai, M. M. Black, and others. 2014. "Reassessing the Value of Vaccines." *The Lancet Global Health* 2 (5): e251–52.

Bartlett, L., E. Weissman, R. Gubin, R. Patton-Molitors, and I. K. Friberg. 2014. "The Impact and Cost of Scaling up Midwifery and Obstetrics in 58 Low- and Middle-Income Countries." *PLoS One* 9 (6): e98550. doi:10.1371/journal.pone.0098550.

Basinga, P., P. J. Gertler, A. Binagwaho, A. L. Soucat, J. Sturdy, and C. M. Vermeersch. 2011. "Effect on Maternal and Child Health Services in Rwanda of Payment to Primary Health-Care Providers for Performance: An Impact Evaluation." *The Lancet* 377 (9775): 1421–28. doi:10.1016/S0140-6736(11)60177-3.

Bellows, B., C. Kyobutungi, M. K. Mutua, C. Warren, and A. Ezeh. 2013. "Increase in Facility-Based Deliveries Associated with a Maternal Health Voucher Programme in Informal Settlements in Nairobi, Kenya." [Research Support, Non-U.S. Gov't]. *Health Policy and Planning* 28 (2): 134–42. doi:10.1093/heapol/czs030.

Bellows, N. M., B. W. Bellows, and C. Warren. 2011. "Systematic Review: The Use of Vouchers for Reproductive Health Services in Developing Countries: Systematic Review." *Tropical Medicine and International Health* 16 (1): 84–96.

Bhutta, Z. A., J. K. Das, N. Walker, A. Rizvi, H. Campbell, and others. 2013. "Interventions to Address Deaths from Childhood Pneumonia and Diarrhoea Equitably: What Works and at What Cost?" *The Lancet* 381 (9875): 1417–29.

Black, R. E., C. G. Victora, S. P. Walker, Z. A. Bhutta, P. Christian, and others. 2013. "Maternal and Child Undernutrition and Overweight in Low-Income and Middle-Income Countries." *The Lancet* 382 (9890): 427–51. doi:10.1016 /S0140-6736(13)60937-X.

Blencowe, H., S. Cousens, F. Bianchi Jassir, L. Say, D. Chou, and others. 2016. "National, Regional, and Worldwide Estimates of Stillbirth Rates in 2015, with Trends from 2000: A Systematic Analysis." *The Lancet Global Health.* doi:http://dx .doi.org/10.1016/S2214-109X(15)00275-2. Epub January 18.

Bosch-Capblanch, X., S. Liaqat, and P. Garner. 2011. "Managerial Supervision to Improve Primary Health Care in Low- and Middle-Income Countries." *Cochrane Database of Systematic Reviews* (9): CD006413. doi:10.1002/14651858 .CD006413.pub2.

Bryce, J., C. G. Victora, J. P. Habicht, J. P. Vaughan, and R. E. Black. 2004. "The Multi-Country Evaluation of the Integrated Management of Childhood Illness Strategy: Lessons for the Evaluation of Public Health Interventions." *American Journal of Public Health* 94 (3): 406–15.

Chachamovich, J. R., E. Chachamovich, H. Ezer, M. P. Fleck, D. Knauth, and E. P. Passos. 2010. "Investigating Quality of Life and Health-Related Quality of Life in Infertility: A Systematic Review." *Journal of Psychosomatic Obstetrics and Gynaecology* 31 (2): 101–10. doi:10.3109/01674 82X.2010.481337.

Christian, P., S. E. Lee, M. Donahue Angel, L. S. Adair, S. E. Arifeen, and others. 2013. "Risk of Childhood Undernutrition Related to Small-for-Gestational Age and Preterm Birth in Low- and Middle-Income Countries." *International Journal of Epidemiology* 42 (5): 1340–55. doi:10.1093/ije/dyt109

Cui, W. 2010. "Mother or Nothing: The Agony of Infertility." *Bulletin of the World Health Organization* 88 (12): 881–82. doi:10.2471/BLT.10.011210.

Das, J. K., R. A. Salam, A. Imdad, Z. Lassi, and Z. A. Bhutta. 2016. "Infant and Young Child Growth." In *Disease Control Priorities* (third edition): Volume 2, *Reproductive, Maternal, Newborn, and Child Health,* edited by R. E. Black, R. Laxminarayan, N. Walker, and M. Temmerman. Washington, DC: World Bank.

Devries, K. M., S. Kishor, H. Johnson, H. Stockl, L. J. Bacchus, and others. 2010. "Intimate Partner Violence during Pregnancy: Analysis of Prevalence Data from 19 Countries." *Reproductive Health Matters* 18 (36): 158–70. doi:10.1016 /S0968-8080(10)36533-5.

Filippi, V., C. Ronsmans, D. Chou, L. Say, and W. Graham. 2016. "Levels and Causes of Maternal Morbidity and Mortality." In *Disease Control Priorities* (third edition): Volume 2, *Reproductive, Maternal, Newborn, and Child Health,* edited by R. E. Black, R. Laxminarayan, N. Walker, and M. Temmerman. Washington, DC: World Bank.

Fox, M. J., R. Martorell, N. Van den Broek, and N. Walker. 2011. "Technical Inputs, Enhancements and Applications of the Lives Saved Tool (LiST)." *BMC Public Health* 11 (Supplement 3).

Garnett, G. P., S. Cousens, T. B. Hallett, R. Steketee, and N. Walker. 2011. "Mathematical Models in the Evaluation of Health Programmes." Review. *The Lancet* 378 (9790): 515–25. doi:10.1016/S0140-6736(10)61505-X.

Grantham-McGregor, S., and International Child Development Committee. 2007. "Early Child Development in Developing Countries. *The Lancet* 369 (9564): 824. doi:10.1016 /S0140-6736(07)60404-8.

Hamer, D. H., E. T. Brooks, K. Semrau, P. Pilingana, W. B. MacLeod, and others. 2012. "Quality and Safety of Integrated Community Case Management of Malaria Using Rapid Diagnostic Tests and Pneumonia by Community Health Workers." *Pathogens and Global Health* 106 (1): 32–39. doi:10.1179/1364859411Y.0000000042.

Horton, S., and C. Levin. 2016. "Cost-Effectiveness of Interventions for Reproductive, Maternal, Newborn, and Child Health." In *Disease Control Priorities* (third edition): Volume 2, *Reproductive, Maternal, Newborn, and Child Health,* edited by R. E. Black, R. Laxminarayan, N. Walker, and M. Temmerman. Washington, DC: World Bank.

Jamison, D. T., J. G. Breman, A. R. Measham, G. Alleyne, M. Claeson, D. B. Evans, P. Jha, A. Mills, and P. Musgrove. 2006. *Disease Control Priorities in Developing Countries,* (second edition). Washington, DC: World Bank and Oxford University Press.

Jamison, D. T., W. Mosley, A. Measham, and J. Bobadilla. 1993. *Disease Control Priorities in Developing Countries,* (first edition). Washington, DC: World Bank and Oxford University Press.

Jones, G., R. W. Steketee, R. E. Black, Z. A. Bhutta, S. S. Morris, and Bellagio Child Survival Study Group. 2003. "How Many Child Deaths Can We Prevent This Year?" *The Lancet* 362 (9377): 65–71.

Kozuki, N., J. Katz, P. Christian, A. C. Lee, L. Liu, and others. 2015. "Comparison of US Birth Weight References and the International Fetal and Newborn Growth Consortium for the 21st Century Standard." *JAMA Pediatrics* 169 (7): e151438. doi:10.1001/jamapediatrics.2015.1438.

Lagarde, M., A. Haines, and N. Palmer. 2009. "The Impact of Conditional Cash Transfers on Health Outcomes and Use of Health Services in Low and Middle Income Countries." *Cochrane Database of Systematic Reviews* 7 (4).

Lagarde, M., and N. Palmer. 2008. "The Impact of User Fees on Health Service Utilization in Low- and Middle-Income Countries: How Strong Is the Evidence?" *Bulletin of the World Health Organization* 86 (11): 839–48.

Lenters, L., K. Wazny, and Z. Bhutta. 2016. "Management of Severe and Moderate Acute Malnutrition in Children." In *Disease Control Priorities* (third edition): Volume 2, *Reproductive, Maternal, Newborn, and Child Health,* edited by R. E. Black, R. Laxminarayan, N. Walker, and M. Temmerman. Washington, DC: World Bank.

Lim, S. S., L. Dandona, J. A. Hoisington, S. L. James, M. C. Hogan, and E. Gakidou. 2010. "India's Janani Suraksha Yojana, a Conditional Cash Transfer Programme to Increase Births in Health Facilities: An Impact Evaluation." *The Lancet* 375 (9730): 2009–23.

Liu, L., K. Hill, S. Oza, D. Hogan, S. Cousens, and others. 2016. "Levels and Causes of Mortality under Age Five." In *Disease Control Priorities* (third edition): Volume 2, *Reproductive, Maternal, Newborn, and Child Health,* edited by

R. E. Black, R. Laxminarayan, N. Walker, and M. Temmerman. Washington, DC: World Bank.

Liu, L., S. Oza, D. Hogan, J. Perin, I. Rudan, and others. 2014. "Global, Regional, and National Causes of Child Mortality in 2000–13, with Projections to Inform Post-2015 Priorities: An Updated Systematic Analysis." [Research Support, Non-U.S. Gov't]. *The Lancet* 385 (9966): 430–40. doi:10.1016/S0140-6736(14)61698-6.

Megiddo, I., A. R. Colson, A. Nandi, S. Chatterjee, S. Prinja, and others. 2014. "Analysis of the Universal Immunization Programme and Introduction of a Rotavirus Vaccine in India with IndiaSim." *Vaccine* 32 (Suppl 1): A151–61.

Nandi, A., A. R. Colson, A. Verma, I. Megiddo, A. Ashok, and R. Laxminarayan. 2015. "Health and Economic Benefits of Scaling up a Home-Based Neonatal Care Package in Rural India: A Modelling Analysis." *Health Policy and Planning*. doi:10.1093/heapol/czv113.

Pattinson, R., K. Kerber, E. Buchmann, I. K. Friberg, M. Belizan, and others. 2011. "Stillbirths: How Can Health Systems Deliver for Mothers and Babies?" *The Lancet* 377 (9777): 1610–23.

Peabody, J. W., R. Shimkhada, S. Quimbo, O. Solon, X. Javier, and C. McCulloch. 2014. "The Impact of Performance Incentives on Child Health Outcomes: Results from a Cluster Randomized Controlled Trial in the Philippines." *Health Policy and Planning* 29 (5): 615–21.

Ponsar, F., M. Van Herp, R. Zachariah, S. Gerard, M. Philips, and G. Jouquet. 2011. "Abolishing User Fees for Children and Pregnant Women Trebled Uptake of Malaria-Related Interventions in Kangaba, Mali." *Health Policy and Planning* 26 (Suppl 2): ii72–83. doi:10.1093/heapol/czr068.

Priedeman Skiles, M., S. L. Curtis, P. Basinga, and G. Angeles. 2013. "An Equity Analysis of Performance-Based Financing in Rwanda: Are Services Reaching the Poorest Women?" *Health Policy and Planning* 28 (8): 825–37.

Prost, A., T. Colbourn, N. Seward, K. Azad, A. Coomarasamy, and others. 2013. "Women's Groups Practising Participatory Learning and Action to Improve Maternal and Newborn Health in Low-Resource Settings: A Systematic Review and Meta-Analysis." *The Lancet* 381 (9879): 1736–46. doi:10.1016/S0140-6736(13)60685-6.

Requejo, J. H., J. Bryce, A. J. Barros, P. Berman, Z. Bhutta, and others. 2015. "Countdown to 2015 and Beyond: Fulfilling the Health Agenda for Women and Children." *The Lancet* 385 (9966): 466–76. doi:10.1016/S0140-6736(14)60925-9.

Sabin, L. L., A. B. Knapp, W. B. MacLeod, G. Phiri-Mazala, J. Kasimba, and others. 2012. "Costs and Cost-Effectiveness of Training Traditional Birth Attendants to Reduce Neonatal Mortality in the Lufwanyama Neonatal Survival Study (LUNESP)." *PLoS One* 7 (4): e35560. doi:10.1371/journal.pone.0035560.

Sachdev, H. P. S., A. Hall, and N. Walker, eds. 2010. "Development and Use of the Lives Saved Tool (LiST): A Model to Estimate the Impact of Scaling up Proven Interventions on Maternal, Neonatal and Child Mortality." *Special issue of International Journal of Epidemiology* 39 (Supplement 1).

Say, L., D. Chou, A. Gemmill, O. Tuncalp, A. B. Moller, and others. 2014. "Global Causes of Maternal Death: A WHO Systematic Analysis." *The Lancet Global Health* 2 (6): e323–333. doi:10.1016/S2214-109X(14)70227-X.

Schmidt, H., L. O. Gostin, and E. J. Emanuel. 2015. "Public Health, Universal Health Coverage, and Sustainable Development Goals: Can They Coexist?" *The Lancet* 386 (9996): 928–30. doi:10.1016/S0140-6736(15)60244-6.

Sedgh, G., S. Singh, and R. Hussain. 2014. "Intended and Unintended Pregnancies Worldwide in 2012 and Recent Trends." *Studies in Family Planning* 45 (3): 301–14. doi:10.1111/j.1728-4465.2014.00393.x.

Shei, A. 2013. "Brazil's Conditional Cash Transfer Program Associated with Declines in Infant Mortality Rates." *Health Affairs* (Millwood) 32 (7): 1274–81.

Singh, S., J. Darroch, and L. Ashford. 2014. *Adding It Up: The Costs and Benefits of Investing in Sexual and Reproductive Health 2014.* New York: Guttmacher Institute.

Singh, S., G. Sedgh, and R. Hussain. 2010. "Unintended Pregnancy: Worldwide Levels, Trends, and Outcomes." *Studies in Family Planning* 41 (4): 241–50.

Singh, S., D. Wulf, R. Hussain, A. Bankole, and G. Sedgh. 2009. *Abortion Worldwide: A Decade of Uneven Progress.* New York: Guttmacher Institute.

Singla, D. R., E. Kumbakumba, and F. E. Aboud. 2015. "Effects of a Parenting Intervention to Address both Maternal Psychological Wellbeing and Child Development and Growth in Rural Uganda: A Community-Based, Cluster Randomised Trial." *The Lancet Global Health* 3 (8): e458–69. doi:10.1016/S2214-109X(15)00099-6.

Spector, J. M., A. Lashoher, P. Agrawal, C. Lemer, G. Dziekan, and others. 2013. "Designing the WHO Safe Childbirth Checklist Program to Improve Quality of Care at Childbirth." *International Journal of Gynaecology and Obstetrics* 122 (2): 164–68.

Stenberg, K., H. Axelson, P. Sheehan, I. Anderson, A. M. Gulmezoglu, and others. 2014. "Advancing Social and Economic Development by Investing in Women's and Children's Health: A New Global Investment Framework." *The Lancet* 383 (9925): 1333–54. doi:10.1016/S0140-6736(13)62231-X.

Stenberg, K., K. Sweeney, H. Axelson, M. Temmerman, and P. Sheehan. 2016. "Returns on Investment in the Continuum of Care for Reproductive, Maternal, Newborn, and Child Health." In *Disease Control Priorities* (third edition): Volume 2, *Reproductive, Maternal, Newborn, and Child Health,* edited by R. E. Black, R. Laxminarayan, N. Walker, and M. Temmerman. Washington, DC: World Bank.

Stevens, G., C. Paciorek, and M. Finucane. 2016. "Levels and Trends in Low Height for Age." In *Disease Control Priorities* (third edition): Volume 2, *Reproductive, Maternal, Newborn, and Child Health,* edited by R. E. Black, R. Laxminarayan, N. Walker, and M. Temmerman. Washington, DC: World Bank.

Stover, J., R. McKinnon, and B. Winfrey. 2010. "Spectrum: A Model Platform for Linking Maternal and Child Survival Interventions with AIDS, Family Planning and Demographic Projections." *International Journal of Epidemiology* 39 (Suppl 1): i7–10. doi:10.1093/ije/dyq016.

Temmerman, M., R. Khosla, Z. A. Bhutta, and F. Bustreo. 2015. "Towards a New Global Strategy for Women's, Children's and Adolescents' Health." Review. *BMJ* 351: h4414. doi:10.1136/bmj.h4414.

Temmerman, M., R. Khosla, L. Laski, Z. Mathews, and L. Say. 2015. "Women's Health Priorities and Interventions." *BMJ* 351: h4147. doi:10.1136/bmj.h4147.

UN (United Nations). 2015. *The Millennium Development Goals Report 2015*. New York: United Nations. http://www.un.org/millenniumgoals/2015_MDG_Report/pdf/MDG%202015%20rev%20(July%201).pdf.

UN IGME (Inter-Agency Group for Child Mortality Estimation). 2015. "Levels & Trends in Child Mortality: Report 2015." UN, New York.

UNPD (United Nations Population Division). 2015. "2015 World Population Prospects." UN, New York.

Verguet, S., Z. D. Olson, J. B. Babigumira, D. Desalegn, K. A. Johansson, and others. 2015. "Health Gains and Financial Risk Protection Afforded by Public Financing of Selected Interventions in Ethiopia: An Extended Cost-Effectiveness Analysis." *The Lancet Global Health* 3 (5): e288-296. doi:10.1016/S2214-109X(14)70346-8.

Verguet, S., R. Laxminarayan, and D. T. Jamison. 2015. "Universal Public Finance of Tuberculosis Treatment in India: An Extended Cost-Effectiveness Analysis." *Health Economics* 24 (3): 318–32.

Victora, C. G., L. Adair, C. Fall, P. C. Hallal, R. Martorell, and others. 2008. "Maternal and Child Undernutrition: Consequences for Adult Health and Human Capital." *The Lancet* 371 (9609): 340–57. doi:10.1016/S0140-6736(07)61692-4.

Villar, J., L. Cheikh Ismail, C. G. Victora, E. O. Ohuma, E. Bertino, and others. 2014. "International Standards for Newborn Weight, Length, and Head Circumference by Gestational Age and Sex: The Newborn Cross-Sectional Study of the INTERGROWTH-21st Project." *The Lancet* 384 (9946): 857–68. doi:10.1016/S0140-6736(14)60932-6.

Walker, N. 2013. "Updates of Assumptions and Methods for the Lives Saved Tool (LiST)." *BMC Public Health* 13 (Supplement 3): S1.

———, C. Fischer Walker, J. Bryce, R. Bahl, S. Cousens, and CHERG Review Groups on Intervention Effects. 2010. "Standards for CHERG Reviews of Intervention Effects on Child Survival." [Research Support, Non-U.S. Gov't].

International Journal of Epidemiology 39 (Suppl 1): i21–31. doi:10.1093/ije/dyq036.

Walker, N., Y. Tam, and I. K. Friberg. 2013. "Overview of the Lives Saved Tool (LiST)." *BMC Public Health* 13 (Suppl 3): S1. doi:10.1186/1471-2458-13-S3-S1.

Walker, S. P., T. D. Wachs, J. M. Gardner, B. Lozoff, G. A. Wasserman, and others. 2007. "Child Development: Risk Factors for Adverse Outcomes in Developing Countries." *The Lancet* 369 (9556): 145–57. doi:10.1016/S0140-6736(07)60076-2.

WHO (World Health Organization). 2012. *WHO Recommendations: Optimizing Health Worker Roles to Improve Access to Key Maternal and Newborn Health Interventions through Task Shifting*. Geneva: WHO.

———. 2015. *Trends in Maternal Mortality: 1990 to 2015: Estimates by WHO, UNICEF, UNFPA, World Bank, and the United Nations Population Division*. Geneva: WHO.

WHO, Department of Reproductive Health and Research, London School of Hygiene and Tropical Medicine, and South African Medical Research Council. 2013. *Global and Regional Estimates of Violence against Women: Prevalence and Health Effects of Intimate Partner Violence and Non-Partner Sexual Violence*. Geneva: WHO. doi:http://www.who.int/reproductivehealth/publications/violence/9789241564625/en/.

Witter, S., A. Fretheim, F. L. Kessy, and A. K. Lindahl. 2012. "Paying for Performance to Improve the Delivery of Health Interventions in Low- and Middle-Income Countries." *Cochrane Database of Systematic Reviews* 2: CD007899. doi:10.1002/14651858.CD007899.pub2.

World Bank. 1993. *World Development Report 1993: Investing in Health*. Oxford: Oxford University Press.

You, D., L. Hug, S. Ejdemyr, P. Idele, D. Hogan, and others. 2015. "Global, Regional, and National Levels and Trends in Under-5 Mortality between 1990 and 2015, with Scenario-Based Projections to 2030: A Systematic Analysis by the UN Inter-agency Group for Child Mortality Estimation." *The Lancet* 386 (10010): 2275–86. doi:10.1016/S0140-6736(15)00120-8.

Young, M., C. Wolfheim, D. R. Marsh, and D. Hammamy. 2012. "World Health Organization/United Nations Children's Fund Joint Statement on Integrated Community Case Management: An Equity-Focused Strategy to Improve Access to Essential Treatment Services for Children." *American Journal of Tropical Medicine and Hygiene* 87 (5 Suppl): 6–10. doi:10.4269/ajtmh.2012.12-0221.

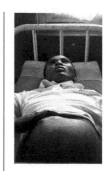

Chapter **2**

Burden of Reproductive Ill Health

Alex Ezeh, Akinrinola Bankole, John Cleland,
Claudia García-Moreno, Marleen Temmerman,
and Abdhalah Kasiira Ziraba

INTRODUCTION

This chapter presents the burden of global reproductive ill health and, where data permit, regional estimates for selected conditions. *Ill health* refers to morbid conditions such as infections and injury and to nonmorbid measures of reproductive health that directly contribute to adverse reproductive health outcomes, including unwanted pregnancies and violence against women. The chapter is organized into six subsections: unintended pregnancies, unsafe abortions, non-sexually transmitted reproductive tract infections (RTIs), infertility, violence against women, and female genital mutilation (FGM). Unintended pregnancies lead to unintended births and induced abortions. Unintended births often occur among young women who are emotionally and physiologically not mature, which has effects on the health of the mother, the pregnancy, and its outcome. Induced abortions in countries where the practice is illegal are often provided in unsafe environments and by untrained personnel, which contribute to the high maternal death from abortion complications. Sexually transmitted infections (STIs) of the reproductive tract receive attention in programming and research, but little attention is focused on other infections that affect fertility and increase the risk of transmission of other infections. Violence against women violates their rights, including limiting access to and use of prevention and treatment services in addition to physical injury and death. FGM causes bodily disfigurement and may present immediate

surgical complications and long-term risk of poor reproductive outcomes, especially during delivery.

Approach to Data Presentation and Limitations

The greatest challenge in undertaking this work is the lack of appropriate data at the global, regional, national, and subnational levels. Even available data are often not adequately disaggregated by important characteristics. Differences in methods and designs adopted by the various studies often limit the comparative value. In many low- and middle-income countries (LMICs), sexual concerns are often not discussed with third parties, which impedes health care seeking. Measuring and quantifying most of these conditions is logistically difficult, and the reliability of responses given by respondents is often poor (Allotey and Reidpath 2002). Because most reproductive conditions are more prevalent during prime ages, missed cases are likely to lead to serious underestimation of the burden of disease as measured by disability-adjusted life years (DALYs) of health lost (AbouZahr and Vaughan 2000).

UNINTENDED PREGNANCIES

Premarital sexual abstinence, prolonged breastfeeding, and abortion all influence fertility; however, contraceptive practice has been the most important driver of

Corresponding author: Alex Ezeh, African Population and Health Research Center, Nairobi, Kenya, and School of Public Health, University of the Witwatersrand, Johannesburg, South Africa, aezeh@aphrc.org.

falling fertility and population growth rates in the past half century. Because of its direct link to family sizes and population change, contraception has a wide range of social, economic, and environmental benefits, in addition to its well-documented health advantages for women and children. It enables women to escape the incessant cycle of pregnancies and infant care and represents progress toward gender equality and enhanced opportunities for women. At the national level, a fall in birth rates brings about declines in dependency ratios and increases potential opportunities for economic growth.

Contraception has wider social and economic benefits, but its immediate purpose is to avoid unintended pregnancies. The majority of these pregnancies stem from the non-use of contraceptive methods among women wishing to avoid or postpone childbearing. This section discusses the measurement of unintended pregnancies, both levels and trends, and reasons for and consequences of unintended births.

Measurement

Measurement of unintended pregnancies is complicated because many are terminated, and these terminations are underreported. Because most induced abortions are from unintended pregnancies, the solution is to combine survey data on unintended births with indirect estimates of abortion incidence available for all subregions and many countries.

Demographic and Health Surveys (DHS) are the main source of data on unintended births. The measurement of unintended births or current pregnancies from this source has been approached in three ways:

- Answers to questions on total desired family size
- Prospective questions on whether another child is wanted
- Retrospective questions on each recent birth to ascertain whether the child was wanted, unwanted, or mistimed by two or more years.

In the first approach, births that exceed total desired family size are defined as unwanted; if they are equal to or less than total desired family size, they are considered wanted. This classification can be expressed as unwanted or wanted fertility rates. No account is taken of mistimed births. A more serious problem stems from the likelihood that desired total family sizes are, in part, a rationalization of actual family sizes, with the consequence that unwanted births are likely to be underestimated.

The second approach is straightforward in prospective studies, but its application is severely limited by the lack of studies. This method has been adapted to single and successive cross-sectional surveys to provide aggregate estimates of unwanted fertility (Casterline and El-Zeini 2007). As with the first approach, mistimed births are ignored.

The third approach uses retrospective questions concerning the wantedness and preferred timing of recent births. It has the advantage of incorporating mistimed as well as unwanted births, but estimates are vulnerable to post factum rationalization due to an understandable reluctance of mothers to report children as unwanted or mistimed. Prospective studies in India, Malawi, Morocco, and Pakistan indicate that a large proportions of births to women who reported at baseline a desire to have no more children were subsequently classified by mothers as wanted or mistimed (Baschieri and others 2013; Jain and others 2014; Speizer and others 2013; Westoff and Bankole 1998). Similarly, an appreciable fraction of births that occur as the result of accidental pregnancy while using a contraceptive method or after abandoning a method are reported as wanted. (Ali, Cleland, and Shaw 2012; Curtis, Evens, and Sambisa 2011; Trussell, Vaughan, and Stanford 1999). These inconsistencies are usually interpreted as the consequence of rationalization, but they may reflect a genuine difference between a more abstract preference before childbirth and a more emotional reaction after the event.

The three approaches to measurement yield very different results. No consensus exists on how best to obtain valid estimates of unintended births, even in the United States, where the topic has attracted considerable attention (Campbell and Mosher 2000; Santelli and others 2003). This section presents results based on the retrospective method because studies using this method are the sole source of global and regional estimates, but the results are presented with the caveat that they may be downwardly biased. Another approach that has been tried, but on a limited scale, is the London Measure of Unplanned Pregnancy (Morof and others 2012; Wellings and others 2013).

Prevalence and Incidence

By combining regional estimates on induced abortion and retrospective survey data on mistimed and unwanted births with allowances for miscarriages, Sedgh, Singh, and Hussain (2014) derive global and regional estimates on the incidence of unintended pregnancies and the proportion of all pregnancies that are unintended (table 2.1). Globally, their prevalence data indicate that 40 percent of all pregnancies in 2012 were unintended. The prevalence of unintended pregnancies is higher, and such pregnancies are more likely to be

Table 2.1 Indicators of Unintended Pregnancies, 2012

| Region | Total number of pregnancies (millions) | Pregnancy rate per 1,000 women ages 15–44 years | | | Percent of pregnancies that are unintended |
		All pregnancies	Intended	Unintended	
Worldwide	213.4	133	80	53	40
More developed	23.4	94	50	44	47
Less developed	190.0	140	85	54	39
Africa	53.8	224	145	80	35
Eastern	19.4	246	138	108	44
Middle	7.8	279	171	108	39
Northern	7.1	144	103	41	29
Southern	1.8	124	55	69	55
Western	17.6	256	191	66	26
Asia	119.7	120	75	46	38
Eastern	36.6	99	62	37	37
South-Central	56.5	134	86	48	36
Southeastern	18.8	127	71	56	44
Western	7.8	141	79	62	44
Europe	14.1	94	52	43	45
Eastern	7.0	110	52	57	52
Northern	1.8	93	58	35	38
Southern	2.4	80	45	35	44
Western	2.8	80	52	27	34
Latin America and the Caribbean	17.8	122	54	68	56
Caribbean	1.3	133	48	84	64
Central America	5.1	125	75	50	40
South America	11.4	120	45	74	62
North America	7.1	100	49	51[a]	51[a]
Oceania	0.9	116	73	43	37

Source: Sedgh, Singh, and Hussain 2014.
Note: In this table, "more developed" comprises Australia, Europe, Japan, New Zealand, and North America. "Less developed" comprises all others.
a. If mistimed births in North America were limited to those that occurred at least two years before they were wanted, as in Africa, Asia, and Latin America and the Caribbean, the unintended pregnancy rate would be 44 percent and the proportion of pregnancies that were unintended in North America would be 42 percent.

terminated, in high-income countries (HICs) than in LMICs. However, when expressed as annual rates per 1,000 women of reproductive age, unintended pregnancies are more common in LMICs.

There is little relationship between the prevalence or incidence of unintended pregnancy and the level of contraceptive use or unmet need. The reason for this apparently counterintuitive observation is that exposure to risk of unintended pregnancy increases as desired family size and fertility fall. In societies in which sexual activity starts early and couples want two or fewer children, the

risk of an unintended pregnancy spans 20 years or more. The use of effective contraception for so many years is a daunting prospect. In societies in which the preference for larger families remains high, as in much of Sub-Saharan Africa, the risk span is shorter. Despite this upward pressure from increasing exposure to risk, unintended pregnancy rates per 1,000 women of reproductive age fell by an estimated 4.8 percent and 5.3 percent in HICs and LMICs, respectively, between 2008 and 2012 (Sedgh, Singh, and Hussain 2014). There was a 5.6 percent decline in Latin America and the Caribbean, and a 6 percent decline in both Asia and Africa. Intended pregnancy rates in LMICs did not change during the period (85 per 1,000 women of reproductive age).

In Sub-Saharan Africa, the proportion of mistimed births is about twice that of unwanted pregnancy among all unplanned births. In Latin America and the Caribbean, mistimed births are about 37 percent higher than unwanted pregnancy as a percentage of all unplanned births (Sedgh, Singh, and Hussain 2014). An application of the standard DHS measure of unwanted fertility, based on total desired family size, shows that unwanted fertility rates are strongly related to household poverty. Averaged across 41 LMICs, the poorest quintile recorded 1.2 unwanted births, compared with about 0.5 such births among the richest quintile (Gillespie and others 2007).

Reasons for Unintended Pregnancies

Approximately 70 percent of unintended pregnancies in LMICs are the direct result of no use or discontinued use of contraceptives; the balance results from accidental pregnancy while using contraception inconsistently or incorrectly and from method failure (Bradley, Croft, and Rutstein 2011; Singh, Darroch, and Ashford 2014). Accordingly, the reasons for unintended pregnancy should be sought primarily in reasons for non-use of contraceptives. In-depth studies confirm survey evidence that health concerns and low perceived risk of conception are genuine and common reasons for non-use but also suggest that lack of knowledge and social obstacles, including fear of others' disapproval, are more important barriers than the survey data imply (Sedgh, and Hussain 2014; Westoff 2012).

Consequences

Insufficient data exist to indicate whether unintended pregnancies carried to term are disadvantaged in health or schooling, compared with intended births. Other effects of unintended pregnancies on family health are easier to document. A reduction in the number of unintended pregnancies is the greatest health benefit of contraception. In 2008, contraception prevented an estimated 250,000 maternal deaths, and an additional 30 percent of maternal deaths could be avoided by fulfillment of the unmet need for contraception (Cleland and others 2012). By preventing high-risk pregnancies, especially in women of high parities, and those that would have ended in unsafe abortion, increased contraceptive use has also reduced the maternal mortality ratio—the risk of maternal death per 100,000 live births—by 26 percent in little more than a decade. The reduction in unintended pregnancies represents major savings in the costs of maternal and neonatal health services (Singh and Darroch 2012).

The reduction of mistimed and unwanted births also improves perinatal outcomes and child survival by lengthening interpregnancy intervals. In LMICs, the risk of prematurity and low birth weight doubles when conception occurs within six months of a previous birth; children born within two years of an older sibling are 60 percent more likely to die in infancy than are those born three years or more after their sibling. In early childhood, children who experience the birth of a younger sibling within two years have twice the risk of death than other children. In high-fertility countries, where most children have younger and older siblings, ensuring an interval of at least two years between births would reduce infant mortality by 10 percent and early childhood deaths by 20 percent (Cleland and others 2012; Cohen and others 2012; Hobcraft, McDonald, and Rutstein 1985; Kozuki and Walker 2013; Kozuki and others 2013).

The reduction of teenage pregnancies is an international priority, both because of the excess risk to maternal health of pregnancy and childbirth before age 18 and because it may curtail schooling and blight aspirations. In most Sub-Saharan African countries, more than 25 percent of women become mothers before age 18 years; equally high probabilities of early childbearing are recorded in Bangladesh, India, the Republic of Yemen, and several countries in Latin America and the Caribbean (Dixon-Mueller 2008). However, the primary cause is early marriage, and first births within marriage are unlikely to be considered unintended.

With respect to perinatal and child health and survival, evidence of an adverse effect of large family sizes is weak (Desai 1995). Excess risk of death is restricted to children of birth order seven or higher, and the relationship between birth order and malnutrition is small and irregular in Sub-Saharan Africa (Mahy 2003; Mukuria, Cushing, and Sangha 2005).

Finally, evidence from Matlab, Bangladesh, suggests the long-term benefits of reduced fertility. In the experimental area in which an early decline in fertility occurred, women had better nutritional status, more assets, and higher earnings than in higher fertility areas. Boys' schooling and girls' nutrition benefited from low fertility (Canning and Schultz 2012).

UNSAFE ABORTION

The World Health Organization (WHO) defines unsafe abortion as the termination of an unwanted pregnancy, either by persons lacking the necessary skills or in an environment lacking minimal medical standards or both.

Unsafe abortion is a major cause of maternal morbidity and mortality, especially in LMICs. About 7 million women are treated for complications from unsafe abortion procedures annually in LMICs (Singh and Maddow-Zimet 2015). Two studies, using different methodologies, indicate that at least 8 percent of maternal mortality is due to unsafe abortion, and the contribution of abortion may be as high as 18 percent of these deaths (Kassebaum and others 2014; Say and others 2014).

Measurement

In countries in which abortion is legally restricted or socially stigmatized, official statistics on abortion are usually nonexistent; those that do exist are typically incomplete and unreliable (Ahman and Shah 2012). Approaches that directly measure unsafe abortion, such as sample surveys and in-depth interviews, are unreliable. Accordingly, efforts to better measure incidence have largely used indirect methods (Ahman and Shah 2012), including surveys of abortion providers, complications statistics, anonymous third-party reports, estimates from experts, and regression equation approaches (Rossier 2003; Singh, Prada, and Juarez 2011).

The WHO's indirect approach involves using available information on unsafe abortion and associated mortality from hospital records and surveys of abortion providers, women's abortion-seeking behavior, postabortion care, and laws regarding abortion to obtain country estimates of unsafe abortion rates. The country-level estimates are then aggregated at the regional and global levels to ensure robust estimates that can potentially offset underestimation or error at the level of individual countries (Ahman and Shah 2012; WHO 2011). The WHO has used this methodology to produce global and regional estimates of unsafe abortion for 1990, 1993, 1996, 2000, 2003, and 2008. These estimates are likely to be conservative (Ahman and Shah 2012).

Much of what is known about the magnitude of unsafe abortion at the country level is from indirect methods, particularly the residual method (Johnston and Westoff 2010), and the Abortion Incidence Complications Methodology (AICM) (Singh, Prada, and Juarez 2011). The AICM relies primarily on data from two surveys: a nationally representative survey of health facilities likely to provide postabortion care, and a purposive sample of health professionals knowledgeable about abortion in the country. The methodology yields estimates of the incidence of unsafe abortion and abortion-related morbidity (table 2.3, columns 1 and 3). The rates tend to be higher in Latin America and the Caribbean than in Asia and Sub-Saharan Africa. Although AICM has been an important source of knowledge in countries with restrictive abortion laws, its limitations include high costs, dependence on a number of assumptions, and reliance on the opinions of health professionals (Juarez, Cabigon, and Singh 2010).

Incidence

An estimated 21.6 million unsafe abortions, or 14 per 1,000 women ages 15–44 years, were performed in 2008 (WHO 2011). These unsafe procedures constituted nearly 49 percent of all abortions, which totaled 43.8 million, or 28 per 1,000 women ages 15–44 years that year (Sedgh and others 2012). Virtually all of the unsafe abortions (98 percent) occurred in LMICs; the highest rates were found in Latin America and the Caribbean (31 per 1,000), followed by Sub-Saharan Africa (28) and Asia (11). The rate of unsafe abortion in HICs is only one per 1,000 (WHO 2011).

The global incidence has remained virtually unchanged since 1995, at 15 per 1,000 women ages 15–44 years in 1995 and 14 per 1,000 in 2003 and 2008 (table 2.2). In LMICs, unsafe abortion is highest among women ages 20–24 years and 25–29 years, with rates of 30 and 31, respectively, per 1,000 women in these age groups (Ahman and Shah 2012). The rate is lowest among women ages 40–44 years (13 per 1,000), and the rate among adolescent women is moderate (16 per 1,000).

Consequences

Maternal Mortality

Unsafe abortion involves health, economic, and social sequelae (Singh and others 2006). The WHO estimates that in 2008, 47,000 women died from unsafe abortion, translating to 30 unsafe abortion deaths per 100,000 live births (WHO 2011). Nearly two-thirds of the deaths (29,000) occurred in Sub-Saharan Africa.

Worldwide, the abortion case fatality rate is 220 per 100,000 unsafe abortions. The rate is highest in Sub-Saharan Africa (460 per 100,000); it is 160 in Asia and 80 in Latin America and the Caribbean. This wide variation across regions is not surprising, since the measure is largely a function of the risks associated with prevalent abortion methods and access to emergency care. Accordingly, while the incidence of unsafe abortion is similar for Sub-Saharan Africa and Latin America and the Caribbean, the procedure is less deadly in Latin America and the Caribbean because of widespread use of medical abortion and better access to health care (WHO 2011). In 2015, the estimated number of maternal deaths worldwide was 303,000 (Alkema and others 2015). According to two more recent parallel studies, the proportion of these deaths that is due to unsafe abortion ranges between

Table 2.2 Trends in Rates of Unsafe Abortion and the Proportion of All Abortions That Are Unsafe: 1995–2008

Region and subregion	2008		2003		1995	
	Rate of unsafe abortion*	Percentage of all abortions that are unsafe	Rate of unsafe abortion*	Percentage of all abortions that are unsafe	Rate of unsafe abortion*	Percentage of all abortions that are unsafe
World	14	49	14	47	15	44
HICs	1	6	2	7	4	9
LMICs	16	56	16	55	18	54
Africa	28	97	29	98	33	99
Asia	11	40	11	38	12	37
Europe	2	9	3	11	6	12
Latin America and the Caribbean	31	95	30	96	35	95
North America	<0.5	<0.5	<0.5	<0.5	<0.5	<0.5
Oceania	2	15	3	16	5	22

Source: Sedgh and others 2012.
Note: HICs = high-income countries; LMICs = low- and middle-income countries.
*Abortions per 1,000 women ages 15–44 years.

Table 2.3 Incidence of Abortion and Complications from Unsafe Abortion in Low- and Middle-Income Countries

Country, date	Annual number of women who had abortions (a)	Abortion rates per 1,000 women (b)	Number of women with complications from unsafe abortion treated in health facilities (c)	Annual rate of complications treated in health facilities per 1,000 women (d)
Africa				
Burkina Faso, 2008 (a)	87,200	25.0	22,900	6.6*
Egypt, Arab Rep. 1996 (b)	324,000	23.0	216,000	15.3
Ethiopia, 2008 (c)	382,450	23.1	52,600	3.2
Kenya, 2013 (d)	464,700	48.0	119,900	12.4*
Malawi, 2009 (e)	67,300	23.0	18,700	6.4*
Nigeria, 1996 (f)	610,000	25.0	142,200	6.1
Rwanda, 2009 (g)	60,000	25.0	16,700	7.0
Uganda, 2002 (h)	296,700	54.0	85,000	16.4
Asia				
Bangladesh, 2010 (i)	647,000	18.2	231,400	6.5
Pakistan, 2002 (j)	890,000	29.0	197,000	7.0
Philippines, 2000 (k)	78,900	27.0	78,150	4.4
Latin America and the Caribbean				
Brazil, 1991 (f)	1,444,000	40.8	288,700	8.1
Chile, 1990 (f)	160,000	50.0	31,900	10.0
Colombia, 2008 (l)	400,400	39.0	93,300	9.0

table continues next page

Table 2.3 Incidence of Abortion and Complications from Unsafe Abortion in Low- and Middle-Income Countries (continued)

Country, date	Annual number of women who had abortions (a)	Abortion rates per 1,000 women (b)	Number of women with complications from unsafe abortion treated in health facilities (c)	Annual rate of complications treated in health facilities per 1,000 women (d)
Dominican Republic, 1990 (f)	82,000	47.0	16,500	9.8
Guatemala, 2003 (m)	65,000	24.0	21,600	8.6
Mexico, 2009 (n)	874,700	33.0	159,000	5.9
Peru, 1989 (f)	271,000	56.1	50,000	. 8.6

Sources: (a) = Sedgh and others 2011; (b) = Henshaw and others 1999; (c) = Singh and others 2010; (d) = African Population and Health Research Center and Ministry of Health Kenya 2013; (e) = Levandowski and others 2013; (f) = Henshaw and others 1999; (g) = Basinga and others 2012; (h) = Singh and others 2005; (i) = Singh and others 2012; (j) = Sathar, Singh, and Fikree 2007; (k) = Juarez and others 2005; (l) = Prada, Biddlecom, and Singh 2011; (m) = Singh, Prada, and Kestler 2006; (n) = Juarez and Singh 2012.
*Figures were not reported in original source; they are derived as d = [(c/a)×100].

8 percent and 18 percent, excluding late maternal death (Kassebaum and others 2014; Say and others 2014).

Abortion-Related Morbidity

Each year, 7 million women receive treatment for complications from unsafe abortions in the developing world (Singh 2006, 2010; Singh and others 2009). The annual rate of treatment after unsafe abortions is 6.9 per 1,000 women of reproductive age, which means 4.6 million women receive needed treatment in Asia, as do 1.6 million in Sub-Saharan Africa and 757,000 in Latin America and the Caribbean (Singh 2006). The incidence and severity of unsafe abortion complications are closely related to the training of the providers and the abortion methods used. A substantial proportion of the procedures are performed by untrained providers, including by pregnant women. In each country in which the AICM has been applied to estimate abortion incidence, a substantial number of women are admitted annually for treatment of complications resulting from unsafe abortions. These estimates are approximations based on the best guesses of health care providers and professionals, as well as on a number of assumptions. Table 2.3 shows abortion rate and abortion complication rate.

Health complications typically associated with unsafe abortion include hemorrhage; sepsis; peritonitis; RTIs; and trauma to the cervix, vagina, uterus, and abdominal organs (Grimes and others 2006; Henshaw and others 2008). Beginning with an effort sparked by a seminal WHO-led study in 1986, a fairly standard method has been developed and used to measure the nature and severity of unsafe abortion complications based on nationally representative surveys (Benson and Crane 2005; Fetters 2010; Figa-Talamanca and others 1986).

Table 2.4 Prevalence of Severe Symptoms from Unsafe Abortion in Low- and Middle-Income Countries

Country, date	Percentage of women with severe symptoms among those presenting with unsafe abortion complications
South Africa, 2000 (a)	10
Malawi, 2009 (b)	21
Ethiopia, 2008 (c)	27
Kenya, 2012 (d)	37
Cambodia, 2005 (e)	42

Sources: (a) = Jewkes and others 2005; (b) = Kalilani-Phiri and others 2015; (c) = Gebreselassie and others 2010; (d) = African Population and Health Research Center and Ministry of Health Kenya 2013; (e) = Fetters and others 2008.

Studies report that among women presenting with unsafe abortion complications in health facilities, the proportion diagnosed with severe symptoms varies widely (table 2.4).

Severe complications, if not well managed, may result in anemia, RTIs, elevated risk of ectopic pregnancy, premature delivery or miscarriage in subsequent pregnancies, and infertility (WHO 2004). Almost 5 million women are living with temporary or permanent disabilities associated with unsafe abortion; more than 3 million of these women suffer from the effects of RTIs, and close to 1.7 million experience secondary infertility (WHO 2007).

Economic and Social Consequences

Unsafe abortion has direct and indirect costs. Direct costs include expenses related to the provision of medical care to women presenting with abortion-related complications, such as cost of medicine, providers' time, and hospital stays. Indirect costs are opportunity costs due to death or disability stemming from the complications.

Direct costs. In 2006, the average direct per-patient costs of treating abortion-related complications were US$130 in Latin America and the Caribbean and US$114 in Sub-Saharan Africa (Vlassoff, Walker, and others 2009). After including indirect costs, per-patient costs of treating postabortion complications in the two regions rose to US$227–US$320.

Indirect costs. A study in Uganda (Sundaram and others 2013) finds that most women treated for unsafe abortion complications experienced one or more adverse effects, including loss of productivity (73 percent); deterioration in household economic circumstances (34 percent); and negative consequences for their children, such as inability to eat well or go to school (60 percent).

Unsafe abortion also has social costs, including social stigma, sanctions, divorce, and spousal and family neglect (Levandowski and others 2012; Moore, Jagwe-Wadda, and Bankole 2011; Rossier 2007; Shellenberg and others 2011).

Unintended pregnancy, unmet need for contraception, and unsafe abortion. Meeting the contraceptive needs of all 225 million women in LMICs who had unmet need for modern contraception in 2014 would have prevented an estimated 52 million unintended pregnancies and averted 24 million abortions, 14 million of which would have been unsafe (Singh, Darroch, and Ashford 2014). Similar associations have been found at the country level (Darroch and others 2009; Sundaram and others 2009; Vlassoff, Sundaram, and others 2009; Vlassoff and others 2011). The demand for family limitation may not be fully satisfied by the use of contraceptives, and some women and couples may resort to abortion. In such situations, both contraceptive use and abortion rates may rise, while fertility declines (Marston and Cleland 2003).

NON-SEXUALLY TRANSMITTED INFECTIONS OF THE REPRODUCTIVE SYSTEM

RTIs may be classified as either transmitted sexually, as with syphilis and gonorrhea, or non-sexually, for example, bacterial vaginosis (BV); others, such as yeast infections, may be both. The focus in this section is on non-STIs of the reproductive tract, specifically two neglected reproductive health morbidities: BV and vulvovaginal candidiasis (VVC). These RTIs are increasingly identified as having substantial public health importance because of the increased risk of STI transmission, including human immunodeficiency virus (HIV) (Cohen and others 2012; Martin and others 1999; Myer and others 2005; Namkinga and others 2005).

Vulvovaginal Candidiasis

VVC is characterized by excessive growth of a normal vaginal flora fungus, candida, often associated with vulval itching, abnormal vaginal discharge, vulval excoriation, and dyspareunia. It is common among women of reproductive age. VVC is relatively more common among women who are pregnant, have poorly controlled diabetes mellitus, or have compromised immunity due to human immunodeficiency virus/acquired immunodeficiency syndrome (HIV/AIDS) or other causes (Buchta and others 2013; de Leon and others 2002; Duerr and others 2003). It is also common in women receiving antibiotic treatment and those using vaginal douching and other forms of vaginal applications (Brown and others 2013; Ekpenyong and others 2012).

Measurement

Measurement of prevalence and incidence of VVC in most settings is challenging. Clinical diagnosis based on symptoms is inadequate owing to the low sensitivity and specificity of criteria used to identify clinically important candida infections. Estimates from such studies cannot be depended upon to generate a reliable epidemiologic profile to act as a basis for public health planning of interventions (Geiger, Foxman, and Gillespie 1995; Rathod and others 2012). In a study of women in India, the positive predictive value for candidiasis was only 19 percent, implying a high likelihood of confusing VVC with BV, since the two are common and may occur together (Rathod and others 2012). However, not all positive laboratory tests for candida constitute clinically important cases of VVC. In response to this challenge, the Centers for Disease Control and Prevention (CDC) has provided diagnostic criteria that include symptoms and laboratory findings (CDC 2010; Ilkit and Guzel 2011). According to these criteria, a patient must have (1) one or more symptoms, such as vaginal itching or discharge; and (2) a positive wet preparation or gram stain or positive culture (CDC 2010).

Given the challenges involved in conducting community-based studies using gynecologic specimens, most studies that have assessed prevalence or incidence have been clinic-based among symptomatic women. Only a few studies have been population based (Ahmad and Khan 2009; Goto and others 2005; Oliveira and others 2007). Estimates derived from clinic-based studies cannot be generalized. Even where community-based studies have been conducted, the tendency is to report the prevalence of candida species recovered from the specimens and symptoms separately; no effort is made to use the criteria that integrate laboratory findings and symptoms to derive the proportion of women with clinically significant candida infection.

Prevalence of Vulvovaginal Candidiasis

The prevalence of VVC varies between subpopulations along characteristics such as age, sexual activity, and socioeconomic status. The proportion of candida species–positive women among women attending clinics with symptoms is generally higher than levels observed in the general population. In some clinic-based studies, results have shown prevalence as high as 40 percent to 60 percent (Ibrahim and others 2013; Nwadioha and others 2013; Okungbowa, Isikhuemhen, and Dede 2003).

Table 2.5 summarizes community-based studies of the prevalence of candida species from vaginal or cervical specimens and of VVC. In the few studies reporting VVC based on clinical and laboratory findings, prevalence seems to be generally less than 10 percent. This result implies that studies and estimates based on only clinical diagnoses tend to overdiagnose, and possibly result in overtreatment of, vaginal candidiasis. The consequences may include unnecessary treatment costs, side effects, and development of resistance to commonly prescribed antifungal drugs.

Consequences of Vulvovaginal Candidiasis

Although VVC might be considered a nuisance, the inflammatory process of VVC puts women at increased risk of transmission of RTIs, including STIs and HIV (Hester and Kennedy 2003; Rathod and others 2012). Against this background, like STIs, VVC should always be managed for the extra benefit of reducing the risk of contracting other STIs. The fact that treatment for VVC is cheap and available over the counter in many countries presents another challenge of overtreatment and potential drug resistance. In most settings, the diagnosis is clinical; however, this diagnosis has a low specificity resulting in cases of BV being treated as VVC, leaving BV untreated.

Bacterial Vaginosis

In BV, normal vaginal *lactobacilli* are replaced by other bacteria, especially *Gardnerella vaginalis* and other anaerobic bacteria (Hay and Taylor-Robinson 1996). There is a link between BV and known risk factors for STIs, including multiple sexual partnerships and early onset of sexual activity (Fethers and others 2008; Foxman 1990; Morris, Rogers, and Kinghorn 2001; Reed and others 2003). Indeed, the debate about whether BV is sexually transmitted or enhanced remains unsettled. Other factors associated with BV include black race (Hay and others 1994; Koumans and others 2007; Ness and others 2003; Wenman and others 2004), use of intrauterine devices (Baeten and others 2001; Madden and others 2012), menses (Eschenbach and others 2000), lack of male circumcision (Gray and others 2009), and douching (Brotman and others 2008).

Measurement

Clinical diagnosis is difficult because symptoms have low predictive values, yet laboratory facilities are not always available, especially in developing countries (Landers and others 2004; Rathod and others 2012). There has been debate on the clinical presentation of BV and isolation of causative bacteria (Hay and Taylor-Robinson 1996).

Table 2.5 Prevalence of Candida Species and Vulvovaginal Candidiasis from Community-Based Studies

Study	Prevalence of candida species (%)	Prevalence of vulvovaginal candidiasis* (%)
Epidemiologic features of vulvovaginal candidiasis among reproductive-age women in India (a)	35.0	7.1
Reproductive tract infections among young married women in Tamil Nadu, India (b)	10.0	10.0
Sexually transmitted infections, bacterial vaginosis, and candidiasis in women of reproductive age in rural Northeast Brazil: a population-based study (c)	12.5	
Prevalence and risk factors for bacterial vaginosis and other vulvovaginitis in a population of sexually active adolescents from Salvador, Bahia, Brazil (d)	22.0	
Sexually transmitted infections in a female population in rural Northeast Brazil: prevalence, morbidity, and risk factors (e)	5.8	
Community-based study of reproductive tract infections among women of the reproductive age group in the Urban Training Centre Area in Hubli Kamataka, India (f)	16.1	
Prevalence of and factors associated with reproductive tract infections among pregnant women in 10 communes in Nghe An Province, Vietnam (g)	17.0	
Prevalence and risk factors for vaginal candidiasis among women seeking primary care for genital infections in Dar es Salaam, Tanzania (h)	45.0	

Sources: (a) = Rathod and others 2012; (b) = Prasad and others 2005; (c) = Oliveira and others 2007; (d) = Mascarenhas, Machado, and others 2012; (e) = de Lima Soares and others 2003; (f) = Balamurugan and Bendigeri 2012; (g) = Goto and others 2005; (h) = Namkinga and others 2005.
*According to Centers for Disease Control and Prevention criteria—one or more symptoms and signs and positive lab test or culture.

The commonly used clinical criteria are the Amsel criteria, with reported sensitivity of more than 90 percent and specificity of more than 75 percent as judged against gram staining (Landers and others 2004). The Nugent Scoring System criteria are considered the gold standard, with better sensitivity and specificity (Mota and others 2000; Nugent, Krohn, and Hillier 1991); however, few studies have used these criteria.

Little systematic effort has been made to estimate the global prevalence of BV. The few systematic reviews that have been conducted reveal that the current evidence is based on small studies (Kenyon, Colebunders, and Crucitti 2013). Estimates from these studies are discussed here in the context of where the study was conducted rather than as global or regional estimates (Kenyon, Colebunders, and Crucitti 2013). International comparisons are difficult because of differences in the populations studied, as well as in the methods used in selecting participants. Also, because of the associations between BV, VVC, pregnancy status, and sexual activity, we only present estimates from studies that include participants from the general adult female population. We exclude those that only focus on pregnant women, those attending sexually transmitted diseases clinics, and those restricted to only sexually experienced women.

Prevalence of Bacterial Vaginosis
Estimates presented here are from studies that use the Nugent Scoring System. A diagnosis of BV is defined as a Nugent score of 7 or higher out of 10 (Nugent, Krohn, and Hillier 1991). Table 2.6 summarizes population-based studies from regions with estimates of BV prevalence.

Although there are no global estimates, it is clear that BV is common and variations exist across countries and subpopulations. The variation within regions makes interpretation of spatial distribution difficult.

Consequences of Bacterial Vaginosis
Although the etiologic mechanism of anaerobic bacteria found in BV-causing pelvic inflammatory disease (PID)

Table 2.6 Prevalence of Bacterial Vaginosis from Population-Based Studies

Region	Country, location, year	Study population	Prevalence of bacterial vaginosis* (%)
Latin America and the Caribbean			
	Brazil, Alagoas, 1997 (a)	Random sample of 341 women	15.3
	Brazil, Serra Pelada, Para, 2004 (b)	Random sample of 209 women	18.7
	Brazil, Pacoti, Ceara, before 2007 (c)	Random sample of 592 women	20.1
	Peru, rural areas, 1997–98 (d)	Random sample of 752 women	40.8
	Peru, Lima, Trujillo, Chiclayo (e)	Random sample of 779 women	26.6
North America			
	United States, NHANES, 2001–04 (f)	Random sample of 3,739 women	29.2
Western Europe			
	Finland, Aland Islands, 1993–2008 (g)	Random sample of 819 women in 1993 and 771 women in 2008	15.6 (1993) 8.6 (2008)
South and Southeast Asia			
	Vietnam, Bavi District, 2006 (h)	Random sample of 1,012 women, excluded menstruating women	11.0
	Vietnam, Haiphong, before 2006 (i)	Random sample of 284 women	27.4
Sub-Saharan Africa			
	The Gambia, Farafenni, 1999 (j)	Random sample of 1,348 women	37.0
	Burkina Faso, Ouagadougou, 2003 (k)	Random sample of 883 women	7.9

Sources: (a) = de Lima Soares and others 2003; (b) = Miranda and others 2009; (c) = Oliveira and others 2007; (d) = Garcia and others 2004; (e) = Jones and others 2007; (f) = Koumans and others 2007; (g) = Eriksson and others 2010; (h) = Lan and others 2008; (i) = Go and others 2006; (j) = Walraven and others 2001; (k) = Kirakoya-Samadoulougou and others 2011.
Note: NHANES = National Health and Nutrition Examination Survey.
*Based on the Nugent Scoring System.

Reproductive, Maternal, Newborn, and Child Health

has not been demonstrated, studies have recovered anaerobic bacteria from PID cases. PID is a major cause of tubal factor secondary infertility, therefore identification and treatment of BV is important (van Oostrum and others 2013). BV is also known to facilitate transmission of other STIs including HIV (Kinuthia and others 2015). Like VVC, clinical diagnosis of BV has low sensitivity and a high likelihood of misdiagnosis and mistreatment; efforts to have a confirmed laboratory diagnosis should always be made. BV has also been associated with miscarriages, premature delivery, and postpartum infection (Nelson and others 2015).

INFERTILITY

Involuntary infertility may bring about much psychological, economic, and social distress to affected individuals, especially in societies in which childbearing is highly expected of any couple. Causes of infertility are many, ranging from ovulation dysfunction, tubal factor (often sequelae), implantation disorders in the uterus, and male factors. Secondary infertility, the more prevalent type, often results from complications following miscarriage, delivery, untreated STI, and induced abortion in low-resource settings (Cates, Farley, and Rowe 1985; Cates, Rolfs, and Aral 1990; Larsen, Masenga, and Mlay 2006). Untreated STIs such as gonorrhea, chlamydia, and PID are responsible for the majority of tubal factor infertility cases (Boivin and others 2007; Bunnell and others 1999; Che and Cleland 2002; Desai, Kosambiya, and Thakor 2003; Heiligenberg and others 2012; Inhorn 2003).

Definition and Measurement

There are disciplinary variations in the definition and operationalization of measurement of infertility, including clinical, epidemiologic, and demographic (Gurunath and others 2011; WHO 2006a; Zegers-Hochschild and others 2009).

The key issues in operationalization of the definition of infertility or childlessness that make comparison and interpretation of estimates from various studies difficult include the following:

• **Exposure to risk of pregnancy as captured by union status, intention of getting pregnant, and contraceptive use:** The nature of a union has implications for frequency and regularity of sexual intercourse, which translates into risk of pregnancy. Similarly, variations occur in measurement of contraceptive use (Gurunath and others 2011).

• **Exposure time:** Sensitivity analysis using DHS data show that using a period of less than five years was likely to result in misclassification of fertile unions as infertile (Mascarenhas, Cheung, and others 2012). Shorter periods of one year help identify individuals and couples who may benefit from earlier intervention; epidemiological studies use two-year time frames that allow the problem of infertility to be quantified at the population level and limit misclassification of either fertile or infertile unions (WHO 2006a).

• **Outcome measure:** The medical literature focuses on failure to achieve or to maintain a clinical pregnancy, which misclassifies women as fertile who have repeat early miscarriage, or endometrial insufficiency resulting in repeat late fetal death or stillbirth. Demographers often use live birth as a more easily measurable outcome that defines childlessness (Gurunath and others 2011). Generally, the clinical definition and its operationalization are best suited for purposes of early diagnosis and management of infertility, whereas the epidemiological definition is best suited for population-level estimates, and demographic definitions for trend analysis.

• **Populations studied:** Some studies have examined women ages 15–44 years and 20–44 years, while others have examined women ages 15–49 years. In countries with high levels of voluntary childlessness, this difference needs to be accounted for because older women (older than age 44 years) may likely be considered infertile although menopausal, and younger women (younger than age 20 years) may likely be considered fertile, yet they may already suffer from tubal factor infertility (Rutstein and Shah 2004; Larsen 2005; Mascarenhas, Cheung, and others 2012).

The definitions of infertility used in the WHO Trend Analysis are as follows:

• *Primary infertility* is the absence of a live birth for women who desire a child, have been in a union for at least five years, and who did not use contraceptives during that time. The prevalence of primary infertility is calculated as the number of women in infertile union divided by the total number of fertile and infertile women.

• *Secondary infertility* is the absence of a live birth for women who desire a child, have been in a union for at least five years since their last live birth, and who did not use contraceptives during that time. The prevalence of secondary infertility is calculated as the number of women in a secondary infertile union divided by all fertile and infertile women who have had at least one live birth.

Prevalence of Primary and Secondary Infertility

The estimates reported here are derived from a global study that evaluates trends, and adjusts downward based on the lowest ranking of the disease as part of the DALY exercise by the Global Burden of Disease group, and reported in the *World Report on Disability* (WHO and World Bank 2011). The WHO, as part of the Global Burden of Disease exercise (Mascarenhas, Flaxman, and others 2012), developed an algorithm that included live birth and a registered desire to have a child. More than 277 health surveys were analyzed to produce trend estimates of infertility at national, regional, and global levels, for the years closest to 1990 and 2010.

The estimates for both primary and secondary infertility are presented by seven regions (high income, Central and Eastern Europe and Central Asia, East Asia and Pacific, Latin America and the Caribbean, North Africa and the Middle East, Sub-Saharan Africa, and South Asia) for the two time frames, 1990 and 2010, for comparative purposes (tables 2.7 and 2.8). Secondary fertility is more prevalent than primary infertility at regional and global levels. Overall, an estimated 48.5 million women worldwide were infertile (involuntarily childless) in 2010. About 1.9 percent of women ages 20–44 years who were exposed to risk of pregnancy had primary infertility, and an additional 10.5 percent had secondary infertility.

Sub-Saharan Africa and South Asia showed declines in the prevalence of primary infertility of 0.8 percentage points and 0.6 percentage points, respectively. Sub-Saharan Africa also recorded a 1.9 percentage point decline in secondary infertility over the period. The only region with an increase in primary infertility was Central and Eastern Europe and Central Asia, where primary infertility went from 1.9 percent in 1990 to 2.3 percent in 2010.

Consequences of Infertility

The consequences of primary and secondary involuntary childlessness in LMICs, where having biological children is highly valued, include stigmatization, economic deprivation, denial of inheritance, divorce, and social isolation (Chachamovich and others 2010; Cui 2010; Dyer and Patel 2012; Fisher and Hammarberg 2012; Hasanpoor-Azghdy, Simbar, and Vedadhir 2014). In many LMICs, family ties are highly valued, and having own biological children is seen as a form of insurance in old age. Women who are unable to bear children feel insecure in their marital unions with respect to inheritance, and they face the possibility of their husbands getting a second wife and divorce.

Prevention and treatment of some of the major causes of infertility, such as STIs, is effective and affordable; treatment of infertility itself is expensive and often inaccessible. Advanced infertility treatment technologies, such as in vitro fertilization, which is the only intervention that can overcome tubal factor infertility, are mainly available in the private sector where the costs are high (Katz and others 2011). Because most affected individuals suffer in silence and the cost of treatment is high, governments have not prioritized the treatment of infertility; insurance either charges high premiums

Table 2.7 Global and Regional Prevalence Estimates for Trend Analysis of Primary Infertility in Women Exposed to the Risk of Pregnancy

Percent

| | Age-standardized prevalence of primary infertility | | | | | |
| | Estimate (percent) | Lower 95% CI | Upper 95% CI | Estimate (percent) | Lower 95% CI | Upper 95% CI |
Region	1990			2010		
Central and Eastern Europe and Central Asia	1.9	1.2	2.7	2.3	1.6	3.4
Sub-Saharan Africa	2.7	2.5	3.0	1.9	1.8	2.1
Middle East and North Africa	2.7	2.3	3.1	2.6	2.1	3.1
South Asia	2.9	2.5	3.3	2.3	1.9	2.7
East Asia and Pacific	1.5	1.3	1.7	1.6	1.3	2.0
Latin America and the Caribbean	1.6	1.4	2.0	1.5	1.2	1.8
High-income	1.9	1.6	2.3	1.9	1.3	2.6
World	2.0	1.9	2.2	1.9	1.7	2.2

Source: Mascarenhas, Flaxman, and others 2012.
Note: CI = confidence interval.

Table 2.8 Global and Regional Prevalence Estimates for Trend Analysis of Secondary Infertility in Women Exposed to the Risk of Pregnancy, Who Have Had a Previous Live Birth

| | Age-standardized prevalence of secondary infertility | | | | | |
| | Estimate (percent) | Lower 95% CI | Upper 95% CI | Estimate (percent) | Lower 95% CI | Upper 95% CI |
Region	1990			2010		
Central and Eastern Europe and Central Asia	16.3	12.0	21.4	18.0	13.8	24.1
Sub-Saharan Africa	13.5	12.5	14.5	11.6	10.6	12.6
Middle East and North Africa	6.7	5.8	7.8	7.2	5.9	8.6
South Asia	11.5	9.7	13.6	12.2	10.1	14.5
East Asia and Pacific[a]	10.1	9.0	11.4	10.9	9.1	13.0
Latin America and the Caribbean	7.3	6.2	8.4	7.5	6.1	9.0
High-income	6.8	5.5	8.4	7.2	5.0	10.2
World[a]	10.2	9.3	11.1	10.5	9.5	11.7

Source: Mascarenhas, Flaxman, and others 2012.
Note: CI = confidence interval.
a. Estimates exclude China.

or does not cover fertility treatment. As a result, cost of treatment of infertility is almost always borne by those affected; in many cases, the available treatment is basic and ineffective (Dyer and Patel 2012).

VIOLENCE AGAINST WOMEN

Violence against women is a serious health problem and a violation of human rights. It has significant impacts on women's health and development, and its consequences are individual as well as intergenerational and societal. Violence affects women's health and well-being, productivity, and ability to bond with and care for their children. Although violence against women has been accepted as an important public health and clinical care issue, it remains unaddressed in the health care policies of many countries.

This section focuses on violence against women and, in particular, on intimate partner violence (IPV) and sexual violence because these are the most common forms of violence experienced globally, and they have important sexual and reproductive health consequences.

Definitions and Measurements

The United Nations Declaration on the Elimination of Violence against Women (1993) defines violence against women[1] as "any act of gender-based violence that results in, or is likely to result in, physical, sexual, or mental harm or suffering to women, including threats of such acts, coercion, or arbitrary deprivation of liberty, whether occurring in public or in private life."

The declaration describes the many forms this violence can take, including the following:

Intimate partner violence (IPV), sexual violence, including abuse of female children, dowry-related violence, killings in the name of "honor," forced marriages, FGM and other traditional practices harmful to women, violence related to exploitation, sexual harassment and intimidation in workplaces, educational institutions, and elsewhere, trafficking, forced prostitution, and violence perpetrated or condoned by the state.

According to Heise and García-Moreno (2002), IPV is behavior by an intimate partner or ex-partner that causes physical, sexual, or psychological harm, including physical aggression, sexual coercion, psychological abuse, and controlling behaviors.

Sexual violence is any sexual act, attempt to obtain a sexual act, or other act directed against a person's sexuality, using coercion, by any person, regardless of their relationship to the victim, in any setting. It includes rape, defined as the physically forced or otherwise coerced penetration of the vulva or anus with a penis, other body part, or object (Jewkes and others 2002).

There are many challenges to measuring violence against women; studies are often not comparable because they use different samples (all women, married women, ever-partnered women, currently partnered), different measures of violence, different time frames (ever, last 12 months, last month). There are also specific ethical and safety concerns related to asking women about partner violence. However, a consensus exists that the best way to measure violence against women is by asking about behavioral acts; standardized methodologies are being developed, particularly for partner violence and sexual violence. Measuring violence against women in conflict settings is even more challenging. Gaps remain in the measurement of other forms such as trafficking, honor killings, and violence in conflict.

The methodology and ethical and safety guidelines developed for the Multi-country Study on Women's Health and Domestic Violence against Women (García-Moreno and others 2005) has contributed substantially to a standardized methodology. They have informed the UN Statistics Division guidelines for measuring violence against women and the violence against women module of the DHS. The past 10 years have seen growing numbers of population-based prevalence surveys using either DHS or the WHO methodology.

In 2013, slightly more than 80 countries had data on IPV; data on nonpartner sexual violence are more limited (WHO, LSHTM, and MRC-SA 2013).

Magnitude of the Problem

Worldwide, 35 percent of women have experienced physical or sexual IPV or nonpartner sexual violence; 38 percent of women who were murdered were murdered by their intimate partners (WHO, LSHTM,

and MRC-SA 2013). Estimates of IPV by World Health Organization region are shown in map 2.1; South-East Asia (37.7 percent), the Eastern Mediterranean (37.0 percent), and Africa (36.6 percent) have the highest rates (WHO, LSHTM, and MRC-SA 2013). A systematic review of sexual violence among women who were refugees and internally displaced people in complex humanitarian emergencies in 14 countries finds that 21 percent of women had experienced sexual violence (both intimate partner and nonpartner) (Vu and others 2014).

Sexual abuse during childhood affects boys and girls. A systematic review of population-based studies suggests that 8.1 percent of women and 5.5 percent of men experienced some form of sexual abuse before age 15 years. The prevalence was higher among women than men in every region (Devries and others 2014).

Violence among young people, including dating violence, is a common problem. The WHO multicountry study finds that the first sexual experience for many women was reported as forced, for example, 17 percent in rural areas of Tanzania, 24 percent in rural Peru, and 30 percent in rural Bangladesh (García-Moreno and others 2005).

Many women do not report their experiences of IPV or sexual violence or seek help for cultural and service-related reasons, including fear of being stigmatized, shame, or nonexistence or lack of trust in services.

Map 2.1 Rates of Intimate Partner Violence, by World Health Organization Region, 2010

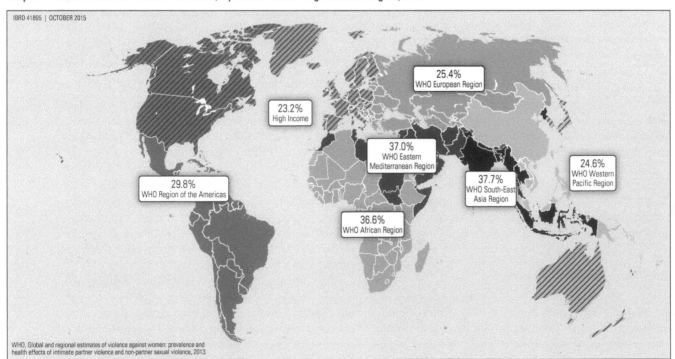

IBRD 41895 | OCTOBER 2015

25.4%
WHO European Region

23.2%
High Income

37.0%
WHO Eastern Mediterranean Region

37.7%
WHO South-East Asia Region

24.6%
WHO Western Pacific Region

29.8%
WHO Region of the Americas

36.6%
WHO African Region

WHO, Global and regional estimates of violence against women: prevalence and health effects of intimate partner violence and non-partner sexual violence, 2013.

Source: WHO 2013.
Note: Regional prevalence rates are presented for each WHO region, including low- and middle-income countries. High-income countries are analyzed separately.

Health and Other Consequences

The direct consequences of violence against women are injury, disability, or death. Indirect consequences include physical, mental, and sexual and reproductive health problems, such as stress-induced physiological changes, substance use, and lack of fertility control and personal autonomy (WHO 2013). Women who experience violence are more likely to have STIs, HIV/AIDS, unintended pregnancies, unsafe abortions, and gynecological problems, compared with women who do not experience such violence (Campbell 2002; Ellsberg and others 2008; Plichta and Falik 2001). Women who have experienced IPV are 1.5 times more likely to have STIs and, in some regions, HIV/AIDS; more than twice as likely to have an abortion; almost twice as likely to report depressive episodes and alcohol use problems; and 4.5 times more likely to have attempted suicide, compared with women who have not been exposed to violence (WHO 2013). IPV has been associated with chronic pelvic pain and other pain syndromes, hypertension, obesity, and other non-communicable diseases (Campbell 2002; Ellsberg and others 2008; Plichta and Falik 2001). Sexual violence is also associated with higher rates of mental health disorders, such as depression and anxiety disorders (WHO 2013).

IPV can begin or persist during pregnancy and result in serious maternal and perinatal health problems. In the WHO multicountry study, between 1 percent and 28 percent of ever-pregnant women reported being physically abused during at least one pregnancy, with most sites falling between 4 percent and 12 percent (García-Moreno and others 2006). Violence during pregnancy is associated with increased risk of miscarriage, premature labor, perinatal death, and low–birth weight babies (Campbell 2002; Fanslow and others 2008; Janssen and others 2003). Women who have experienced IPV are 16 percent more likely to have a low–birth weight baby (WHO 2013). IPV during pregnancy is also significantly associated with adverse health behaviors during pregnancy, including smoking, alcohol and substance abuse, and delay in prenatal care, even after controlling for other mediating factors (Campbell 2002).

Violence against women can also lead to death from suicide; homicide, including in the name of honor, usually committed by family members for cultural reasons; female infanticide; maternal death from unsafe abortion; and deaths from HIV/AIDS. Up to 38 percent of murders of women are committed by their partners, compared with 6 percent of murders of men (Stöckl and others 2013).

Sexual abuse during childhood is associated with higher rates of sexual risk taking, substance use, and additional victimization. Each of these behaviors increases the risks of subsequent health problems.

There are often long-term intergenerational health consequences for those who witness violence, especially children, with negative consequences for their health and development. IPV is associated with increased mortality in infants and children younger than age five years (Ahmed, Koenig, and Stephenson 2006; Asling-Monemi, Tabassum, and Persson 2008; Boy and Salihu 2004), and with behavioral problems among children, as well as low educational attainment. Health systems and health care providers can play a critical role in identification, assessment, treatment, documentation, referral, and follow-up; this role needs to be integrated into national health programs and policies (WHO 2013).

FEMALE GENITAL MUTILATION

FGM comprises all procedures that involve the partial or total removal of external genitalia or other injury to the female genital organs for nonmedical reasons (OHCHR and others 2008). Although FGM is internationally recognized as a violation of human rights, and legislation to prohibit the procedure has been put in place in many countries, the practice has still been documented in many African countries and several regions in Asia and the Middle East (OHCHR and others 2008). Some forms of FGM have also been reported in other countries, including among certain ethnic groups in Central and South America, as well as among some migrants living in HICs (Yoder, Abderrahim, and Zhuzhini 2004). The importance of FGM from a public health perspective arises from the fact that, in addition to medical and psychological complications, the practice violates human rights and child rights, given that it is almost always carried out among minors (Yoder and Wang 2013).

Measurement

Data on FGM at the population level have become increasingly available, mainly from population-based surveys that include questions on the practice among women ages 15–49 years and their daughters, such as the DHSs and the UNICEF Multiple Indicator Cluster Surveys (MICS) (Yoder and Wang 2013; Yoder, Abderrahim, and Zhuzhini 2004). Before the DHSs, there were no national population-level data on FGM. Currently, many Sub-Saharan African countries have national-level prevalence data, as do some in the Middle East, including the Republic of Yemen and Iraq (Yoder and Wang 2013).

The prevalence of FGM is calculated from survey questions in the following areas:

- Circumcision status of respondents
- Information on the event among those who were circumcised
- Circumcision status of one's daughters
- Women's and men's opinions of the practice.

Although the phrasing and level of depth of inquiry vary by country, the key question used to estimate prevalence is often phrased, "Have you (yourself) been circumcised?" The current global estimate of FGM is derived from weighted averages of FGM prevalence among girls ages 0–14 years and girls and women ages 15–49 years, using DHS, MICS, and Household Health Survey data. The number of girls and women who have been cut was calculated using 2011 demographic figures produced by the UN Population Division (UNPD 2013). The number of cut women ages 50 years and older is based on FGM prevalence in women ages 45–49 (UNICEF 2013).

Prevalence of Female Genital Mutilation

An estimated 125 million girls and women concentrated in 29 countries in the Middle East and Sub-Saharan Africa have undergone FGM (UNICEF 2013). The global estimate of FGM is unknown because the exact number of those with FGM among migrants from countries with the practice is unknown. Although prevalence estimates among migrants have been computed in some host countries, the overall burden is unknown (Dorkenoo, Morison, and Macfarlane 2007; Dubourg and others 2011; Exterkate 2013).

Table 2.9 shows the national prevalence estimates of FGM in 29 countries by age category and place of residence. The prevalence varies across countries from as low as less than 5 percent in Cameroon, Ghana, Niger, Togo, and Uganda, to more than 90 percent in Djibouti, the Arab Republic of Egypt, Guinea, and Somalia. With the exception of Chad, Iraq, Mali, Nigeria, and the Republic of Yemen, the prevalence of FGM is higher in rural areas than in urban areas. In most countries, older age groups have higher prevalence of FGM.

Consequences of Female Genital Mutilation

FGM is painful, traumatic, and emotionally distressful. Immediate and long-term health consequences include gynecological complications, such as the following:

- Structural complications of the genitourinary system, such as vaginal stenosis, urethral strictures, labial fusion, and fistulae involving the genital tract

- Postprocedural complications of the skin and subcutaneous tissue, such as keloids, sebaceous cysts, scars and fibrosis, and nonhealing ulcers
- Disorders of the urinary system, such as acute or chronic urinary tract infections, meatus, urinary crystals, pyelonephritis, urinary retention and incontinence, and kidney failure
- Infections
- Hemodynamic complications, such as hemorrhage, hypovolemic or septic shock, and anemia
- Procedural and everyday life difficulties, such as gynecological examination, cytology testing, evacuation of the uterus postabortion, intrauterine device placement, and tampon usage
- Pain associated with the female genital organs or menstrual cycle, such as hematocolpos, vulvodynia, dyspareunia, acute or chronic lower abdominal pain, hypersensitivity of the genital area, and clitoral neuroma
- Injury of neighboring organs and structures, such as the urethra, bladder, urinary meatus, vaginal wall, anus, and rectum
- Death.

FGM has been associated with obstetric complications. Studies, including a large WHO study in African countries, show that women with FGM are significantly more at risk of cesarean section, postpartum hemorrhage, episiotomy, extended maternal hospital stay, resuscitation of infants, low–birth weight infants, and inpatient perinatal death (Kaplan and others 2013; Lovel, McGettigan, and Mohammed 2000; WHO 2006b).

Several sexual and mental health complications are also associated with FGM, including sexual aversion and lack of sexual enjoyment or desire, vaginal dryness, orgasmic dysfunction, nonorganic vaginismus, apareunia, posttraumatic stress disorder, depression, somatization disorder, neurasthenia, anxiety disorders, specific phobias, psychosomatic disorders, and eating disorders (Berg, Denison, and Rappaport 2010).

Although health care professionals are aware of FGM and some of its health consequences, their ability to identify and manage complications remains suboptimal (WHO 2001). Moreover, some health care providers still consider certain forms of FGM as not harmful; some perform medical FGM (Ali 2012). The WHO has condemned medicalization of FGM and recognizes that its cessation is an essential component of the human rights–based approach.

Table 2.9 Prevalence of Female Genital Mutilation among Girls and Women

Country (data source)	Reference year	FGM prevalence among girls and women (%)	FGM prevalence among girls and women by age and residence (%)									
			Age category							Residence	
			15–19	20–24	25–29	30–34	35–39	40–44	45–49	Urban	Rural
Benin (DHS)	2006	13	8	10	14	14	16	17	16	9	15
Burkina Faso (DHS and MICS)	2010	76	58	70	78	83	85	88	89	69	78
Cameroon (DHS)	2004	1	0.4	3	2	1	1	2	2	1	2
Central African Republic (MICS)	2010	24	18	22	25	26	28	30	34	18	29
Chad (MICS)	2010	44	41	43	46	45	46	45	47	46	44
Côte d'Ivoire (MICS)	2006	36	28	34	38	43	44	41	40	34	39
Djibouti (MICS)	2006	93	90	94	93	96	95	93	94	93	96
Egypt, Arab Rep. (DHS)	2008	91	81	87	94	95	96	96	96	85	96
Eritrea (DHS)	2002	89	78	88	91	93	93	94	95	86	91
Ethiopia (DHS)	2005	74	62	73	78	78	81	82	81	69	76
The Gambia (MICS)	2010	76	77	77	78	75	73	75	79	75	78
Ghana (MICS)	2011	4	2	2	3	4	6	7	6	3	5
Guinea (DHS)	2005	96	89	95	97	97	99	98	100	94	96
Guinea-Bissau (MICS/RHS)	2010	50	48	49	51	50	49	54	50	41	57
Iraq (MICS)	2011	8	5	8	9	9	10	9	10	9	6
Kenya (DHS)	2008–09	27	15	21	25	30	35	40	49	17	31
Liberia (DHS)	2007	66	44	58	68	70	73	78	85	45	81
Mali (MICS)	2010	89	88	88	88	89	90	89	89	89	88
Mauritania (MICS)	2011	69	66	66	67	71	72	76	75	57	81
Niger (DHS/MICS)	2006	2	2	2	2	2	3	3	3	2	2

table continues next page

Table 2.9 Prevalence of Female Genital Mutilation among Girls and Women (continued)

Country (data source)	Reference year	FGM prevalence among girls and women (%)	Age category								Residence	
			15–19	20–24	25–29	30–34	35–39	40–44	45–49	Urban	Rural
Nigeria (MICS)	2011	27	19	22	26	30	32	35	38	33	24
Senegal (DHS/MICS)	2010–11	26	24	24	26	25	29	27	29	23	28
Sierra Leone (MICS)	2010	88	80	87	92	93	96	95	96	81	92
Somalia (MICS)	2006	98	97	98	98	99	99	98	99	97	98
Sudan (SHHS)	2010	88	84	87	90	88	90	90	89	84	90
Tanzania (DHS)	2010	15	7	11	12	19	22	22	22	8	17
Togo (MICS)	2010	4	1	2	4	5	6	5	7	3	5
Uganda (DHS)	2011	1	1	1	2	2	1	2	2	1	1
Yemen, Rep. (DHS)	1997	23	19	22	21	23	24	25	25	26	22

Source: UNICEF 2013.
Note: DHS = Demographic and Health Survey; FGM = female genital mutilation; MICS = Multiple Indicator Cluster Survey; RHS=Reproductive Health Survey; SHHS = Sudan Household Health Survey.

CONCLUSIONS

This chapter focuses on selected reproductive health diseases and their predisposing factors that lead to morbidity and mortality but that are generally neglected in research and public health programming. Although the data remain scant, these conditions are clearly pervasive; some are predisposing factors for other conditions.

Part of the challenge to policy makers is in measurement. Variations in definitions and reference populations affect the comparability of data. Unwanted pregnancies, abortions, infertility, infections of the reproductive tract, and violence against women are associated with stigmatization, especially in LMICs, and are often underreported or misreported in surveys and health care facilities. There are few global, regional, or national estimates of some of these conditions. Some estimates are based on indirect methods, and questions arise about their validity.

Most of these conditions have cost-effective interventions. Most unwanted pregnancies can be averted through the provision of proven family-planning technologies; safe abortion services are associated with low complication rates. Treatment for RTIs is available and affordable, yet many women never receive treatment, predisposing them to the risk of other infections, including HIV/AIDS. Violence against women is equally prevalent; while preventive interventions pose challenges, health systems can do much more for prevention, provision of care and services, and mitigation of consequences.

The poor integration and mainstreaming of these cost-effective interventions in public health prevention and management programs exacerbates their public health impacts. The counterargument might be that the burden of these conditions and their economic costs are vague, and no concrete evidence exists for advocacy within and across countries and regions. However, the evidence of the substantial burden of violence against women has yet to translate into significant policy and programmatic action to address the problem in many LMICs.

NOTES

World Bank Income Classifications as of July 2014 are as follows, based on estimates of gross national income (GNI) per capita for 2013:

- Low-income countries (LICs) = US$1,045 or less
- Middle-income countries (MICs) are subdivided:
  a) lower-middle-income = US$1,046–US$4,125
  b) upper-middle-income (UMICs) = US$4,126–US$12,745
- High-income countries (HICs) = US$12,746 or more.

For consistency and ease of comparison, *DCP3* is using the World Health Organization's Global Health Estimates (GHE) for data on diseases burden, except in cases where a relevant data point is not available from GHE. In those instances, an alternative data source is noted.

1. Violence against women is also referred to as *gender-based violence* because most of the violence that women experience is rooted in gender inequality. More recently, however, gender-based violence has come to be understood by some as also including violence against men and on the basis of sexual orientation or gender identity.

REFERENCES

AbouZahr, C., and J. P. Vaughan. 2000. "Assessing the Burden of Sexual and Reproductive Ill health: Questions Regarding the Use of Disability-Adjusted Life Years." *Bulletin of the World Health Organization* 78 (5): 655–66.

African Population and Health Research Center and Ministry of Health Kenya. 2013. *Incidence and Complications of Unsafe Abortion in Kenya: Key Findings of a National Study.* Nairobi, Kenya.

Ahmad, A., and A. U. Khan. 2009. "Prevalence of Candida Species and Potential Risk Factors for Vulvovaginal Candidiasis in Aligarh, India." *European Journal of Obstetrics and Gynecology Reproductive Biology* 144 (1): 68–71.

Ahman, E., and I. H. Shah. 2012. "Generating National Unsafe Abortion Estimates: Challenges and Choices." In *Methodologies for Estimating Abortion Incidence and Abortion-Related Morbidity: A Review*, edited by S. Singh, L. Remez, and A. Tartaglione, 13–20. New York: Guttmacher Institute.

Ahmed, S., M. A. Koenig, and R. Stephenson. 2006. "Effects of Domestic Violence on Perinatal and Early-Childhood Mortality: Evidence from North India." *American Journal of Public Health* 96 (8): 1423–28.

Ali, A. A. 2012. "Knowledge and Attitudes of Female Genital Mutilation among Midwives in Eastern Sudan." *Reproductive Health* 9: 23.

Ali, M., J. Cleland, and I. H. Shah. 2012. *Causes and Consequences of Contraceptive Discontinuation: Evidence from 60 Demographic and Health Surveys.* Geneva: World Health Organization.

Alkema, L. D. Chou, D. Hogan, S. Zhang, A.-B. Moller, and others. "Global, Regional, and National Levels and Trends in Maternal Mortality between 1990 and 2015, with Scenario-Based Projections to 2030: A Systematic Analysis by the UN Maternal Mortality Estimation Inter-Agency Group." *The Lancet.* Epub November 13, 2015. doi:10.1016/S0140-6736(15)00838-7.

Allotey, P. A., and D. D. Reidpath. 2002. "Objectivity in Priority Setting Tools in Reproductive Health: Context and the DALY." *Reproductive Health Matters* 10 (20): 38–46.

Asling-Monemi, K., N. R. Tabassum, and L. A. Persson. 2008. "Violence against Women and the Risk of Under-Five

Mortality: Analysis of Community-Based Data from Rural Bangladesh." *Acta Paediatrica* 97 (2): 226–32.

Baeten, J. M., P. M. Nyange, B. A. Richardson, L. Lavreys, B. Chohan, and others. 2001. "Hormonal Contraception and Risk of Sexually Transmitted Disease Acquisition: Results from a Prospective Study." *American Journal of Obstetrics and Gynecology* 185 (2): 380–85.

Balamurugan, S. S., and N. Bendigeri. 2012. "Community-Based Study of Reproductive Tract Infections among Women of the Reproductive Age Group in the Urban Health Training Centre Area in Hubli, Karnataka." *Indian Journal of Community Medicine* 37 (1): 34–38.

Baschieri, A., J. Cleland, K. Machiyama, S. Floyd, A. L. N. Dube, and others. 2013. "Fertility Intentions, Child Growth and Nutrition in Northern Malawi." Paper presented at IUSSP International Population Conference, Busan, August.

Basinga, P., A. M. Moore, S. Singh, L. Remez, F. Birungi, and L. Nyirazinyoye. 2012. *Unintended Pregnancy and Induced Abortion in Rwanda: Causes and Consequences.* New York: Guttmacher Institute.

Benson, J., and B. Crane. 2005. "Incorporating Health Outcomes into Cost Estimates of Unsafe Abortion." Background paper prepared for workshop on research on the economic impact of abortion-related morbidity and mortality, Guttmacher Institute, New York.

Berg, R. C., E. Denison, and F. A. Rappaport. 2010. *Psychological, Social and Sexual Consequences of Female Genital Mutilation/ Cutting (FGM/C): A Systematic Review on Quantitative Studies.* Report from Kunnskapssenteret nr 13-2010, Nasjonalt kunnskapssenter for helsetjenesten, Oslo.

Boivin, J., L. Bunting, J. A. Collins, and K. G. Nygren. 2007. "International Estimates of Infertility Prevalence and Treatment-Seeking: Potential Need and Demand for Infertility Medical Care." *Human Reproduction* 22 (6): 1506–12.

Boy, A., and H. M. Salihu. 2004. "Intimate Partner Violence and Birth Outcomes: A Systematic Review." *International Journal of Fertility and Women's Medicine* 49 (4): 159–64.

Bradley, S. E. K., T. N. Croft, and S. O. Rutstein. 2011. *The Impact of Contraceptive Failure on Unintended Births and Induced Abortions: Estimates and Strategies for Reduction.* DHS Analytical Studies 22, Macro International Inc., Calverton, MD.

Brotman, R. M., M. A. Klebanoff, T. R. Nansel, W. W. Andrews, J. R. Schwebke, and others. 2008. "A Longitudinal Study of Vaginal Douching and Bacterial Vaginosis—A Marginal Structural Modeling Analysis." *American Journal of Epidemiology* 168 (2): 188–96.

Brown, J. M., K. L. Hess, S. Brown, C. Murphy, A. L. Waldman, and M. Hezareh. 2013. "Intravaginal Practices and Risk of Bacterial Vaginosis and Candidiasis Infection among a Cohort of Women in the United States." *Obstetrics and Gynecology* 121 (4): 773–80.

Buchta, V., V. Matula, J. Kestřánek, M. Vejsová, L. Křivčíková, and J. Spaček. 2013. "[Is Diabetes Mellitus a Risk Factor in Genital Yeast Infections?]." *Ceska Gynekologie* 78 (6): 537–44.

Bunnell, R. E., L. Dahlberg, R. Rolfs, R. Ransom, K. Gershman, and others. 1999. "High Prevalence and Incidence of Sexually Transmitted Diseases in Urban Adolescent Females

Despite Moderate Risk Behaviors." *Journal of Infectious Diseases* 180 (5): 1624–31.

Campbell, A. A., and W. D. Mosher. 2000. "A History of the Measurement of Unintended Pregnancies and Births." *Maternal and Child Health* 4 (3): 163–69.

Campbell, J. C. 2002. "Health Consequences of Intimate Partner Violence." *The Lancet* 359 (9314): 1331–36.

Canning, D., and T. P. Schultz. 2012. "The Economic Consequences of Reproductive and Family Planning." *The Lancet* 380 (9837): 65–71.

Casterline, J., and L. El-Zeini. 2007. "The Estimation of Unwanted Fertility." *Demography* 44 (4): 729–45.

Cates, W., Jr., T. M. Farley, and P. J. Rowe. 1985. "Worldwide Patterns of Infertility: Is Africa Different?" *The Lancet* 2 (8455): 596–98.

Cates, W., Jr., R. T. Rolfs, and S. O. Aral. 1990. "Sexually Transmitted Diseases, Pelvic Inflammatory Disease, and Infertility: An Epidemiologic Update." *Epidemiologic Reviews* 12: 199–220.

CDC (Centers for Disease Control and Prevention). 2010. *Sexually Transmitted Diseases Treatment Guidelines, 2010.* Morbidity and Mortality Weekly Report 59 (RR-12).

Chachamovich, J. R., E. Chachamovich, E. Ezer, M. P. Fleck, D. Knauth, and E. P. Passos. 2010. "Investigating Quality of Life and Health-Related Quality of Life in Infertility: A Systematic Review." *Journal of Psychosomatic Obstetrics and Gynaecology* 31 (2): 101–10.

Che, Y., and J. Cleland. 2002. "Infertility in Shanghai: Prevalence, Treatment Seeking and Impact." *Journal of Obstetrics and Gynaecology* 22 (6): 643–48.

Cleland, J., A. Conde-Agudelo, H. Peterson, J. Ross, and A. Tsui. 2012. "Contraception and Health." *The Lancet* 380 (9837): 149–56.

Cohen, C. R., J. R. Lingappa, J. M. Baeten, M. O. Ngayo, C. A. Spiegel, and others. 2012. "Bacterial Vaginosis Associated with Increased Risk of Female-to-Male HIV-1 Transmission: A Prospective Cohort Analysis among African Couples." *PLoS Medicine* 9 (6): e1001251.

Cui, W. 2010. "Mother or Nothing: The Agony of Infertility." *Bulletin of the World Health Organization* 88 (12): 881–82.

Curtis, S., E. Evens, and W. Sambisa. 2011. "Contraceptive Discontinuation and Unintended Pregnancy: An Imperfect Relationship." *International Perspectives on Sexual and Reproductive Health* 37 (2): 58–66.

Darroch, J. E., S. Singh, H. Bal, and J. V. Cabigon. 2009. "Meeting Women's Contraceptive Needs in the Philippines, In Brief." Guttmacher Institute, New York.

de Leon, E. M., S. J. Jacober, J. D. Sobel, and B. Foxman. 2002. "Prevalence and Risk Factors for Vaginal Candida Colonization in Women with Type 1 and Type 2 Diabetes." *BMC Infectious Diseases* 2: 1.

de Lima Soares, V., A. M. de Mesquita, F. G. Cavlacante, Z. P. Silva, V. Hora, and others. 2003. "Sexually Transmitted Infections in a Female Population in Rural North-East Brazil: Prevalence, Morbidity and Risk Factors." *Tropical Medicine and International Health* 8 (7): 595–603.

Desai, S. 1995. "When Are Children from Large Families Disadvantaged? Evidence from Cross-National Surveys." *Population Studies* 49 (2): 195–210.

Desai, V. K., J. K. Kosambiya, and H. G. Thakor. 2003. "Prevalence of Sexually Transmitted Infections and Performance of STI Syndromes against Aetiological Diagnosis, in Female Sex Workers of Red Light Area in Surat, India." *Sexually Transmitted Infections* 79 (2): 111–15.

Devries, K. M., J. Y. T. Mak, L. Bacchus, S. Lim, M. Petzold, and others. 2014. "Childhood Sexual Abuse and Suicidal Behavior: A Meta-Analysis." *Pediatrics* 133 (5): e1331–e1334.

Dixon-Mueller, R. 2008. "How Young Is Too Young? Comparative Perspectives on Adolescent Sexual, Marital and Reproductive Transitions." *Studies in Family Planning* 39 (4): 247–62.

Dorkenoo, E., L. Morison, and A. Macfarlane. 2007. *A Statistical Study to Estimate the Prevalence of Female Genital Mutilation in England and Wales: Summary Report.* London: Foundation for Women's Health, Research and Development (FORWARD).

Dubourg, D., F. Richard, E. Leye, S. Ndame, T. Rommens, and others. 2011. "Estimating the Number of Women with Female Genital Mutilation in Belgium." *European Journal of Contraceptive and Reproductive Health Care* 16 (4): 248–57.

Duerr, A., C. M. Heilig, S. F. Meikle, S. Cu-Uvin, R. S. Klein, and others. 2003. "Incident and Persistent Vulvovaginal Candidiasis among Human Immunodeficiency Virus-Infected Women: Risk Factors and Severity." *Obstetrics and Gynecology* 101 (3): 548–56.

Dyer, S. J., and M. Patel. 2012. "The Economic Impact of Infertility on Women in Developing Countries: A Systematic Review." *Facts, Views and Visions, Issues in Obstetrics, Gynaecology, and Reproductive Health* 4 (2): 102–09.

Ekpenyong, C. E., E. C. Inyang-etoh, E. O. Ettebong, U. P. Akpan, J. O. Ibu, and N. E. Daniel. 2012. "Recurrent Vulvovaginal Candidosis among Young Women in South Eastern Nigeria: The Role of Lifestyle and Health-Care Practices." *International Journal of STD and AIDS* 23 (10): 704–09.

Ellsberg, M., H. A. Jansen, L. Heise, C. H. Watts, C. García-Moreno, and others. 2008. "Intimate Partner Violence and Women's Physical and Mental Health in the WHO Multi-Country Study on Women's Health and Domestic Violence: An Observational Study." *The Lancet* 371 (9619): 1165–72.

Eriksson, K., A. Adolfsson, U. Forsum, and P. G. Larsson. 2010. "The Prevalence of BV in the Population on the Aland Islands during a 15-Year Period." *APMIS* 118 (11): 903–8.

Eschenbach, D. A., S. S. Thwin, D. L. Patton, T. M. Hooton, A. E. Stapleton, and others. 2000. "Influence of the Normal Menstrual Cycle on Vaginal Tissue, Discharge, and Microflora." *Clinical Infectious Diseases* 30 (6): 901–07.

Exterkate, M. 2013. *Female Genital Mutilation in the Netherlands: Prevalence, Incidence and Determinants.* Utrecht, Netherlands: Pharos.

Fanslow, J., M. Silva, A. Whitehead, and E. Robinson. 2008. "Pregnancy Outcomes and Intimate Partner Violence in New Zealand." *Australia and New Zealand Journal of Obstetrics and Gynaecology* 48 (4): 391–97.

Fethers, K. A., C. K. Fairley, J. S. Hocking, L. C. Gurrin, and C. S. Bradshaw. 2008. "Sexual Risk Factors and Bacterial Vaginosis: A Systematic Review and Meta-Analysis." *Clinical Infectious Diseases* 47 (11): 1426–35.

Fetters, T. 2010. "Prospective Approach to Measuring Abortion-Related Morbidity: Individual-Level Data on Postabortion Patients." In *Methodologies for Estimating Abortion Incidence and Abortion-Related Morbidity: A Review*, edited by S. Singh, L. Remez, and A. Tartaglione. New York: Guttmacher Institute; Paris: International Union for the Scientific Study of Population.

Fetters, T. S. Vonthanak, C. Picardo, and T. Rathavy. 2008. "Abortion-Related Complications in Cambodia." *BJOG: An International Journal of Obstetrics and Gynaecology* 115 (8): 957–68; discussion 968.

Figa-Talamanca, I., T. A. Sinnathuray, K. Yusof, C. K. Fong, V. T. Palan, and others. 1986. "Illegal Abortion: An Attempt to Assess Its Cost to the Health Services and Its Incidence in the Community." *International Journal of Health Services* 16 (3): 375–89.

Fisher, J. R., and K. Hammarberg. 2012. "Psychological and Social Aspects of Infertility in Men: An Overview of the Evidence and Implications for Psychologically Informed Clinical Care and Future Research." *Asian Journal of Andrology* 14 (1): 121–29.

Foxman, B. 1990. "The Epidemiology of Vulvovaginal Candidiasis: Risk Factors." *American Journal of Public Health* 80 (3): 329–31.

Garcia, P. J., S. Chavez, B. Feringa, M. Chiappe, L. Weili, and others. 2004. "Reproductive Tract Infections in Rural Women from the Highlands, Jungle, and Coastal Regions of Peru." *Bulletin of the World Health Organization* 82 (7): 483–92.

García-Moreno, C., H. A. Jansen, M. Ellsberg, L. Heise, and C. Watts. 2005. *WHO Multi-Country Study on Women's Health and Domestic Violence against Women: Initial Results on Prevalence, Health Outcomes and Women's Responses.* Geneva: World Health Organization.

———. 2006. "Prevalence of Intimate Partner Violence: Findings from the WHO Multi-Country Study on Women's Health and Domestic Violence." *The Lancet* 368 (9543): 260–69.

Gebreselassie, H., T. Fetters, S. Singh, A. Abdella, Y. Gebrehiwot, and others. 2010. "Caring for Women with Abortion Complications in Ethiopia: National Estimates and Future Implications." *International Perspectives on Sexual and Reproductive Health* 36 (1): 6–15.

Geiger, A. M., B. Foxman, and B. W. Gillespie. 1995. "The Epidemiology of Vulvovaginal Candidiasis among University Students." *American Journal of Public Health* 85 (8 Pt. 1): 1146–48.

Gillespie, D., S. Ahmed, A. Tsui, and S. Radloff. 2007. "Unwanted Fertility among the Poor: An Inequity?" *Bulletin of the World Health Organization* 85 (2): 100–7.

Go, V. F., V. M. Quan, D. D. Celentano, L. H. Moulton, and J. M. Zenilman. 2006. "Prevalence and Risk Factors for Reproductive Tract Infections among Women in Rural Vietnam." *Southeast Asian Journal of Tropical Medicine and Public Health* 37 (1): 185–89.

Goto, A., Q. V. Nguyen, N. M. Pham, K. Kato, T. P. Cao, and others. 2005. "Prevalence of and Factors Associated with Reproductive Tract Infections among Pregnant Women in Ten Communes in Nghe An Province, Vietnam." *Journal of Epidemiology* 15 (5): 163–72.

Gray, R. H., G. Kigozi, D. Serwadda, F. Makumbi, F. Nalugodo, and others. 2009. "The Effects of Male Circumcision on Female Partners' Genital Tract Symptoms and Vaginal Infections in a Randomized Trial in Rakai, Uganda." *American Journal of Obstetrics and Gynecology* 200 (1): 42. e1–7.

Grimes, D. A., J. Benson, S. Singh, M. Romero, B. Ganatra, and others. 2006. "Unsafe Abortion: The Preventable Pandemic." *The Lancet* 368 (9550): 1908–19.

Gurunath, S., Z. Pandian, R. A. Anderson, and S. Bhattacharya. 2011. "Defining Infertility—A Systematic Review of Prevalence Studies." *Human Reproduction Update* 17 (5): 575–88.

Hasanpoor-Azghdy, S. B., M. Simbar, and A. Vedadhir. 2014. "The Emotional-Psychological Consequences of Infertility among Infertile Women Seeking Treatment: Results of a Qualitative Study." *Iran Journal of Reproductive Medicine* 12 (2): 131–38.

Hay, P. E., R. F. Lamont, D. Taylor-Robinson, D. J. Morgan, C. Ison, and J. Pearson. 1994. "Abnormal Bacterial Colonisation of the Genital Tract and Subsequent Preterm Delivery and Late Miscarriage." *BMJ* 308 (6924): 295–98.

Hay, P. E., and D. Taylor-Robinson. 1996. "Defining Bacterial Vaginosis: To BV or not to BV, that Is the Question." *International Journal of STD and AIDS* 7 (4): 233–35.

Heiligenberg, M., B. Rijnders, M. F. Schim van der Loeff, H. J. de Vries, W. I. van der Meijden, and others. 2012. "High Prevalence of Sexually Transmitted Infections in HIV-Infected Men during Routine Outpatient Visits in the Netherlands." *Sexually Transmitted Diseases* 39 (1): 8–15.

Heise, L., and C. García-Moreno. 2002. "Violence by Intimate Partners." In *World Report on Violence and Health*, edited by E. G. Krug, L. L. Dahlberg, J. A. Mercy, A. B. Zwi, and R. Lozano, 87–122. Geneva: World Health Organization.

Henshaw, S. K., I. Adewole, S. Singh, A. Bankole, B. Oye-Adeniran, and R. Hussain. 2008. "Severity and Cost of Unsafe Abortion Complications Treated in Nigerian Hospitals." *International Family Planning Perspectives* 34 (1): 40–50.

Henshaw, S. K., S. Singh, A. Bankole, B. Oye-Adeniran, and R. Hussain. 1999. "The Incidence of Abortion Worldwide." *International Family Planning Perspectives* 25: S30–38.

Hester, R. A., and S. B. Kennedy. 2003. "Candida Infection as a Risk Factor for HIV Transmission." *Journal of Women's Health* 12 (5): 487–94.

Hobcraft, J., J. McDonald, and S. O. Rutstein. 1985. "Demographic Determinants of Infant and Child Mortality." *Population Studies* 39 (3): 363–85.

Ibrahim, S. M., M. Bukar, Y. Mohammed, B. M. Audu, and H. M. Ibrahim. 2013. "Prevalence of Vaginal Candidiasis among Pregnant Women with Abnormal Vaginal Discharge in Maiduguri." *Nigerian Journal of Medicine* 22 (2): 138–42.

Ilkit, M., and A. B. Guzel. 2011. "The Epidemiology, Pathogenesis, and Diagnosis of Vulvovaginal Candidosis: A Mycological Perspective." *Critical Reviews in Microbiology* 37 (3): 250–61.

Inhorn, M. C. 2003. "Global Infertility and the Globalization of New Reproductive Technologies: Illustrations from Egypt." *Social Science and Medicine* 56 (9): 1837–51.

Jain, A., A. Mahmood, Z. A. Sathar, and I. Masood. 2014. "Unmet Need and Unwanted Childbearing in Pakistan: Evidence from a Panel Survey." *Studies in Family Planning* 45 (2): 277–99.

Janssen, P. A., V. L. Holt, N. K. Sugg, I. Emanuel, C. M. Critchlow, and A. D. Henderson. 2003. "Intimate Partner Violence and Adverse Pregnancy Outcomes: A Population-Based Study." *American Journal of Obstetrics and Gynecology* 188 (5): 1341–47.

Jewkes, R., H. Brown, K. Dickson-Tetteh, J. Levin, and H. Rees. 2002. "Prevalence of Morbidity Associated with Abortion before and after Legalisation in South Africa." *BMJ* 324 (7348): 1252–53.

Jewkes, R., H. Rees, K. Dickson, H. Brown, and J. Levin. 2005. "The Impact of Age on the Epidemiology of Incomplete Abortions in South Africa after Legislative Change." *BJOG* 112 (3): 355–59.

Johnston, H. B., and C. F. Westoff. 2010. "Examples of Model-Based Approaches to Estimating Abortion." In *Methodologies for Estimating Abortion Incidence and Abortion-Related Morbidity: A Review*, edited by S. Singh, L. Remez, and A. Tartaglione. New York: Guttmacher Institute; Paris: International Union for the Scientific Study of Population.

Jones, F. R., G. Miller, N. Gadea, R. Meza, S. Leon, and others. 2007. "Prevalence of Bacterial Vaginosis among Young Women in Low-Income Populations of Coastal Peru." *International Journal of STD and AIDS* 18 (3): 188–92.

Juarez, F., J. Cabigon, S. Singh, and R. Hussain. 2005. "The Incidence of Induced Abortion in the Philippines: Current Level and Recent Trends." *International Family Planning Perspectives* 31 (3): 140–49.

Juarez, F., J. Cabigon, and S. Singh. 2010. "The Sealed Envelope Method of Estimating Induced Abortion: How Much of an Improvement?" In *Methodologies for Estimating Abortion Incidence and Abortion-Related Morbidity: A Review*, edited by S. Singh, L. Remez, and A. Tartaglione. New York: Guttmacher Institute.

Juarez, F., and S. Singh. 2012. "Incidence of Induced Abortion by Age and State, Mexico, 2009: New Estimates Using a Modified Methodology." *International Perspectives on Sexual and Reproductive Health* 38 (2): 58–67.

Kalilani-Phiri, L., H. Gebreselassie, B. A. Levandowski, E. Kichingale, F. Kachale, and G. Kangaude. 2015. "The Severity of Abortion Complications in Malawi." *International Journal of Gynecology and Obstetrics* 128 (2): 160–64.

Kaplan, A., M. Forbes, I. Bonhoure, M. Utzet, M. Martin, and others. 2013. "Female Genital Mutilation/Cutting in The Gambia: Long-Term Health Consequences and Complications during Delivery and for the Newborn." *International Journal of Women's Health* 5: 323–31.

Kassebaum, N. J., A. Bertozzi-Villa, M. S. Coggeshall, K. A. Shackelford, C. Steiner, and others. 2014. "Global, Regional, and National Levels and Causes of Maternal Mortality during 1990–2013: A Systematic Analysis for the Global Burden of Disease Study 2013." *The Lancet* 384 (9947): 980–1004.

Katz, P., J. Showstack, J. F. Smith, R. D. Nachtigall, S. G. Millstein, and others. 2011. "Costs of Infertility Treatment: Results from an 18-Month Prospective Cohort Study." *Fertility and Sterility* 95 (3): 915–21.

Kenyon, C., R. Colebunders, and T. Crucitti. 2013. "The Global Epidemiology of Bacterial Vaginosis: A Systematic Review." *American Journal of Obstetrics and Gynecology* 209 (6): 505–23.

Kinuthia, J., A. L. Drake, D. Matemo, B. A. Richardson, C. Zeh, and others. 2015. "HIV Acquisition during Pregnancy and Postpartum Is Associated with Genital Infections and Partnership Characteristics." *AIDS* 29 (15): 2025–33.

Kirakoya-Samadoulougou, F., N. Nagot, M. C. Defer, S. Yaro, P. Fao, and others. 2011. "Epidemiology of Herpes Simplex Virus Type 2 Infection in Rural and Urban Burkina Faso." *Sexually Transmitted Diseases* 38 (2): 117–23.

Koumans, E. H., M. Sternberg, C. Bruce, G. McQuillan, J. Kendrick, and others. 2007. "The Prevalence of Bacterial Vaginosis in the United States, 2001–2004; Associations with Symptoms, Sexual Behaviors, and Reproductive Health." *Sexually Transmitted Diseases* 34 (11): 864–69.

Kozuki, N., A. C. Lee, M. F. Silveira, C. G. Victora, L. Adair, and others. 2013. "The Associations of Birth Intervals with Small-for-Gestational-Age, Preterm, and Neonatal and Infant Mortality: A Meta-Analysis." *BMC Public Health* 13 (Suppl 3): S3.

Kozuki, N., and N. Walker. 2013. "Exploring the Association between Short/Long Preceding Birth Intervals and Child Mortality: Using Reference Birth Interval Children of the Same Mother as Comparison." *BMC Public Health* 13 (Suppl 3): S6.

Lan, P. T., C. S. Lundborg, H. D. Phuc, A. Sihavong, M. Unemo, and others. 2008. "Reproductive Tract Infections Including Sexually Transmitted Infections: A Population-Based Study of Women of Reproductive Age in a Rural District of Vietnam." *Sexually Transmitted Infections* 84 (2): 126–32.

Landers, D. V., H. C. Wiesenfeld, R. P. Heine, M. A. Krohn, and S. L. Hillier. 2004. "Predictive Value of the Clinical Diagnosis of Lower Genital Tract Infection in Women." *American Journal of Obstetrics and Gynecology* 190 (4): 1004–10.

Larsen, U. 2005. "Research on Infertility: Which Definition Should We Use?" *Fertility and Sterility* 83 (4): 846–52.

Larsen, U., G. Masenga, and J. Mlay. 2006. "Infertility in a Community and Clinic-Based Sample of Couples in Moshi, Northern Tanzania." *East African Medical Journal* 83 (1): 10–17.

Levandowski, B. A., L. Kalilani-Phiri, F. Kachle, P. Awah, G. Kangaude, and C. Mhango. 2012. "Investigating Social Consequences of Unwanted Pregnancy and Unsafe Abortion in Malawi: The Role of Stigma." *International Journal of Gynaecology and Obstetrics* 118 (Suppl 2): S167–71.

Levandowski, B. A., C. Mhango, E. Kuchingale, J. Lunguzi, H. Katengeza, and others. 2013. "The Incidence of Induced Abortion in Malawi." *International Perspectives on Sexual and Reproductive Health* 39 (2): 88–96.

Lovel, H., C. McGettigan, and Z. Mohammed. 2000. *A Systematic Review of the Health Complications of Female Genital Mutilation Including Sequelae in Childbirth.* Geneva: World Health Organization.

Madden, T., J. M. Grentzer, G. M. Secura, J. E. Allsworth, and J. F. Peipert. 2012. "Risk of Bacterial Vaginosis in Users of the Intrauterine Device: A Longitudinal Study." *Sexually Transmitted Diseases* 39 (3): 217–22.

Mahy, M. 2003. *Childhood Mortality in the Developing World: A Review of Evidence from the Demographic and Health Surveys.* Demographic and Health Surveys Comparative Reports 4. Calverton, MD: ORC Macro.

Marston, C., and J. Cleland. 2003. "Relationships between Contraception and Abortion: A Review of the Evidence." *International Family Planning Perspectives* 29 (1): 6–13.

Martin, H. L., B. A. Richardson, P. M. Nyange, L. Lavreys, S. L. Hillier, and others. 1999. "Vaginal *Lactobacilli*, Microbial Flora, and Risk of Human Immunodeficiency Virus Type 1 and Sexually Transmitted Disease Acquisition." *Journal of Infectious Diseases* 180 (6): 1863–68.

Mascarenhas, M. N., H. Cheung, C. D. Mathers, and G. A. Stevens. 2012. "Measuring Infertility in Populations: Constructing a Standard Definition for Use with Demographic and Reproductive Health Surveys." *Population Health Metrics* 10: 17.

Mascarenhas, M. N., S. R. Flaxman, T. Boerma, S. Vanderpoel, and G. A. Stevens. 2012. "National, Regional, and Global Trends in Infertility Prevalence since 1990: A Systematic Analysis of 277 Health Surveys." *PLoS Medicine* 9 (12): e1001356.

Mascarenhas, R. E. M., M. S. C. Machado, B. F. Costa e Silva, R. F. Pimentel, T. T. Ferreira, and others. 2012. "Prevalence and Risk Factors for Bacterial Vaginosis and other Vulvovaginitis in a Population of Sexually Active Adolescents from Salvador, Bahia, Brazil." *Infectious Diseases in Obstetrics and Gynecology* 2012: 378640.

Miranda, A. E., P. R. Mercon-de-Vargas, C. E. Corbett, J. F. Corbett, and R. Dietze. 2009. "Perspectives on Sexual and Reproductive Health among Women in an Ancient Mining Area in Brazil." *Revista Panamericana de Salud Publica* 25 (2): 157–61.

Moore, A. M., G. Jagwe-Wadda, and A. Bankole. 2011. "Mens' Attitudes about Abortion in Uganda." *Journal of Biosocial Science* 43 (1): 31–45.

Morof, D., J. Steinauer, S. Haider, S. Liu, P. Darney, and G. Barrett. 2012. "Evaluation of the London Measure of Unplanned Pregnancy in a United States Population of Women." *PLoS One* 7 (4): e35381.

Morris, M. C., P. A. Rogers, and G. Kinghorn. 2001. "Is Bacterial Vaginosis a Sexually Transmitted Infection?" *Sexually Transmitted Infections* 77 (1): 63–68.

Mota, A., E. Prieto, V. Carnall, and F. Exposto. 2000. "[Evaluation of Microscopy Methods for the Diagnosis of Bacterial Vaginosis]." *Acta Medica Portuguesa* 13 (3): 77–80.

Mukuria, A., J. Cushing, and J. Sangha. 2005. *Nutritional Status of Children: Results from the Demographic and Health Surveys 1994–2001.* DHS Comparative Report 10. Calverton, MD: ORC Macro.

Myer, L., L. Denny, R. Telerant, M. Souza, T. C. Wright Jr., and L. Kuhn. 2005. "Bacterial Vaginosis and Susceptibility to HIV Infection in South African Women: A Nested Case-Control Study." *Journal of Infectious Diseases* 192 (8): 1372–80.

Namkinga, L. A., M. I. Matee, A. K. Kivaisi, and C. Moshiro. 2005. "Prevalence and Risk Factors for Vaginal Candidiasis among Women Seeking Primary Care for Genital Infections in Dar es Salaam, Tanzania." *East African Medical Journal* 82 (3): 138–43.

Nelson, D. B., A. L. Hanlon, B. Wu, C. Liu, and D. N. Fredricks. 2015. "First Trimester Levels of BV-Associated Bacteria and Risk of Miscarriage among Women Early in Pregnancy." *Maternal and Child Health Journal* 19 (12): 2682–87.

Ness, R. B., S. Hillier, H. E. Richter, D. E. Soper, C. Stamm, and others. 2003. "Can Known Risk Factors Explain Racial Differences in the Occurrence of Bacterial Vaginosis?" *Journal of the National Medical Association* 95 (3): 201–12.

Nugent, R. P., M. A. Krohn, and S. L. Hillier. 1991. "Reliability of Diagnosing Bacterial Vaginosis Is Improved by a Standardized Method of Gram Stain Interpretation." *Journal of Clinical Microbiology* 29 (2): 297–301.

Nwadioha, S. I., E. O. Nwokedi, J. Egesie, and H. Enejuo. 2013. "Vaginal Candidiasis and Its Risk Factors among Women Attending a Nigerian Teaching Hospital." *Nigerian Postgraduate Medical Journal* 20 (1): 20–23.

OHCHR, UNAIDS, UNDP, UNECA, UNESCO, and others. 2008. *Eliminating Female Genital Mutilation: An Interagency Statement.* Geneva: World Health Organization.

Okungbowa, F. I., O. S. Isikhuemhen, and A. P. Dede. 2003. "The Distribution Frequency of Candida Species in the Genitourinary Tract among Symptomatic Individuals in Nigerian Cities." *Revista Iberoamicana de Micologia* 20 (2): 60–63.

Oliveira, F. A., V. Pfleger, K. Lang, J. Heukelbach, I. Miralles, and others. 2007. "Sexually Transmitted Infections, Bacterial Vaginosis, and Candidiasis in Women of Reproductive Age in Rural Northeast Brazil: A Population-Based Study." *Memorias do Instituto Oswaldo Cruz* 102 (6): 751–56.

Plichta, S. B., and M. Falik. 2001. "Prevalence of Violence and Its Implications for Women's Health." *Women's Health Issues* 11 (3): 244–58.

Prada, E., A. Biddlecom, and S. Singh. 2011. "Induced Abortion in Colombia: New Estimates and Change between 1989 and 2008." *International Perspectives on Sexual and Reproductive Health* 37 (3): 114–24.

Prasad, J. H., S. Abraham, K. M. Kurz, V. George, M. K. Lalitha, and others. 2005. "Reproductive Tract Infections among Young Married Women in Tamil Nadu, India." *International Family Planning Perspectives* 31 (2): 73–82.

Rathod, S. D., J. D. Klausner, K. Krupp, A. L. Reingold, and P. Madhivanan. 2012. "Epidemiologic Features of Vulvovaginal Candidiasis among Reproductive-Age Women in India." *Infectious Diseases in Obstetrics and Gynecology* 859071. doi:10.1155/2012/859071.

Reed, B. D., P. Zazove, C. L. Pierson, D. W. Gorenflo, and J. Horrocks. 2003. "Candida Transmission and Sexual Behaviors as Risks for a Repeat Episode of Candida Vulvovaginitis." *Journal of Womens Health (Larchmont)* 12 (10): 979–89.

Rossier, C. 2003. "Estimating Induced Abortion Rates: A Review." *Studies in Family Planning* 34 (2): 87–102.

———. 2007. "Abortion: An Open Secret? Abortion and Social Network Involvement in Burkina Faso." *Reproductive Health Matters* 15 (30): 230–38.

Rutstein, S. O., and I. H. Shah. 2004. *Infecundity, Infertility, and Childlessness in Developing Countries.* DHS Comparative Reports 9. Calverton, MD: ORC Macro and the World Health Organization.

Santelli, J., R. Rochat, K. Hatfield-Timajchy, B. C. Gilbert, K. Curtis, and others. 2003. "The Measurement and Meaning of Unintended Pregnancy." *Perspectives on Sexual and Reproductive Health* 35 (2): 94–101.

Sathar, Z. A., S. Singh, and F. F. Fikree. 2007. "Estimating the Incidence of Abortion in Pakistan." *Studies in Family Planning* 38 (1): 11–22.

Say, L., D. Chou, A. Gemmill, O. Tunçalp, A.-B. Moller, and others. 2014. "Global Causes of Maternal Death: A WHO Systematic Analysis." *The Lancet Global Health* 2 (6): e323–33.

Sedgh, G., and R. Hussain. 2014. "Reasons for Contraceptive Non-Use among Women with an Unmet Need for Contraception in Developing Countries: A Comprehensive Analysis of Levels and Trends." *Studies in Family Planning* 42 (2): 151–169.

Sedgh, G., C. Rossier, I. Kaboré, A. Bankole, and M. Mikulich. 2011. "Estimating Abortion Incidence in Burkina Faso Using Two Methodologies." *Studies in Family Planning* 42 (3): 147–54.

Sedgh, G., S. Singh, I. H. Shah, E. Ahman, S. K. Henshaw, and A. Bankole. 2012. "Induced Abortion: Incidence and Trends Worldwide from 1995 to 2008." *The Lancet* 379 (9816): 625–32.

Sedgh, G., S. Singh, and R. Hussain. 2014. "Intended and Unintended Pregnancies Worldwide in 2012 and Recent Trends." *Studies in Family Planning* 45 (3): 301–14.

Shellenberg, K. M., A. M. Moore, A. Bankole, F. Juarez, A. K. Amideyi, and others. 2011. "Social Stigma and Disclosure about Induced Abortion: Results from an

Exploratory Study." *Global Public Health* 6 (Suppl 1): S111–25.

Singh, S. 2006. "Hospital Admissions Resulting from Unsafe Abortion: Estimates from 13 Developing Countries." *The Lancet* 368 (9550): 1887–92.

———. 2010. "Global Consequences of Unsafe Abortion." *Women's Health (London, England)* 6 (6): 849–60.

Singh, S., and J. E. Darroch. 2012. *Adding It Up: Costs and Benefits of Contraceptive Services—Estimates for 2012*. New York: Guttmacher Institute and United Nations Population Fund.

———, and L. S. Ashford. 2014. *Adding It Up: The Costs and Benefits of Investing in Sexual and Reproductive Health*. New York: Guttmacher Institute.

Singh, S., T. Fetters, H. Gebreselassie, A. Abdella, Y. Gebrehiwot, and others. 2010. "The Estimated Incidence of Induced Abortion in Ethiopia, 2008." *International Perspectives on Sexual and Reproductive Health* 36 (1): 16–25.

Singh, S., A. Hossain, I. Maddow-Zimet, H. Ullah Bhuiyan, M. Vlassoff, and R. Hussain. 2012. "The Incidence of Menstrual Regulation Procedures and Abortion in Bangladesh, 2010." *International Perspectives on Sexual and Reproductive Health* 53 (3).

Singh, S., F. Juarez, J. Cabigon, H. Ball, R. Hussain, and J. Nadeau. 2006. *Unintended Pregnancy and Induced Abortion in the Philippines: Causes and Consequences*. New York: Guttmacher Institute.

Singh, S., and I. Maddow-Zimet. 2015. "Facility-Based Treatment for Medical Complications Resulting from Unsafe Pregnancy Termination in the Developing World, 2012: A Review of Evidence from 26 Countries." *BJOG*. doi/10.1111/1471-0528.13552.

Singh, S., E. Prada, and F. Juarez. 2011. "The Abortion Incidence Complications Method: A Quantitative Technique." In *Methodologies for Estimating Abortion Incidence and Abortion-Related Morbidity: A Review*, edited by S. Singh, L. Remez, and A. Tartaglione. New York: Guttmacher Institute.

Singh, S., E. Prada, and E. Kestler. 2006. "Induced Abortion and Unintended Pregnancy in Guatemala." *International Family Planning Perspectives* 32 (3): 136–45.

Singh, S., E. Prada, F. Mirembe, and C. Kiggundu. 2005. "The Incidence of Induced Abortion in Uganda." *International Family Planning Perspectives* 31 (4): 183–91.

Singh, S., G. Sedgh, and R. Hussain. 2010. "Unintended Pregnancy: Worldwide Levels, Trends, and Outcomes." *Studies in Family Planning* 41 (4): 241–50.

Singh, S., D. Wulf, R. Hussain, A. Bankole, and G. Sedgh. 2009. *Abortion Worldwide: A Decade of Uneven Progress*. New York: Guttmacher Institute.

Speizer, I. S., L. M. Calhoun, T. Hoke, and R. Sengupta. 2013. "Measurement of Unmet Need for Family Planning: Longitudinal Analysis of the Impact of Fertility Desires on Subsequent Childbearing Behaviors among Urban Women from Uttar Pradesh, India." *Contraception* 88 (4): 553–60.

Stockl, H., K. Devries, A. Rotstein, N. Abrahams, J. Campbell, and others. 2013. "The Global Prevalence of Intimate Partner Homicide: A Systematic Review." *The Lancet* 382 (9895): 859–65.

Sundaram, A., M. Vlassoff, A. Bankole, L. Remez, and Y. Gebrehiwot. 2009. "Benefits of Meeting the Contraceptive Needs of Ethiopian Women." In Brief, Guttmacher Institute, New York.

Sundaram, A., M. Vlassoff, F. Mugisha, A. Bankole, S. Singh, and others. 2013. "Documenting the Individual- and Household-Level Cost of Unsafe Abortion in Uganda." *Perspectives on Sexual and Reproductive Health* 39 (4): 174–84.

Trussell, J., B. Vaughan, and J. Stanford. 1999. "Are All Contraceptive Failures Unintended Pregnancies?" *Family Planning Perspectives* 31 (5): 246–47.

UNICEF (United Nations Children's Fund). 2013. *Female Genital Mutilation/Cutting: A Statistical Overview and Exploration of the Dynamics of Change*. New York: UNICEF.

UNPD (United Nations Population Division). 2013. "World Population Prospects: The 2012 Revision." Department of Economic and Social Affairs, Population Division, United Nations, New York.

van Oostrum, N., P. De Sutter, J. Meys, and H. Verstraelen. 2013. "Risks Associated with Bacterial Vaginosis in Infertility Patients: A Systematic Review and Meta-Analysis." *Human Reproduction* 28 (7): 1809–15.

Vlassoff, M., A. Sundaram, A. Bankole, L. Remez, and F. Mugisha. 2009. "Benefits of Meeting the Contraceptive Needs of Ugandan Women." In Brief, Guttmacher Institute, New York.

Vlassoff, M., A. Sundaram, A. Bankole, L. Remez, and D. Yugbare. 2011. "Avantages liés à la satisfaction des besoins en matière de contraception moderne au Burkina Faso." In Brief, Guttmacher Institute, New York.

Vlassoff, M., D. Walker, J. Shearer, D. Newlands, and S. Singh. 2009. "Estimates of Health Care System Costs of Unsafe Abortion in Africa and Latin America." *International Perspectives on Sexual and Reproductive Health* 35 (3): 114–21.

Vu, A., A. Adam, A. Wirtz, K. Pham, L. Rubenstein, and others. 2014. "The Prevalence of Sexual Violence among Female Refugees in Complex Humanitarian Emergencies: A Systematic Review and Meta-Analysis." *PLoS Currents Disasters* 1.

Walraven, G., C. Scherf, B. West, G. Ekpo, K. Paine, and others. 2001. "The Burden of Reproductive-Organ Disease in Rural Women in The Gambia, West Africa." *The Lancet* 357 (9263): 1161–67.

Wellings, K., K. G. Jones, C. H. Mercer, C. Tanton, S. Clifton, and others. 2013. "The Prevalence of Unplanned Pregnancy and Associated Factors in Britain: Findings from the Third National Survey of Sexual Attitudes and Lifestyles (Natsal-3)." *The Lancet* 382 (9907): 1807–16.

Wenman, W. M., M. R. Joffres, I. V. Tataryn, and the Edmonton Perinatal Infections Group. 2004. "A Prospective Cohort Study of Pregnancy Risk Factors and Birth Outcomes in Aboriginal Women." *CMAJ* 171 (6): 585–89.

Westoff, C. F. 2012. *Unmet Need for Modern Contraceptive Methods*. DHS Analytical Studies 28. Calverton, MD: ICF International.

————, and A. Bankole. 1998. "The Time Dynamics of Unmet Need: An Example from Morocco." *International Family Planning Perspectives* 24 (1): 12–24.

WHO (World Health Organization). 2001. *Management of Pregnancy, Childbirth and Postpartum Period in the Presence of Female Genital Mutilation.* Geneva: WHO.

————. 2004. *Unsafe Abortion: Global and Regional Estimates of the Incidence of Unsafe Abortion and Associated Mortality in 2000.* Geneva: WHO.

————. 2006a. *Reproductive Health Indicators: Guidelines for Their Generation, Interpretation and Analysis for Global Monitoring.* Geneva: WHO.

————. 2006b. "Female Genital Mutilation and Obstetric Outcome: WHO Collaborative Prospective Study in Six African Countries." Study Group on Female Genital Mutilation and Obstetric Outcome. *The Lancet* 367 (9525): 1835–41.

————. 2007. *Unsafe Abortion: Global and Regional Estimates of the Incidence of Unsafe Abortion and Associated Mortality in 2003.* Geneva: WHO.

————. 2011. *Unsafe Abortion: Global and Regional Estimates of the Incidence of Unsafe Abortion and Associated Mortality in 2008.* Geneva: WHO.

————. 2013. *Responding to Intimate Partner Violence and Sexual Violence against Women: WHO Clinical and Policy Guidelines.* Geneva: WHO.

————. 2014. *Trends in Maternal Mortality: 1990 to 2013. Estimates by WHO, UNICEF, UNFPA, The World Bank and the United Nations Population Division.* Geneva: WHO.

WHO and World Bank. 2011. *World Report on Disability 2011.* Geneva: WHO.

WHO, LSHTM (London School of Hygiene and Tropical Medicine), and MRC-SA (South Africa Medical Research Council). 2013. *Global and Regional Estimates of Violence against Women: Prevalence and Health Effects of Intimate Partner Violence and Non-Partner Sexual Violence.* Geneva: WHO.

Yoder, P. S., N. Abderrahim, and A. Zhuzhini. 2004. *Female Genital Cutting in the Demographic Health Surveys: A Critical and Comparative Analysis.* DHS Comparative Reports 7. Calverton, MD: ORC Macro.

Yoder, P. S., and S. Wang. 2013. *Female Genital Cutting: The Interpretation of Recent DHS Data.* DHS Comparative Reports 33. Calverton, MD: ICF International.

Zegers-Hochschild, F., G. D. Adamson, J. de Mouzon, O. Ishihara, R. Mansour, and others. 2009. "The International Committee for Monitoring Assisted Reproductive Technology (ICMART) and the World Health Organization (WHO) Revised Glossary on ART Terminology, 2009." *Human Reproduction* 24 (11): 2683–87.

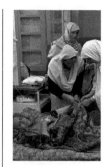

Chapter 3

Levels and Causes of Maternal Mortality and Morbidity

Véronique Filippi, Doris Chou, Carine Ronsmans,
Wendy Graham, and Lale Say

INTRODUCTION

In September 2000, 189 world leaders signed a declaration on eight Millennium Development Goals (MDGs) to improve the lives of women, men, and children in their respective countries (United Nations General Assembly 2000). Goal 5a calls for the reduction of maternal mortality by 75 percent between 1990 and 2015. Goal 5a was supplemented by MDG 5b on universal access to contraception. MDGs 5a and 5b have been important catalysts for the reductions in maternal mortality levels that have been achieved in many settings.[1]

Despite substantial progress, challenges remain. The majority of low-income countries (LICs), particularly in Sub-Saharan Africa and postconflict settings, have not made sufficient progress to meet MDG 5a. The post-2015 agenda on sustainable development is broader than the MDG agenda, with a greater number of nonhealth goals and a strong focus on inequity reduction; the new agenda includes an absolute reduction in maternal mortality as a marker of progress.[2] This new indicator is expected to be framed as targets for preventable maternal deaths (Bustreo and others 2013; Gilmore and Camhe Gebreyesus 2012).

The International Classification of Diseases (ICD-10) defines maternal death as "[The] death of a woman while pregnant or within 42 days of the end of pregnancy, irrespective of the duration and site of the pregnancy, from any cause related to or aggravated by the pregnancy or its management, but not from accidental or incidental causes" (WHO 2010, 156). Subsequent guidance on the classification of causes includes nine groups of underlying causes (box 3.1) (WHO 2012).

Despite the increased global focus on maternal mortality as a public health issue, little detailed knowledge is available on the levels of maternal mortality and morbidity and the causes of their occurrence. A large proportion of maternal deaths occur in settings in which vital registration is deficient and many sick women do not access services. To obtain data on population levels of maternal mortality in these settings, special surveys are needed, including the following (Abouzahr 1999):

- Reproductive Age Mortality Studies, which investigate all reproductive age deaths
- Demographic and Health Surveys, which interview women and men about their siblings' survival in adulthood to identify deaths of sisters during or following pregnancy (the siblings are from the same mother) (Ahmed and others 2014)
- Smaller studies, which use the indirect sisterhood method
- National investigations, which add questions to censuses
- Verbal autopsy studies, which provide information on causes and circumstances of deaths.

Corresponding author: Véronique Filippi, London School of Hygiene & Tropical Medicine, Veronique.Filippi@lshtm.ac.uk.

Maternal death studies require large sample sizes; recent national-level data are often nonexistent, and maternal mortality tracking relies principally on mathematical models. This lack of data has led to a repeated call for countries to improve their vital registration systems and to strengthen other mechanisms for informing intervention strategies, such as the maternal death surveillance and response system proposed within the new accountability framework (WHO 2013). Accountability remains a central part of United Nations Secretary General Ban Ki-Moon's updated global strategy to accelerate progress for women's, children's, and adolescent's health (http://www.everywomaneverychild.org/global-strategy-2). The accountability framework, developed under the 2010 global strategy to accelerate women's and children's health, included recommendations for improvements in resource tracking; international and national oversight; and data monitoring, including maternal mortality (Commission on Information and Accountability for Women's and Children's Health 2011).

Information on maternal morbidity is frequently collected in hospital studies, which are only representative of patients who seek care. Community-based studies are rare in LICs and suffer from methodological limitations, particularly when they rely on self-reporting of obstetric complications. Self-reporting is known not to agree sufficiently with medical diagnoses to estimate prevalence. In particular, studies validating retrospective interview surveys find that women without medical diagnoses of complications during labor frequently reported symptoms of morbidity during surveys, a phenomenon that can lead to an overestimation of prevalence (Ronsmans and others 1997; Souza and others 2008). In addition, community-based studies have focused on direct obstetric complications; little is known about the nature and incidence of many indirect complications that are aggravated by pregnancy. For example, reliable population-based estimates of the occurrence of asthma during pregnancy do not exist in LICs.

This chapter addresses the extent and nature of maternal mortality and morbidity and serves as a backdrop to subsequent chapters on obstetric interventions in LICs. It introduces the determinants of maternal mortality and morbidity and their strategic implications. The next section uses the most recent estimates from the World Health Organization (WHO) to show that women face a higher risk of maternal death in Sub-Saharan Africa. It discusses the recent findings of a WHO meta-analysis that show that the most important direct causes are hemorrhage, hypertension, abortion, and sepsis; however, the proportion of deaths due to indirect causes is increasing in most parts of the world. The chapter then focuses on pregnancy-related complications, including nonfatal illnesses such as antenatal and postpartum depression, using the findings from systematic reviews conducted by the Child Health Epidemiology Reference Group. The most common contributors to maternal morbidity are probably anemia and depression at the community level, but prolonged and obstructed labor results in the highest burden of disease because of fistulas (IHME 2013). The chapter discusses the broader determinants of maternal morbidity and mortality, and then concludes by making the links with the interventions highlighted in chapter 7 in this volume (Gülmezoglu and others 2016).

MATERNAL MORTALITY LEVELS AND TRENDS

The WHO, in collaboration with the United Nations Children's Fund, the United Nations Population Fund, the World Bank Group, and the United Nations Population Division, publishes global estimates of maternal mortality, which are excerpted in this chapter (WHO 2015). A complete description of the methodology and underlying data and statistical model can be found in the publication and online.[3] In this chapter, the latest estimate is for 2015. Whenever an estimate includes trend data between two points, updates of those estimates typically supersede previously published figures. Readers are directed to the WHO's Reproductive Health and Research web page on maternal mortality to access the latest published data.[4]

Maternal Mortality Ratio Levels and Trends, 1990–2015

Globally, the total number of maternal deaths decreased by 43 percent from 532,000 in 1990 to 303,000 in 2015. The global maternal mortality ratio (MMR) declined by 44 percent, from 385 maternal deaths per 100,000 live births in 1990 to 216 in 2015—an average annual decline of 2.3 percent (WHO 2015).

All MDG regions experienced a decline in the MMR between 1990 and 2015. The highest reduction was in Eastern Asia (72 percent), followed by Southern Asia (67 percent), South-Eastern Asia (66 percent), Northern Africa (59 percent), Oceania (52 percent), Caucasus and Central Asia (52 percent), Latin America and the Caribbean (50 percent), Sub-Saharan Africa (45 percent), and Western Asia (43 percent). Although the Caucasus and Central Asia experienced a relatively low level of decline, its already low MMR of 69 maternal deaths per 100,000 live births in 1990 suggests that a different set of more finely tuned strategies might be required to respond to the challenge of achieving the same rate of decline as other regions with higher 1990 MMRs, with possibly a stronger focus on improved fertility control (Shelburne and Trentini 2010).

Despite an initial increase in maternal mortality in regions highly affected by human immunodeficiency virus/acquired immunodeficiency syndrome (HIV/AIDS), evidence suggests that maternal mortality due to HIV/AIDS peaked in 2005 and showed signs of decline in 2010 and 2015, most likely because of the increased availability of antiretroviral medication. Of the 183 countries included in this exercise, 9 countries that had high levels of maternal mortality in 1990 are categorized as having met the MDG goal of having reduced maternal mortality by 75 percent. They are Maldives (90 percent reduction in MMR); Bhutan (84 percent); Cambodia (84 percent); Cabo Verde (84 percent); the Islamic Republic of Iran (80 percent); Timor-Leste (80 percent); Lao People's Democratic Republic (78 percent); Rwanda (78 percent); and Mongolia (76 percent).

An additional 39 countries are characterized as having made a 50 percent reduction in maternal mortality; 21 countries have made insufficient progress; and 26 made no progress.

These estimates should be viewed in context; accurate data on maternal mortality are lacking for the majority of countries. The range of uncertainty indicates that the true total number of maternal deaths in 2015 could plausibly be as low as 291,000 and as high as 349,000. Similarly, the global MMR plausibly ranges from 207 to 249 maternal deaths per 100,000 live births.

Disproportionate Burden in Low- and Middle-Income Countries

Low- and middle-income countries (LMICs, as defined by the World Bank) account for 99 percent (300,000) of global maternal deaths. The MMR in these regions (242 per 100,000) is 14 times higher than that in high-income countries (HICs, as defined by the World Bank (17 per 100,000). Most maternal deaths occur in MDG regions Sub-Saharan Africa (201,000) and South Asia (66,000). Sub-Saharan Africa alone accounts for 66 percent of maternal deaths and has the highest MMR, at 546 maternal deaths per 100,000 live births. By MDG region, Eastern Asia has the lowest rate among developing regions, at 27 maternal deaths per 100,000 live births. Of the remaining developing regions, four had low MMRs: Caucasus and Central Asia (33), Northern Africa (70), Western Asia (91), and Latin America and the Caribbean (67). Three had moderate MMRs: South-Eastern Asia (110), Southern Asia (176), and Oceania (187). The adult lifetime risk of maternal mortality—the probability that a 15-year-old woman will die eventually from a maternal cause—in Sub-Saharan Africa is the highest at 1 in 36; this number is in contrast to 1 in 150 in Oceania; 1 in 210 in Southern Asia; 1 in 380 in South-Eastern Asia; and 1 in 4,900 in developed regions. The global adult lifetime risk of maternal mortality is 1 in 180.

At the country level, two countries, Nigeria and India, account for more than one-third of all global maternal deaths in 2015, with an approximate 58,000 (uncertainty interval [UI] 42,000 to 84,000) maternal deaths (19 percent) and 45,000 (UI 36,000 to 56,000) maternal deaths (15 percent), respectively. Ten countries account for nearly 59 percent of global maternal deaths. In addition to Nigeria and India, they are the Democratic Republic of Congo (22,000; UI 16,000 to 33,000), Ethiopia (11,000; UI 7,900 to 18,000), Pakistan (9,700; UI 6,100 to 15,000), Tanzania (8,200; UI 5,800 to 12,000), Kenya (8,000; UI 5,400 to 12,000), Indonesia (6,400; UI 4,700 to 9,000), Uganda (5,700; UI 4,100 to 8,200), and Bangladesh (5,500; UI 3,900 to 8,800). Of the 183 countries and territories in this analysis, Sierre Leone and Chad have the highest adult lifetime risk of maternal mortality, 1 in 17 and 1 in 18, respectively.

MEDICAL CAUSES OF MATERNAL DEATHS

Most maternal deaths do not have well-defined causes. Nevertheless, using the available data, nearly 73.0 percent of all maternal deaths between 2003 and 2009 were attributable to direct obstetric causes; deaths due to indirect causes accounted for 27.5 percent (95 percent confidence interval 19.7–37.5) of all deaths. The major causes of maternal mortality are as follows (Say and others 2014):

- Hemorrhage, 27.1 percent (95 percent confidence interval 19.9–36.2); more than 72.6 percent of deaths from hemorrhage were classified as postpartum hemorrhage

- Hypertension, 14.0 percent (95 percent confidence interval 11.1–17. 4)
- Sepsis, 10.7 percent (95 percent confidence interval 5.9–18.6)
- Abortive outcomes, 7.9 percent (95 percent confidence interval 4.7–13.2)
- Embolism and other direct causes, 12.8 percent.

Three causes of death—unsafe abortions, obstructed labor, and indirect causes—are of considerable programmatic interest but are particularly difficult to capture. The first case, unsafe abortions, is discussed further in chapter 2 of this volume (Ezeh and others 2016).

Deaths from Abortions

Say and others (2014) estimate that 7.9 percent (95 percent confidence interval 4.7–13.2) of all maternal deaths were due to abortive outcomes, including spontaneous or induced abortions and ectopic pregnancies. This share is lower than in previous assessments, which estimated mortality due to unsafe abortion at 13 percent (WHO 2011b).

Ectopic Pregnancy

Although ectopic pregnancy can have very serious mortality consequences, and there have been reports of increased incidence, it remains a rare event at less than 2 per 100 deliveries (Stulberg and others 2013). This condition has a high case fatality rate where urgent surgical care is not available. However, no systematic review of its global prevalence has been published since the 1980s.

Induced Abortions

In classifying maternal deaths due to abortion, and more specifically to unsafe abortion, which is defined as the termination of an unintended pregnancy "performed by persons lacking the necessary skills or in an environment not in conformity with minimal clinical standards, or both" (WHO 1993; Ganatra and others 2014, 155), there is a particular risk for misclassification that may lead to underreporting. ICD-10 does not have a specific code for unsafe abortion; accordingly, deaths attributed to unsafe abortion are often documented within special studies. Even where induced abortion is legal, the religious and cultural values in many countries can mean that women do not disclose abortion attempts, and relatives or health care professionals do not report these deaths as such. Underregistration of deaths may be the result of the stigmatization of abortion, which may result in intentional misclassification by providers where abortion is restricted.

Deaths from Obstructed Labor

Obstructed labor is commonly considered to be or diagnosed as a clinical cause of maternal death. However, as a death classification, it may be hard to capture because deaths occurring after obstructed labor and its consequences may be coded under hemorrhage or sepsis. This practice is especially an issue in settings in which verbal autopsies are used to determine cause of death, because verbal autopsy methods vary; lack of consistent case definitions and confusion regarding hierarchical assignment of causes affect the validity of the study data. In total, complications of delivery accounted for 2.8 percent (95 percent confidence interval 1.6–4.9), and obstructed labor accounted for 2.8 percent (95 percent confidence interval 1.4–5.5) of all maternal deaths globally, both reported within the "other direct" category, which totals to 9.6 percent (95 percent confidence interval 6.5–14.3).

Deaths from Indirect Causes

The review found that the indirect causes of maternal death, when combined, are the most common cause of maternal death. A breakdown of deaths due to indirect causes suggests that more than 70 percent are from preexisting medical conditions, including HIV/AIDS, exacerbated by pregnancy. Information on the number and proportion of maternal deaths related to HIV/AIDS alone is presented in box 3.2. However, these estimates should be considered with caution, given the phenomenon of misattribution of indirect maternal causes of death. Underestimation of 20 percent to 90 percent of maternal deaths has been described in a number of settings. In Austria, misclassification was significantly higher for indirect deaths (81 percent, 95 percent confidence interval 64–91 percent) than for direct deaths (28 percent, 95 percent confidence interval 21 percent to 36 percent); in the United Kingdom, indirect deaths may account for up to 74 percent of underreported maternal deaths from 2003 to 2005 (Karimian-Teherani and others 2002; Lewis 2007).

Global Distribution of Maternal Deaths

The global distribution of maternal deaths is influenced by the two regions, Sub-Saharan Africa and Southern Asia, that account for the majority of all maternal deaths (WHO 2014b). Although estimated regional cause-of-death distributions are uncertain for many

Proportions of Considered AIDS-Related Indirect Maternal Deaths

Assessing maternal deaths among human immuno-deficiency virus (HIV)–infected women is a separate but related estimation process. Worldwide in 2015, 4,700 maternal deaths were attributed to HIV (an indirect cause of maternal deaths because the condition usually preexists pregnancy, and this cause of death is not specific to pregnant women); 4,000 (85 percent) of these deaths were in Sub-Saharan Africa. The MDG region of Southern Asia was a distant second, with 310 deaths. The proportion of maternal deaths attributed to HIV was highest in Sub-Saharan Africa (2.0 percent) and Latin America and the Caribbean (1.5 percent). Without HIV, the MMR for Sub-Saharan Africa would be 535 maternal deaths per 100,000 live births, rather than 510.

The proportion of HIV-attributable maternal deaths is 10 percent or more in five countries: South Africa (32 percent), Swaziland (19 percent), Botswana (18 percent), Lesotho (13 percent), and Mozambique (11 percent).

AIDS-related indirect maternal deaths accounted for 1.6 percent of global maternal deaths. Underreporting and misclassification of indirect maternal deaths due to HIV/AIDS are a particular issue in death certificate coding and when countries rely on verbal autopsies to ascertain cause of death. This imprecision highlights the need for review of deaths of HIV-infected women temporal to pregnancy; the women may die from HIV or with HIV while pregnant. As methods for global maternal death estimation evolve, the evidence for the parameters needed to estimate indirect maternal HIV deaths and further clarification on the use of ICD-10 codes will standardize and improve our understanding of maternal and HIV death tallies.

---

causes, point estimates show substantial differences across regions. Hemorrhage accounted for 36.9 percent (95 percent confidence interval 24.1 percent to 51.6 percent) of deaths in northern Africa, compared with 16.3 percent (95 percent confidence interval 11.1 percent to 24.6 percent) in developed regions. Hypertensive disorders were a significant cause of death in Latin American and the Caribbean, accounting for 22.1 percent (95 percent confidence interval 19.9 percent to 24.6 percent) of all maternal deaths in the region.

Almost all sepsis deaths occurred in developing regions, and the percentage of deaths was highest at 13.7 percent (95 percent confidence interval 3.3 percent to 35.9 percent) in Southern Asia. Only a small proportion of deaths are estimated to result from abortion in Eastern Asia, 0.8 percent (95 percent confidence interval 0.2 percent to 2.0 percent), where access to abortion is generally less restricted. Latin America and the Caribbean and Sub-Saharan Africa have higher proportions of deaths in this category than the global average, 9.9 percent (95 percent confidence interval 8.1 percent to 13.0 percent) and 9.6 percent (95 percent confidence interval 5.1 percent to 17.2 percent), respectively. Another direct cause, embolism, accounted for more deaths than the global average in South-Eastern Asia and Eastern Asia, 12.1 percent (95 percent confidence interval 3.2 percent to 33.4 percent) and 11.5 percent (95 percent confidence interval 1.6 percent to 40.6 percent), respectively.

The proportion of deaths due to indirect causes was highest in Southern Asia, 29.3 percent (95 percent confidence interval 12.2 percent to 55.1 percent), followed by Sub-Saharan Africa, 28.6 percent (95 percent confidence interval 19.9 percent to 40.3 percent); indirect causes also accounted for nearly 25.0 percent of the deaths in the developed regions. The overall proportion of HIV/AIDS maternal deaths is highest in Sub-Saharan Africa, 6.4 percent (95 percent confidence interval 4.6 percent to 8.8 percent).

Trends in Maternal Death Causes

The continued dearth of basic information in most countries of the developing region, where most of the deaths occur, impedes the ability to address the question of changes in causes of maternal deaths over time. In determining trends in causes of maternal deaths, it is reasonable to conclude that the proportion of indirect deaths is increasing in all regions. The actual indirect causes differ in that HIV/AIDS deaths are highest in Sub-Saharan Africa; other medical causes are highest in developed regions and Eastern Asia.

MEDICAL CAUSES OF MATERNAL MORBIDITY

Definition of Maternal Morbidity

The WHO Maternal Morbidity Working Group defines maternal morbidity as "any health condition attributed to and/or aggravated by pregnancy and childbirth that has a negative impact on the woman's wellbeing" (Firoz and others 2013, 795). The working group emphasizes the wide range of indirect conditions in the morbidity that women experience during pregnancy, delivery, or postpregnancy by listing more than 180 diagnoses and dividing them into 14 organ dysfunction categories, ranging from obstetric to cardiorespiratory and rheumatology conditions.

The negative impact of pregnancy-related ill health is highlighted on the basis of subsequent disabilities, including how severely the woman's functional status is affected and for how long. The origins of maternal morbidity occur during pregnancy, but the sequelae might take several months to manifest themselves. Capturing the negative impact of morbidities requires a longer reference period than used for the death definition.

Perceived Morbidity

Where women are not able to access services easily, surveys are conducted to measure their health status. Accurate diagnoses are difficult to make in survey conditions without confirmation from a clinical examination, laboratory reports, or medical records (Ronsmans and others 1997). However, surveys provide evidence of women's experience of health and morbidity during pregnancy. Overall, many women complain about ill health in pregnancy and the puerperium. Studies of self-reports in low-income settings typically find that more than 70 percent of women report signs or symptoms of pregnancy-related complications (Lagro and others 2003). In a Nepal study, women reported, on average, three to four days per week with symptoms of illness during pregnancy (Christian and others 2000). The type of symptoms reported varied according to gestational age, with nausea and vomiting more common in early pregnancy, and swelling of the hands and face more common toward the end of pregnancy. Counterintuitive changes in self-reported ill health have been described for the postpartum period, with anticipated declines in symptoms over time sometimes followed by increases (Filippi and others 2007; Saurel-Cubizolles and others 2000); self-perceived ill health is not simply a result of biological changes but also of social support and influences.

Severity of Conditions

Maternal health specialists have tried since the 1990s to distinguish between women with severe and less severe conditions in the measurement of morbidity (Stones and others 1991). Maternal deaths are relatively rare events, and these specialists believe that cases at the very severe end of the maternal morbidity spectrum have two useful characteristics: they are more frequent than maternal deaths, and they share similar characteristics to maternal deaths, including some common risk factors. Women who nearly died during pregnancy, labor, or postpregnancy, but survived, usually because of chance or good hospital care, are maternal "near-misses" (WHO 2011a). Depending on the definitions used and on the country and hospital settings, maternal near-misses occur for 0.05 percent to 15.0 percent of hospitalized women (Tuncalp and others 2012). The WHO has developed operational definitions of near-misses to facilitate comparisons between settings (WHO 2011a).

Nevertheless, it is worth noting that the cause patterns of maternal mortality, near-misses, and less severe morbidity differ, depending on the case fatality of certain conditions and the ease of halting the progression of disease (Pattinson and others 2003).

Principal Morbidity Diagnoses

The principal medical causes of mortality are also important morbidity diagnoses, but they are not the only ones to consider. To this list must be added other contributing factors, such as depression and anemia, because of their frequency or severity. We must also add the sequelae of difficult labor, such as incontinence, fistulas, and prolapse. A further consideration is the presence of comorbidities, such as obstructed labor followed by infection, that complicate management, diagnosis, and classification.

Figure 3.1 illustrates a conceptual framework of the ways in which different maternal conditions interact. Long-term health sequelae are associated with certain diagnoses in pregnancy. For example, neglected obstructed and prolonged labors are associated with obstetric fistulas. The conceptual framework also includes medical risk factors. One of these, obesity, has become a global epidemic and has been linked with increasing levels of hypertension and diabetes. The management of pregnancy and childbirth, including cesarean section, is also a risk factor for future problems, for example, placenta previa. Female genital mutilation, particularly in its most severe form, is associated with adverse maternal and perinatal outcomes, including postpartum hemorrhage and emergency cesarean (WHO 2006).

Figure 3.1 Conceptual Framework of Maternal Health

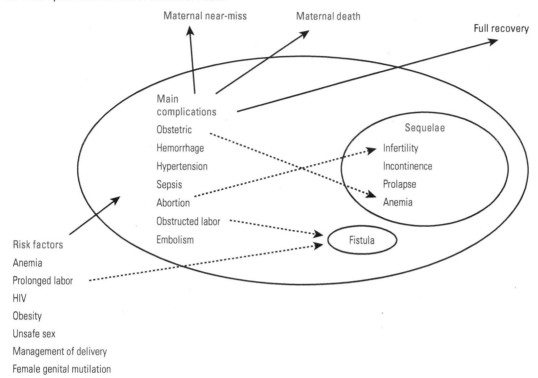

This section focuses on 11 groups of diagnoses that can lead to direct obstetric deaths or associated long-term ill health: abortion, hypertensive disease, obstetric hemorrhage, infection, prolonged and obstructed labor, anemia, postpartum depression, postpartum incontinence, fistula, postpartum prolapse, and HIV/AIDS. Other important indirect conditions that we do not consider are discussed in other *DCP3* volumes, including volume 6 on *HIV/AIDS, STIs, Tuberculosis, and Malaria*. Figures 3.2 and 3.3 summarize the prevalence of the considered conditions.

Abortion

Morbidity with abortive outcomes comprises several diagnoses, including ectopic pregnancy, abortion, and miscarriage, as well as other abortive conditions (WHO 2013) (box 3.3).

Induced abortion is a safe procedure, safer than childbirth when performed in a suitable environment and with the right method. Among unsafe abortions, the morbidity burden is large. Information on the incidence of unsafe abortion and subsequent outcomes at the population level is particularly challenging to obtain because of fear of disclosure. On the basis of estimates derived from hospital data (adjusted for bias), an estimated 22 million unsafe abortions occur each year

worldwide (WHO 2011b); of these, 5 million women are subsequently hospitalized (Singh 2006), most because of hemorrhage (44 percent of admitted cases) or infections (24 percent) (Adler and others 2012a). On average, 237 women experience a severe maternal morbidity associated with induced abortion for every 100,000 live births in countries where abortion is unsafe (Adler and others 2012b). Evidence indicates that the morbidity patterns associated with unsafe abortion are being transformed by the rapid growth of the medical abortion market, with the incidence of severe morbidity episodes declining more rapidly than the incidence of less severe episodes (Singh, Monteiro, and Levin 2012).

Hypertensive Disease

Women in pregnancy or the puerperium can suffer from preeclampsia, eclampsia, and chronic hypertension. Eclampsia and preeclampsia tend to occur more frequently in the second half of pregnancy; less commonly, they can occur up to six weeks after delivery. Medication can alleviate the symptoms and their negative effects, but the only cure is expedited delivery. The etiology of the condition remains unclear.

One systematic review reported that the global prevalence of preeclampsia is 4.6 percent (95 percent confidence interval 2.7 percent to 8.2 percent), and

Figure 3.2 Prevalence of Direct Obstetric Complications

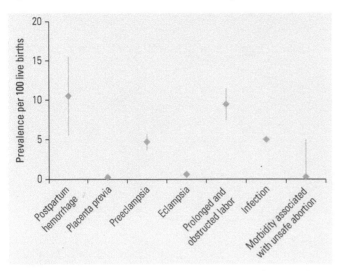

Sources: Based on Abalos and others 2013; Adler and Filippi, unpublished; Calvert and others 2012; Cresswell and others 2013; Dolea and Stein 2003.

Figure 3.3 Prevalence of Severe Direct Obstetric Complications

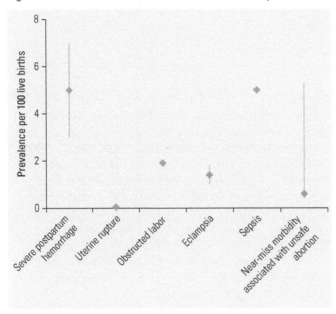

Sources: Based on Abalos and others 2013; Adler and others 2012a; Adler and Filippi, unpublished; Calvert and others 2012; Hofmeyr and others 2005.

the prevalence of eclampsia is 1.4 percent (95 percent confidence interval 1.0 percent to 2.0 percent) (Abalos and others 2013). The review finds evidence of regional variations, with Sub-Saharan Africa having the highest incidence of both conditions. Preeclampsia and eclampsia are more common among women in their first pregnancy, women who are obese, women with preexisting hypertension, and women with diabetes. All of these characteristics are increasingly more common in pregnant populations. Preeclampsia and eclampsia

are associated with perinatal deaths, placental abruption, and cardiovascular disease in later life in the mother.

Obstetric Hemorrhage

Women can experience anomalous or excessive bleeding because of an early pregnancy loss, a placental implantation abnormality, or an abnormality in the process of childbirth. The systematic review by Cresswell and others (2013) finds a global prevalence of 0.5 percent for placenta previa (95 percent confidence interval 0.4 percent to 0.6 percent). An equivalent systematic review for placental abruption has not been published, but most papers on this condition suggest an approximate prevalence of 1 percent (Ananth and others 1999).

Postpartum hemorrhage is a major cause of maternal morbidity worldwide. A systematic review finds a global prevalence of blood loss equal to or greater than 500 milliliters in 10.8 percent of vaginal deliveries (95 percent confidence interval 9.6 percent to 12.1 percent) (Calvert and others 2012); the prevalence of severe hemorrhage (equal to or greater than 1,000 milliliters) was 2.8 percent (95 percent confidence interval 2.4 percent to 3.2 percent). The review includes many study settings in which active management of the third stage of labor is practiced. The prevalence of postpartum hemorrhage in home deliveries is probably higher. Postpartum hemorrhage is associated with anemia, which can persist for several months after birth (Wagner and others 2012).

The incidence of hemorrhage has increased in HICs in recent years (Mehrabadi and others 2013). This trend has been linked to changes in risk factors, such as pregnancies at older ages, obesity, and previous cesarean delivery, as well as to better data capture systems (Kamara and others 2013). These risk factors are increasingly more common in LICs as well.

Pregnancy-Related Infection

Puerperal sepsis causes the greatest concern of all pregnancy-related infections because of its severity. No review of the prevalence of sepsis has been published since the work in the early 2000s for the Global Burden of Diseases (Dolea and Stein 2003). In this review, Dolea and Stein calculate that the incidence of sepsis ranged from 2.7 to 5.2 per 100 live births according to world region. A community-based study in India finds that the incidence of puerperal sepsis in the first week postpartum was 1.2 percent after home delivery and 1.4 percent after facility-based delivery. The incidence of fever was higher at 4 percent overall in the same Indian study (Iyengar 2012). Another study in India finds a high incidence of puerperal infections at home (10 percent) and of fever (12 percent), but the study uses broader

Definitions of Obstetric Causes of Maternal Morbidities and Deaths

Abortive outcomes include abortion, miscarriage, ectopic pregnancy, and other abortive conditions (WHO 2013). Abortive outcomes take place before 28 weeks during pregnancy, but this time definition varies among countries, with lower cut-offs of 24 weeks also used.

Preeclampsia is characterized by high blood pressure and protein in the urine; women are diagnosed with **eclampsia** when the preeclampsia syndrome is associated with convulsions.

Obstetric hemorrhage refers to anomalous or excessive bleeding because of an early pregnancy loss, a placental implantation abnormality (including placenta previa or placental abruption), or because of an abnormality in the process of childbirth.

Pregnancy-related infections include puerperal sepsis, infections of the genitourinary tract in pregnancy, other puerperal infections, and infections of the breast associated with childbirth (WHO 2013).

Prolonged labor is labor lasting more than 12 hours, in spite of good uterine contractions and good cervix dilation. In **obstructed labor**, the fetal descent is impaired by a mechanical barrier in the birth canal, despite good contractions (WHO 2008). Causes of obstructed labor include cephalopelvic disproportion, abnormal presentation, fetal abnormality, and abnormality of the reproductive tract.

Sources: WHO 2008, 2013.

definitions and followed women for only 28 days (Bang and others 2004). Risk factors for infections include HIV/AIDS and cesarean section.

Prolonged and Obstructed Labor

An unpublished systematic review by Adler and others located only 16 published population-based studies of obstructed and prolonged labor worldwide since 2000. The studies could not be combined through meta-analysis to obtain a global prevalence because of high heterogeneity, which was largely attributed to differences in case definitions. However, the median prevalence was estimated to be 1.9 per 100 deliveries for obstructed labor, and 8.7 per 100 deliveries for combined obstructed and prolonged labor. A systematic review of articles from 1997 to 2002 reporting on uterine rupture finds extremely low prevalence in the community setting (median 0.053, range 0.016 to 0.30 per hundred pregnant women), but it included a study with self-reporting, which tends to overestimate the prevalence of rare conditions (Hofmeyr, Say, and Gülmezoglu 2005).

Anemia

Anemia—which occurs when the number of red cells or hemoglobin (Hb) concentration has reached too low a level in the blood—is a commonly diagnosed condition during pregnancy or the postpartum period.

Its main symptoms include excessive fatigue; it can contribute to or lead directly to a maternal death when Hb concentration has reached particularly low levels. Anemia has many different causes, including blood loss; infection-related blood cell destruction; and deficient red blood cell production because of sickle cell disease, parasitic diseases such as hookworm or malaria, or nutritional deficiency, including iron deficiency.

During pregnancy, anemia is diagnosed when Hb levels are below the threshold of 11 grams/deciliter. Anemia is classified as severe when the levels reach 7 grams/deciliter. Anemia is well-documented in low-income settings thanks to the ease with which lay fieldworkers can collect hemoglobin levels in survey conditions. Using 257 population-based data sets for 107 countries, Stevens and others (2013) estimate that globally 38.0 percent (95 percent confidence interval 34 percent to 43 percent) of pregnant women have anemia, and 0.9 percent (95 percent confidence interval 0.6 percent to 1.3 percent) have severe anemia. Pregnant women in Central and West Africa appear particularly affected (56.0 percent are anemic, and 1.8 percent are severely so). However, global prevalence trends have improved since 1995 (Stevens and others 2013). The review by Wagner and others (2012) demonstrates that women who suffer severe blood loss during childbirth may remain anemic for several months during the postpartum period.

Postpartum Depression

Mental health disorders during pregnancy and the postpartum period include conditions of various severity and etiology, ranging from baby blues to postpartum depression and puerperal psychosis, as well as posttraumatic stress disorders linked, for example, to the death of a baby. The most common of these disorders is depression, which is associated with pregnancy-related deaths by suicide and with developmental delays in children.

Most studies detect depression through screening questionnaires for psychological distress; the most widely used tool is the Edinburgh Postnatal Depression Scale, which has been translated into many languages and used in many different cultures. These screening questionnaires are not equivalent to clinical diagnoses by medical providers; rather, they indicate a high probability of depression among those who have high scores.

Depression is a well-studied area, with a number of systematic reviews and meta-analyses, supported by large numbers of papers, although only a small proportion of these articles are from LMICs. Fisher and others (2012) calculate that in LMICs, the prevalence of depression and anxiety was 16 percent (95 percent confidence interval 15 percent to 17 percent) during pregnancy and 20 percent (95 percent confidence interval 19 percent to 21 percent) during the postpartum period. Halbreich and Karkun (2006), who conducted the most comprehensive systematic review to date from a geographical perspective, find a broader range of prevalence of depression (0 percent to 60 percent). They attribute this wide range to cultural differences in the reporting and in the understanding of depression, as well as differences in tools and other methodological approaches. They also conclude, in view of the wide ranges in the estimates, that the prevalence of depression is high and that the widely cited prevalence of 10 percent to 15 percent is not representative of the actual global prevalence.

Incontinence

Incontinence is any involuntary loss of urine. The most common form of urinary incontinence during and after childbirth is stress urinary incontinence, which consists of involuntary leakages on exertion or effort.

Little information is available on the incidence of incontinence in the postpartum period in LMICs. Walker and Gunasekera (2011) find four studies of reproductive-age women published between 1985 and 2010, in which the prevalence ranged from 5 percent to 32 percent. Another systematic review calculates the mean pooled estimates for all types of incontinence during the first three months postpartum to be 33 percent for parous women and 29 percent for primiparous women (Thom and Rortveit 2010). In addition, they find that

the risk was higher for vaginal birth (31 percent) than for cesarean birth (15 percent), as reported in several case control studies. Although the authors of this paper attempted to obtain information for all countries, no papers from LICs were included.

Obstetric Fistula

Obstetric fistula results in the continuous loss of urine or fecal matter, occurring both day and night (Polan and others 2015). It has been described as a condition worse than death in view of its medical manifestation, treatment difficulties, and social consequences (Lewis Wall 2006). It occurs when labor is obstructed, and contractions continue with the baby's head stuck in the pelvis or vagina; cesarean section is usually required to deliver the baby (Lewis Wall 2012). As a result of the severe delay in delivery and continuous pressure of the fetal head on maternal tissues, blood flow is blocked, resulting in necrosis. This condition leaves abnormal gaps (or communications) between the vagina and bladder or rectum, allowing urine or stool to pass continuously through the vagina. The meta-analysis by Adler and others (2013) of the incidence of fistula in LMICs finds a pooled incidence of 0.09 (95 percent confidence interval 0.01–0.25) per 1,000 recently pregnant women. Another recent meta-analysis of Demographic and Health Survey data finds a lifetime prevalence of 3 cases per 1,000 women of reproductive age (95 percent credible intervals 1.3–5.5) in Sub-Saharan Africa (Maheu-Giroux and others 2015). The condition is extremely rare in HICs, where there are few delays in obtaining good quality maternity care.

Postpartum Vaginal or Uterine Prolapse

Pelvic organ prolapse is defined as the symptomatic "descent of one or more of: the anterior vaginal wall, the posterior vaginal wall, and the apex of the vagina or vault" (Haylen and others 2010, 8). In lay terms, it is when a "descent of the pelvic organs results in the protrusion of the vagina, uterus, or both" (Jelovsek, Maher, and Barber 2007, 1027). Incidence increases with age, parity, and body mass index; hard physical labor is also a risk factor. Prolapse is among the Global Burden of Disease's most common sequelae, with a prevalence of about 9.28 percent. Few population-based incidence studies measure prolapse after childbirth. There is a lack of agreement as to what constitutes a significant prolapse; a grading system exists, but it requires clinical interpretation. In Burkina Faso, 26 percent of women with uncomplicated facility-based deliveries received a diagnosis of prolapse in the postpartum period (Filippi and others 2007). In The Gambia, a population-based study with physical examinations finds that 46 percent of women ages 15–54 years had prolapse, and 14 percent had moderate or severe prolapse (Scherf and others 2002). Severe prolapse affects quality of life and is associated with depression (Zekele and others 2013).

HIV/AIDS

A positive HIV status is linked to an increased risk of death in pregnant and nonpregnant women (Zaba and others 2013). A recent systematic review suggests that HIV-infected women had eight times the risk of a pregnancy-related death, compared with uninfected women; the excess mortality attributable to HIV/AIDS among HIV-infected pregnant and postpartum women was close to 1,000 deaths per 100,000 pregnant women. The excess mortality attributable to HIV in pregnant women is much smaller than in nonpregnant women, however, probably because women who become pregnant tend to be healthier. A review that investigates the interaction between HIV/AIDS status and direct obstetric complications shows that women who are HIV-positive are 3.4 times more likely to develop sepsis (Calvert and Ronsmans 2013). The evidence of positive links for hypertensive diseases of pregnancy, dystocia, and hemorrhage was variable.

Global Burden of Diseases

The prevalence of conditions, as well as the prevalence, severity or disability weight, and the duration of their respective sequelae, are key factors in establishing the burden of various conditions in a population and in prioritizing them. Some conditions are noteworthy, for example, uterine rupture, because they are very severe and are associated with high risk of death in the mother or the baby. A few severe conditions, for example, fistula, despite being rare, can last a very long time and severely affect women's quality of life.

The WHO Global Health Estimates and IHME Global Burden of Disease estimates suggest that the absolute number of disability-adjusted life years associated with maternal conditions have decreased, owing to lower maternal mortality rates, but the number of years lived with disabilities has increased (Vos and others 2012; WHO 2014a). The increase in disabilities is mostly due to obstructed labor, hypertension, and indirect conditions (Vos and others 2012); it is also due to the high population growth rate, which means that the total number of women of reproductive age is rising.

Major Pregnancy-Related Complications

A longitudinal study shows that women who initially survived severe complications were more likely to die

within the next five years than other women (Storeng and others 2012). Many of these deaths occur in subsequent pregnancies, indicating that a small number of women, often those with chronic illnesses, accumulate pregnancy-related risks. What proportion of women suffer a major complication during pregnancy, taking into account various comorbidities? Researchers at Columbia University has suggested 15 percent prevalence as a benchmark for their indicators of met need for complications (Paxton, Maine, and Hijab 2003). This number has not been validated, except possibly by a study in India (Bang and others 2004). If all of the acute direct complications with nonabortive outcomes mentioned in this chapter (Ronsmans and others 2002) were mutually exclusive, the total prevalence could be as high as 31 percent.

BROADER DETERMINANTS OF MATERNAL MORTALITY AND MORBIDITY

This section presents an overview of the broader determinants of maternal mortality and morbidity and highlights the specificities of maternal health by introducing an established conceptual framework and other classification approaches. Determinants include individual risk factors, such as age and parity; characteristics of the social, legal, and economic contexts; and the physical environment, for example, water sources and geographical accessibility.

Significant Individual Risk Factors

Descriptive studies have demonstrated that women face the highest risk of pregnancy-related death and severe morbidity (Hurt and others 2008) when they are very young or older (Blanc, Winfrey, and Ross 2013) when they are expecting their first baby or when they have had many pregnancies, when they live far away from health facilities, or when they do not benefit from support from their families and friends (Mbizvo and others 1993). Table 3.1 illustrates some of the main determinants of maternal mortality and how they influence women's chances of survival during pregnancy or childbirth.

We consider two additional important facets of maternal mortality when discussing determinants and interventions to reduce deaths.

- The risk of maternal deaths has two components: the risk of getting pregnant, which is a risk related to fertility and its control or lack of control; and the obstetric risk of developing a complication and dying while pregnant or in labor. The obstetric risk is highest

Table 3.1 Examples of Risk Factors and Pathways of Influence

Individual nonmedical risk factors

Age	Women at the extreme ends of the reproductive age range (younger than age 20 years and older than age 35 years) have a higher risk of death for both physiological and sociocultural reasons; the largest number of deaths might be in the middle group, because this is when most births occurs.
Parity	Higher risks of complications and death are associated with first pregnancy and more than three to five pregnancies. Women in their first pregnancies have longer duration of labor; women with multiple pregnancies are more likely to suffer postpartum hemorrhage.
Unintended pregnancies	Unwanted pregnancy is a risk factor for unsafe abortion, lack of social support, and domestic violence. Women who continue with their pregnancies are less likely to plan for childbirth and more likely to commit suicide (Ahmed and others 2004).
Marital status	Single women who are pregnant often lack support from their partners or their families and are more likely to try to induce an abortion or to run into financial and other logistical difficulties when seeking care for labor.
Women's education	Women who are educated know where to obtain effective services and are more likely to request these services.
Husbands' education	The husband's educational level is often a more important determinant of maternal mortality than the woman's education (Evjen-Olsen and others 2008).
Ethnicity and religion	In high-income countries, women from black or migrant communities are more likely to die during pregnancy for cultural and medical reasons, including chronic ill health. Women from certain religious groups may seek medical advice from their religious leaders or deliver in places of worship.
Poverty	Money is often required to travel or to deliver safely. Emergency cesarean section is a very expensive procedure, which can lead to delays in seeking care and in catastrophic expenditures.
Obesity and other nutritional factors	Obese or anemic women are more likely to die in childbirth. Obese women face increased risk due to comorbid conditions, such as diabetes, hypertension, or cardiac problems; it is also technically more difficult to provide them with clinical care. Severely anemic women cannot tolerate hemorrhage to the same degree as women with higher hemoglobin levels.
Past obstetric history	Past stillbirths and emergency cesarean are predictors of complications and deaths.

Social and economic context

Women's status	Often measured using education as a proxy, women's status indicators help to assess the extent to which women can make decisions on their own and the extent to which women and their decisions are valued. Many proxy variables have been used to measure women's status, including age at marriage, financial decision-making power, and women's opinions on domestic violence (Gabrysch and Campbell 2009).
Legality of reproductive health services	Where abortion laws are restrictive, women are more likely to have unsafe abortions. The current focus is on delegating certain procedures to midlevel providers to ensure that more women have access to safe and effective services.
Conflict	Extremely high levels of maternal mortality have been reported where infrastructure and communication systems have been destroyed, for example, in Afghanistan and Somalia.

Physical environment and health systems characteristics

Staff and facilities	The number, quality, and distribution of staff members are important risk factors for mortality; it is difficult to predict which women will have complications, and women are more likely to die in home births. Skilled birth attendance is often the most significant risk factor in maternal mortality models. Women who live at a distance from facilities are much more likely to delay seeking care and to experience multiple referrals.
Transportation network	Patient access to transportation and problematic topography are risk factors for long duration of the second tier of delays. (See section on "Three Delays Model.")
Water and sanitation	The availability and quality of water and sanitation (WATSAN) are key factors at the community level; they influence direct risks of diarrheal diseases and other water-borne infections in pregnant and parturient women, as does personal hygiene before and after delivery (Shordt, Smet, and Herschderfer 2012). WATSAN can indirectly pose risks to women's health if they carry heavy water receptacles or are subjected to violence at public water collection points or latrines. In health care facilities, WATSAN affects the hygiene practices of providers during childbirth, such as hand washing and environmental cleaning, with attendant increased risks of maternal and newborn nosocomial infections (Hussein and others 2011).
Quality of care and accountability	As more women deliver with skilled providers, the quality of care in facilities becomes increasingly important. The accountability of the health sector is a new focus of interventions to improve the quality of care. The availability of blood is one of the most important determinants of the quality of care received by women who are severely ill (Graham, McCaw-Binns, and Munjanja 2013).

Note: See Gabrysch and Campbell (2009) for further examples of risk factors.

at the time of delivery. The determinants of these risks share many similarities, but also have specific characteristics.

- Although the overall risks of maternal death are highest among young adolescents and older women of reproductive age, the highest number of deaths is in the middle group of women around age 25 years.

Three Delays Model

Conceptual models guide research and practice and help in the determination of how best to reduce adverse outcomes, by grouping determinants and highlighting their linkages with events in the pathway from health to death. The three delays model (Thaddeus and Maine 1994), attractive because of its simplicity and action-oriented presentation, is based on the following premises:

- Maternal complications are mostly emergencies.
- Maternal complications cannot be predicted with sufficient accuracy.
- Maternal deaths are largely preventable through tertiary prevention (preventing deaths among women who have been diagnosed with a complication).

At the 1987 launch of the Safe Motherhood Initiative, maternal health experts discussed how long a woman would have to have a particular complication before she would die, if untreated. They agreed that for the most frequent complications, women with postpartum hemorrhage had less than 2 hours before death; for antepartum hemorrhage, eclampsia, obstructed labor, and sepsis, the times would be 12 hours, 2 days, 3 days, and 6 days, respectively.

The model has three levels of delay:

- The first delay is the elapsed time between the onset of a complication and the recognition of the need to transport the patient to a facility.
- The second delay is the elapsed time between leaving the home and reaching the facility.
- The third delay is the elapsed time from presentation at the facility to the provision of appropriate treatment.

Each delay has a distinctive set of determinants. The determinants of the first delay are related to the individual circumstances of the women and their families, who must first recognize that care is needed and then be able to access transport or money to travel to facilities. The determinants of the second delay concern the physical environment, the type of transport, and the quality of the roads, as well as the performance of the referral system between facilities. The determinants of the third delay are related to quality of care, such as the number and training of staff members and the availability of blood supplies and essential equipment. Although the actions and characteristics of women and families can influence the length of the third delay, for example, by helping to mobilize elements of the surgical kits for cesarean delivery by purchasing missing supplies in pharmacies (Gohou and others 2004), most of the determinants of the third delay are related to service provision.

The three delays model has weaknesses. It does not include the concept of primary prevention (avoid pregnancy) and secondary prevention (avoid complications once pregnant). It ignores family planning, noncommunicable chronic diseases, antenatal care, and postpartum care. Implicitly, it also assumes that complications arise at home, where women intend to give birth, whereas increasing numbers of women deliver in facilities (Filippi and others 2009). In addition, it does not consider the newly identified "fourth delay," which arises when women are discharged unwell or chronically ill from facilities and die at home during the postpregnancy period or in the next pregnancy (Pacagnella and others 2012; Storeng and others 2012).

Rights-Based Approach

The rights-based approach to understanding the determinants of maternal health is primarily concerned with the legal, cultural, and social context of service accessibility and delivery; it has been gaining a higher profile with the introduction of MDG 5b in 2007. It began with the observation that most maternal deaths are avoidable, as illustrated by the wide divergence in lifetime risks of maternal death (the probability that a 15-year-old woman will die of a pregnancy related cause) between HICs (one in 3,700) and LMICs (one in 160) (WHO 2014a), and between rich and poor women; that a considerable evidence-based literature exists with respect to effective clinical interventions; and that the reduction of maternal mortality is firmly embedded in women's ability to control the occurrence and timing of pregnancy (Freedman 2001).

Most maternal deaths are not simply biological phenomena; many are in part explained by the lack of freedom and entitlements experienced by women and service providers, as well as by the lack of accountability of providers, health systems, and countries toward women and their families (Freedman 2001; PMNCH 2013). The concept of *freedom* refers to the right of women to control their bodies, including their reproductive options, and to have access to acceptable and effective family planning services, including safe abortions. *Entitlements* are concerned with access to good quality services, which must be evidence based and respectful and emphasize equity in access for all women who need care, whether they are rich or poor, married or single.

The accessibility and availability of good quality family planning and legal abortion services are key determinants of maternal mortality in many LICs. Quantitative models suggest that preventing pregnancy with contraception has a bigger role to play in reducing maternal mortality than does inducing abortion when pregnant with an unintended pregnancy (Singh and Darroch 2012). However, although access to safe abortion techniques has become easier with the availability of medical abortion, including on the black market from drug sellers or the Internet in countries where abortion is illegal, many women still die because they cannot access safe abortion services (Ganatra and others 2014). The distal determinants of fertility and unwanted pregnancy are broadly similar to the distal determinants of maternal health, with their emphasis on culture, poverty, and education, but their proximate determinants are somewhat different, with a focus on fecundability and marriage patterns (Bongaarts 1978) and, in the case of unwanted pregnancies, an emphasis on the needs of younger and unattached women.

Several studies, mostly qualitative, highlight episodes of rampant disrespect and abuse of pregnant women or women in labor in some maternity units (Hassan-Bitar and Wick 2007; Silal and others 2012). Groundbreaking research is taking place with the TRAction Project in Kenya and Tanzania to delineate the different forms of disrespect and abuse, understand their origins, and quantitatively document their frequency.[5] Lack of respectful care could mean that women do not seek care when they need it, or do not seek it as quickly as they should, and could contribute to deaths of mothers and babies.

Finally, it is important to be aware that in HICs and LMICs, violence is sometimes one of the most frequent causes of death during pregnancy and childbirth (Ganatra, Coyaji, and Rao 1998; Glazier and others 2006).

Health System Factors

The maternal mortality level is one of the best criteria for assessing the relative performance of health systems. One example of a coverage indicator of the continuum of care is skilled birth attendance, which is particularly inequitable. While women rely on a functioning health system to access and use professional care, this indicator has shown large differences between the richest and the poorest women (WHO and UNICEF 2012). Health system classifications are helpful in highlighting the barriers or in facilitating the factors that many women meet when they seek care during pregnancy, childbirth, or emergency situations. These classifications complement the three delays model because they go beyond emergency obstetric care. The WHO health system building blocks offer a starting point for classifying health system determinants and include the following:

- Quality of service delivery and referral system
- Number, distribution, and training of the types of providers required, including midwives and obstetrician-gynecologists
- Completeness and responsiveness of the health information system, including the adequacy of the Maternal Death Surveillance and Response (WHO 2013)
- Ease of access to essential medications, such as magnesium sulfate, misoprostol, and oxytocin, and the supplies necessary for blood transfusions
- Leadership and financing, a particularly relevant issue in several Sub-Saharan African countries that have ended user fees
- Governance, including the capacity of authorities at various levels of the health system to put policies and management systems in place so that women's health can improve.

All of these building blocks are determinants of the coverage and quality of care that women receive across the continuum of care. Country case studies describe the relative importance of these building blocks or equivalent groupings in understanding progress in maternal health (McPake and Koblinsky 2009). The equitable distribution of staff and the adequacy of blood supplies appear to be issues in most settings in LICs. Coverage of one visit for antenatal care is very high; the median coverage level is 88 percent among the Countdown Countries for which data are available (Countdown Countries comprise 75 countries where 95 percent of the world's maternal and child deaths occur). Progress has also been made for skilled birth attendance since 1990 (median coverage of 57 percent), emergency obstetric care (as measured, for example, by the cesarean section rate, and by the density of emergency obstetric care facilities per birth or population), and postnatal care for mothers (median coverage of 41 percent). However, large urban-rural and wealth inequities remain, particularly in countries that have made the least progress since the 1990s (Cavallaro and others 2013; WHO and UNICEF 2012).

Intersectoral Issues

The health sector does not exist in isolation; in developing and implementing effective policies, its interactions with other sectors, such as education, finance, water, and transport, must be considered. For example, the well-documented decline in maternal mortality in Bangladesh may be related to the availability of emergency obstetric care interventions and fertility decline, but it is also likely to be linked to the increased participation of women in the labor force. Several ecological studies of maternal mortality have shown the relationship between maternal mortality and skilled birth attendance, as well as to gross national product, health care expenditures, female literacy, population density, and access to clean water (Buor and Bream 2004; Montoya, Calvert, and Filippi 2014).

Observational studies have shown inadequate levels of hygiene in many maternity facilities (Benova, Cumming, and Campbell 2014), with direct health impacts on mothers, newborns, and care providers (Mehta and others 2011). The reasons are multifactorial and include poor infrastructure; inadequate equipment and supplies; and poor practices by care providers and cleaners as a result of inadequate knowledge, attitudes, motivation, and supervision (Campbell and others 2015). Interventions to address these constraints go beyond the health sector, particularly for water and sanitation (Shordt, Smet, and Herschderfer 2012). Timely access to care and the difficulties in obtaining motorized transport, as well as challenging topography and inadequate and poorly maintained roads, are important barriers to care. Gabrysch and others (2011) demonstrate that in Zambia, the odds of women being able or choosing to deliver in a health facility decreased by 29 percent with every doubling of distance between their home and the closest facility. They conclude that if all Zambian women lived within 5 kilometers of health facilities, 16 percent of home deliveries could be averted.

A Lifecycle Perspective

Safe motherhood programs traditionally consider each pregnancy to be a separate event. Emerging evidence from cohort studies of near-miss patients suggests that women who have suffered severe obstetric complications have increased mortality risks for several years and have a higher risk of complications in subsequent pregnancies. It is important to be able to identify these women and offer them medical support for an extended postpartum period and in subsequent pregnancies (Assarag and others 2015; Storeng and others 2012).

CONCLUSIONS

This chapter summarizes available data on the levels and trends of maternal mortality and morbidity and their main determinants. Mathematical modeling indicates that maternal mortality is declining in most countries, that women face the highest risk of death in the MDG region of Oceania and Sub-Saharan Africa, and that deaths due to direct causes—such as hemorrhage and hypertension—continue to be the main causes in Latin America and the Caribbean and in Sub-Saharan Africa. The proportion of hemorrhage and hypertension deaths found globally remains high despite established interventions to prevent and treat direct causes of maternal death (see chapter 7), such as active management of the third stage of labor. With the data available, it is not possible to determine if this high proportion is the result of a failure to implement policies and therefore quality of care, if there is a shift toward antepartum hemorrhage, or if misclassifications of abortion and obstructed labor are erroneously increasing the hemorrhage category.

Role of Indirect Causes

The data presented in this chapter also suggest that the proportion of maternal deaths due to indirect causes is increasing in most parts of the world. In addition, although the proportion of women who have a serious morbidity remains a hotly debated topic by epidemiologists, we estimate that approximately 30 percent of women may have a serious condition during pregnancy, childbirth, or the postpartum period. The main strategies used to date to reduce maternal mortality are based on the understanding that most complications are emergencies and that most deaths occur during a very short period around childbirth. Accordingly, the focus has been on reducing delays for emergency care, as well as on preventive measures, such as facilitating access to skilled birth attendance and reproductive rights. Complementary strategies are needed to address the indirect causes of death and the broader burden of maternal morbidity, in particular, given that the sequelae of maternal morbidity can last a long time.

Health program managers and policy makers need to continue to encourage women to deliver in health facilities, where complications can be prevented by appropriate care and where women can receive lifesaving interventions. At the same time, the gaps in coverage of effective interventions for indirect causes of death according to their distribution in various settings have significant implications for the complexity of service delivery in light of the urgent need to accelerate the rate of decline in maternal mortality and, ultimately, to stop all preventable deaths. Primary health care may have a greater role in the future in improving the health outcomes of pregnant and recently delivered women.

Quality of Health Care Services

In addition, if the post-2015 agenda is to emphasize universal access to essential interventions, the perceived and technical quality of the health care services provided becomes even more crucial in the fight against maternal mortality and morbidity, given their consequences for both demand for and supply of services. Thus, the international community emphasizes the development and implementation of a palette of quality-of-care interventions, including clinical audits, childbirth checklists, maternal deaths surveillance and response, and interventions to increase awareness around respectful care.

Need for Better Data

Finally, we conclude with a call for action for better data. Although the global attention to maternal mortality has engendered more studies and attempts to measure it, the quality, regularity, and ability of the results to robustly show differentials have not improved dramatically, especially routine sources of information such as vital registration. We remain largely dependent on research and mathematical modeling. The paucity of information on maternal morbidity is an even greater issue. At the community level, data on direct obstetric complications are almost nonexistent; the burden of ill health associated with some conditions, such as sepsis and ectopic pregnancies, has not been reviewed for many years. Better population-based sources for local-level decision making are essential to achieving improved outcomes.

NOTES

World Bank Income Classifications as of July 2014 are as follows, based on estimates of gross national income (GNI) per capita for 2013:

- Low-income countries (LICs) = US$1,045 or less
- Middle-income countries (MICs) are subdivided:
  a) lower-middle-income = US$1,046–US$4,125
  b) upper-middle-income (UMICs) = US$4,126–US$12,745
- High-income countries (HICs) = US$12,746 or more.

For consistency and ease of comparison, DCP3 is using the World Health Organization's Global Health Estimates (GHE) for data on diseases burden, except in cases where a relevant data point is not available from GHE. In those instances, an alternative data source is noted.

1. This chapter uses World Bank regions in discussions based on income level, and Milllennium Development Goal (MDG) regions otherwise. See http://mdgs.un.org/unsd /mdg/Host.aspx?Content=Data/REgionalGroupings .htm for the MDG regional groupings.
2. See website of the Open Working Group on Sustainable Development Goals at http://sustainabledevelopment .un.org/owg.html.
3. See http://www.who.int/reproductivehealth/publications /monitoring/maternal-mortality-2015/en/.
4. This data can be found at http://www.who.int /reproductivehealth/publications/monitoring/maternal -mortality-2015/en/.
5. http://www.urc-chs.com/news?newsItemID=324.

REFERENCES

Abalos, E., C. Cuesta, A. L. Grosso, D. Chou, and L. Say. 2013. "Global and Regional Estimates of Preeclampsia and Eclampsia: A Systematic Review." *European Journal of Obstetrics and Gynecology and Reproductive Biology* 170 (1): 1–7.

Abouzahr, C. 1999. "Measuring Maternal Mortality: What Do We Need to Know?" In *Safe Motherhood Initiatives: Critical Issues*, edited by M. Berer and T. K. Sundari Ravindran. London: Reproductive Health Matters.

Adler, A., and V. Filippi. Unpublished. "Prevalence of Obstructed Labour: A Systematic Review." Report, London School of Hygiene & Tropical Medicine, United Kingdom.

Adler, A. J., V. Filippi, S. L. Thomas, and C. Ronsmans. 2012a. "Incidence of Severe Acute Maternal Morbidity Associated with Abortion: A Systematic Review." *Tropical Medicine and International Health* 17 (2): 177–90.

———. 2012b. "Quantifying the Global Burden of Morbidity due to Unsafe Abortion: Magnitude in Hospital-Based Studies and Methodological Issues." *International Journal of Gynecology and Obstetrics* 118 (2): S65–77.

Adler, A., V. Filippi, C. Calvert, and C. Ronsmans. 2013. "Estimating the Prevalence of Fistula: A Systematic Review and a Meta-Analysis." *BMC Pregnancy and Childbirth* 13: 246.

Ahmed, M. K., J. van Ginneken, A. Razzaque, and N. Alam. 2004. "Violent Deaths among Women of Reproductive Age in Rural Bangladesh." *Social Science and Medicine* 59 (2): 311–19.

Ahmed, S., L. Qingfend, C. Scrafford, and T. W. Pullum. 2014. *An Assessment of DHS Maternal Mortality Data and Estimates.* DHS Methodological Report 13. Rockville, MD: ICF International.

Ananth, C. V., G. S. Berkowitz, D. A. Savitz, and R. H. Lapinski. 1999. "Placental Abruption and Adverse Perinatal Outcomes." *Journal of the American Medical Association* 282 (17): 1646–51.

Assarag, B., B. Dujardin, A. Essolbi, I. Cherkaoui, and V. De Brouwere. 2015. "Consequences of Severe Obstetric Complications on Women's Health in Morocco: Please, Listen to Me!" *Tropical Medicine and International Health* 20 (11): 1406–14.

Bang, R. A., A. T. Bang, M. H. Reddy, M. D. Deshmukh, S. B. Baitule, and others. 2004. "Maternal Morbidity during Labour and the Puerperium in Rural Homes and the Need for Medical Attention: A Prospective Observational Study in Gadchiroli, India." *BJOG* 111 (3): 231–38.

Benova, L., O. Cumming, and O. M. R. Campbell. 2014. "Systematic Review and Meta-Analysis: Association between Water and Sanitation Environment and Maternal Mortality." *Tropical Medicine and International Health* 19 (4): 368–87.

Blanc, A. K., W. Winfrey, and J. Ross. 2013. "New Findings for Maternal Mortality Age Patterns: Aggregated Results for 38 Countries." *PLoS One* 8 (4): e59864.

Bongaarts, J. 1978. "A Framework for Analysing the Proximate Determinants of Fertility." *Population and Development Review* 4 (1): 105–32.

Buor, D., and K. Bream. 2004. "An Analysis of the Determinants of Maternal Mortality in Sub-Saharan Africa." *Journal of Womens Health* 13 (8): 926–38.

Bustreo, F., L. Say, M. Koblinsky, T. W. Pullum, M. Temmerman, and others. 2013. "Ending Preventable Maternal Deaths: The Time Is Now." *The Lancet Global Health* 1 (4): E176–77.

Calvert, C., S. Thomas, C. Ronsmans, K. Wagner, A. Adler, and V. Filippi. 2012. "Identifying Regional Variation in Maternal Haemorrhage: A Systematic Review and Meta-Analysis." *PLoS One* 7 (7).

Calvert, C., and C. Ronsmans. 2013. "The Contribution of HIV to Pregnancy-Related Mortality: A Systematic Review and a Meta-Analysis." *AIDS* 27 (10): 1631.

Campbell, O. M. R., L. Benola, G. Gon, K. Afsana, and O. Cumming. 2015. "Getting the Basic Rights—The Role of Water, Sanitation and Hygiene in Reproductive Health: A Conceptual Framework." *Tropical Medicine and International Health* 20 (82): 252–67.

Cavallaro, F. L., J. A. Cresswell, G. Franca, C. Victora, A. Barros, and others. 2013. "Trends in Caesarean Delivery by Country and Wealth Quintile: Cross Sectional Surveys in Southern Asia and Sub-Saharan Africa." *Bulletin of the World Health Organization* 91 (12): 914–22.

Christian, P., K. P. West, S. K. Khatry, J. Katz, S. C. Leclerq, and others. 2000. "Vitamin A and B-Carotene Supplementation Reduces Symptoms of Illness in Pregnant and Lactating Nepali Women." *Journal of Nutrition* 130 (11): 2675–82.

Commission on Information and Accountability for Women's and Children's Health. 2011. *Keeping Promises, Measuring Results.* Geneva: WHO.

Cresswell, J. A., C. Ronsmans, C. Calvert, and V. Filippi. 2013. "Prevalence of Placenta Praevia by World Region: A Systematic Review and Meta-Analysis." *Tropical Medicine and International Health* 18 (6): 712–14.

Dolea, C., and C. Stein. 2003. *Burden of Maternal Sepsis in the Year 2000. Evidence and Information for Policy.* Geneva: WHO.

Evjen-Olsen, B., S. G. Hinderaker, R. T. Lie, P. Bergsjo, P. Gasheka, and G. Kvale. 2008. "Risk Factors for Maternal Death in the Highlands of Rural Northern Tanzania: A Case-Control Study." *BMC Public Health* 8: 52.

Ezeh, A., A. Bankole, J. Cleland, C. Garcia-Moreno, M. Temmerman, and A. K. Ziraba. 2016. "Burden of Reproductive Ill Health." In *Disease Control Priorities* (third edition): Volume 2, *Reproductive, Maternal, Newborn, and Child Health*, edited by R. Black, R. Laxminarayan, M. Temmerman, and N. Walker. Washington, DC: World Bank.

Filippi, V., R. Ganaba, R. F. Baggaley, T. Marshall, K. T. Storeng, and others. 2007. "Health of Women after Severe Obstetric Complications in Burkina Faso: A Longitudinal Study." *The Lancet* 370 (9595): 1329–37.

Filippi, V., F. Richard, I. Lange, and F. Ouattara. 2009. "Identifying Barriers from Home to the Appropriate Hospital through Near-Miss Audits in Developing Countries." *Best Practice & Research Clinical Obstetrics & Gynaecology* 23 (3): 389–400.

Firoz, T., D. Chou, P. von Dadelszen, P. Agrawal, R. Vanderkruik, and others. 2013. "Measuring Maternal Health: Focusing on Maternal Morbidity." *Bulletin of the World Health Organization* 91 (10): 794–96.

Fisher, J., M. Cabral de Mello, V. Patel, A. Rahman, T. Tran, and others. 2012. "Prevalence and Determinants of Common Perinatal Disorders in Women in Low- and Lower-Middle-Income Countries: A Systematic Review." *Bulletin of the World Health Organization* 90: 139–49.

Freedman, L. P. 2001. "Using Human Rights in Maternal Mortality Programs: From Analysis to Strategy." *International Journal of Gynecology and Obstetrics* 75 (1): 51–60.

Gabrysch, S., and O. M. R. Campbell. 2009. "Still Too Far to Walk: Literature Review of the Determinants of Delivery Service Use." *BMC Pregnancy and Childbirth* 9: 34.

Gabrysch, S., S. Cousens, J. Cox, and O. M. R. Campbell. 2011. "The Influence of Distance and Level of Care on Delivery Care in Rural Zambia: A Study of Linked National Data and Geographic Information System." *PLoS Medicine* 8 (1).

Ganatra, B. R., K. J. Coyaji, and V. N. Rao. 1998. "Too Far, Too Little, Too Late: A Community-Based Case-Control Study of Maternal Mortality in Rural West Maharashtra, India." *Bulletin of the World Health Organization* 76 (6): 591–98.

Ganatra, B., O. Tuncalp, H. B. Johnston, B. R. Johnson, A. M. Gulmezoglu, and others. 2014. "From Concept to Measurement: Operationalizing WHO's Definition of Unsafe Abortion." *Bulletin of the World Health Organization* 92: 155.

Gilmore, K., and T. A. Camhe Gebreyesus. 2012. "What Will It Take to Eliminate Preventable Maternal Deaths?" *The Lancet* 386 (9837): 87–88.

Glazier, A., M. Gulmezoglu, G. P. Schmid, C. G. Moreno, and P. F. A. Van Look. 2006. "Sexual and Reproductive Health: A Matter of Life and Death." *The Lancet* 368 (9547): 1595–607.

Gohou, V., C. Ronsmans, L. Kacou, K. Yao, K. Bohousso, and others. 2004. "Responsiveness to Life-Threatening Obstetric Emergencies in Two Hospitals in Abidjan, Côte d'Ivoire." *Tropical Medicine and International Health* 9 (3): 406–15.

Graham, W., S. McCaw-Binns, and S. Munjanja. 2013. "Translating Coverage Gains into Health Gains for All Women and Children: The Quality Care Opportunity." *PLoS Medicine* 10 (1).

Gülmezoglu, A. M., T. A. Lawrie, N. Hezelgrave, O. T. Oladoppo, J. P. Souza, and others. 2016. "Interventions to Reduce Maternal and Newborn Morbidity and Mortality." In *Disease Control Priorities* (third edition): Volume 2,

Reproductive, Maternal, Newborn, and Child Health, edited by R. Black, R. Laxminarayan, M. Temmerman, and N. Walker. Washington, DC: World Bank.

Halbreich, U., and S. Karkun. 2006. "Cross-Cultural and Social Diversity of Prevalence of Postpartum Depression and Depressive Symptoms." *Journal of Affective Disorders* 91 (2–3): 97–111.

Hassan-Bitar, A., and L. Wick. 2007. "Evoking the Guardian Angel: Childbirth Care in a Palestinian Hospital." *Reproductive Health Matters* 15 (30): 103–13.

Haylen, B. T., D. de Ritter, R. M. Freeman, S. E. Swift, B. Berghmans, and others. 2010. "An International Urogynecological Association (IUGA)/International Continence Society (ICS) Joint Report on the Terminology for Female Pelvic Floor Dysfunction." *Neurourology and Urodynamics* 21 (1): 5–26.

Hofmeyr, G. J., L. Say, and A. Gülmezoglu. 2005. "WHO Systematic Review of Maternal Mortality and Morbidity: The Prevalence of Uterine Rupture." *BJOG* 112 (9): 1221–28.

Hurt, L., N. Alam, G. Dieltens, N. Aktar, and C. Ronsmans. 2008. "Duration and Magnitude of Mortality after Pregnancy in Rural Bangladesh." *International Journal of Epidemiology* 37 (2): 397–404.

Hussein, J., D. V. Malavankar, S. Sharma, and L. D'Ambruoso. 2011. "A Review of Health System Infection Control Measured in Developing Countries: What Can Be Learned to Reduce Maternal Mortality." *Global Health* 7: 14.

IHME (Institute for Health Metrics and Evaluation). 2013. *The Global Burden of Disease: Generating Evidence, Guiding Policy.* Seattle, WA: IHME.

Iyengar, K. 2012. "Early Postpartum Maternal Morbidity among Rural Women in Rajasthan, India: A Community Based-Study." *Journal of Health Population and Nutrition* 30 (2): 213–25.

Jelovsek, J. E., C. Maher, and J. M. Barber. 2007. "Pelvic Organ Prolapse." *The Lancet* 369 (9566): 1027–38.

Kamara, M., J. J Henderson, D. A. Doherty, J. E. Dickinson, and C. E. Pennell. 2013. "The Risk of Placenta Accreta Following Primary Elective Caesarean Delivery: A Case-Control Study." *BJOG* 120 (7): 879–86.

Karimian-Teherani, D., G. Haidinger, T. Waldhoer, A. Beck, and C. Vutuc. 2002. "Under-Reporting of Direct and Indirect Obstetrical Deaths in Austria, 1980–98." *Acta Obstetricia et Gynecologica Scandinavica* 81 (4): 323–27.

Lagro, M., A. Liche, T. Mumba, R. Ntbeka, and J. van Roosmalen. 2003. "Postpartum Health among Rural Zambian Women." *African Journal of Reproductive Health* 7 (3): 41–48.

Lewis, G. ed. 2007. *Saving Mothers' Lives: Reviewing Maternal Deaths to Make Motherhood Safer 2003–2005.* The Seventh Report of the Confidential Enquiries into Maternal Deaths in the United Kingdom. London: CEMACH.

Lewis Wall, L. 2006. "Obstetric Vaginal Fistula as an International Public Health Problem." *The Lancet* 368 (9542): 1201–09.

———. 2012. "A Framework for Analyzing the Determinants of Obstetric Fistula Formation." *Studies in Family Planning* 43 (4): 255–72.

Maheu-Giroux, M., V. Filippi, S. Samadoulougou, M.C. Castro, N. Maulet, and others. 2015. "Prevalence of Symptoms of Vaginal Fistula in 19 Sub-Saharan Africa Countries: A Meta-Analysis of National Household Survey Data." *The Lancet Global Health* 3 (5): e271–78.

Mbizvo, M. T., S. Fawcus, G. Lindmark, and L. Nystrom. 1993. "Maternal Mortality in Rural and Urban Zimbabwe: Social and Reproductive Factors in an Incident Case-Referent Study." *Social Sciences and Medicine* 36 (9): 1197–205.

McPake, B., and M. Koblinsky. 2009. "Improving Maternal Survival in South Asia: What Can We Learn from Case Studies?" *Journal of Health Population and Nutrition* 27 (2): 93–107.

Mehrabadi, A., J. A. Hutcheon, L. Lee, M. S. Kramer, R. M. Liston, and others. 2013. "Epidemiological Investigation of a Temporal Increase in Atonic Postpartum Haemorrhage: A Population-Based Retrospective Study." *BJOG* 120 (7): 853–62.

Mehta, R., D. V. Mavalankar, K. Ramani, S. Sharma, and J. Hussein. 2011. "Infection Control in Delivery Care Units, Gujarat, India: A Needs Assessment." *BMC Pregnancy and Childbirth* 11: 37.

Montoya, A., C. Calvert, and V. Filippi. 2014. "Explaining Differences in Maternal Mortality Levels in Sub-Saharan African Hospitals: A Systematic Review and Meta-Analysis." *International Health* 6 (1): 1–11.

Pacagnella, R. C., J. G. Cecatti, M. J. Osis, and J. P. Souza. 2012. "The Role of Delays in Severe Maternal Morbidity and Mortality: Expanding the Conceptual Framework." *Reproductive Health Matters* 20 (39): 155–63.

Pattinson, R., E. Buchmann, G. Mantel, M. Schoon, and H. Rees. 2003. "Can Enquiries into Severe Acute Maternal Morbidity Act as a Surrogate for Maternal Death Enquiries?" *BJOG* 110 (10): 889–93.

Paxton, A., D. Maine, and N. Hijab. 2003. "AMDD Workbook. Using the UN Process Indicators of Emergency Obstetric Services: Questions and Answers." Averting Death and Disability Program, Columbia University, Mailman School of Public Health.

PMNCH (Partnership for Maternal, Newborn and Child Health). 2013. *Human Rights and Accountability.* Knowledge Summaries 23: Women's and Children's Health. Geneva: PMNCH.

Polan, M. L., A. Sleemi, M. M. Bedane, S. Lozo, and M. A. Morgan. 2015. "Obstetric Fistula." In *Disease Control Priorities* (3rd edition): Volume 1, chapter 6, *Essential Surgery*, edited by H. T. Debas, P. Donkor, A. Gawande, D. T. Jamison, M. E. Kruk, and C. N. Mock. Washington, DC: World Bank.

Ronsmans, C., E. Achadi, S. Cohen, and A. Zarri. 1997. "Women's Recall of Obstetric Complications in South Kalimantan, Indonesia." *Studies in Family Planning* 28 (3): 204–14.

Ronsmans, C., O. M. R. Campbell, J. McDermott, and M. Koblinsky. 2002. "Questioning the Indicators of Need for Obstetric Care." *Bulletin of the World Health Organization* 80: 317–24.

Saurel-Cubizolles, M.-J., P. Romito, N. Lelong, and P.-Y. Ancell. 2000. "Women's Health after Childbirth: A Longitudinal Study in France and Italy." *BJOG* 107 (10): 1202–09.

Say, L., D. Chou, A. Gemmill, O. Tuncalpo, A.-B. Moller, and others. 2014. "Global Causes of Maternal Death: A WHO Systematic Analysis." *The Lancet Global Health* 2 (6): e323–33.

Scherf, C., L. Morison, A. Fiander, G. Ekpo, and G. Walraven. 2002. "Epidemiology of Pelvic Organ Prolapse in Rural Gambia, West Africa." *BJOG* 109 (4): 431–36.

Shelburne, R. C., and C. Trentini. 2010. "After the Financial Crisis: Achieving the Millennium Goals in Europe, the Caucasus and Central Asia." Discussion Paper Series 2010.1, United Nations Economic Commission for Europe, Geneva.

Shordt, K., E. Smet, and K. Herschderfer. 2012. *Getting It Right: Improving Maternal Health through Water, Sanitation & Hygiene.* Simavi: Haarlem.

Silal, S. P., L. Penn-Kekana, B. Harris, S. Birch, and D. McIntyre. 2012. "Exploring Inequalities in Access to and Use of Maternal Health Services in South Africa." *BMC Health Services Research* 12: 120.

Singh, S. 2006. "Hospital Admissions Resulting from Unsafe Abortions: Estimates from 13 Developing Countries." *The Lancet* 368 (9550): 1887–92.

———, and J. E. Darroch. 2012. *Adding It Up: Costs and Benefits of Contraceptive Services: Estimates for 2012.* New York: Guttmacher Institute and UNFPA.

Singh, S., M. Monteiro, and J. Levin. 2012. "Trends in Hospitalization for Abortion-Related Complications in Brazil, 1992–2009: Why the Decline in Numbers and Severity?" *International Journal of Gynaecology and Obstetrics* 118 (2): S99–106.

Souza, J. P., M. A. Parpinelli, E. Amaral, and J. G. Cecatti. 2008. "Population Surveys Using Validated Questionnaires Provided Useful Information on the Prevalence of Maternal Morbidities." *Journal of Clinical Epidemiology* 61 (2): 169–76.

Stevens, G. A., M. M. Finucane, L. M. De-Regil, C. J. Paciorek, S. R. Flaxman, and others. 2013. "Global, Regional, and National Trends in Haemoglobin Concentration and Prevalence of Total and Severe Anaemia in Children and Pregnant and Non-Pregnant Women for 1995–2011: A Systematic Analysis of Population-Representative Data." *The Lancet Global Health* 1 (1): E16–25.

Stones, W., W. Lim, F. Al-Azzawi, and M. Kelly. 1991. "An Investigation of Maternal Morbidity with Identification of Life-Threatening 'Near-Miss' Episodes." *Health Trends* 23 (1): 13–15.

Storeng, K. T., S. Drabo, R. Ganaba, J. Sundby, C. Calvert, and others. 2012. "Mortality after Near-Miss Complications in Burkina Faso: Medical, Social and Health-Care Factors." *Bulletin of the World Health Organization* 90 (6): 418–25.

Stulberg, D. B., L. R. Cain, I. Dahlquist, and D. S. Lauderdale. 2013. "Ectopic Pregnancy Rates in the Medicaid Population." *American Journal of Obstetrics and Gynecology* 208 (4): 274.

Thaddeus, S., and D. Maine. 1994. "Too Far to Walk: Maternal Mortality in Context." *Social Sciences and Medicine* 38 (8): 1091–110.

Thom, D. H., and G. Rortveit. 2010. "Prevalence of Postpartum Urinary Incontinence: A Systematic Review." *Acta Obstetricia et Gynecologica Scandinavica* 89 (12): 1511–22.

Tuncalp, O., M. Hindin, J. P. Souza, D. Chou, and L. Say. 2012. "The Prevalence of Maternal Near-Miss: A Systematic Review." *BJOG* 119 (6): 653–61.

United Nations General Assembly. 2000. "United Nations Millennium Declaration." United Nations General Assembly, New York. http://www.un.org/millennium /declaration/ares552e.htm.

Vos, T., A. Flaxman, M. Naghavi, R. Lozano, C. Michaud, and others. 2012. "Years Lived with a Disability (YLDs) for 1160 Sequelae of 289 Diseases and Injuries 1990–2010: A Systematic Analysis for the Global Burden of Disease Study 2010." *The Lancet* 380 (9859): 2163–96.

Wagner, K., C. Ronsmans, S. L. Thomas, C. Calvert, A. Adler, and others. 2012. "Women Who Experience Obstetric Haemorrhage Are at Higher Risk of Anaemia, in Both Rich and Poor Countries." *Tropical Medicine and International Health* 17 (1): 9–22.

Walker, G. J. A., and P. Gunasekera. 2011. "Pelvic Organ Prolapse and Incontinence in Developing Countries: Review of Prevalence and Risk Factors." *International Urogynecology Journal* 22 (2): 127–35.

WHO (World Health Organization). 1993. *The Prevention and Management of Unsafe Abortion.* Report of a Technical Working Group. Geneva: WHO.

———. 2006. "Female Genital Mutilation and Obstetric Outcome: WHO Collaborative Prospective Study in Six African Countries." WHO Study Group on Female Genital Mutilation and Obstetric Outcome. *The Lancet* 367 (9525): 1835–41.

———. 2008. *Managing Prolonged and Obstructed Labor.* Geneva: WHO.

———. 2010. *ICD-10: International Classification of Diseases and Related Health Problems.* 10th Revision, Vol. 2, Instruction Manual. Geneva: WHO.

———. 2011a. *Evaluating the Quality of Care for Severe Pregnancy Complications: The WHO Near-Miss Approach for Maternal Health.* Geneva: WHO.

———. 2011b. *Unsafe Abortion: Global and Regional Estimates of Incidence of Unsafe Abortion and Associated Mortality in 2008.* Sixth edition. Geneva: WHO.

———. 2012. *The WHO Application of ICD-10 to Deaths during Pregnancy, Childbirth and the Puerperium: ICD-MM.* Geneva: WHO.

———. 2013. *Maternal Death Surveillance and Response Technical Guidance: Information for Action to Prevent Maternal Death.* Geneva: WHO.

———. 2014a. "Global Health Estimates for Deaths by Cause, Age, and Sex for Years 2000–2012." WHO, Geneva. http:// www.who.int/healthinfo/global_burden_disease/en/.

———. 2014b. *Trends in Maternal Mortality: 1990 to 2013. Estimates by WHO, UNICEF, UNFPA, the World Bank and the United Nations Population Division.* Geneva: WHO.

———. 2015. *Trends in Maternal Mortality: 1990 to 2015. Estimates by WHO, UNICEF, UNFPA, the World Bank and the United Nations Population Division.* Geneva: WHO.

WHO and UNICEF (United Nations Children's Fund). 2012. *Countdown to 2015, Maternal, Newborn, and Child Survival.*

Building a Future for Women and Children: The 2012 Report. Geneva: WHO and UNICEF.

Zaba, B., C. Calvert, M. Marston, R. Isingo, J. Nakiyingi-Miiro, and others. 2013. "Effect of HIV Infection on Pregnancy-Related Mortality in Sub-Saharan Africa: Secondary Analyses of Pooled Community-Based Data from the Network for Analysing Longitudinal Population-Based HIV/AIDS Data on Africa (ALPHA)." *The Lancet* 381 (9879): 1763–71.

Zekele, B. M., T. A. Ayele, M. A. Woldetsadik, T. A. Bisetegn, and A. A. Adane. 2013. "Depression among Women with Obstetric Fistula, and Pelvic Organ Prolapse in Northwest Ethiopia." *BMC Psychiatry* 13: 236.

Chapter 4

Levels and Causes of Mortality under Age Five Years

Li Liu, Kenneth Hill, Shefali Oza, Dan Hogan,
Yue Chu, Simon Cousens, Colin Mathers,
Cynthia Stanton, Joy Lawn, and Robert E. Black

INTRODUCTION

This chapter reviews recent estimates of levels and distributions by cause of death of children under age five years, including stillbirths. We focus on 2000–15 and present results by World Bank region. We introduce an innovation by including information on stillbirths, defined as deaths from the 28th week of gestation. The standard convention has been to use live birth as the starting point of risk measurement, as in Millennium Development Goal 4 (MDG 4) to reduce mortality under age five years by two-thirds from 1990 to 2015 (UN 2000). However, substantial proportions of stillbirths are preventable given adequate obstetric care, and would, if prevented, increase the number of live births. We argue that including stillbirths in summary measures of child mortality provides a more inclusive assessment of health service provision than the standard convention.

Data on levels and trends of mortality before age five years are taken from the 2015 report by the United Nations Inter-Agency Group on Mortality Estimation (IGME) (You and others 2015). Data on levels and trends of causes of mortality under age five years are taken from the latest estimates produced by the World Health Organization (WHO) and UNICEF's (United Nations Children's Fund) Child Health Epidemiology Reference Group (Liu and others, forthcoming).

LEVELS AND TRENDS OF MORTALITY UNDER AGE FIVE YEARS, 2000–15

Mortality rates among young children are the best single indicator of child health in low- and middle-income countries (LMICs), and they are often also used as indicators of general social and economic development. The most widely used measure of child mortality in recent years has been the under-five mortality rate (U5MR), defined as the probability of dying between live birth and age five years; this measure was adopted as the primary target for MDG 4 (UN 2013). However, like all summary measures, the U5MR conceals age detail and patterns of mortality—and mortality change—in the first month and year of life that are of epidemiological and programmatic interest. In this chapter, we include stillbirths as part of the risk of dying under age five years, and the pregnancies at risk as all those that reach 28 weeks gestation (described as "viable fetuses"). We introduce a new measure, the total under-five mortality rate, or TU5MR, defined as the probability of dying between the 28th week of pregnancy and the fifth birthday.

We present estimates both as probabilities of dying and in the form of numbers of deaths and for age ranges 28 weeks to live birth, live birth to 27 days, 28 days to one year, and one year to five years. The probabilities of dying for these age ranges correspond to the conventional stillbirth, neonatal, postneonatal, and child

Corresponding author: Li Liu, The Institute for International Programs, Johns Hopkins Bloomberg School of Public Health, Baltimore, MD, USA; lliu26@jhu.edu.

mortality rates. We also present estimates of the broadest measure of child mortality risk, the TU5MR.

As a result of using this new conceptualization, we have to combine information from two sources, one for stillbirths and the other for mortality following a live birth, and make some approximations along the way. However, the approximations are relatively minor and do not affect the overall picture of recent levels and trends in TU5MR.

Sources

The estimates presented in this section are based on separate estimation exercises, one for the stillbirth rate and one for mortality of live-born children to age five years. For mortality of live-born children, we use the estimates by the IGME (You and others 2015); the methodology used by the IGME to arrive at estimates is described elsewhere (Alkema and others 2014). We present the probabilities of dying from live birth and the ratio of numbers of deaths to live births for World Bank regions for 2000 and 2015.

The derivation of stillbirth rates and numbers of stillbirths is less direct. The most recent systematic analysis of stillbirth rates provides estimates for MDG regions for 1995 and 2009 (Cousens and others 2011). We use the rate of change in the stillbirth rate between 1995 and 2009 for each MDG region to interpolate to 2000 and extrapolate to 2015. We then assume that these rates for MDG regions, suitably aggregated, closely approximate those for World Bank regions for those years. Specifically, to approximate the World Bank region of East Asia and Pacific, we combine the MDG regions of East Asia, South-East Asia, and Oceania; for the World Bank region of Middle East and North Africa, we combine the MDG regions of Western Asia and North Africa; and for the World Bank region of Europe and Central Asia, we combine the Commonwealth of Independent States (CIS) Europe and CIS Asia.

To estimate numbers of stillbirths, we use the relationship between rates and numbers of events. The neonatal mortality rate (NMR) is calculated as the number of neonatal deaths (ND) divided by the number of live births, so given the number of ND and the NMR, we can calculate the number of live births. The stillbirth mortality rate (SBR) is calculated as the number of stillbirths divided by the sum of the number of stillbirths and live births. We can estimate the number of stillbirths from the NMR, ND, and SBR as follows:

$$SB = ND \times SBR/[NMR \times (1 - SBR)].$$

These numbers are not affected by differences in numbers of live births between MDG and World Bank regions,

only by possible differences in stillbirth rates, which are likely to be minor, given the close overlap of the regions.

Results

Table 4.1 shows probabilities of dying for the four age ranges and for the TU5MR. Globally, the TU5MR declined from 95.4 per 1,000 viable fetuses in 2000 to 59.1 in 2015, an annual average rate of reduction (ARR) of 3.2 percent (table 4.2). For LMICs, the TU5MR declined from 105.9 in 2000 to 65.2 in 2015, and the decline for high-income countries (HICs) was from 14.3 to 9.7. The ARR was somewhat faster in the LMICs (3.2 percent) than in the HICs (2.6 percent), so the risk ratio for LMICs to HICs declined from 7.4 to 6.7 over the period; the absolute difference narrowed much more sharply, from 92 to 56 per 1,000 viable fetuses. In both years, there is large variation across regions. HICs had the lowest risks, about one-third that of the next best region, Latin America and the Caribbean. Sub-Saharan Africa had the highest risk, with the TU5MR remaining substantially greater than 100 per 1,000 in both years, more than 10 times the risk in HICs. The region with the second-highest risk in both years was South Asia, although its TU5MR fell to less than 100 in 2015; its disadvantage relative to HICs declined only slightly, however, from 8.3 to 7.9. The remaining regions had rather similar TU5MRs, between 44 and 59 per 1,000 in 2000 and between 26 and 36 in 2015, slightly narrowing their disadvantage relative to HICs.

At the global level, the neonatal period has the highest age-specific risk in both 2000 and 2015. This is also the case for LMICs as a group and for all regions individually, except Sub-Saharan Africa in 2000 and East Asia and Pacific in 2015. For all LMICs, and particularly for Sub-Saharan Africa, the age range of lowest risk shifts from stillbirths in 2000 to ages one to five years in 2015. South Asia's lowest risk is in the postneonatal group in 2000; for all other regions, the lowest risk in both years is from ages one to five years. The absolute difference between the highest and lowest risk among age ranges decreased by more than 90 percent from 2000 to 2015. The mortality rate estimate for Sub-Saharan Africa is 2.4 times that of the next highest region (South Asia), for both postneonatal and ages one to five years, despite similar neonatal and stillbirth rates.

Table 4.2 shows the ARR in probabilities of dying between 2000 and 2015 for the age ranges and regions shown in table 4.1. As noted, the ARR for TU5MR globally was 3.2 percent, somewhat less than the rate needed (4.4 percent) to achieve the MDG 4 target for the conventional U5MR. If we apply the MDG 4 target for U5MR to the TU5MR, the only region to

Table 4.1 Probabilities of Dying per 1,000 Pregnancy Completions from the 28th Week of Pregnancy to Age Five Years, 2000 and 2015

World Bank region	2000					2015				
	28 weeks gestation to birth	Birth to 27 days	28 days to 1 year	1–5 years	TU5MR	28 weeks gestation to birth	Birth to 27 days	28 days to 1 year	1–5 years	TU5MR
Low- and middle-income countries	22.8	33.0	25.0	25.1	105.9	19.1	20.7	13.7	11.7	65.2
East Asia and Pacific	15.2	21.0	12.2	9.1	57.5	9.2	8.9	5.9	3.0	27.0
Europe and Central Asia	10.0	19.7	14.9	7.6	52.2	8.1	10.6	7.1	2.6	28.4
Latin America and the Caribbean	10.8	15.1	12.8	5.7	44.4	7.6	9.6	6.2	2.9	26.2
Middle East and North Africa	14.8	22.2	13.4	9.1	59.4	11.4	13.8	6.7	3.6	35.7
South Asia	28.9	44.9	21.3	23.9	119.0	25.3	29.2	11.4	10.6	76.5
Sub-Saharan Africa	30.0	39.6	51.5	56.3	177.4	27.2	27.8	26.8	25.2	107.0
High-income countries	3.6	5.7	3.2	1.7	14.3	2.8	3.7	2.1	1.0	9.7
World	20.6	29.9	22.5	22.4	95.4	17.3	18.9	12.4	10.5	59.1

Sources: Based on Cousens and others 2011; and 2015 UN Inter-Agency Group for Child Mortality Estimation (IGME).
Note: TU5MR = total under-5 mortality rate.

Table 4.2 Annual Rates of Reduction in Probabilities of Dying per 1,000 Pregnancy Completions from the 28th Week of Pregnancy to Age Five Years, between 2000 and 2015

World Bank region	2000–15				
	28 weeks gestation to birth	Birth to 27 days	28 days to 1 year	1–5 years	TU5MR
Low- and middle-income countries	1.18	3.11	4.01	5.09	3.23
East Asia and Pacific	3.35	5.72	4.84	7.40	5.04
Europe and Central Asia	1.40	4.13	4.94	7.15	4.06
Latin America and the Caribbean	2.34	3.02	4.83	4.51	3.52
Middle East and North Africa	1.74	3.17	4.62	6.18	3.39
South Asia	0.89	2.87	4.17	5.42	2.95
Sub-Saharan Africa	0.65	2.36	4.35	5.36	3.37
High-income countries	1.68	2.88	2.81	3.54	2.59
World	1.16	3.06	3.97	5.05	3.19

Sources: Based on Cousens and others 2011; and 2015 UN Inter-Agency Group for Child Mortality Estimation (IGME).
Note: TU5MR = total under-5 mortality rate.

exceed the MDG 4 target ARR was East Asia and Pacific (5.0 percent), although LMIC countries of Europe and Central Asia (4.1 percent) came fairly close. All other regions, with ARRs ranging between 2.6 percent and 3.5 percent, performed well below the MDG target. Globally and in all regions, declines were slowest for stillbirths, averaging only about 1 percent per year in the aggregate, and highest for child mortality rates except for Latin America and the Caribbean; rates of decline

for postneonatal mortality exceeded the TU5MR, on average, in most regions. It is interesting to note how similar the rates of decline are for postneonatal mortality risks and risks between ages one and five years on the one hand, and how different stillbirth rates of decline are from declines of risk after birth, on the other hand. The ARR of mortality risk after the neonatal period was very close to or greater than the rate of reduction required to achieve the primary MDG 4 target in all LMICs; failure

Table 4.3 Numbers of Deaths from the 28th Week of Pregnancy to Age Five Years, 2000 and 2015 *(thousands)*

World Bank region	2000					2015				
	28 weeks gestation to birth	Birth to 27 days	28 days to 1 year	1–5 years	TU5MR	28 weeks gestation to birth	Birth to 27 days	28 days to 1 year	1–5 years	TU5MR
Low- and middle- income countries	2,639	3,826	2,891	2,906	12,262	2,420	2,625	1,735	1,478	8,256
East Asia and Pacific	420	581	337	252	1,591	279	270	178	89	816
Europe and Central Asia	39	78	59	30	206	36	47	31	12	126
Latin America and the Caribbean	111	156	132	59	458	71	90	58	27	246
Middle East and North Africa	102	154	93	63	412	105	128	62	34	328
South Asia	1,130	1,755	834	932	4,651	925	1,065	416	389	2,795
Sub-Saharan Africa	836	1,103	1,437	1,569	4,945	1,003	1,025	990	928	3,946
High-income countries	54	86	49	25	213	44	58	33	16	152
World	2,693	3,912	2,940	2,931	12,476	2,464	2,682	1,768	1,494	8,408

Sources: Based on Cousens and others 2011; and 2015 UN Inter-Agency Group for Child Mortality Estimation (IGME).
Note: TU5MR = total under-5 mortality rate.

Table 4.4 Annual Rates of Reduction in Numbers of Deaths from the 28th Week of Pregnancy to Age Five Years, 2000 and 2015

World Bank region	2000–15				
	28 weeks gestation to birth	Birth to 27 days	28 days to 1 year	1–5 years	TU5MR
Low- and middle-income countries	0.58	2.51	3.41	4.51	2.64
East Asia and Pacific	2.73	5.12	4.26	6.94	4.45
Europe and Central Asia	0.63	3.37	4.19	6.30	3.28
Latin America and the Caribbean	2.99	3.66	5.47	5.29	4.15
Middle East and North Africa	−0.19	1.24	2.72	4.18	1.51
South Asia	1.33	3.33	4.64	5.83	3.40
Sub-Saharan Africa	−1.21	0.49	2.49	3.50	1.50
High-income countries	1.31	2.64	2.51	2.85	2.27
World	0.59	2.52	3.39	4.49	2.63

Sources: Based on Cousens and others 2011; and 2015 UN Inter-Agency Group for Child Mortality Estimation (IGME).
Note: TU5MR = total under-5 mortality rate.

to achieve the target rate of decline overall was the result of relatively slower declines for stillbirths (especially) and neonatal mortality.

The numbers of deaths by age range are a product of risk (probability of dying) and numbers at risk (whether population, births, or viable fetuses). Table 4.3 shows estimated numbers of deaths by age range, region, and year. The number of deaths between 28 weeks of gestation and age five declined from 12.5 million in 2000 to 8.4 million in 2015, a decline of 2.6 percent per year (table 4.4). Globally, the numbers of deaths are highest in the neonatal period in both years, followed by the

postneonatal period in 2000 but by stillbirths in 2015. The numbers of deaths declined for all regions and for all age ranges, except for stillbirths in Sub-Saharan Africa and the Middle East and North Africa, which increased at 1.21 percent and 0.19 percent per year, respectively, reflecting slowly increasing risks, especially in Sub-Saharan Africa. The numbers of deaths under age five years declined fastest in Latin America and the Caribbean and in East Asia and Pacific; the slowest rate of decline, by a substantial margin, was in Sub-Saharan Africa and the Middle East and North Africa (1.5 percent in both regions); the third-slowest were HICs (2.2 percent).

During this period, there was a marked concentration of global deaths before the fifth birthday in Sub-Saharan Africa, with the proportion increasing from 40 percent to 47 percent; the proportion of child deaths between the ages of one and five years increased from 54 percent to 62 percent. Approximately 98 percent of deaths occurred in LMICs in all age groups in both 2000 and 2015. In East Asia and Pacific and South Asia, which are the two regions with shares of global deaths under age five years of more than 10 percent, the proportion declined, from 13 percent to 10 percent and from 37 percent to 33 percent, respectively.

Estimates of stillbirth rates have not been developed by gender of the fetus, but estimates are available of the conventional U5MR by gender. For LMICs overall in 2013, the ratio of boys to girls U5MR was about 1.08, but this average conceals substantial regional variation. For Europe and Central Asia, Latin America and the Caribbean, East Asia and Pacific, and HICs, the ratio ranged from 1.19 to 1.26; for Sub-Saharan Africa and the Middle East and North Africa, the ratio was about 1.15, but was less than 1.0 in South Asia, indicating a disadvantage for girls (results not shown). The numbers of deaths by gender of child reflect both differences in risk by gender and differences in gender ratios at birth, such that the overall ratio for LMICs of deaths of boys to deaths of girls under age five years is 1.17; this rate varies from 1.08 in South Asia to about 1.30 in East Asia and Pacific (elevated by the very high sex ratio at birth in China), Europe and Central Asia, Latin America and the Caribbean, and HICs. As a general rule (Hill and Upchurch 1995), the ratio of boys to girls U5MR tends to rise as overall U5MR declines until it reaches values of less than about 25 per 1,000 live births, so the ratio for LMICs is likely to increase in coming decades.

Discussion and Policy Implications

A major advance in the discussion of child mortality change in this chapter is the inclusion of stillbirths in overall mortality before age five years; this change adds 2.5 million deaths before age five, many of them preventable given existing interventions, to the global total in 2015. We see this as important because some overlap exists between the infrastructure and interventions to prevent stillbirths and those to reduce neonatal deaths.

Our analysis shows that both mortality risks and numbers of deaths under age five years declined substantially from 2000 to 2015, and that all four age ranges benefited in all regions. However, the global pace of decline was still slower than that required to achieve the MDG 4 target. This disappointing rate of decline was due to slow progress in reducing stillbirth and neonatal

mortality rates (annual rates of decline of 1.2 percent[1] and 3.1 percent, respectively, at the global level) and a shift in at-risk populations away from lower mortality to higher mortality regions, particularly in Sub-Saharan Africa. Population estimates (UN 2015) indicate that the proportion of global births in Sub-Saharan Africa increased from 20.1 percent in 2000 to 25.3 percent in 2015, and this trend is expected to continue. Another characteristic of under-five mortality in Sub-Saharan Africa is the high child mortality rate (ages one to five years) relative to other age ranges.

Further reductions in child mortality accordingly face several challenges:

- First, faster reductions in stillbirth rates and neonatal mortality rates are needed. In both cases, progress will require greater contact with effective health systems around childbirth, with higher proportions of deliveries taking place in well-equipped facilities with high quality of care; the development of such facilities will be expensive.
- Second, faster declines must be achieved at all ages under five years in Sub-Saharan Africa; given a continuing trend toward higher proportions of births in the region, declines in risk must reach at least the LMIC average so as not to be a brake on global progress; some preliminary evidence (You and others 2015) suggests that rates of decline are accelerating in some countries in the region.
- Finally, the high mortality risk of children between their first and fifth birthdays is a concern, particularly in Sub-Saharan Africa. Progress has been substantial in this age range, but risks remain high; in some regions, injury risks are actually increasing (Liu and others, forthcoming).

Child mortality reduction benefits from some tailwinds however. An increasing proportion of births will occur in urban areas, with lower mortality risks (Fink and Hill 2013). The numbers of births are likely to stop increasing in regions other than Sub-Saharan Africa; in some regions, the numbers are already falling, which will affect the numbers of child deaths, although not the rates. Falling fertility will also somewhat reduce the risk profile of births, with smaller proportions of high parity births and births to older mothers; falling fertility does, however, increase the proportion of one high risk group, first births, and it appears to have limited impact on birth intervals (Hill and Liu 2013). One of the most widely recognized factors associated with child mortality decline is maternal education (Hill and Liu 2013), and the educational profile of women in LMICs is improving rapidly; cohorts with high proportions of women with secondary or higher education, the levels with the strongest associations with reduced child mortality, are now approaching the peak years of reproduction.

A final positive factor is likely to be continued economic growth, which, according to some forecasts, may differentially favor Sub-Saharan Africa; much may depend, however, on how the gains in income growth are distributed among populations.

LEVELS AND TRENDS OF CAUSES OF MORTALITY UNDER AGE FIVE YEARS, 2000–15

Both probabilities of dying and numbers of deaths under age five years declined substantially from 2000 to 2015. At the global level, however, the declines failed to reach the MDG 4 targets, and acceleration is needed at the global, regional, and national levels beyond 2015. Progress can be accelerated by using reliable information about the distribution of deaths by cause and by scaling up cause-specific interventions (Bhutta and others 2008; Darmstadt and others 2005; Jones and others 2003; Lawn and others 2011). To guide global and national programs and research efforts, information about the distribution of causes of child deaths should be routinely updated. To assess the lasting effects of child health interventions and assist the development of long-term child survival strategies, time trends of child deaths by cause that are derived using consistent methods are needed.

This chapter focuses on major child deaths from the 28th week of pregnancy to age five years, so we discuss causes of both stillbirths and deaths from live birth to age five years. Because there is only moderate overlap between the causes of death in late pregnancy and in the neonatal period, we will first discuss cause structures of stillbirths, and then the causes of death after a live birth.

National data on causes of stillbirth are not available for either HICs or LMICs. As of 2011, more than 35 stillbirth classification systems had been published in the literature, the majority of them developed to describe the 2 percent of stillbirths occurring in HICs. These classification systems generally require fetal surveillance, advanced diagnostics, and post mortem examination, making their use in resource-constrained settings impractical (Lawn and others 2011). Even if data exist, unexplained stillbirths have been shown to account for 15 percent to 71 percent of stillbirths, limiting the usefulness of the data, especially for comparative purposes. Flenady and others (2009, 10) state that restricting reporting to the underlying cause of stillbirth is "challenging, (and often inappropriate), due to the complexity of the clinical situation in which the fetus dies." For this reason, data are also needed on contributing causes

and factors associated with stillbirth, two aspects of the International Classification of Diseases that are particularly weak.

With respect to deaths in childhood, the Child Health Epidemiology Reference Group has published a series of estimates of the distribution of causes of child death since 2005, during which time estimation methods and the quality and quantity of input data have improved (Black and others 2010; Bryce and others 2005; Johnson and others 2010; Lawn, Wilczynska-Ketnede, and Cousens 2006; Liu and others 2012; Liu and others 2015; Liu and others, forthcoming; Morris, Black, and Tomaskovic 2003). We report here estimates of the distribution of child deaths by cause among live births in 2015 and time trends of child deaths by cause since 2000 (Liu and others 2015).

Data and Methods

In LMICs, data on stillbirths by cause are sparse and generally based on classification systems that rely on maternal history and health and intrapartum events, and less frequently, on placental histopathology and other tests. Such classification systems have been judged to be suboptimal and are not recommended (Flenady and others 2009). Given that approximately 40 percent of births in LMICs are managed at home and that limited stillbirth data are recorded even at health facilities, the WHO and collaborators have developed a stillbirth verbal autopsy, validated in Ghana (Edmond and others 2008), India (Aggarwal, Jain, and Kumar 2011), and Pakistan (Nausheen and others 2013), with the goal of establishing population-based cause-of-stillbirth data. Other endeavors to expand the available data on the causes of stillbirth include a probabilistic model to predict likely causes of stillbirth based on verbal autopsy questions (Vergnano and others 2011) and the use of birth attendants as respondents for stillbirth verbal autopsy (Engmann and others 2012).

Accordingly, given the current state of cause-of-stillbirth data, for the purposes of this chapter, global estimates of the percent of stillbirths occurring after the onset of labor are presented. Where cause data are weak, categorizing stillbirths by time of death (antepartum versus intrapartum) is helpful in that many intrapartum deaths are term fetuses who should survive if born alive; these deaths are often associated with poor quality care (Lawn and others 2011). In addition, selected data are presented to illustrate common causes of stillbirth from HICs and LMICs.

A detailed description of the input data and estimation methods for the cause-of-death distribution among live-born children has been published elsewhere

(Liu and others 2012; Liu and others 2015; Liu and others, forthcoming).

Results

Table 4.5 shows the percentage of stillbirths occurring during the intrapartum period by world region based on the results of a systematic review of the literature (Lawn and others 2011). Globally, 45 percent of stillbirths occur during labor, ranging from 14 percent in HICs, to 16 percent in the Middle East and North Africa, and 23–56 percent in LMICs (Lawn and others 2011).

Table 4.6 summarizes the distribution of single causes of stillbirth and contributing conditions from areas within six HICs using the Cause of Death and Associated Conditions classification system that was judged favorably for retention of stillbirth information in an evaluation of stillbirth classification systems (Flenady and others 2009). The six countries include Australia, Canada, the Netherlands, Norway, the United Kingdom, and the United States. Stillbirth is defined in table 4.6 as a fetal death at a gestational age of 22 weeks or more, or 500 or more grams birth weight. The leading causes of death are "unknown" (30 percent), followed by placental pathology (29 percent) and infection (12 percent). Fewer than 10 percent of stillbirths were attributed to any one of the remaining five causes. However, although only 7 percent of stillbirths were attributed to maternal conditions as the single cause, maternal causes contributed to 24 percent of stillbirths, and placental pathologies contributed to more than 50 percent of all stillbirths. Using this data-intensive classification system, intrapartum conditions, defined narrowly as extreme prematurity

Table 4.5 Estimates of the Percentage of Stillbirths during the Intrapartum Period, by Region, 2008

World region	Estimated intrapartum stillbirths (%)
Low- and middle-income countries	44.3
East Asia and Pacific	24.0
Europe and Central Asia	20.0
Latin America and the Caribbean	23.1
Middle East and North Africa	16.4
South Asia	56.6
Sub-Saharan Africa	46.5
High-income countries	13.7
World	43.7

Source: Adapted from Lawn and others (2011) to reflect regions consistent with those used elsewhere in this chapter.

Table 4.6 Distribution of Single Causes of Stillbirth and Percentage of Contributing Causes in Six High-Income Countries Using the Cause of Death and Associated Conditions Classification System
Percent

Single cause of stillbirth		Contributing causes of death	
Unknown	30	Lacking or despite documentation and autopsy results	30
Placental pathologies	29	Infection or inflammation, abruption or retroplacental hematoma, infarction and thrombi, circulatory disorders, transfusion or feto-maternal hemorrhage, small-for-gestation placenta, villous or vascular maldevelopment	59
Infection	12	Unspecified, Group B streptococci	14
Cord	9	Knots, loops, abnormal insertion, focal anomaly, generalized anomaly, infection or inflammation	17
Maternal	7	Unspecified, hypertensive disorder, cervix insufficiency, hematology, diabetes, autoimmune disease	24
Congenital abnormalities	6	Unspecified, cardiovascular or lymphatic, triploidies	11
Fetal	4	Unspecified	7
Intrapartum	3	Extreme prematurity, asphyxia of unknown cause	5
Associated perinatal	n.a.	Small for gestational age, oligohydramnios, preterm premature rupture of the membranes, multiples, antepartum hemorrhage, suboptimal care	26
Associated maternal	n.a.	Smoking, maternal body mass index ≥ 30 kg/m^2, obstetric history	10
Total	*100*		

Source: Flenady and others 2009.

Note: kg/m^2 = kilograms per square meter; n.a. = not applicable. High-income countries for this table comprise Australia, Canada, the Netherlands, Norway, the United Kingdom, and the United States.

Table 4.7 Distribution of Causes of Stillbirth during the Antepartum and Intrapartum Periods in Kintampo, Ghana, 2003–04
Percent

	Antepartum period	Intrapartum period
Congenital abnormalities	1.7	0.8
Maternal disease	14.0	0.0
Obstetric complications	0.0	59.3
Maternal hemorrhage	4.1	4.8
Other	22.8	3.6
Unexplained	57.4	31.5
Total (N)	100 (413)	100 (248)

Source: Edmond and others 2008.

Table 4.8 Distribution of Causes of Stillbirth in a Hospital in Chandigarh, India, 2006–08

Causes of stillbirth determined via clinical assessment	Percent
Congenital malformations	12.0
Underlying maternal illness	12.9
Pregnancy-induced hypertension	30.7
Antepartum hemorrhage	15.6
Obstetric complications	8.4
Multiple pregnancy	2.2
Asphyxia not explained by any maternal condition	1.8
Other specific fetal problem	4.0
Unexplained stillbirth	10.2
Unexplained small size for gestational date	0.0
Unexplained preterm birth (< 37 weeks)	2.2
Total (N)	100 (225)

Source: Aggarwal, Jain, and Kumar 2011.

and asphyxia from unknown cause, were responsible for only 3 percent of stillbirths in these HICs. Nine percent of stillbirths occurred during the intrapartum period (data not shown), although the cause of most of them stemmed from the antepartum period.

Table 4.7 presents the percentage distribution of causes of stillbirth occurring during the antepartum and intrapartum periods in rural Ghana (Edmond and others 2008). Data were collected via verbal autopsy among women who delivered at home and at health facilities, with stillbirth defined as fetal death at 28 or more weeks of gestation. More than 37.5 percent of stillbirths occurred during the intrapartum period. More than half of antepartum stillbirths were unexplained (57.4 percent), making interpretation of the remaining categories difficult. Among intrapartum stillbirths, 31.5 percent were unexplained and 59.3 percent were attributed to obstetric complications.

Table 4.8 presents hospital-based cause-of-stillbirth data from Chandigarh, India, based on clinical and laboratory information and following standard obstetric guidelines. Stillbirth is defined here as a birth for which no fetal heart sounds were heard during labor and the neonatologist perceived no signs of life upon physical examination after birth. Findings indicate that 30.6 percent of stillbirths occurred during the intrapartum period; 80.0 percent were attributed to the five major causes of stillbirth, with pregnancy-induced hypertension the leading cause (30.7 percent). Only 10.2 percent were classified as "unexplained" (Aggarwal, Jain, and Kumar 2011).

Among the 5.9 million deaths of live-born children who died in the first five years of life in 2015, 45.1 percent (2.7 million) occurred in the neonatal period (table 4.3). The three leading causes of deaths are preterm birth complications (1.056 million, 17.8 percent), pneumonia

(0.922 million, 15.5 percent), and intrapartum-related events or birth asphyxia (0.689 million, 11.6 percent) (table 4.9). Other important causes include diarrhea (0.526 million, 8.9 percent), congenital malformation (0.505 million, 8.5 percent), sepsis or meningitis (0.525 million, 8.8 percent), and injury (0.331 million, 5.6 percent).

The burden of mortality by cause in live-born children younger than age five years varied widely across the regions in 2015 (figure 4.1). Nearly half (49.5 percent, 2.943 million) of deaths in children younger than age five years were in Sub-Saharan Africa, which included 96.4 percent (0.294 million) of global child deaths due to malaria and 90.6 percent (0.077 million) of global child deaths due to HIV/AIDS. South Asia had the highest number of any region of neonatal deaths in live-born children (1.065 million deaths, 57.0 percent). Preterm birth complications were the leading cause in this region, responsible for 24.8 percent, or 0.465 million deaths under age five years.

The Democratic Republic of Congo, Ethiopia, India, Nigeria, and Pakistan collectively accounted for about half the total number of global under age five years deaths (48.3 percent, 2.871 million) and neonatal deaths (50.8 percent, 1.362 million) in 2015. In India, 1.2 million children younger than age five years died in 2015; more than half of them (57.9 percent, 0.696 million) died in the first 28 days of life. Major causes of death included preterm birth complications (0.321 million, 26.7 percent), pneumonia (0.180 million, 15.0 percent), and intrapartum-related complications (0.142 million, 11.9 percent). Angola, the Democratic Republic of Congo, India, Nigeria, and Pakistan were the top five countries with the most pneumonia deaths and the most diarrhea deaths. For intrapartum-related complications, Ethiopia replaced Angola on the list. For preterm birth complications, China replaced Angola. Burkina Faso, the Democratic Republic of Congo, Côte d'Ivoire, Mali, and Nigeria had the most malaria deaths.

Compared with 2000, approximately 4 million fewer deaths under age five years occurred in 2015. Deaths from pneumonia, diarrhea, and malaria decreased the most in absolute terms, by 680,000, 663,000 million, and 419,000 million, respectively. Collectively, the three causes were responsible for 43.9 percent of the absolute reduction in under age five years deaths in 2000–15.

In 2000–15, child mortality rates of all the causes decreased, albeit at differing rates. In neonates, the burden of preterm birth complications decreased from 1.242 million in 2000 to 0.946 million in 2015, with the associated mortality rate falling by 2.4 percent per year. Intrapartum-related deaths decreased from 1.040 to 0.635 million, with the mortality rate declining at an average ARR of 3.9 percent. Neonatal sepsis or meningitis decreased from 0.529 million in 2000 to 0.410 million in 2015, a rate of 2.3 percent per year. Neonatal tetanus decreased from 0.164 million to 0.034 million at 10.9 percent per year. For children who died between the ages of 1 and 59 months, trends in numbers and rates of death by cause were highly variable from 2000 to 2015. Pneumonia deaths in this age group decreased from 1.44 million to 0.76 million, with the pneumonia-specific mortality rate dropping an average of 4.8 percent per year. Diarrhea deaths decreased from 1.172 million to 0.509 million, a 6.1 percent decrease in the mortality rate per year during this period. Malaria deaths declined from 0.725 million in 2000 to 0.306 million in 2015, with the malaria-specific mortality rate dropping 6.3 percent per year. Measles mortality fluctuated, in part due to outbreaks, but overall it decreased from 0.481 million to 0.074 million, a rate of 13.1 percent per year.

In 2000–15, the U5MR decreased at varying rates across regions. HICs and South Asia had the slowest reductions, at an average ARR of 3.0 percent and 3.8 percent, respectively. In Sub-Saharan Africa, the pneumonia-specific mortality rate among children ages 1–59 months decreased at an annual rate of 4.2 percent. The ARR for preterm birth complications was only 1.3 percent among children ages 1–59 months (0.3 percent among children under age five). The malaria-specific mortality rate decreased 7.6 percent annually. Measles had the highest ARR at an average of 16.5 percent. In South

Table 4.9 Estimated Numbers of Deaths by Cause among Live-Born Children Younger than Age Five Years, 2015

Causes	Estimated number (millions)	Cause-specific mortality rate (per 1,000 live births)
Neonates ages 0–27 days		
Preterm birth complications[a]	0.946	6.770
Intrapartum-related events[b]	0.635	4.547
Sepsis or meningitis[c]	0.410	2.937
Congenital abnormalities[d]	0.299	2.139
Other conditions[e]	0.177	1.268
Pneumonia[f]	0.162	1.159
Tetanus	0.035	0.247
Diarrhea[g]	0.017	0.125
Children ages 1–59 months		
Pneumonia[f]	0.760	5.443
Other conditions[e]	0.655	4.691
Diarrhea[g]	0.509	3.643
Injury	0.331	2.367
Malaria	0.306	2.193
Congenital abnormalities[d]	0.206	1.471
Meningitis[c]	0.115	0.826
Preterm birth complications[a]	0.110	0.790
AIDS	0.086	0.614
Measles	0.074	0.531
Intrapartum-related events[b]	0.054	0.388
Pertussis	0.054	0.387

Source: Liu and others, forthcoming.
Note: Other conditions among children ages 1–59 months include congenital malformation, causes originating during the perinatal period, cancer, pertussis, severe malnutrition, and other specified causes. Intrapartum-related events were formerly referred to as "birth asphyxia." AIDS = acquired immunodeficiency syndrome.
a. Estimated number of preterm deaths in children younger than age five years overall including the neonatal period is 1.056 million.
b. Estimated number of intrapartum-related events deaths in children younger than age five years overall including the neonatal period is 0.689 million.
c. Estimated number of sepsis or meningitis deaths in children younger than age five years overall including the neonatal period is 0.526 million.
d. Estimated number of congenital abnormalities deaths in children younger than age five years overall including the neonatal period is 0.504 million.
e. Estimated number of other conditions deaths in children younger than age five years overall including the neonatal period is 0.832 million.
f. Estimated number of pneumonia deaths in children younger than age five years overall including the neonatal period is 0.922 million.
g. Estimated number of diarrhea deaths in children younger than age five years overall including the neonatal period is 0.526 million.

Asia, the mortality rates for pneumonia and diarrhea among children ages 1–59 months decreased on average by 5.6 percent and 6.1 percent per year, respectively. However, the mortality rate attributable to neonatal

Figure 4.1 Causes of Childhood Deaths among Live-Born Children Younger than Age Five Years, by World Bank Region, 2015

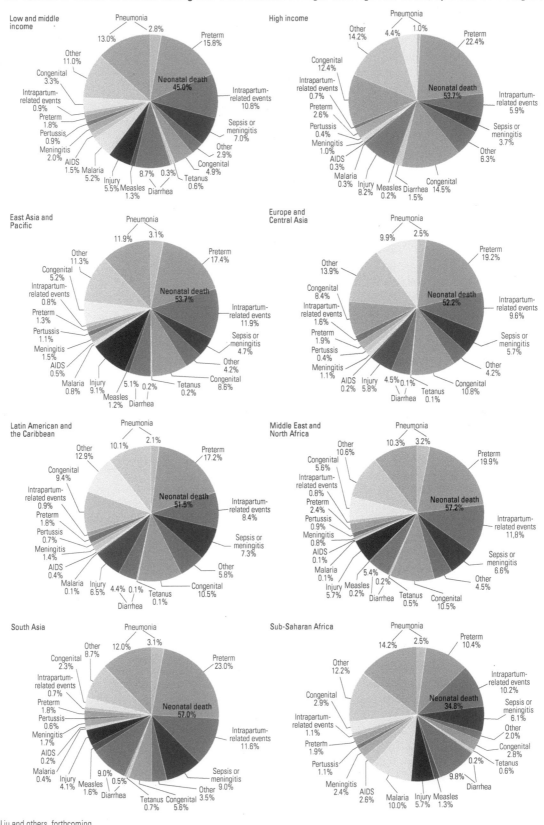

Source: Liu and others, forthcoming.
Note: AIDS = acquired immunodeficiency syndrome.

preterm births fell little, on average only 1.3 percent. At the country level, varying trends in cause-specific death rates were seen in 2000–15 (data are not shown).

Discussion and Policy Implications

Our estimate of 2.5 million stillbirths based on an extrapolation of previous estimates is very similar to a new estimate for 2015 of 2.6 million (Blencowe and others, forthcoming). The numbers have been declining by 0.6 percent annually since 2000 and showing the lowest rate of decline of the four age groups constituting TU5MR. Although cause-of-stillbirth data are sparse and lack comparability, it is clear that the percentage of intrapartum stillbirths is two to four times higher in LMICs than HICs and that continued improvements in the implementation of evidence-based obstetric care require policy prioritization to prevent the majority of these deaths. Equally important is the need for consensus on a cause-of-stillbirth classification system that can be used in high- and low-resource settings to monitor trends and assess program effectiveness. Although probabilities of stillbirth are eight or more times higher in South Asia and Sub-Saharan Africa than in HICs, many stillbirths in HICs are considered potentially preventable, particularly among disadvantaged women, requiring greater outreach for antenatal care and improved living standards. Research to address antepartum stillbirths and stillbirths associated with extreme prematurity and infection are priorities in high-income settings (Flenady and others 2009).

Among the 5.9 million live-born children who died before reaching their fifth birthday in 2015, 45.1 percent died in the neonatal period. Preterm birth complications and pneumonia remained the top killers in this age group. Intrapartum-related events became the third leading cause of child deaths globally. Other important leading causes of child deaths include diarrhea, congenital malformation, neonatal sepsis or meningitis, injury, and malaria.

From 2000 to 2015, substantial reductions in deaths under age five years were seen at the global level. However, the pace of reduction varied by cause. Pneumonia, diarrhea, and malaria collectively contributed nearly half of the total reduction. Other major causes, such as preterm birth complications, declined at a much slower rate globally and nearly stalled in South Asia.

Scale-up of proven interventions to prevent and treat childhood infectious diseases and leading neonatal conditions is urgently needed to maintain and accelerate the pace of improving child survival worldwide (Liu and others 2015). Improving quality care at birth, such as better implementation of neonatal resuscitation, antenatal corticosteroids, and kangaroo mother care, is a key strategy in reducing neonatal deaths due to intrapartum-related complications and preterm birth complications (Bhutta and others 2014). Scaling up new vaccines, such as *Haemophilus influenza* type B, pneumococcus, and rotavirus vaccines has the potential to further reduce pneumonia and diarrhea (Bhutta and others 2013; Walker and others 2013). Additional implementation research is urgently needed to understand how to better scale up coverage and quality of these interventions (Requejo and others 2015). Social interventions to improve child survival are as important as cause-specific interventions. Examples include improving family planning programs to help couples achieve their desired family size by minimizing unintended pregnancies and increasing women's education (Cleland and others 2012; Gakidou and others 2010).

Causes of 3.5 percent of deaths under age five years among live-born children were directly derived based on vital registration data and 6.4 percent from a model using vital registration data; causes for 90.1 percent were derived using verbal autopsy data (Liu and others, forthcoming). Verbal autopsy as a distinct scientific area has been improving substantially yet remains subject to inherent limitations (Anker 1997; Fottrell and Byass 2010; Murray and others 2011). Estimates produced by sophisticated modeling cannot and should not replace any existing and future data collection efforts to generate context-specific information, given that the strengths and limitations of the local data collection process are fully accessible and well understood. Furthermore, national civil registration and vital statistics systems need to be further strengthened and invested in more heavily to deliver on the promise of improved and reliable health statistics. Ultimately, evidence-based policy making and program planning can only be optimized if full openness and transparency can be achieved in the evidence-generating process (Sutherland 2013).

CONCLUSION

We present in this chapter a new concept of TU5MR, which is a composite measure of mortality occurring between 28 weeks gestation and age five years. Within this age group, child survival efforts should focus on stillbirth and neonatal mortality, as well as preterm birth complications, pneumonia, and intrapartum-related complications. More information is needed to better understand levels and causes of stillbirth. To end preventable child deaths in a generation and attain the ambitious Sustainable Development Goals, child survival needs to remain front and center on the global development agenda.

NOTES

World Bank Income Classifications as of July 2014 are as unnumbered note 1 as follows, based on estimates of gross national income (GNI) per capita for 2013:

- Low-income countries (LICs) = US$1,045 or less
- Middle-income countries (MICs) are subdivided:
  a) lower-middle-income = US$1,046 to US$4,125
  b) upper-middle-income (UMICs) = US$4,126 to US$12,745
- High-income countries (HICs) = US$12,746 or more.

1. A constant annual rate of decline was assumed when interpolating and extrapolating to derive stillbirth rates for 2000 and 2015 from 1995 and 2009 estimates, respectively. However, if the reduction of stillbirth rates has been accelerating in this period, we could have underestimated the annual rate of decline of stillbirth rates.

REFERENCES

Aggarwal, A. K., V. Jain, and R. Kumar. 2011. "Validity of Verbal Autopsy for Ascertaining the Causes of Stillbirth." *Bulletin of the World Health Organization* 89 (1): 31–40.

Alkema, L., J. R. New, J. Pedersen, and D. You. 2014. "Child Mortality Estimation 2013: An Overview of Updates in Estimation Methods by the United Nations Inter-Agency Group for Child Mortality Estimation." *PLoS One* 9 (7): e101112. doi: http://dx.doi.org/10.1371/journal .pone.0101112.

Anker, M. 1997. "The Effect of Misclassification Error on Reported Cause-Specific Mortality Fractions from Verbal Autopsy." *International Journal of Epidemiology* 26 (5): 1090–96.

Bhutta, Z. A., T. Ahmed, R. E. Black, S. Cousens, K. Dewey, and others. 2008. "What Works? Interventions for Maternal and Child Undernutrition and Survival." *The Lancet* 371 (9610): 417–40.

Bhutta, Z. A., J. K. Das, R. Bahl, J. E. Lawn, R. A. Salam, and others. 2014. "Can Available Interventions End Preventable Deaths in Mothers, Newborn Babies, and Stillbirths, and at What Cost?" *The Lancet* 384 (9940): 347–70.

Bhutta, Z. A., J. K. Das, N. Walker, A. Rizvi, H. Campbell, and others. 2013. "Interventions to Address Deaths from Childhood Pneumonia and Diarrhoea Equitably: What Works and at What Cost?" *The Lancet* 381 (9875): 1417–29.

Black, R. E., S. Cousens, H. L. Johnson, J. E. Lawn, I. Rudan, and others. 2010. "Global, Regional, and National Causes of Child Mortality in 2008: A Systematic Analysis." *The Lancet* 375 (9730): 1969–87.

Bryce, J., C. Boschi-Pinto, K. Shibuya, R. E. Black, and WHO Child Health Epidemiology Reference Group. 2005. "WHO Estimates of the Causes of Death in Children." *The Lancet* 365 (9465): 1147–52.

Cleland, J., A. Conde-Agudelo, H. Peterson, J. Ross, and A. Tsui. 2012. "Contraception and Health." *The Lancet* 380 (9837): 149–56.

Cousens, S., H. Blencowe, C. Stanton, D. Chou, S. Ahmed, and others. 2011. "National, Regional, and Worldwide Estimates of Stillbirth Rates in 2009 with Trends since 1995: A Systematic Analysis." *The Lancet* 377 (9774): 1319–30.

Darmstadt, G. L., Z. A. Bhutta, S. Cousens, T. Adam, N. Walker, and others. 2005. "Evidence-Based, Cost-Effective Interventions: How Many Newborn Babies Can We Save?" *The Lancet* 365 (9463): 977–88.

Edmond, K. M., M. A. Quigley, C. Zandoh, S. Danso, C. Hurt, and others. 2008. "Aetiology of Stillbirths and Neonatal Deaths in Rural Ghana: Implications for Health Programming in Developing Countries." *Paediatric and Perinatal Epidemiology* 22 (5): 430–37.

Engmann, C., A. Garces, I. Jehan, J. Ditekemena, M. Phiri, and others. 2012. "Birth Attendants as Perinatal Verbal Autopsy Respondents in Low- and Middle-Income Countries: A Viable Alternative?" *Bulletin of the World Health Organization* 90 (3): 200–08.

Fink, G., and K. Hill. 2013. "Urbanization and Child Mortality—Evidence from Demographic and Health Surveys." Background paper prepared for Commission on Investing in Health. Harvard School of Public Health, Cambridge, MA.

Flenady, V., J. F. Frøen, H. Pinar, R. Torabi, E. Saastad, and others. 2009. "An Evaluation of Classification Systems for Stillbirth." *BMC Pregnancy and Childbirth* 9 (1): 24.

Fottrell, E., and P. Byass. 2010. "Verbal Autopsy: Methods in Transition." *Epidemiologic Reviews* 32 (1): 38–55.

Gakidou, E., K. Cowling, R. Lozano, and C. J. Murray. 2010. "Increased Educational Attainment and Its Effect on Child Mortality in 175 Countries between 1970 and 2009: A Systematic Analysis." *The Lancet* 376 (9745): 959–74.

Hill, K., and L. Liu. 2013. "Challenges and Opportunities for Further Reductions in Infant and Child Mortality." Expert Paper 2013/11, United Nations Population Division, New York.

Hill, K., and D. M. Upchurch. 1995. "Gender Differences in Child Health: Evidence from the Demographic and Health Surveys." *Population and Development Review* 21 (1): 127–51.

Johnson, H. L., L. Liu, C. Fischer-Walker, and R. E. Black. 2010. "Estimating the Distribution of Causes of Death among Children Age 1–59 Months in High-Mortality Countries with Incomplete Death Certification." *International Journal of Epidemiology* 39 (4): 1103–14.

Jones, G., R. W. Steketee, R. E. Black, Z. A. Bhutta, S. S. Morris, and others. 2003. "How Many Child Deaths Can We Prevent This Year?" *The Lancet* 362 (9377): 65–71.

Lawn, J. E., H. Blencowe, R. Pattinson, S. Cousens, R. Kumar, and others. 2011. "Stillbirths: Where? When? Why? How to Make the Data Count?" *The Lancet* 377 (9775): 1448–63.

Lawn, J. E., K. Wilczynska-Ketende, and S. N. Cousens. 2006. "Estimating the Causes of 4 Million Neonatal Deaths in the Year 2000." *International Journal of Epidemiology* 35 (3): 706–18.

Liu, L., H. L. Johnson, S. Cousens, J. Perin, S. Scott, and others. 2012. "Global, Regional, and National Causes of Child Mortality: An Updated Systematic Analysis for 2010 with Time Trends since 2000." *The Lancet* 379 (9832): 2151–61.

Liu, L., S. Oza, D. Hogan, J. Perin, I. Rudan, and others. 2015. "Global, Regional, and National Causes of Child Mortality in 2000–13, with Projections to Inform Post-2015 Priorities: An Updated Systematic Analysis." *The Lancet* 385 (9966): 430–40.

Liu, L., S. Oza, D. Hogan, Y. Chu, J. Perin, and others. Forthcoming. *National, Regional and Global Causes of Child Mortality in 2000–2015: Reflecting on the MDG 4 and Embarking on the SDG 3.2.*

Morris, S. S., R. E. Black, and L. Tomaskovic. 2003. "Predicting the Distribution of Under-Five Deaths by Cause in Countries without Adequate Vital Registration Systems." *International Journal of Epidemiology* 32 (6): 1041–51.

Murray, C. J., A. D. Lopez, R. Black, R. Ahuja, S. M. Ali, and others. 2011. "Population Health Metrics Research Consortium Gold Standard Verbal Autopsy Validation Study: Design, Implementation, and Development of Analysis Datasets." *Population Health Metrics* 9 (1): 27.

Nausheen, S., S. B. Soofi, K. Sadiq, K. A. Habib, A. Turab, and others. 2013. "Validation of Verbal Autopsy Tool for Ascertaining the Causes of Stillbirth." *PLoS One* 9 (8): 10.

Requejo, J. H., J. Bryce, A. J. Barros, P. Berman, Z. Bhutta, and others. 2015. "Countdown to 2015 and Beyond: Fulfilling the Health Agenda for Women and Children." *The Lancet* 385 (9966): 466–76.

Sutherland, W. J. 2013. "Review by Quality Not Quantity for Better Policy." *Nature* 503 (7475): 167.

UN (United Nations). 2000. *United Nations Millennium Declaration: Resolution Adopted by the General Assembly.* 55/2. New York: United Nations.

———. 2013. *The Millennium Development Goals Report 2013.* New York: United Nations.

———. 2015. *World Population Prospects: The 2015 Revision.* New York: DoEaSA, Population Division, UN. DVD.

Vergnano, S., E. Fottrell, D. Osrin, P. N. Kazembe, C. Mwansambo, and others 2011. "Adaptation of a Probabilistic Method (InterVA) of Verbal Autopsy to Improve the Interpretation of Cause of Stillbirth and Neonatal Death in Malawi, Nepal, and Zimbabwe." *Population Health Metrics* 9: 48.

Walker, C. L. F., I. Rudan, L. Liu, H. Nair, E. Theodoratou, and others. 2013. "Global Burden of Childhood Pneumonia and Diarrhoea." *The Lancet* 381 (9875): 1405–16.

You, D., L. Hug, S. Ejdemyr, and J. Beise. 2015. *Levels and Trends in Child Mortality. Report 2015. Estimates Developed by the UN Inter-Agency Group for Child Mortality Estimation.* New York: United Nations Children's Fund.

Chapter 5

Levels and Trends in Low Height-for-Age

Gretchen A. Stevens, Mariel M. Finucane, and
Christopher J. Paciorek

INTRODUCTION

Children's nutritional status influences their survival, cognitive development, and lifelong health (Adair and others 2013; Black and others 2013; Grantham-McGregor and others 2007; Olofin and others 2013). Inadequate nutrition, together with infections, results in restricted linear growth. Stunting, or low height-for-age, is an indicator of overall nutritional status (Black and others 2013; WHO 2013) and an important cause of morbidity and mortality in infants and children (Black and others 2013; Olofin and others 2013).

Stunting caused an estimated 14 percent to 17 percent of mortality in children under age five years in 2011, accounting for 1.0 million to 1.2 million deaths (Black and others 2013). The World Health Assembly endorsed the target of reducing the number of children with stunting by 40 percent by 2025, compared with the 2010 baseline (World Health Assembly 2012). According to the World Health Organization (WHO), rates of stunting reduction need to be accelerated to meet this target (World Health Assembly 2012).

Country-level information on trends in child height-for-age is needed for priority setting, planning, and program evaluation. Stunting estimates are made at the regional level for all world regions by UNICEF, WHO, and World Bank (2012, 2014). This chapter presents a set of country-level estimates by the Nutrition Impact Model Study (NIMS) for 1985–2011 (Stevens and others 2012). The NIMS collaboration estimates trends in the complete distributions of child height-for-age by country, including stunting prevalence. Paciorek and others (2013) extend this body of work to separately estimate children's height-for-age distribution in urban and rural areas, by country and year. Separate estimates for urban and rural areas allow strategies that target children in each setting to be prioritized.

METHODS

We present published estimates of the height-for-age distribution from the NIMS study (Paciorek and others 2013; Stevens and others 2012). We accessed population-representative data on the height of children under age five years from nationally or regionally representative household surveys, including Demographic and Health Surveys and Multiple Indicator Cluster Surveys, as follows:

- We obtained these data as anonymized individual anthropometric measurements, if accessible, or as summary statistics from the WHO's Global Database on Child Growth and Malnutrition (de Onis and Blossner 2003), or from preliminary reports not yet included in the WHO's database.
- For data obtained as individual observations, we extracted information on urban or rural place of residence for each observation. We calculated height-for-age z-scores (HAZ) using the 2006 WHO child

Corresponding author: Gretchen A. Stevens, Department of Health Statistics and Information Systems, World Health Organization, Geneva; stevensg@who.int.

growth standards for each individual measurement (WHO 2006).

- For data obtained as summary statistics, we extracted the summary statistic for the entire population covered by each data source, usually at the national level, and, where possible, separately for urban and rural areas.

- In cases for which only summarized statistics were calculated using the 1977 National Center for Health Statistics reference, regression equations were developed to convert these estimates to the 2006 WHO child growth standards (Stevens and others 2012). Our final data set included measured heights of more than 7.7 million children under age five years.

Despite the extensive data search, there were gaps in data availability; an average of 4.5 data sources were available for each country over the 26 years in the study period. We therefore developed Bayesian hierarchical mixture models to estimate the complete distribution of childhood HAZ for each country and year, from which we calculated summary statistics such as mean HAZ and the prevalence of stunting. The inputs for our model were individual-level records and summary statistics. Two statistical analyses were conducted:

- An analysis of HAZ distribution in 141 low- and middle-income countries (LMICs) for each year from 1985 to 2011

- An analysis of HAZ distribution in urban and rural areas in the same 141 LMICs for each year from 1985 to 2011.

In the first model, estimates for each country-year were informed by data from that country-year itself, if available, and by data from other years in the same country and in other countries, especially those in the same region with data in similar periods. This hierarchical model shares information to a greater degree where data are nonexistent or weakly informative (for example, because they have a small sample size), and to a lesser degree in data-rich countries and regions. We modeled trends over time both as a linear trend and as a smooth nonlinear trend. The estimates were informed by time-varying covariates that help predict HAZ, including maternal education, national income (natural logarithm of per capita gross domestic product [GDP] in inflation-adjusted U.S. dollars), proportion of the population in urban areas, and an aggregate metric of access to basic health care. Finally, the model accounted for the fact that data did not cover the entire country; data that did not cover the complete age range

of 0–59 months may have more variation relative to the true levels than nationally representative data and data that covered the full range of ages. Estimates by sex were not made because little difference was found between male and female stunting prevalence (Stevens and others 2012).

For the second analysis, the statistical model was extended to make separate estimates for urban and rural children. The urban-rural difference in HAZ distribution was allowed to vary by country and year. Both analyses were also carried out for children's weight-for-age distribution, not reported here.

Public health professionals usually report the prevalence of stunting (as defined by the WHO as HAZ below −2), rather than other metrics, such as mean HAZ or the prevalence of severe stunting (HAZ below −3). In this chapter, we report mean HAZ, prevalence of stunting (HAZ below −2), and prevalence of severe stunting (HAZ below −3).

GLOBAL AND REGIONAL TRENDS

Global Trends

In LMICs the prevalence of stunting has declined and mean HAZ has improved since 1985. In 1985, 47.2 percent (95 percent uncertainty interval 44.0–50.3) of children under age five years were moderately or severely stunted; this rate improved to 29.9 percent (27.1–32.9) in 2011 (figure 5.1). Mean HAZ increased during the same period, from −1.86 (−2.01 to −1.72) to −1.16 (−1.29 to −1.04).

Despite large improvements, many children remain stunted. In 2011, 314 million (95 percent uncertainty interval 296 million to 331 million) children had HAZ below −1, a moderate improvement from 367 million (352 million to 379 million) in 1985. Of the children with HAZ below −1 in 2011, 46 percent had HAZ between −1 and −2, 31 percent had HAZ between −2 and −3, and 23 percent had HAZ below −3.

Regional Trends

Although child height improved in LMICs as a whole, progress was less consistent at the regional level (figure 5.1). East Asia and Pacific and South Asia show the largest improvements in mean HAZ, increasing by about 0.4 per decade. Mean HAZ also increased to a lesser extent in Europe and Central Asia, the Middle East and North Africa, and Latin America and the Caribbean (increases of 0.20–0.23 per decade). However, children's height in Sub-Saharan Africa showed inconsistent progress. In Sub-Saharan Africa, stunting prevalence may

Figure 5.1 Trends in Mean Height-for-Age Z-Score and Stunting Prevalence, by Region, 1985–2011

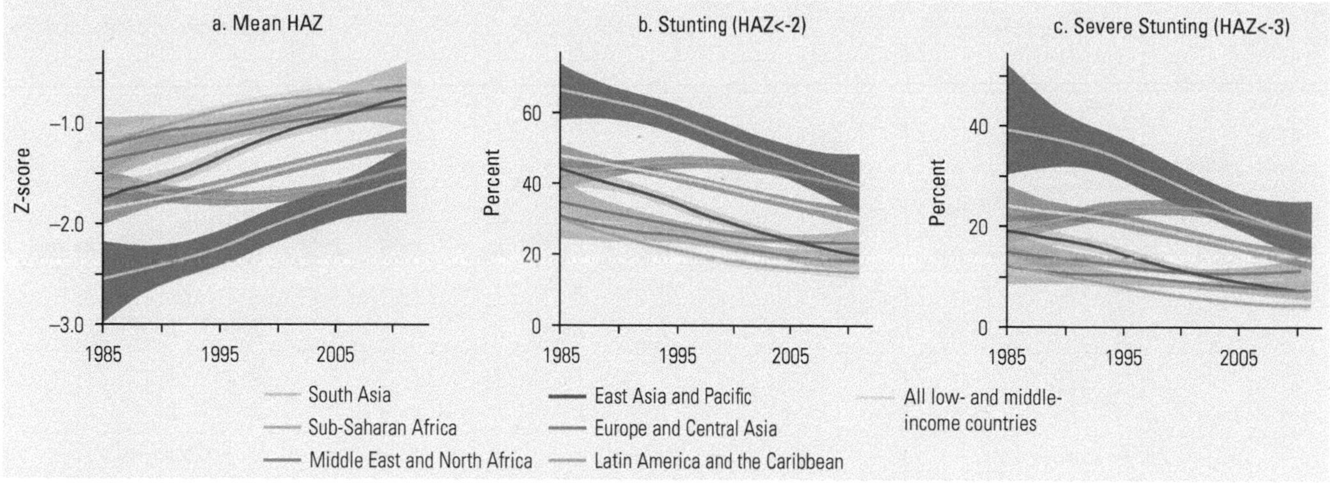

a. Mean HAZ   b. Stunting (HAZ<-2)   c. Severe Stunting (HAZ<-3)

— South Asia   — East Asia and Pacific   — All low- and middle-income countries
— Sub-Saharan Africa   — Europe and Central Asia
— Middle East and North Africa   — Latin America and the Caribbean

Source: Stevens and others 2012.
Note: Shaded areas show the 95 percent uncertainty interval. HAZ = height-for-age z-scores.

have increased from 41.4 percent (95 percent uncertainty interval 37.3–45.6) in 1985 to more than 45 from 1995 to 1999; it subsequently decreased to 37.7 percent (35.3–40.2) by 2011.

In 1985, mean HAZ was higher and the prevalence of stunting was lower in urban areas than in rural areas in all regions (figure 5.2). Urban and rural mean HAZ and prevalence of stunting largely improved at the same pace; the urban-rural gaps in mean HAZ and prevalence of stunting were, in most cases, maintained during the period. Nevertheless, some improvements were observed. In Europe and Central Asia and the Middle East and North Africa, both the absolute and relative gaps in the prevalence of stunting decreased. In Europe and Central Asia, the gap between urban and rural prevalence of stunting fell from 15 percent in 1985 to 7 percent, the narrowest gap observed, in 2011.

The most impressive improvement in children's height occurred in China, followed by Vietnam, Bangladesh, India, Bhutan, Brazil, Nepal, and Tunisia; in these countries, mean HAZ increased by 0.35–0.51 per decade. In most of these high-performing countries, the urban-rural gap in mean HAZ also declined; the exceptions are China, Vietnam, and with large uncertainty, Jamaica. HAZ may have deteriorated in 17 countries between 1985 and 2011, nearly all in Sub-Saharan Africa and the Oceania region of East Asia and Pacific; most had large uncertainties, with the exception of estimated declines in Côte d'Ivoire and Niger. Overall, the rate of improvement in mean HAZ was positively correlated with a reduction in urban-rural inequality in mean HAZ.

Improvement in mean HAZ at the national level can be divided into three components:

- Improvement in mean HAZ in rural children
- Improvement in mean HAZ in urban children
- Increases in the proportion of children in urban areas.

Figure 5.3 shows each component's contribution in each region. In East Asia and Pacific and in South Asia, both predominantly rural regions in 1985 (less than 30 percent urban) and in 2011 (less than 50 percent urban), improvements in rural HAZ contributed 68 percent or more of the overall improvement in HAZ. In contrast, in Latin America and the Caribbean, a predominantly urban region (66 percent urban in 1985, increasing to 78 percent urban by 2011), urban improvements contributed more than 70 percent of the overall improvement.

Height-for-Age in 2011

Despite large improvements in HAZ in most regions, only a few countries have mean HAZ and stunting prevalence that approach the ideal of a mean HAZ of at least zero and stunting prevalence of 2.3 percent (maps 5.1, 5.2, 5.3). Chile, Jamaica, and Kuwait have mean HAZ greater than 0 and a prevalence of stunting of less than 5 percent, as do urban areas of China.

The majority of stunted children still live in rural areas. These stunted children live mainly in South Asia (52 million [uncertainty interval 42 million to 62 million]) and Sub-Saharan Africa (37 million [35 million to 40 million]). In rural areas in Afghanistan,

Figure 5.2 Trends in Urban and Rural Prevalence of Stunting, by Region, 1985–2011

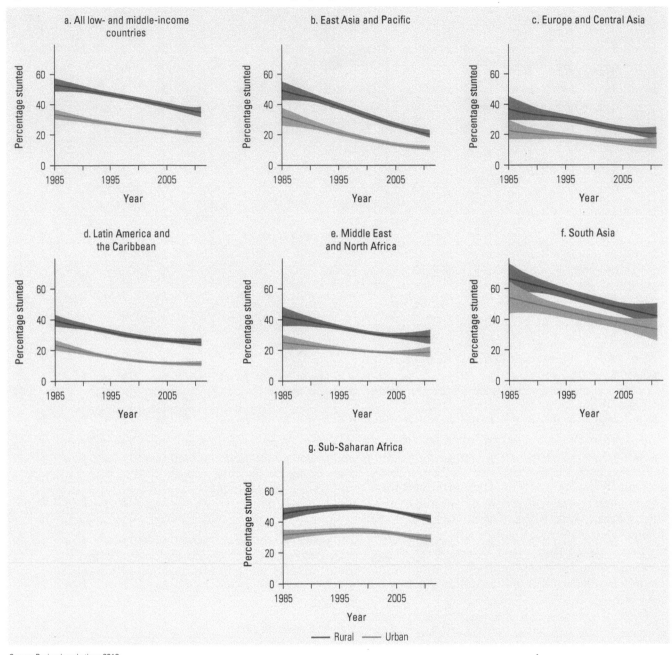

Source: Paciorek and others 2013.
Note: Shaded areas show the 95 percent uncertainty interval of the trend.

Burundi, Guatemala, Niger, Timor-Leste, and the Republic of Yemen, more than 50 percent of the children under age five years were stunted in 2011.

Nevertheless, as urbanization increases, a rising percentage of stunted children live in urban areas—from 23 percent in 1985 to 31 percent in 2011 (figure 5.4). In 2011, 18 million (uncertainty interval 14 million to 22 million) stunted children lived in urban South Asia

and 15 million (14 million to 16 million) in urban Sub-Saharan Africa.

IMPLICATIONS FOR PRIORITY SETTING

Stunting has received increased attention as a primary indicator of children's nutritional status. It has been included as one of three health status indicators by the

Commission on Information and Accountability for Women's and Children's Health, together with maternal mortality ratios and mortality in children under age five years (WHO 2013). The Scaling-Up Nutrition initiative provides a catalyst for implementing effective nutrition interventions at the population level, and the WHO's target to reduce the number of stunted children provides a goal (World Health Assembly 2012). Other anthropometric indicators, such as wasting and severe wasting, provide complementary information on acute nutritional situations (box 5.1).

Figure 5.3 Contributions of Urban Improvement, Urbanization, and Rural Improvement to Overall Improvements in Mean HAZ, 1985–2011

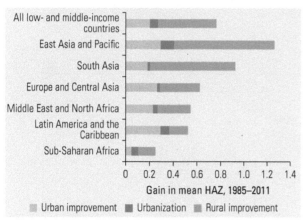

Source: Paciorek and others 2013.
Note: HAZ = height-for-age z-scores.

Stunting prevalence and mean HAZ have improved globally and in most regions, although progress has been uneven in Sub-Saharan Africa. Improvements in HAZ at the national level have generally not been accompanied by reductions in the gap between urban and rural stunting or between stunting in poorer and wealthier populations (Restrepo-Méndez and others 2014). South Asia and Sub-Saharan Africa, the regions with the highest rates of stunting and severe stunting, also have the highest rates of child mortality (UNICEF 2014; WHO 2013). Because children's nutrition, as measured by linear growth, is protective (Olofin and others 2013), it is important to prioritize programs that target these areas.

Children's linear growth is restricted when they do not receive sufficient nutrition (through nonexclusive breastfeeding or inappropriate complementary feeding) or when they lose nutrients during sickness. Both situations have a range of contributing factors. Food insufficiency, poor water and sanitation, and limited access to high-quality primary care are all associated with household and community poverty; all may lead to poor growth outcomes (WHO 2014a). However, interventions such as nutrition education and diarrhea case management can mitigate low height-for-age (Bhutta and others 2008; Bhutta and others 2013).

We previously found that reductions in stunting were consistent with a shift of the entire distribution of HAZ (Stevens and others 2012). This finding implies that, for the past two and a half decades, the primary

Map 5.1 Prevalence of Stunting by Country, 2011

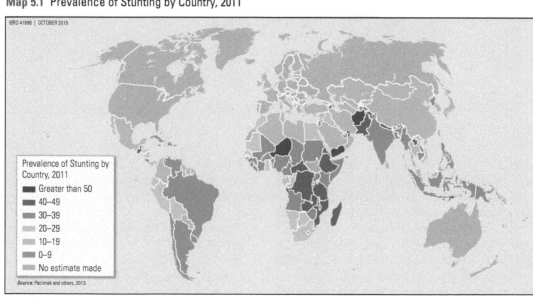

Source: Stevens and others 2012.

Map 5.2 Prevalence of Stunting by Country: Urban Areas, 2011

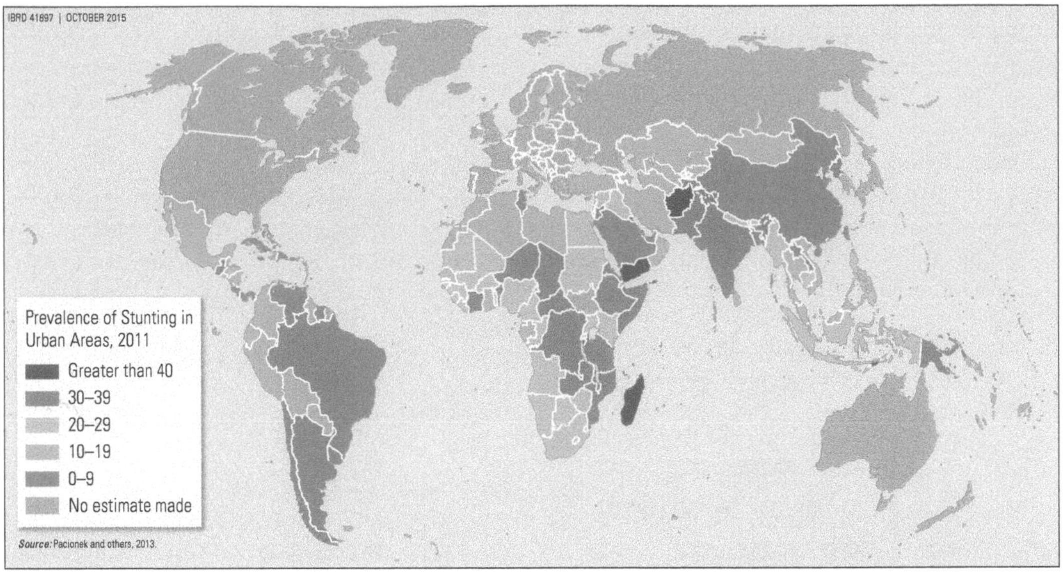

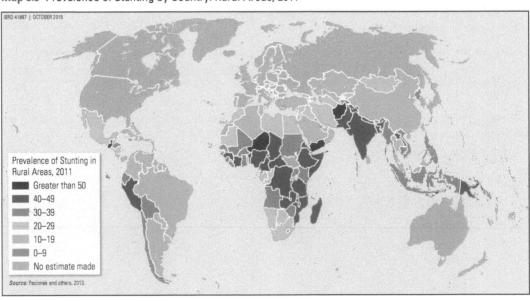

Source: Paciorek and others 2013.

Map 5.3 Prevalence of Stunting by Country: Rural Areas, 2011

Source: Paciorek and others 2013.

mechanism for improvement has been population improvements rather than targeted interventions. These population improvements include enhanced health promotion, such as breastfeeding and complementary feeding; improved environmental and sanitary conditions; increased availability and affordability of nutritious foods; and improved income and education levels. Because the burden of stunting is still largely in rural areas, evaluating potential interventions' expected benefits for rural children is appropriate.

Although the relative importance of various population forces is uncertain, several lessons have emerged from the research:

- Growth in national income seems to have a positive effect on child nutrition but may be insufficient, perhaps because improving nutritional status requires more equitable income distribution and increased investments in health care and nutrition programs (Anand and Ravallion 1993; Haddad and

Figure 5.4 Number of Stunted Children, by Region and Urban or Rural Residence, 1985–2011

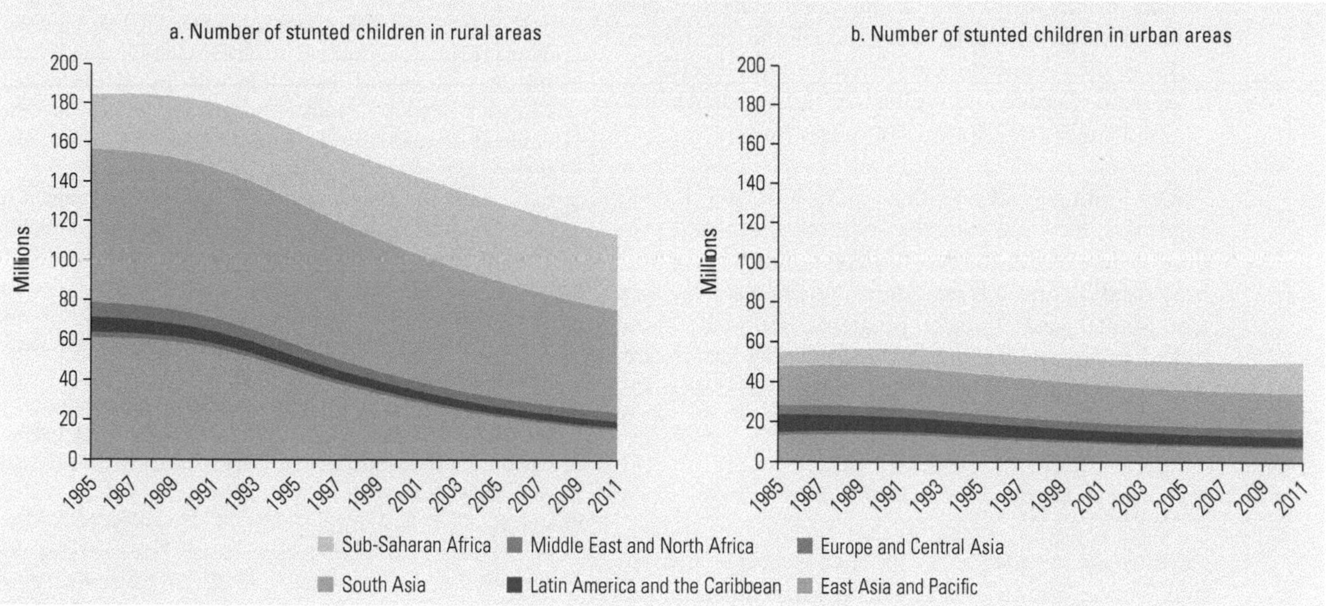

a. Number of stunted children in rural areas

b. Number of stunted children in urban areas

Sub-Saharan Africa Middle East and North Africa Europe and Central Asia

South Asia Latin America and the Caribbean East Asia and Pacific

Source: Paciorek and others 2013.

Box 5.1

Global Patterns in Wasting or Low Weight-for-Height

Child wasting may be caused by acute illness, inappropriate feeding, or insufficient feeding. The World Health Assembly endorsed a target goal of reducing and maintaining childhood wasting to less than 5 percent by 2025 (World Health Assembly 2012). The global prevalence of wasting in 2013 was 7.7 percent (uncertainty interval 6.6 percent to 8.9 percent), and the global prevalence of severe wasting was 2.6 percent (uncertainty interval 2.1 percent to 3.2 percent) (UNICEF, WHO, and World Bank 2014). According to these estimates, the prevalence of wasting and severe wasting were highest in the World Bank regions (in decreasing order) of South Asia, Sub-Saharan Africa, and the Middle East and

North Africa, with estimated regional prevalence of wasting ranging between 15 percent and 7 percent.

Of the 102 countries for which data on severe wasting from 2006 to 2012 were available, 51 had at least one survey with a severe wasting prevalence of 2 percent or higher. Of the 110 countries reporting data on wasting in the same period, 64 reported prevalence of wasting greater than 5 percent in at least one survey. In nine countries—Bangladesh, Benin, Chad, Djibouti, India, Niger, Papua New Guinea, South Sudan, and Timor-Leste—the most recent survey data (excluding data before 2006) indicate a prevalence of wasting greater than 15 percent (WHO 2014b).

---

others 2003; Ravallion 1990; Smith and Haddad 2002; Subramanyam and others 2011).

- Macroeconomic shocks, structural adjustment, and trade policy reforms have been implicated in the worsening nutritional status in Sub-Saharan Africa in the 1980s and 1990s (Cooper Weil and others 1990;

Pongou, Salomon, and Ezzati 2006). The adverse effects on nutrition were greatest in poorer households, especially in rural areas, transmitted through lower household earnings and assets, reduced food subsidies, and reduced health care use (Cooper Weil and others 1990; Pongou, Salomon, and Ezzati 2006).

In contrast, programs that improve income, nutrition, and health care among the poor generally also improve growth outcomes, especially in children of lower socioeconomic status (Bhutta and others 2013; Fernald, Gertler, and Neufeld 2008; Lagarde, Haines, and Palmer 2007; Rivera and others 2004).

These findings indicate that child nutrition is best improved through equitable economic growth, pro-poor primary care, and nutrition programs that support breastfeeding and appropriate complementary feeding. Conditional cash transfer programs, especially those linked to nutrition education and primary health care, offer the potential to help target and deliver these interventions (Bassett 2008).

CONCLUSIONS

Prioritizing improvements in HAZ in rural areas of high-burden countries is an essential component of initiatives to improve child health and nutrition. Achieving this goal may occur through policies that improve households' economic status and food security; provide more equitable access to interventions and services, such as clean water and sanitation; encourage breastfeeding and complementary feeding using local foods; and offer case management of diarrhea and other infectious diseases (Bhutta and others 2013; Sanchez and Swaminathan 2005; WHO 2014a).

A second essential component of improvement initiatives is the development and implementation of complementary policies and programs for children in urban settings. An increasing share of undernourished children live in cities; these children are susceptible to economic shocks that affect food prices and may face different barriers to accessing adequate nutrition than rural children.

NOTES

World Bank Income Classifications as of July 2014 are as follows, based on estimates of gross national income (GNI) per capita for 2013:

- Low-income countries (LICs) = US$1,045 or less
- Middle-income countries (MICs) are subdivided:
  a) lower-middle-income = US$1,046 to US$4,125
  b) upper-middle-income (UMICs) = US$4,126 to US$12,745
- High-income countries (HICs) = US$12,746 or more.

The authors alone are responsible for the views expressed in this chapter and they do not necessarily represent the views, decisions, or policies of the institutions with which they are affiliated.

REFERENCES

Adair, L. S., C. H. Fall, C. Osmond, A. D. Stein, R. Martorell, and others. 2013. "Associations of Linear Growth and Relative Weight Gain during Early Life with Adult Health and Human Capital in Countries of Low and Middle Income: Findings from Five Birth Cohort Studies." *The Lancet* P382 (9891): 525–34.

Anand, S., and M. Ravallion. 1993. "Human Development in Poor Countries: On the Role of Private Incomes and Public Services." *Journal of Economic Perspectives* 7 (1): 133–50.

Bassett, L. 2008. "Can Conditional Cash Transfer Programs Play a Greater Role in Reducing Child Undernutrition?" Social Protection Discussion Paper 0835, World Bank, Washington, DC.

Bhutta, Z. A., T. Ahmed, R. E. Black, S. Cousens, K. Dewey, and others. 2008. "What Works? Interventions for Maternal and Child Undernutrition and Survival." *The Lancet* 371 (9610): 417–40.

Bhutta, Z. A., J. K. Das, A. Rizvi, M. F. Gaffey, N. Walker, and others. 2013. "Evidence-Based Interventions for Improvement of Maternal and Child Nutrition: What Can Be Done and at What Cost?" *The Lancet* 382 (9890): 452–77.

Black, R. E., C. G. Victora, S. P. Walker, Z. A. Bhutta, P. Christian, and others. 2013. "Maternal and Child Undernutrition and Overweight in Low-Income and Middle-Income Countries." *The Lancet* 382 (9890): 427–51.

Cooper Weil, D., A. Alicbusan, J. Wilson, M. Reich, and D. Bradley. 1990. *The Impact of Development Policies on Health: A Review of the Literature.* Geneva: World Health Organization.

de Onis, M., and M. Blossner. 2003. "The World Health Organization Global Database on Child Growth and Malnutrition: Methodology and Applications." *International Journal of Epidemiology* 32 (4): 518–26.

Fernald, L. C., P. J. Gertler, and L. M. Neufeld. 2008. "Role of Cash in Conditional Cash Transfer Programmes for Child Health, Growth, and Development: An Analysis of Mexico's Oportunidades." *The Lancet* 371 (9615): 828–37.

Grantham-McGregor, S., Y. B. Cheung, S. Cueto, P. Glewwe, L. Richter, and others. 2007. "Developmental Potential in the First 5 Years for Children in Developing Countries." *The Lancet* 369 (9555): 60–70.

Haddad, L., H. Alderman, S. Appleton, L. Song, and Y. Yohannes. 2003. "Reducing Child Malnutrition: How Far Does Income Growth Take Us?" *World Bank Economic Review* 17 (1): 107–31.

Lagarde, M., A. Haines, and N. Palmer. 2007. "Conditional Cash Transfers for Improving Uptake of Health Interventions in Low- and Middle-Income Countries: A Systematic Review." *Journal of the American Medical Association* 298 (16): 1900–10.

Olofin, I., C. M. McDonald, M. Ezzati, S. Flaxman, R. E. Black, and others. 2013. "Associations of Suboptimal Growth with All-Cause and Cause-Specific Mortality in Children under Five Years: A Pooled Analysis of Ten Prospective Studies." *PLoS One* 8 (5): e6636.

Paciorek, C. J., G. A. Stevens, M. L. Finucane, and M. Ezzati. 2013. "Children's Height and Weight in Rural and Urban Populations in Low-Income and Middle-Income Countries: A Systematic Review." *The Lancet Global Health* 1 (5): e300–e309.

Pongou, R., J. A. Salomon, and M. Ezzati. 2006. "Health Impacts of Macroeconomic Crises and Policies: Determinants of Variation in Childhood Malnutrition Trends in Cameroon." *International Journal of Epidemiology* 35 (3): 648–56.

Ravallion, M. 1990. "Income Effects on Undernutrition." *Economic Development and Cultural Change* 38 (3): 489–515.

Restrepo-Méndez, M. C., A. J. D. Barros, R. E. Black, and C. G. Victora. 2014. "Time Trends in Socio-Economic Inequalities in Stunting Prevalence: Analyses of Repeated National Surveys." *Public Health Nutrition* 18 (12) 2097–104. doi:10.1017/S1368980014002924.

Rivera, J. A., D. Sotres-Alvarez, J. P. Habicht, T. Shamah, and S. Villalpando. 2004. "Impact of the Mexican Program for Education, Health, and Nutrition (Progresa) on Rates of Growth and Anemia in Infants and Young Children: A Randomized Effectiveness Study." *Journal of the American Medical Association* 291 (21): 2563–70.

Sanchez, P. A., and M. S. Swaminathan. 2005. "Hunger in Africa: The Link between Unhealthy People and Unhealthy Soils." *The Lancet* 365 (9457): 442–44.

Smith, L. C., and L. Haddad. 2002. "How Potent Is Economic Growth in Reducing Undernutrition? What Are the Pathways of Impact? New Cross-Country Evidence." *Economic Development and Cultural Change* 51 (1): 55–76.

Stevens, G. A., M. M. Finucane, C. J. Paciorek, S. R. Flaxman, R. A. White, and others. 2012. "Trends in Mild, Moderate, and Severe Stunting and Underweight, and Progress towards MDG 1 in 141 Developing Countries: A Systematic Analysis of Population Representative Data." *The Lancet* 380 (9844): 824–34.

Subramanyam, M. A., I. Kawachi, L. F. Berkman, and S. V. Subramanian. 2011. "Is Economic Growth Associated with Reduction in Child Undernutrition in India?" *PLoS Medicine* 8 (3): e1000424.

UNICEF (United Nations Children's Fund). 2014. *Levels and Trends in Child Mortality.* New York: UNICEF.

UNICEF, WHO, and World Bank. 2012. *UNICEF-WHO-World Bank Joint Child Malnutrition Estimates.* Geneva: WHO.

———. 2014. *UNICEF-WHO-The World Bank: 2013 Joint Child Malnutrition Estimates: Levels and Trends.* Geneva: WHO. http://www.who.int/nutgrowthdb/estimates2013/en/.

WHO (World Health Organization). 2006. *WHO Child Growth Standards Length/Height-for-Age, Weight-for-Age, Weight-for-Length, Weight-for-Height and Body Mass Index-for-Age: Methods and Development.* Geneva: WHO.

———. 2013. *Global Health Observatory: Health Equity Monitor.* Geneva: WHO.

———. 2014a. "Global Nutrition Targets 2025: Stunting Policy Brief." WHO/NMH/NHD/14.3, WHO, Geneva.

———. 2014b. *World Health Statistics 2014.* Geneva: WHO.

World Health Assembly. 2012. "Comprehensive Implementation Plan on Maternal, Infant and Young Child Nutrition." World Health Organization, Geneva.

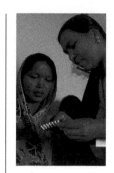

Chapter 6

Interventions to Improve Reproductive Health

John Stover, Karen Hardee, Bella Ganatra, Claudia García
Moreno, and Susan Horton

INTRODUCTION

Health systems and individuals can take a number of
actions to safeguard reproductive health. These actions
differ from many other health interventions in that the
motivation for their use is not necessarily limited to
better health and involves cultural and societal norms.
Irrespective of these additional considerations, these
interventions have important health implications. This
chapter describes four areas of intervention:

- Family planning
- Adolescent sexual and reproductive health
- Unsafe abortion
- Violence against women.

Each of these areas involves the delivery of specific
health services to prevent or alleviate health risks; each
also involves the complex social and cultural issues that
affect the widespread implementation and use of the
services.

FAMILY PLANNING

Rationales for Family Planning Programs

Family planning has been a major development success
over the past half century, with global fertility rates falling from more than six children per woman during her
lifetime in the 1960s to less than three children in the

1990s. Family planning offers a range of potential benefits that encompass economic development, maternal
and child health, education, and women's empowerment
(Bongaarts and others 2012). Furthermore, family planning is cost-effective. The United Nations (UN) estimates
that for every US$1 spent on family planning, from US$2
to US$6 can be saved from the reduced numbers of peo-
ple needing other public services, such as immunizations,
health care, education, and sanitation (UN Population
Division 2009).

Support for voluntary family planning has been
based on several rationales, including the following
(Habumuremyi and Zenawi 2012):

- Population and development, the so-called demo-
  graphic rationale
- Maternal and child health
- Human rights and equity
- Environment and sustainable development.

Demographic Rationale

The population and development rationale for family
planning emerged in the 1960s amid a concern that rates
of rapid population growth would hinder economic
growth in low- and middle-income countries (LMICs)
and affect the ability of these countries to improve the
well-being of their citizens. This rationale has been
in and out of favor (Birdsall, Kelly, and Sinding 2001;
Bongaarts and others 2012; NAS 1986). Recent evidence

Corresponding author: John Stover, Vice President and founder of Avenir Health, Glastonbury, Connecticut, United States, JStover@avenirhealth.org.

shows positive links between slower population growth and economic development—at least in the initial phase of the demographic transition, when countries enjoy a demographic dividend, if other economic and human capital policies are in place. The demographic dividend allows countries to take advantage of a beneficial dependency ratio between the working-age population and the groups who need support, that is, children and the elderly (Bloom, Canning, and Sevilla 2003). It is important to have supportive economic policies and labor regulations in place to reap the potential benefits of the demographic dividend; many countries in Sub-Saharan Africa need to coordinate development of their economic and reproductive health policies to fully realize this effect.

Maternal and Child Health Rationale

The improved health of mothers and children has long been a rationale for the provision of family planning (Seltzer 2002). In the 2009 round of the Family Planning Effort Index, measured periodically since 1972, women's health was the dominant justification for family planning programs, followed by reducing unwanted fertility (Ross and Smith 2011). These reasons ranked higher than fertility reduction, economic development, and reduction of childbearing among unmarried youth. Contraception can serve as an effective primary prevention strategy in LMICs to reduce maternal mortality (Ahmed and others 2012). By one estimate, increases in contraceptive use from 1990 to 2008 contributed to 1.7 million fewer maternal deaths (Ross and Blanc 2012). Reductions in fertility rates accounted for 53 percent of the decline in maternal deaths; lower maternal mortality rates per birth accounted for 47 percent of the decline (Ross and Blanc 2012).

Family planning can have significant effects on the health of children. Analysis of data from Demographic and Health Surveys (DHS) from 52 countries showed that children born within two years of a previous birth have a 60 percent increased risk of infant death, and those within two to three years have a 10 percent increased risk of infant death, compared with children born after an interval of three or more years from the last sibling (Rutstein and others 2008). These analyses have confirmed the usefulness of program initiatives to promote healthy timing and spacing of births.

Human Rights and Equity Rationale

The right of couples and individuals to decide freely and responsibly on the number and spacing of their children was articulated at the 1968 International Conference on Human Rights (UN 1968). Subsequent international population conferences in 1974, 1984, and 1994 reaffirmed this right (Singh 2009).

The human rights rationale has focused on sexual reproductive health and rights, with family planning implicitly included. Efforts are underway to more explicitly define a rights-based approach to implementing voluntary family planning programming (Hardee and others 2014). Ensuring equity is a fundamental principal of human rights–based programming. Wealth quintiles analysis has shown that wealthier women have lower fertility rates and better access to family planning than poorer women. Gillespie and others (2007), in a study of 41 countries, find that although variations were observed among countries, the number of unwanted births in the poorest quintile was more than twice that in the wealthiest quintile, at 1.2 and 0.5, respectively.

Environment and Sustainable Development Rationale

A resurgence of interest in global population dynamics is linked to growing attention to environmental issues, climate change, and concerns about food security (Engelman 1997; Jiang and Hardee 2011; Martine and Schensul 2013; Moreland and Smith 2012; Royal Society 2012). Although global population growth is slowing, the momentum built into past population trends means that the world's population will continue to grow. The world's population surpassed 7 billion in 2012; the 2013 UN Population Division projection estimates that it could grow to 9.6 billion by the middle of the century and level off at about 10.9 billion by the end of the century under their low scenario, or it could grow to more than 16 billion by the end of the century under their high scenario. According to the United Nations Population Fund (UNFPA), "Whether future demographic trends work for or against sustainable development will depend on policies that are put in place today" (UNFPA 2013, 5). If the unmet need for family planning services were satisfied in all countries, world population growth would fall between the UN's low and medium projections (Moreland, Smith, and Sharma 2010).

Health Consequences of High Fertility

High fertility affects the health of mothers and children in several ways. Unwanted pregnancies may lead to unsafe abortions, which are associated with elevated risks of maternal mortality. All births carry some risk of maternal mortality, so women with a large number of births have higher lifetime risk of dying from maternal causes. The World Health Organization's (WHO's) Global Health Estimates reports that there were 303,000 maternal deaths in 2015; 300,000 of these deaths occurred in LMICs (WHO 2015). The maternal mortality ratio

(MMR) in LMICs averages about 242 maternal deaths per 100,000 live births. At that rate, a woman with seven births has a 2 percent chance of dying from maternal causes, compared with 0.5 percent for a woman with two births. In Sub-Saharan Africa, where the MMR is 546, the risk of death increases to almost 5 percent for a women with seven births (WHO 2014a, 2014b, 2015).

The risk of maternal mortality is particularly high for older women; it is typically two to three times higher for women over age 40 years who give birth than for those ages 35–39 years (Blanc, Winfrey, and Ross 2013). High-parity births (fourth and higher births) may also carry an increased risk. Family planning can reduce maternal mortality by reducing the number of times a woman is exposed to the risk and by helping women avoid high-risk births. From 1990 to 2005, family planning may have averted more than 1.5 million maternal deaths through lower fertility rates and reductions in the MMR due to fewer high-parity births to older women (Stover and Ross 2009).

Family planning also influences child survival rates. Child mortality rates are generally higher for high-risk births, typically defined as births of order four (a woman's fourth birth) and above, births occurring less than 24 months after a previous birth, and births to mothers who are less than age 18 years or more than age 35 years. Short birth intervals, young age of mother at birth, and parity greater than three are associated with greater chances of births that are preterm, low birth weight, and small for gestational age (Kozuki, Lee, Silveira, Sania, and others 2013; Kozuki, Lee, Silveira, Victora, and others 2013). DHS data show the risk of child mortality by birth characteristic. Mortality rates are about 50 percent higher for closely spaced births and births to mothers under age 18 years. The largest effects occur when multiple risk factors are combined. Mortality increases by 150 percent to 300 percent for births with short intervals to very young mothers and those with high parity and short birth intervals. Family planning affects the distribution of births by risk factor. On average, the percentage of births with any one of these avoidable risk factors drops from about 73 percent when the national total fertility rate is greater than seven to 25 percent at a total fertility rate of less than two. As figure 6.1 shows, the greatest change from a high to a low total fertility rate is in the proportion of births that are high parity and have multiple risk factors.

Contraceptive Methods

A wide variety of contraceptive methods are available to women and men (table 6.1). These include permanent methods, that is, female and male sterilization, for couples who know that they do not want any more children; long-acting reversible contraceptives (such as intrauterine devices [IUDs], implants, and injections) for couples who do not want more children in the near term but may want more later; temporary methods (such as oral contraceptives and condoms) that provide short-term protection; and nonmedical methods (such as fertility awareness methods, lactational amenorrhea, and withdrawal) for couples who do not want to use a contraceptive agent or device or who do not have access to them.

Women and men report a number of factors that are important to them in choosing methods (WHO 1997). Among the key factors that allow potential users to match contraceptive methods to their needs are effectiveness, duration of effectiveness, and reversibility. Other major considerations include side effects, ease of use, ability to hide use from a partner, and familiarity with the method. Some women are also concerned about whether the method regulates menstruation or causes amenorrhea.

Although the number of approved methods is quite large, in practice couples in most countries have limited options. Ross and Stover (2013) analyze data from the Family Planning Effort Index scores to show the number of methods available over time in 80 countries. The Family Planning Effort Index measures, among other things, the percentage of the population that has ready and easy access to contraceptive methods (Ross and Smith 2011). If a method is considered to be available when more than 50 percent of the population has access, then potential users had access to 3.5 methods in 2009, up from 2 methods in 1982.

Globally, female sterilization is used by the largest share of couples (figure 6.2) and dominates the method mix in Asia, Latin America and the Caribbean, and North America. The second most popular method is the IUD, which has the largest share of users in Asia. Oral contraceptives have a significant share of users in most regions, except Asia. The highest share for injectables is in Latin America and the Caribbean and in Sub-Saharan Africa.

Although cost and demand play roles in determining method availability, the most important factors affecting availability in many settings are religious and cultural factors and program factors. Figure 6.3 shows the wide variation in method mix across a selection of countries with total contraceptive prevalence between 45 percent and 75 percent. In Bangladesh, Morocco, and Zimbabwe, oral contraceptives account for 50 percent or more of all contraceptive use; in Brazil and India, sterilization is the preferred option. In the Arab Republic of Egypt and other Muslim countries, the IUD is the most popular form of long-acting contraceptive.

Figure 6.1 Distribution of Births by Risk Factor by Total Fertility Rate

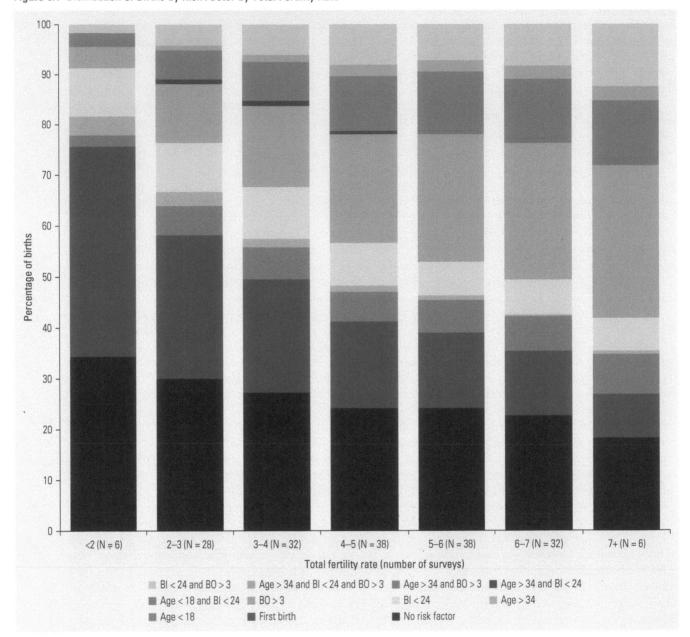

Source: Demographic and Health Surveys from 1980 to 2012.
Note: Age = mother's age at time of birth; BI = birth interval; BO = birth order.

The method mix in Kenya has evolved, and injectables are now the most popular form of contraception. In Turkey and Ukraine, for example, withdrawal and condoms are used most often; high rates of abortion compensate for the lower effectiveness of these methods (UN Population Division 2013b). In countries with limited access to health clinics, community-based distribution (CBD) and social marketing are used to reach a large portion of the population, resulting in greater reliance on methods appropriate for those delivery channels, such as oral contraceptives, injectables, and condoms. In countries with higher access to medical providers, physician-supplied methods, such as IUDs, may be preferred.

More than 180 new contraceptive methods are in various stages of research and development (http://pipeline.ctiexchange.org/products/table).

Table 6.1 Contraceptive Methods

Method	Types	Duration	Effectiveness[a] (percent)	CYP factor
Sterilization	Female sterilization	Permanent	99	10–13 per sterilization
	Male sterilization	Permanent	99	10–13 per sterilization
Implants	Implanon	3 years	99	2.5 per implant
	Sino-Implant	4 years	99	3.2 per implant
	Jadelle	5 years	99	3.8 per implant
Intrauterine devices	Copper-T-380A	10 years	99	4.6 per insertion
	Levonorgestrel-releasing intrauterine device	5 years	99	3.3 per insertion
Injectables	Depo-Provera	3 months	93	4 injections per CYP
	Noristerat	2 months	93	6 injections per CYP
	Cyclofem	1 month	93	13 injections per CYP
Oral contraceptives	Many brands	One month per cycle	90	15 cycles per CYP
Condoms	Male	One sex act	79	120 units per CYP
	Female	One sex act	75	120 units per CYP
Spermicides	Vaginal foaming tablets	One sex act	67	120 tablets per CYP
Emergency contraception		One unprotected sex act	75	20 doses per CYP
Monthly vaginal ring or patch		One month	90	15 units per CYP
Diaphragm		One sex act	88	—
Lactational amenorrhea		6 months	99	4 active users per CYP
Fertility-awareness methods	Standard days, Two Day Ovulation, Symptothermal	One sex act	72	1.5 CYP per trained adopter
Withdrawal		One sex act	75	—

Source: USAID: http://www.usaid.gov/what-we-do/global-health/family-planning/couple-years-protection-cyp.
Note: — = not available; CYP = couple-years of protection.
a. Effectiveness estimates are drawn from Trussel (2011).

Although many will never reach the market, some have the potential to address current barriers to use for some users. Several new methods that may address some limitations in current methods are becoming available. Sino-implant (II), a subdermal contraceptive implant consisting of two silicone rods with 75 milligrams of levonorgestrel, provides four years of protection. Although similar to other implants already on the market, Sino-implant (II) is considerably less expensive and could potentially expand the availability of implants. It is registered for use in about 20 countries. Sayana Press, an injectable contraceptive (Depo-Provera) with a duration of three month, is packaged in a Uniject system that allows subcutaneous injection. The main advantage of this system is that field workers can easily administer it without the need for users to visit clinics. It is expected to appeal to programs that rely on community workers to reach large numbers of users. In the longer term, it may even be labeled for self-injection.

Organization of Family Planning Programs

Global Initiatives

Family planning programming has been guided by global initiatives for decades, including through decennial population conferences in 1974 in Bucharest, 1984 in Mexico City, and 1994 in Cairo, as well as global frameworks, including the 2000 Millennium Development Goals (MDGs). The twentieth anniversary of the 1994 International Conference on Population and Development (ICPD) has passed, and the UN recently adopted the post-2015 development agenda. The ICPD positioned family planning within a broad context of

Figure 6.2 Global Distribution of Contraceptive Methods, 2012

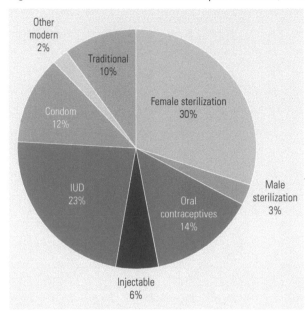

Source: Biddlecom and Kantorova 2013.
Note: IUD = intrauterine device.

reproductive health and human rights. Both the ICPD and the SDGs now include targets and indicators related to universal access to reproductive health. Attention to shortages of contraceptives led to the 2001 Istanbul conference, "Meeting the Reproductive Health Challenge: Securing Contraceptives, and Condoms for HIV/AIDS Prevention," which resulted in the establishment of the Reproductive Health Supplies Coalition (http://www.rhsupplies.com).

In 2010 the UN Secretary General launched Every Woman Every Child, a global effort to provide catalytic support to achieve MDGs 4, 5, and 6 by 2015 (http://www.everywomaneverychild.org/about). The Ouagadougou Declaration, to which eight West African countries agreed in 2011, called for countries to accelerate the implementation of national strategies for reproductive health and family planning and to address the unmet needs of populations (FP Ouagadougou Partnership 2014). The 2012 London Summit on Family Planning resulted in pledges of resources to reach an additional 120 million new users with voluntary family planning services by 2020 (Bill & Melinda Gates Foundation and DFID 2012).

Figure 6.3 Share of Contraceptive Users by Method, Selected Countries

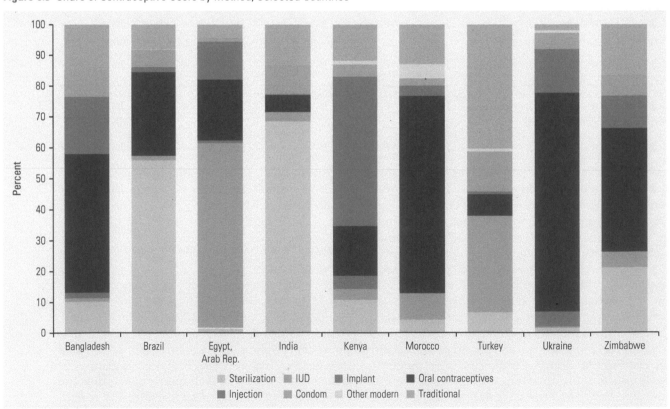

Source: Demographic and Health Surveys, latest available survey for each country.
Note: IUD = intrauterine device.

Services Delivery

Family planning is delivered through a variety of programs and services. In 2011, 91 percent of governments in LMICs surveyed by the UN reported that they provide direct support for family planning, an increase from 64 percent in 1976 (UN 2011). Currently, a focus on total market approaches includes all service modalities—public, private, and nongovernmental organizations—to expand the reach of family planning services and meet the needs of the diverse clientele across countries (Barnes, Vail, and Crosby 2012). Initiatives to identify the ingredients of successful family planning programs (Richey and Salem 2008) and high-impact practices in family planning (www.fphighimpactpractices.org/), and approaches to scaling up services and ensuring equitable access (Amadou and others 2013; Simmons and Shiffman 2007), are shaping service delivery programming. Scaling-up approaches include task-shifting (Janowitz, Stanback, and Boyer 2012) and innovative financing schemes.

Public, nongovernmental, and commercial providers. Funding for public family planning programs comes from a variety of sources. Many middle-income countries fund contraceptive services, along with all other health services, out of tax revenues. Low-income countries often rely on donor funding for commodities, training, research, policy reform, evaluation, and service delivery outside the health facility. Donors that have supported family planning programs include bilateral donors such as the United States Agency for International Development and the U.K. Department for International Development; multilateral donors such as the United Nations Population Fund; and foundations such as the Bill & Melinda Gates Foundation. This support usually takes the form of commodities and funding of nongovernmental organizations to provide specific services. Many LMICs have provided line items in their budgets for family planning commodities. Even in low-income countries, national governments provide most of the funds for infrastructure and personnel.

Integration with other sectors. Family planning services are usually integrated with other health services. Activities for outreach, advocacy, the building of political commitment, and resource mobilization are often integrated with other development priorities, such as HIV prevention and treatment, child immunization, and environmental protection.

Community-based programming. Community-based programming has been part of family planning programs since the 1970s. CBD was designed to extend the reach of clinics to serve clients who were unable to travel to clinics or who did not know about clinic services for family planning. CBD programs focused on rural areas and trained community members to provide family planning information and selected resupply methods. Under various names, including *community-based distributor, community health worker,* and *health extension worker,* this cadre of staff has delivered information and selected services to families' doorsteps, providing access for women with limited mobility and those at a distance from clinical services. These workers, for example, the Accredited Social Health Activists in India, at times accompany clients to health facilities for clinical methods of contraception.

A review of the evidence shows that CBD has increased access to and use of contraception in Sub-Saharan Africa (Phillips, Greene, and Jackson 1999). Bongaarts and others (2012) report that CBD resulted in increases in contraceptive acceptance and use on the order of 15 percent to 25 percent. In Bangladesh, the Matlab program achieved a 25 percent reduction in fertility during an eight-year period among women who were visited every two weeks by trained community health workers (Koenig and others 1987). A study in Madagascar finds that individuals who had direct communication with community health workers were 10 times more likely to use contraceptives than individuals who did not (Stoebenau and Valente 2003). Community-based health workers have successfully reached underserved populations, including unmarried women, those with less supportive husbands, and indigenous women (Malarcher and others 2011; Prata and others 2005).

Community-based programming is considered to be a high-impact practice in family planning (HIP 2012), and interest is growing. To rapidly scale up access to a range of public health services, including family planning, Ethiopia in 2003 began to deploy more than 30,000 health extension workers at the community level. Ethiopia's health extension workers are partially credited with achieving that country's rapid increase in its contraceptive prevalence rate, from 13.9 percent in 2005 to 27.3 percent in 2011 (USAID/Africa Bureau and others 2013).

Social marketing. Social marketing has been part of family planning programming since the 1960s, when it was first used to link social good with marketing approaches to raise awareness and promote condom use (Chandy and others 1965). Social marketing combines the "4Ps" of marketing—product, price, place, and promotion—to increase use by population groups. Social marketing in family planning programs makes contraceptive products accessible and affordable through private-sector outlets, most notably, pharmacies and shops, while using commercial marketing techniques to achieve behavioral change goals (HIP 2012).

Using a variety of models, family planning social marketing has been used most widely to promote condoms and oral contraceptives, with strong evidence of impact (Chapman and Astatke 2003; Madhavan and Bishai 2010; Sweat and others 2012). It has also been used to promote injectables, emergency contraception, and the Standard Days Method (CycleBeads®). In 1990, social marketing contributed an estimated 7.4 million couple-year protection (CYP), growing to 23.4 million in 2000 and 53.4 million in 2010 (DKT International 2011), more than a sevenfold increase during the 20-year time span.

Social franchising. Social franchising has been used to increase the share of the private commercial sector in family planning. From the first social franchises for family planning that Sangini started in Nepal in 1994 and Greenstar in Pakistan in 1995, the use of this approach has grown globally and includes PROSALUD in Bolivia and Blue Star in Ghana. An extension of social marketing, social franchises use the same techniques as commercial franchises—standardized, high-quality services, offered by trained providers under a franchise name.

Social franchising for family planning supports fee-based provision of a range of clinical contraceptive methods and broader reproductive health services. Fees can be paid with cash, vouchers, or other mechanisms. An analysis of the effect of social franchising on contraceptive use in four countries finds that "franchising has a positive association with both general and family planning client volumes, and the number of family planning brands available," with client satisfaction varying across settings (Stephenson and others 2004, 2053). A 2010 assessment of evaluations of social franchising concludes that the studies demonstrate strong evidence that social franchising increases the uptake of family planning services, and moderate evidence that it increases use by poor populations (Madhavan and Bishai 2010).

Mobile services. Mobile services have been used to extend access to long-acting and permanent contraceptive methods to remote populations using trained providers (Bakamjian 2008). A 2010 evaluation of mobile outreach services operated by Marie Stopes International in Ethiopia, Myanmar, Pakistan, Sierra Leone, and Vietnam to provide IUDs and implants finds that women were generally satisfied with the services, would use the mobile services again, and would recommend the services to others (Eva and Ngo 2010). In Nepal, mobile services are a key component of the government's program to reach remote areas. Government-run mobile clinics provide 20 percent of voluntary female sterilization procedures

and more than 33 percent of voluntary male sterilization procedures (Ministry of Health and Population [Nepal], New ERA, and Macro International Inc. 2012). For mobile services to provide optimal care, it is important that adequate follow-up care be available.

mHealth. Family planning programming has made use of a range of media, including radio and television, to raise awareness and spread messages about services (Bertrand and others 2006). These conventional uses of information and communication technologies are being supplemented by use of wireless technology, most notably cell phones. mHealth is reaching clients with information and financing mechanisms and measures to strengthen services, including providing training and support to health workers, addressing commodity logistics, and monitoring and evaluation. These mHealth initiatives are building on the rapidly growing use of wireless technology. A 2012 review of information and communication technologies for family planning and reproductive health noted that such initiatives "range from using SMS [short message service] and text messages to give information on family planning methods to women mobile users; to wireless solutions that update and connect rural health workers to web-based distance learning programs; to mobile phones and PC [personal computer] solutions that help to manage health data, drug supplies, patient medical records, and the health workforce" (AIDSTAR-Two 2012, 32). mHealth initiatives are relatively new, and few have been well evaluated; most are in pilot phases, with little current evidence of scale up.

Results-based financing. Use of results-based financing, known by many names, including *performance-based financing* and *performance-based incentives*, is a rising trend in health programming. Given the history of misuse of incentive payments in family planning (Norman 2013), careful consideration of which aspects of performance are to be rewarded is critical. Performance payments that focus on improving access to family planning services and reducing financial and other barriers are appropriate. For example, reasonable reimbursement to compensate for the costs of obtaining a voluntary sterilization are allowable. However, paying clients to accept contraception or to accept certain methods are not. Similarly, offering incentives to providers to achieve target numbers of users or specific methods is not condoned (Eichler and others 2010).

Vouchers. Performance-based financing for family planning has included vouchers for services and conditional cash transfers. Vouchers can increase access for poor and marginalized populations to specific reproductive services and products at qualified outlets at subsidized prices (Bongaarts and others 2012). A systematic review of the evidence on vouchers in LMICs finds 13 programs that fit the systematic review criteria; of these, all evaluations reported positive findings, indicating that voucher programs increased the use of reproductive health services, improved quality of care, and improved population health outcomes (Bellows, Bellows, and Warren 2011). However, most voucher programs are small, and additional research is needed to evaluate their impact.

Conditional cash transfers. Conditional cash transfer (CCT) programs can include family planning, although such programs should not make contraceptive use a condition for acceptance into the program. CCTs are relatively new and require more research on their effects on family planning decision making. For example, Brazil's Bolsa Família CCT, which reaches 12 million families with payments going through women, resulted in significantly increased women's decision-making power related to contraception but only in urban areas (De Brauw and others 2013). In Mexico's Oportunidades program, contraceptive use increased more among the beneficiaries in communities with the CCT program, compared with women in communities in which the program had not been initiated (Feldman and others 2009). Nicaragua's CCT, Red de Protección Social, is credited with increasing birth spacing among beneficiaries (Todd, Winters, and Stecklov 2010).

Cost-Effectiveness of Family Planning

A systematic literature search identified seven studies on cost-effectiveness of contraceptives published since 2000; one additional study was obtained from a supplemental search adding the term "couple-year protection" as an economic term. The literature on cost-effectiveness of family planning is well established, given that lending and aid for family planning has been available since at least the 1970s. Recent studies focus on the cost-effectiveness of extending benefits to underserved countries and on newer family planning methods.

Four studies use cost per life-year saved, examining primarily the benefits to the mother's health from pregnancies averted; the other four use cost per CYP. The four studies focusing on mother's health (Afghanistan, India, and two from Nigeria; see Horton, Wu, and Brouwer 2015) conclude that modern contraceptives are very cost-effective in that cost per life-year saved was less than per capita gross domestic product (GDP).

The four studies using CYP as an outcome examined somewhat disparate policies. Seamans and Harner-Jay (2007) conclude that using more modern methods of vasectomy compared with older methods reduced the cost per CYP in three countries, provided that clinics do a large enough volume of procedures to maintain quality. Abbas, Khan, and Khan (2013); Nakhaee and others (2002); and Onwujekwe and others (2013) examine the expansion of modern contraceptive use in countries with limited access. Abbas, Khan, and Khan (2013) conclude that the public services in Pakistan are high cost per CYP compared with other countries; Nakhaee and others (2002) rank the cost effectiveness of various methods for the Islamic Republic of Iran; and Onwujekwe and others (2013) conclude that willingness to pay exceeds costs for methods other than female condoms in Nigeria.

ADOLESCENT SEXUAL AND REPRODUCTIVE HEALTH

The public health outcomes of adolescent pregnancy are profound. Adolescents ages 15–19 years are twice as likely to die during pregnancy and childbirth than women older than age 20 years; those under age 15 years are five times more likely to die during pregnancy or childbirth (WHO 2011). Complications of pregnancy and childbirth are the leading cause of death for adolescent girls ages 15–19 years in LMICs. Adolescents undergo an estimated 3.2 million unsafe abortions every year (UNFPA 2013). The social outcomes of adolescent pregnancy are also profound, with girls' potential remaining unfulfilled and their basic human rights denied (Hindon and Fatusi 2009; UNFPA 2013; WHO 2011).

Programming for Adolescents

Providing adolescents with the means to attain high standards of health, in ways that ensure equality, nondiscrimination, privacy, and confidentiality, is an integral part of respecting and protecting globally accepted human rights (Ringheim 2007; UNFPA 2012). Ensuring that adolescents have access to sexual and reproductive health services requires extending the availability, accessibility, acceptability, and quality of the information and the services (Hardee and others 2013). Helping adolescents make a healthy transition to adulthood involves programs to protect them from unintended pregnancy, sexually transmitted infections (STIs), and poor reproductive health outcomes. These programs can enable young people to delay sexual activity, to protect themselves from pregnancy and STIs once they do initiate sexual activity, and to ensure that sex is not coerced.

The range of interventions suggested include strengthening the enabling environment, and providing information and services and support programs to build resilience and assets.

Enabling Environment

Provide legal protection. Although the need for strong legal protection for adolescents is clear, few interventions have been documented or evaluated. Still, laws protecting against child marriage and against rape and other forms of gender-based violence clearly need to be developed and implemented (Lee-Rife and others 2012; WHO 2011). Laws requiring parental consent for adolescents to access HIV testing discourage adolescents from knowing their HIV status and accessing treatment in a timely fashion.

Reduce gender-inequitable norms and violence. Norms about acceptable behavior for males and females strongly influence the socialization of children and adolescents; gender disparities become more evident as children near adolescence (UNICEF 2011). Gender norms tend to dictate that girls should be sexually submissive, while boys should be sexually adventurous; these norms promote the acceptance of gender-based violence, place girls at risk of unintended pregnancy, and put both girls and boys at risk for HIV (Gay and others 2011). Gender norms that accept gender-based violence are harmful to the lives and reproductive health of adolescents.

Keep girls and boys in school. Staying in school provides a protective effect. Girls who stay in school are less likely to become pregnant, less likely to marry at a young age (Lloyd and Young 2009; UNFPA 2013), and more likely to use contraception. Staying in school also provides a protective effect against HIV acquisition (Bradley and others 2007; Hargreaves and others 2008). Interventions to abolish school fees have enabled adolescents to attend or to stay in school (Burns, Mingat, and Rakotomalala 2003; Deininger 2003; UNICEF 2005; World Bank and UNICEF 2009).

CCTs show the potential to enable girls to stay in school (Baird and others 2012), but context is important. Recent studies in South Africa show an effect of cash transfers on herpes simplex virus type 2 (HSV-2) but no effect on HIV incidence (Karim and others 2015; Pettifor and others 2015). Community-based programming (CBP) to encourage girls to stay in school can also be effective (Erulkar and Muthengi 2009).

Information and Services

Offer age-appropriate comprehensive sex education. Ensuring that young people have the appropriate information to plan to protect themselves—before their first sexual experience—is vitally important.

As the late Doug Kirby stated, young people around the world are seeking access to reliable information on reproductive health and answers for their questions and concerns about sexuality. "They need information not only about physiology and a better understanding of the norms that society has set for sexual behavior, but they also need to acquire the skills necessary to develop healthy relationships and engage in responsible decision-making about sex, especially during adolescence when their emotional development accelerates" (Kirby 2011).

Evidence shows that comprehensive sex education with specific characteristics regarding content and pedagogy, taught by trained teachers, can affect behavior, including delaying sexual debut, decreasing number of sexual partners, and increasing the use of condoms or other contraceptives (Grunseit and others 1997; Mavedzenge, Doyle, and Ross 2011; UNESCO 2009). It is important to include a discussion of gender norms that can put both male and female adolescents at risk (Barker and others 2010; Pulerwitz and others 2006).

Use mass media. Multiple mass media approaches have been used to inform adolescents about sexual and reproductive health issues, particularly AIDS and HIV (UNFPA 2013). Evaluated media approaches include entertainment-education, social marketing, and media channels (television, radio, magazines, and the Internet) (Gurman and Underwood 2008). Newer social media approaches are promising, but their effects have yet to be evaluated.

A systematic review of the effectiveness of 24 mass media interventions on HIV-related knowledge, attitudes, and behaviors finds that such programs generally produced small to moderate changes (Bertrand and others 2006). Outcomes included increased knowledge and behavioral changes, such as reduction in high-risk behavior, increased communication, and increased condom use. A similar review by Gurman and Underwood (2008), which focuses specifically on media interventions for adolescents, finds similar outcomes, although the review highlights the paucity of results in the literature pertaining to gender-specific and youth-focused interventions.

Gurman and Underwood (2008) offer four lessons from their review:

- Ensure that the intervention is appropriate for the intended audience.
- Design interventions that go beyond the individual level to include contextual factors, such as improving communication with caring adults, changing gender norms, and linking to services.

- Include a range of media, as well as interpersonal communication.
- Plan for the evaluation at the beginning of the program.

Provide adolescent-friendly contraceptive services. The importance of providing adolescents and youth with services that are tailored to their special needs has long been recognized (Senderwitz 1999). Rather than stand-alone youth-friendly services or separate spaces within services for adolescents, current programming is focusing on mainstreaming adolescent-friendly contraceptive services with existing family planning services. Four components of adolescent-friendly contraceptive services are important to reducing the common barriers adolescents face in accessing services (box 6.1).

Interventions in China, Ghana, India, Kenya, Nicaragua, Tanzania, Uganda, and Zimbabwe have shown that providing one or more of the components of adolescent-friendly contraceptive services can increase use of contraceptives or condoms (Decker and Montagu 2007; Kanesathasan and others 2008; Karim and others 2009; Kim and others 2001; Lou and others 2004; Meuwissen, Gorter, and Knottnerus 2006; Williams and others 2007).

Youth centers, however, have not been found to be an effective and efficient programming strategy for reaching youth (Zuurmond, Geary, and Ross 2012).

Expand access to and promotion of the use of condoms and other contraceptives. Ensuring access to and regular use of condoms and other contraceptives is an essential element in programs to protect youth from unintended pregnancies and STIs. The use of condoms to guard against STIs can provide the added benefit of safeguarding fertility (Brady 2003). Promoting condoms for pregnancy prevention, as well as for prevention of HIV and other STIs, could increase condom use for safe sex among young people (Agha 2003). An analysis of survey data from 18 Sub-Saharan African countries finds that use of condoms for pregnancy prevention rose significantly in 13 of 18 countries between 1993 and 2001. Condom use among young Sub-Saharan African women increased by an average annual rate of 1.4 percent, with 58.5 percent of the users reporting that they were motivated by a desire to prevent pregnancy (Cleland, Ali, and Shah 2006).

Evidence suggests that if condom use is established during adolescence, it is more likely to be sustained in the long term (Schutt-Aine and Maddaleno 2003). A study of sexually active youth in Ethiopia, 75 percent of whom were female, finds that once young people started to use condoms, they were more likely to continue to use them (Molla, Astrøm, and Berhane 2007). Still, a review of 28 studies of HIV prevention in Sub-Saharan Africa finds that the effect of interventions on condom use at last sexual activity were generally greater in males than in females, suggesting that "women still experience marked difficulties in negotiating condom use or assuming full control over their sexual activity" (Michielsen and others 2010, 1201).

A gender-transformative approach could be to ensure that all adolescent girls receive fertility awareness training, for example, using CycleSmar™ or using CycleBeads® as they begin menstruation as a teaching tool to empower them to know and understand their reproductive cycles and to understand when they can get pregnant (IRH, n.d.a). A new study is underway to study the effects of fertility awareness on contraceptive use (IRH, n.d.b).

Implement programs for out-of-school and married adolescents. Most programming for adolescents is school- or health facility–based, yet millions of children and adolescents are not in school. UNESCO estimates that 57 million children of primary school age and 69 million children of lower-secondary school age do not attend school (UNESCO 2013; UNFPA 2013). Mass media approaches and CBP show promise in reaching out-of-school adolescents, although programming for this group is challenging (Bhuiya and others 2004).

Building Resilience and Assets

Programs to improve life skills and build resilience to risk factors among adolescents have shown promising results (Askew and others 2004; Erulkar and others 2004; Kanesathasan and others 2008; Kim and others 2001; Mathur, Mehta, and Malhotra 2004; Meekers, Stallworthy, and Harris 1997). These programs, which focus on building protective factors to promote success rather than eliminating factors associated with failure,

---

Box 6.1

Components of Adolescent-Friendly Contraceptive Services:

- Train providers to provide nonjudgmental services that promote gender-equitable norms and encourage healthy decision making by adolescents.
- Enforce confidentiality and ensure audio and visual privacy.
- Offer a wide range of contraceptive methods.
- Provide no-cost or subsidized services.

Source: HIP, forthcoming.

have included a mix of community awareness and engagement of community leaders; assistance to link adolescents with significant adults in their lives, most notably parents; provision of safe spaces for adolescents; and provision of information, services, and the building of skills. Cuidate, a sexual-risk-reduction program in Mexico, provides a six-hour training program for parents and adolescents. After four years, the adolescent program participants were more likely to be older at first sexual activity and to use a condom or other contraceptive at first sexual activity, compared with the control group (Villarruel and others 2010).

UNSAFE ABORTION

Interventions to Reduce Unsafe Abortion

Although the need for abortion can be reduced if the need for contraceptive options is better addressed, the need for safe abortion care will remain. Contraceptive methods do fail; women often become pregnant in circumstances in which the use of contraception may not be possible or where sex is nonconsensual. Medical or other circumstances for the woman could change even after she becomes pregnant.

Abortion in early pregnancy (less than nine weeks) performed with appropriate techniques by trained personnel is one of the safest medical procedures, with a case fatality rate of 0.6 per 100,000 procedures (Raymond and Grimes 2012); this rate is 14 times lower than the risk of death associated with childbirth. Complications increase with increasing gestation, but the termination of pregnancy remains a safe procedure.

Safe and Simple Technologies

The WHO recognizes vacuum aspiration (manual and electric) up to 12–14 weeks of gestation, and dilation and evacuation beyond that stage, as safe and appropriate surgical procedures. Medical abortion using the sequential combination of mifepristone, followed by misoprostol, is recommended as a safe and effective method that can be used at any stage of pregnancy, although doses and specific protocols change as gestation advances. Vacuum aspiration can be provided on an outpatient basis at the primary care level; medical abortion up to nine weeks is a process rather than a procedure and can be managed as an outpatient primary care service, with some of the medications taken by women at home (WHO 2012).

Access to Technologies

Although simple, safe, and effective medical interventions already exist, appropriate technology is of little benefit if it is not used by providers and is not accessible to women. Therein lies the challenge. Legal restrictions on the circumstances under which abortions are permitted or who can provide them; critical health workforce shortages, particularly in South Asia and Sub-Saharan Africa; lack of training opportunities for providers; conscientious objection to care provision on the part of some providers; and the social, cultural, and political stigma around abortion all make it difficult to ensure access to safe abortion care. Despite the availability of vacuum aspiration for more than 40 years, the use of sharp curettage (dilation and curettage) is still common in many countries. The WHO no longer recommends dilation and curettage because it has more complications, often needs general anesthesia, and has higher costs for women and health facilities (WHO 2012). Similarly, although both mifepristone and misoprostol are included in the WHO's model list of essential medicines, mifepristone is not registered or available across most of Latin America and the Caribbean and Sub-Saharan Africa (Gynuity 2013).

Promising Approaches

Services to the full extent of the law. Although laws vary, all but six countries allow legal abortion in some circumstances, most often to save the life of the woman and often when pregnancy is the result of rape or incest (UN Population Division 2013a). Whatever the legal context, the treatment of women with complications is legal, and evacuation in case of incomplete abortion is a signal function of basic emergency obstetric care. Interpreting and implementing laws to their full extent and keeping the health of women center stage can make safer care more accessible.

Expanding the pool of providers. A systematic review of the evidence shows that both vacuum aspiration and medical abortion can be safely provided by non-physician providers (Renner, Brahmi, and Kapp 2013). Many countries allow clinical associates, midwives, or nurses to treat incomplete abortion using manual vacuum aspiration; several, including Vietnam, allow them to provide induced abortion as well. Bangladesh has had a mature program with auxiliary workers providing menstrual regulation for more than 40 years (Johnston and others 2011). Because medical abortion is a relatively newer technology, fewer countries have yet moved to decentralize care; it is well-suited to a wider provider base since it does not need surgical skills. Ethiopia and Ghana both allow midwives to provide medical abortions, and Nepal has incrementally progressed to allowing midwives, then nurses, and more recently, auxiliary nurses working at lower-level facilities to provide medical abortions, demonstrating the feasibility even in low-resource settings.

In many contexts, a pharmacy is the first and sometimes only health care contact for a woman with an unintended pregnancy. Although results have not always been successful, interventions to provide pharmacy workers with accurate information, minimize harm, or develop referral linkages with other authorized providers have potential and need to be further explored (Sneeringer and others 2012). Similarly, community health workers can play a role in assessing eligibility, making appropriate referrals, and helping women determine the need for follow-up care.

Where mifepristone is not available. If mifepristone is not available, misoprostol, an inexpensive anti-ulcer medicine with other obstetric and gynecological uses, is usually more readily accessible and can be used alone to terminate a pregnancy. The failure rate is higher than when used in combination with mifepristone, but it is still safe and effective, and is a WHO-recommended option (WHO 2012). Important gains in reducing the morbidity and mortality from unsafe abortions have been made, especially in Latin America and the Caribbean, with the use of this strategy.

Innovations. The use of telemedicine to provide medical abortions can help bring needed care to women who do not have physical access (Gomperts and others 2012; Grindlay, Lane, and Grossman 2013; Grossman and others 2011). Decreasing the need for clinic visits through approaches that allow telephone follow-up or self-assessment of the abortion process using semi-quantitative pregnancy tests (Lynd and others 2013) is another promising innovation. mHealth approaches with text messaging can help support women through the abortion process, providing information and reminders about medications, side effects, and postabortion contraception. The risk-reduction model pioneered in Uruguay combines provision of information and post-abortion care; this approach can be legally implemented even in countries with restrictive legal environments (Fiol and others 2012).

Information and attitudes. Even where abortion is legal, women are often unaware of how and where to access it (Adinma and others 2011; Banerjee and others 2013; Thapa, Sharma, and Khatiwada 2014). Approaches to empowering women with knowledge using inter-personal communication, drama, theater, radio, wall signage, and mass media communication have all had some success; understanding the local context and appropriately tailoring the approach is critical (Banerjee

and others 2013; Bingham and others 2011). Telephone help lines can provide confidential sources of information and support. Social networking and Internet-based information are becoming increasingly important in providing accurate information; however, empowering women to be able to detect misinformation and avoid dangers, like the sale of spurious medical abortion agents, is also needed.

Addressing the stigma and taboos around sexuality, unintended pregnancies, and abortion is important, as is providing women with the information and skills to negotiate traditional gender roles and inequities. Providers need medically accurate information and the skills to be able to clarify internal values and provide care to women in a nonjudgmental way.

Postabortion contraception. Although the evidence on its overall impact on maternal mortality has not been well studied, ensuring effective and seamless linkages among abortion care, contraceptive information, voluntary counseling, and onsite availability of contraception is an important strategy for increasing the use of post-abortion contraception and helping women prevent subsequent unintended pregnancies (Tripney, Kwan, and Bird 2013). However, ensuring that contraceptive acceptance does not become coercive or a precondition to getting abortion care is also needed.

A multifaceted approach is needed. An excellent example is seen in Nepal, where legal reform followed by proactive efforts to scale up services has yielded rich dividends and already shows some evidence of a decline in serious morbidity from unsafe abortion (Henderson and others 2013; Samandari and others 2012).

Conclusion. A combination of approaches that include sexuality education and women's contraceptive needs to reduce the need for abortion, the provision of safe abortion services, and the availability of treatment for complications to attenuate morbidity and reduce the mortality from unsafe abortions—grounded in a framework of human rights—can collectively minimize the burden of the consequences of unsafe abortion. Safe abortion has been shown to be cost-effective (see *DCP3*, volume 1, *Essential Surgery*, chapter 18 [Prinja and others 2015]).

VIOLENCE AGAINST WOMEN

What Can the Health Sector Do?

Primary prevention of violence is critically important, but it is also necessary to provide care and support for the many women who already face violence. Early identification and response can play an important role in secondary prevention by mitigating the consequences of violence and reducing the risk of further violent episodes. Early identification and response can also contribute to primary prevention by identifying and supporting the children of women who suffer domestic violence. Evidence suggests that early intervention is likely to have a positive impact on later risk behaviors and health problems among children and adolescents. It can also contribute to reducing the social and economic costs of such violence. (Bott, Morrison, and Ellsberg 2005; García Moreno and others 2014). (See *DCP3* volume 7, *Injury Prevention and Environmental Health*, Mercy and others, forthcoming, for further discussion of interpersonal violence)

Although violence against women has been accepted as a critical public health and clinical care issue, the health care policies of many countries still do not address it. The critical role that the health system and health care providers can play in identification, assessment, treatment, crisis intervention, documentation, referral, and follow-up is poorly understood or poorly accepted within national health programs and policies (WHO 2013; WHO 2014c). Women who have been subjected to violence often seek health care for their injuries, even if they may not disclose the associated abuse or violence, and a health care provider is likely to be the first professional contact for survivors of intimate partner violence or sexual assault. Women also identify health care providers as the professionals they would most trust with the disclosure of abuse (Feder and others 2006). Reproductive health care providers are particularly well positioned given that most women will at some point consult them for contraception, antenatal care, and delivery.

Responding to Intimate Partner Violence and Sexual Violence

The WHO clinical and policy guidelines (WHO 2013) summarize the evidence for clinical interventions for intimate partner violence and for sexual violence against women. They also review the evidence for service delivery and training on these issues for health care providers and make evidence-based recommendations to improve the response of the health sector to violence against women.

Health professionals can provide assistance to women suffering from violence by facilitating disclosure, offering support and referral, gathering forensic evidence—particularly in cases of sexual violence—and providing the appropriate medical services and follow-up care. Health care providers who come into contact with women facing intimate partner violence need to be able to recognize the signs and respond appropriately and safely. Women exposed to violence require comprehensive, gender-sensitive health care services that address the physical and mental health consequences of their experience and aid their recovery. Women may also require crisis intervention services to prevent further harm. Treating cases of rape includes providing emergency contraception and prophylaxis for HIV and other STIs; psychological first-line support; and access to safe abortion and longer-term mental health care support, if needed. In addition to providing immediate medical services, the health sector is a potentially crucial gateway to providing assistance through referral to specific services for violence against women—or other aid that women may require at a later date, such as social welfare and legal aid. In all circumstances, all health care providers should be trained to provide a minimum first-line supportive response (WHO 2013, 2014b).

The WHO recommendations are addressed to health care providers because they are in a unique position to address the health and psychosocial needs of women who live with or who have experienced violence. They also seek to inform health policy makers or program managers in charge of planning and implementing health care services and those designing curricula.

The health sector can also play an advocacy role by supporting research to document the impact and extent of the problem, raise awareness, and establish links in the multisectoral response that is needed to address this serious health risk for women.

CONCLUSIONS

Significant progress in improving reproductive health has been made in some areas. Family planning has expanded worldwide through new approaches and new methods. A renewed commitment to family planning among donors and national governments has stimulated wider coverage of services accompanied by greater emphasis on quality and human rights. A new focus on adolescent sexual health has spurred interest in better ways to reach adolescents with effective messages and services. New approaches to reducing gender-based violence have been tested and the lessons learned have been distilled in clinical and policy guidelines.

However, much remains to be done. In spite of the advances in family planning, in 35 countries fewer than 30 percent of women of reproductive age use modern contraception. Choice of methods is still limited in many countries, even some with high levels of contraceptive prevalence, because of lack of access, provider biases, and other program factors. Although good options for safe abortion exist, these services remain unavailable in many countries because of legal barriers, lack of training, and stigma. We have more information about how to reach adolescents with effective services and how to reduce gender-based violence. The major challenge is how to more widely implement those programs that have been proven to be safe, effective, and affordable.

NOTE

World Bank Income Classifications as of July 2014 are as follows, based on estimates of gross national income (GNI) per capita for 2013:

- Low-income countries (LICs) = US$1,045 or less
- Middle-income countries (MICs) are subdivided:
  a) lower-middle-income = US$1,046 to US$4,125
  b) upper-middle-income (UMICs) = US$4,126 to US$12,745
- High-income countries (HICs) = US$12,746 or more.

REFERENCES

Abbas, K., A. A. Khan, and A. Khan. 2013. "Costs and Utilization of Public Sector Family Planning Services in Pakistan." *Journal of the Pakistan Medical Association* 63 (4 Suppl 3): S33–9.

Adinma, E. D., J. I. Adinma, J. Ugboaja, C. Iwuoha, A. Akiode, and others. 2011. "Knowledge and Perception of the Nigerian Abortion Law by Abortion Seekers in South-Eastern Nigeria." *Journal of Obstetrics and Gynaecology* 31 (8): 763–76.

Agha, S. 2003. "The Impact of a Mass Media Campaign on Personal Risk Perception, Perceived Self-Efficacy and on Other Behavioral Predictors." *AIDS Care* 15 (6): 749–62.

Ahmed, S., Q. Li, L. Liu, and A. Tsui. 2012. "Maternal Deaths Averted by Contraceptive Use: An Analysis of 172 Countries." *The Lancet* 380 (9837): 111–25.

AIDSTAR-Two. 2012. *The Use of Information and Communication Technology in Family Planning, Reproductive Health and Other Health Programs: A Review of Trends and Evidence.* Cambridge, MA: Management Sciences for Health.

Amadou, B., J. Curran, L. Wilson, N. A. Dagadu, V. Jennings, and others. 2013. "Guide for Monitoring Scale up of Health Practices and Innovations." Manual. MEASURE Evaluation PRH, Chapel Hill, NC.

Askew, I., J. Chege, C. Njue, and S. Radeny. 2004. "A Multi-Sectoral Approach to Providing Reproductive Health Information and Services to Young People in Western Kenya: Kenya Adolescent Reproductive Health Project." FRONTIERS Project, Population Council, Washington, DC.

Baird, S. J., R. S. Garfein, C. T. McIntosh, and B. Ozler. 2012. "Effect of a Cash Transfer Programme for Schooling on Prevalence of HIV and Herpes Simplex Type 2 in Malawi: A Cluster Randomised Trial." *The Lancet* 379 (9823): 1320–29.

Bakamjian, L. 2008. "Linking Communities to Family Planning and LAPM via Mobile Services." Presentation at the Flexible Fund Partner's Meeting, Washington, DC. EngenderHealth, New York.

Banerjee, S. K., K. L. Andersen, J. Warvadekar, and E. Pearson. 2013. "Effectiveness of a Behavior Change Communication Intervention to Improve Knowledge and Perceptions about Abortion in Bihar and Jharkhand, India." *International Perspectives on Sexual and Reproductive Health* 39 (3): 142–51.

Barker, G., C. Ricardo, M. Nascimento, A. Olukoya, and C. Santos. 2010. "Questioning Gender Norms with Men to Improve Health Outcomes: Evidence of Impact." *Global Public Health* 5 (5): 539–53.

Barnes, J., J. Vail, and D. Crosby. 2012. "Total Market Initiatives for Reproductive Health. Strengthening Health Outcomes through the Private Sector Project." Abt Associates, Bethesda, MD.

Bellows, N. M., B. W. Bellows, and C. Warren. 2011. "The Use of Vouchers for Reproductive Health Services in Developing Countries: A Systematic Review." *Tropical Medicine and International Health* 16 (1): 84–96.

Bertrand, J., K. O'Reilly, J. Denison, R. Anhang, and M. Sweat. 2006. "Systematic Review of the Effectiveness of Mass Communication Programs to Change HIV/AIDS-Related Behaviors in Developing Countries." *Health Education Research* 21 (4): 567–97.

Bhuiya, I., U. Rob, A. H. Chowdhury, L. Rahman, N. Haque, and others. 2004. "Improving Adolescent Reproductive Health in Bangladesh." FRONTIERS, Population Council, Washington, DC.

Biddlecom, A., and V. Kantorova. 2013. "Global Trends in Contraceptive Method Mix and Implications for Meeting Demand for Family Planning." Presented in Session 81 at the meeting of the Population Association of America, New Orleans, April 11–13.

Bill & Melinda Gates Foundation and DFID (UK Department for International Development). 2012. "Landmark Summit Puts Women at Heart of Global Health Agenda." Press Release. http://www.londonfamilyplanningsummit.co.uk /1530%20FINAL%20press%20release.pdf.

Bingham, A., J. K. Drake, L. Goodyear, C. Y. Gopinath, A. Kaufman, and others. 2011. "The Role of Interpersonal Communication in Preventing Unsafe Abortion in Communities: The Dialogues for Life Project in Nepal." *Journal of Health Communication* 16 (3): 245–63.

Birdsall, N., A. C. Kelly, and S. W. Sinding, eds. 2001. *Population in the Developing World Matters: Demography, Economic Growth and Poverty.* Oxford: Oxford University Press.

Blanc, A. K., W. Winfrey, and J. Ross. 2013. "New Findings for Maternal Mortality Age Patterns: Aggregated Results for 38 Countries." *PLoS One* 8 (4): e59864. doi:10.1371/journal .pone.0059864.

Bloom, D. E., D. Canning, and J. Sevilla. 2003. *The Demographic Dividend: A New Perspective on the Economic Consequences of Population Change.* Santa Monica, CA: Population Matters, RAND.

Bongaarts, J., J. Cleland, J. Townsend, J. Bertrand, and M. Das Gupta. 2012. *Family Planning in the 21st Century: Rationale and Design.* New York, NY: Population Council.

Bott, S., A. Morrison, and M. Ellsberg. 2005. "Preventing and Responding to Gender-Based Violence in Middle- and Low-Income Countries: A Global Review and Analysis." World Bank, Washington, DC.

Bradley, H., A. Bedada, H. Brahmbhatt, A. Kidanu, D. Gillespie, and others. 2007. "Educational Attainment and HIV Status among Ethiopian Voluntary Counseling and Testing Clients." *AIDS and Behavior* 11 (5): 736–42.

Brady, M. 2003. "Preventing Sexually Transmitted Infections and Unintended Pregnancy, and Safeguarding Fertility: Triple Protection Needs of Young Women." *Reproductive Health Matters* 11 (22): 134–41.

Burns, B., A. Mingat, and R. Rakotomalala. 2003. *Achieving Universal Primary Education by 2015: A Chance for Every Child.* Washington, DC: World Bank.

Chandy, K. T., T. R. Balakrishman, J. M. Kantawalla, K. Mohan, N. P. Sen, and others. 1965. "Proposals for Family Planning Promotion: A Marketing Plan." *Studies in Family Planning* 1 (6): 7–12.

Chapman, S., and H. Astatke. 2003. "Review of DFID Approach to Social Marketing. Annex 5: Effectiveness, Efficiency, and Equity in Social Marketing, and Appendix to Annex 5: The Social Marketing Evidence Base." DFID Health Systems Resource Centre, London.

Cleland, J., M. Ali, and I. Shah. 2006. "Trends in Protective Behavior among Single vs. Married Young Women in Sub-Saharan Africa: The Big Picture." *Reproductive Health Matters* 14 (28): 17–22.

De Brauw, A., D. O. Gilligan, J. Hoddinott, and S. Roy. 2013. "The Impact of Bolsa Família on Women's Decision-Making Power." *World Development* 59: 487–504.

Decker, M., and D. Montagu. 2007. "Reaching Youth through Franchise Clinics: Assessment of Kenyan Private Sector Involvement in Youth Services." *Journal of Adolescent Health* 40: 280–82.

Deininger, K. 2003. "Does Cost of Schooling Affect Enrollment by the Poor? Universal Primary Education in Uganda." *Economics of Education Review* 22 (3): 291–305.

DHS (Demographic and Health Surveys. Data from multiple surveys and years. http://www.statcompiler.com.

DKT International. 2011. "1990–2010 Contraceptive Social Marketing Statistics." DKT International, Washington, DC.

Eichler, R., B. Seligman, A. Beith, and J. Wright. 2010. *Performance-Based Incentives: Ensuring Voluntarism in Family Planning Initiatives.* Bethesda, MD: Health Systems 20/20 Project, Abt Associates Inc.

Engelman, R. 1997. *Why Population Matters: International Edition.* Washington, DC: Population Action International.

Erulkar, A. S., L. Ettyang, C. Onoka, F. K. Nyagah, and A. Muyonga. 2004. "Behavior Change Evaluation of a Culturally Consistent Reproductive Health Program for Young Kenyans." *International Family Planning Perspectives* 30 (2): 58–67.

Erulkar, A. S., and E. Muthengi. 2009. "Evaluation of Berhane Hewan: A Program to Delay Child Marriage in Rural Ethiopia." *International Perspectives on Sexual and Reproductive Health* 35 (1): 6–14.

Eva, G., and T. D. Ngo. 2010. *MSI Mobile Outreach Services: Retrospective Evaluations from Ethiopia, Myanmar, Pakistan, Sierra Leone and Vietnam.* London: Marie Stopes International.

Feder, G. S., M. Hutson, J. Ramsay, and A. R. Taket. 2006. "Women Exposed to Intimate Partner Violence: Expectations and Experiences When They Encounter Health Care Professionals: A Meta-Analysis of Qualitative Studies." *Archives of Internal Medicine* 166 (1): 22–37.

Feldman, B. S., A. M. Zaslavsky, M. Ezzati, K. E. Peterson, and M. Mitchell. 2009. "Contraceptive Use, Birth Spacing, and Autonomy: An Analysis of the Oportunidades Program in Rural Mexico." *Studies in Family Planning* 40 (1): 51–62.

Fiol, V., L. Briozzo, A. Labandera, V. Recchi, and M. Piñeyro. 2012. "Improving Care of Women at Risk of Unsafe Abortion: Implementing a Risk-Reduction Model at the Uruguayan-Brazilian Border." *International Journal of Gynaecology and Obstetrics* 118 (Suppl 1): S21–27.

FP Ouagadougou Partnership. 2014. *Family Planning: Francophone West Africa on the Move—A Call to Action.* Family Planning Ouagadougou Partnership. http://www.prb.org/pdf12/ouagadougou-partnership_en.pdf.

García Moreno, C., C. Zimmerman, A. Morris-Gehring, L. Heise, A. Amin, and others. 2014. "Addressing Violence against Women: A Call to Action." *The Lancet* 385 (9978): 1685–95. doi:10.1026/S0140-6736(14)61830-4

Gay, J., K. Hardee, M. Croce-Galis, and C. Hall. 2011. "What Works to Meet the Sexual and Reproductive Health Needs of Women Living with HIV/AIDS?" *Journal of the International AIDS Society* 14 (56). doi: 10.1186/1758-2652-14-56.

Gillespie, D., S. Ahmed, A. Tsui, and S. Radloff. 2007. "Unwanted Fertility among the Poor: An Inequity?" *Bulletin of the World Health Organization* 85 (2): 100–7.

Gomperts, R., S. Petwo, K. Jelinksa, L. Steen, K. Gemzell-Danielsson, and others. 2012. "Regional Differences in Surgical Intervention Following Medical Termination of Pregnancy Provided by Telemedicine." *Acta Obstetricia Gynecologica Scandinavica* 91 (2): 226–31.

Grindlay, K., K. Lane, and D. Grossman. 2013. "Women and Health Providers' Experiences with Medical Abortion Provided through Telemedicine: A Qualitative Study." *Women's Health Issues* 23 (2): e117–22.

Grossman, D., K. Grindlay, T. Buchacker, K. Lane, and K. Blanchard. 2011. "Effectiveness and Acceptability of Medical Abortion Provided through Telemedicine." *Obstetrics and Gynecology* 118 (2 pt 1): 296–303.

Grunseit, A., S. Kippax, P. Aggleton, M. Baldo, and G. Slutkin. 1997. "Sexuality Education and Young People's Sexual Behavior: A Review of Studies." *Journal of Adolescent Research* 12 (4): 421–53.

Gurman, T. A., and C. Underwood. 2008. "Using Media to Address Adolescent Sexual Health: Lessons Learned Abroad." In *Managing the Media Monster. The Influence of Media (from Television to Text Messages) on Teen Sexual Behavior and Attitude,* edited by J. D. Brown. Washington, DC: National Campaign to End Teen and Unplanned Pregnancy.

Gynuity. 2013. "Map of Mefepristone Approvals." http://gynuity.org/downloads/mapmife_en.pdf.

Habumuremyi, P. D., and M. Zenawi. 2012. "Making Family Planning a National Development Priority." *The Lancet* 380 (9837): 78–80.

Hardee, K., J. Kumar, K. Newman, L. Bakamjian, S. Harris, and others. 2014. "Voluntary, Human Rights-Based Family Planning: A Conceptual Framework." *Studies in Family Planning* 45 (1): 1–18.

Hardee, K., K. Newman, L. Bakamjian, J. Kumar, S. Harris, and others. 2013. "Voluntary Family Planning Programs that Respect, Protect, and Fulfill Human Rights: A Conceptual Framework." Futures Group, Washington, DC.

Hargreaves, J. R., L. A. Morison, J. C. Kim, C. P. Bonell, J. D. H. Porter, and others. 2008. "The Association between School Attendance, HIV Infection and Sexual Behaviour among Young People in Rural South Africa." *Journal of Epidemiology and Community Health* 62 (2): 113–19.

Henderson, J., M. Puri, M. Blum, C. C. Harper, A. Rana, and others. 2013. "Effects of Abortion Legalization in Nepal, 2001–2010." *PLoS One* 8 (5): e64755.

Hindon, M., and A. O. Fatusi. 2009. "Adolescent Sexual and Reproductive Health in Developing Countries: An Overview of Trends and Interventions." *International Perspectives on Sexual and Reproductive Health* 35 (2): 58–62.

HIP (High Impact Practices for Family Planning). 2012. "Community Health Workers: Bringing Family Planning Services to Where People Live." USAID, Washington, DC. http://www.fphighimpactpractices.org/resources/community-health-workers-bringing-family-planning-services-where-people-live-and-work.

———. Forthcoming. "Making Existing Contraceptive Services Adolescent Friendly." USAID, Washington, DC. http://www.fphighimpactpractices.org.

Horton, S., D. C. N. Wu, and E. Brouwer. 2015. "Methodology and Results for Systematic Search, Cost and Cost-Effectiveness Analysis." Working Paper, *Disease Control Priorities*, 3rd edition, Volume 2. http://www.dcp-3.org/resources/working-papers.

IRH (Institute for Reproductive Health). n.d.a. "CycleSmartTM CycleBeads." Brochure. Georgetown University, Washington, DC. http://irh.org/resource-library/cyclesmart-cyclebeads-brochure/.

———. n.d.b. "IRH Awarded Fertility Awareness 'Fact Project' by USAID." Institute for Reproductive Health, Georgetown University, Washington, DC. http://irh.org/blog/irh-awarded-fertility-awareness-fact-project-by-usaid/.

Janowitz, B., J. Stanback, and B. Boyer. 2012. "Task Sharing in Family Planning." *Studies in Family Planning* 43 (1): 47–62.

Jiang, L., and K. Hardee. 2011. "How Do Recent Population Trends Matter to Climate Change?" *Population Research and Policy Review* 30: 287–312.

Johnston, H. B., A. Schurmann, E. Oliveras, and H. H. Akhter. 2011. "Scaled Up and Marginalized: A Review of Bangladesh's Menstrual Regulation Programme and Its Impact." In *Social Determinants Approaches to Public Health: From Concept to Practice*, edited by E. Blas, J. Sommerfeld, and A. S. Kurup, 9–24. Geneva: World Health Organization.

Kanesathasan, A., L. J. Cardinal, E. Pearson, S. Gupta, S. Mukherjee, and A. Malhotra. 2008. "Catalyzing Change: Improving Youth Sexual and Reproductive Health through DISHA, an Integrated Program in India." International Centre for Research on Women, Washington, DC.

Karim, Q. A., K. Leasek, A. Kharsany, H. Humphries F. Ntombela, and others. 2015. "Impact of Conditional Cash Incentives of HSV-2 and HIV Prevention in Rural South African High School Students: Results of the CAPRISA 007 Cluster Randomized Controlled Trial." International AIDS Conference, Vancouver, July 19–22.

Karim, A., T. Williams, L. Patkykewish, D. Ali, C. Colvin, and others. 2009. "The Impact of African Youth Alliance Program on the Sexual Behavior of Young People in Uganda." *Studies in Family Planning* 40 (4): 289–306.

Kim, Y. M., A. Kols, R. Nyakauru, C. Marangwanda, and P. Chibatamoto. 2001. "Promoting Sexual Responsibility among Young People in Zimbabwe." *International Family Planning Perspectives* 27 (1): 11–19.

Kirby, D. 2011. "Sex Education: Access and Impact on Sexual Behaviour of Young People." UN/POP/EGM-AYD/2011/07, United Nations Population Division, New York.

Koenig, M. A., J. F. Phillips, R. S. Simmons, and M. A. Khan. 1987. "Trends in Family Size Preferences and Contraceptive Use in Matlab, Bangladesh." *Studies in Family Planning* 18 (3): 117–27.

Kozuki, N., A. C. Lee, M. F. Silveira, A. Sania, J. P. Vogel, and others. 2013. "The Associations of Parity and Maternal Age with Small-for-Gestational-Age, Preterm, and Neonatal and Infant Mortality: A Meta-Analysis." *BMC Public Health* 13 (Suppl 3): S2. http://www.biomedcentral.com/1471-2458/13/S3/S2.

Kozuki, N., A. C. Lee, M. F. Silveira, C. G. Victora, L. Adair, and others. 2013. "The Associations of Birth Intervals with Small-for-Gestational Age, Preterm and Neonatal, and Infant Mortality: A Meta-Analysis." *BMC Public Health* 13 (Suppl 3): S3. http://www.biomedcentral.com/1471-2458/13/S3/S3.

Lee-Rife, S., A. Malhotra, A. Warner, and A. M. Glinski. 2012. "What Works to Prevent Child Marriage: A Review of the Evidence." *Studies in Family Planning* 43 (4): 287–303.

Lloyd, C., and J. Young. 2009. *New Lessons: The Power of Educating Adolescent Girls*. New York: Population Council.

Lou, C., B. Wang, Y. Shen, and E. Gao. 2004. "Effects of a Community-Based Sex Education and Reproductive Health Service Program on Contraceptive Use of Unmarried Youths in Shanghai." *Journal of Adolescent Health* 33: 433–40.

Lynd, K., J. Blum, N. Ngoc, T. Shochet, P. D. Blumenthal, and others. 2013. "Simplified Medical Abortion Using a Semi-Quantitative Pregnancy Test for Home Based Follow Up." *International Journal of Gynecology and Obstetrics* 121 (2): 144–48.

Madhavan, S., and D. Bishai. 2010. "Private Sector Engagement in Sexual and Reproductive Health and Maternal and Neonatal Health: A Review of the Evidence." Human Development Resource Center, DFID, London.

Malarcher, S., O. Meirik, E. Lebetkin, I. Shah, J. Spieler, and others. 2011. "Provision of DMPA by Community Health

Workers: What the Evidence Shows." *Contraception* 83 (6): 495–503.

Martine, G., and D. Schensul, eds. 2013. *The Demography of Adaptation to Climate Change*. New York, London, and Mexico City: UNFPA, IIED, and El Colegio de Mexico.

Mathur, S., M. Mehta, and A. Malhotra. 2004. "Youth Reproductive Health in Nepal: Is Participation the Answer?" International Center for Research on Women, Washington, DC.

Mavedzenge, S. N., A. Doyle, and D. Ross. 2011. "HIV Prevention in Young People in Sub-Saharan Africa: A Systematic Review." *Journal of Adolescent Health* 49 (6): 568–86.

Meekers, D., G. Stallworthy, and J. Harris. 1997. "Changing Adolescents' Beliefs about Protective Sexual Behavior: The Botswana Tsa Banana Program." Working Paper 3, Population Services International, Research Division, Washington, DC.

Mercy, J., S. Hilis, A. Butchart, M. Bellis, C. Ward, and others. "Interpersonal Violence: Global Impact and the Paths to Prevention." Forthcoming. In *Disease Control Priorities* (third edition): Volume 7, *Intentional Injury and Environmental Health*, edited by C. N. Mock, R. Nugent, and O. Kobusingye. Washington, DC: World Bank.

Meuwissen, L. E., A. C. Gorter, and A. J. Knottnerus. 2006. "Impact of Accessible Sexual and Reproductive Health Care on Poor and Underserved Adolescents in Managua, Nicaragua: A Quasi-Experimental Intervention Study." *Journal of Adolescent Health* 38 (1): 56.

Michielsen, K., M. Chersich, S. Luchters, P. De Koker, R. Van Rossem, and others. 2010. "Effectiveness of HIV Prevention for Youth in Sub-Saharan Africa: Systematic Review and Meta-Analysis of Randomized and Non-Randomized Trials." *AIDS* 24 (8): 1193–202.

Ministry of Health and Population [Nepal], New ERA, and Macro International Inc. 2012. *Demographic and Health Survey 2011*. Kathmandu, Nepal: Ministry of Health and Population, New ERA, and ICF International, Calverton, Maryland.

Molla, M., A. Astrøm, and Y. Berhane. 2007. "Applicability of the Theory of Planned Behavior to Intended and Self-Reported Condom Use in a Rural Ethiopian Population." *AIDS Care* 19 (3): 425–31.

Moreland, S., and E. Smith. 2012. "Modeling Climate Change, Food Security, and Population Change. Pilot-Testing the Model in Ethiopia." USAID, MEASURE Evaluation PRH, and the David and Lucile Packard Foundation, Chapel Hill, NC.

Moreland, S., E. Smith, and S. Sharma. 2010. "World Population Prospects and Unmet Need for Family Planning." Futures Group, Washington, DC.

Nakhaee, N., A. R. Mirahmadizadeh, H. A. Gorji, and M. Mohammadi. 2002. "Assessing the Cost-Effectiveness of Contraceptive Methods in Shiraz, Islamic Republic of Iran." *Eastern Mediterranean Health Journal* 8: 55–63.

NAS (National Academy of Sciences). 1986. *Population Growth and Economic Development: Policy Questions. Committee on Population, National Research Council*. Washington, DC: National Academy Press.

Norman, C. 2013. "Utilizing Incentives for Global Family Planning and Reproductive Health Services Update: Altruistic or Euphemism for Population Control?" Master's Thesis, Global Studies Program, Brandeis University, Waltham, MA.

Onwujekwe, O., C. Ogbonna, O. Ibe, and B. Ozochukwu. 2013. "Willingness-to-Pay and Benefit-Cost of Modern Contraceptives in Nigeria." *International Journal of Gynecology and Obstetrics* 122: 94–98.

Pettifor, A., C. MacPhail, A. Selon, X. Gomez-Olive, J. Hughes, and others. 2015 "HPTN 068 Conditional Cash Transfer to Prevent Infection among Young Women in South Africa: Results of a Randomized Controlled Trial." International AIDS Conference, Vancouver, July 19–22.

Phillips, J. F., W. L. Greene, and E. F. Jackson. 1999. "Lessons from Community-Based Distribution of Family Planning in Africa." Working Paper 121, Population Council, New York. http://www.popcouncil.org/pdfs/wp/121.pdf.

Prata, N., F. Vahidnia, M. Potts, and I. Dries-Daffner. 2005. "Revisiting Community-Based Distribution Programs: Are They Still Needed?" *Contraception* 72 (6): 402–7.

Prinja, S., A. Nandi, S. Horton, X. Levin, and R. Laxminarayan. 2015. "Costs, Effectiveness, and Cost-Effectiveness of Selected Surgical Procedures and Platforms." In *Disease Control Priorities* (third edition): Volume 1, *Essential Surgery*, edited by H. T. Debas, P. Donkor, A. Gawande, D. T. Jamison, M. E. Kruk, and C. N. Mock. Washington, DC: World Bank.

Pulerwitz, J., G. Barker, M. Segundo, and M. Nascimento. 2006. *Promoting More Gender-Equitable Norms and Behaviors among Young Men as an HIV/AIDS Prevention Strategy*. Washington, DC: Horizons Program, Population Council.

Raymond, E. G., and D. A. Grimes. 2012. "The Comparative Safety of Legal Induced Abortion and Childbirth in the United States." *Obstetrics and Gynecology* 119 (2 Pt 1): 215–19.

Renner, R., D. Brahmi, and N. Kapp. 2013. "Who Can Provide Effective and Safe Termination of Pregnancy Care? A Systematic Review." *BJOG* 120 (1): 23–31.

Richey, M., and R. M. Salem. 2008. *Elements of Success in Family Planning*. Population Reports Series J (57), INFO Project, Johns Hopkins Bloomberg School of Public Health, Baltimore.

Ringheim, K. 2007. "Ethical and Human Rights Perspectives on Providers' Obligation to Ensure Adolescents' Rights to Privacy." *Studies in Family Planning* 38 (4): 245–52.

Ross, J., and A. K. Blanc. 2012. "Why Aren't There More Maternal Deaths? A Decomposition Analysis." *Maternal Child Health Journal* 16 (2): 456–63. doi:10.1007/s10995-011-0777-x.

Ross, J., and E. Smith. 2011. "Trends in National Family Planning Programs, 1999, 2004 and 2009." *International Perspectives on Sexual and Reproductive Health* 37 (3): 125–33.

Ross, J., and J. Stover. 2013. "Use of Modern Contraception Increases When More Methods Become Available: Analysis of Evidence from 1982–2009." *Global Health: Science and Practice* 1 (2): 203–12. doi:10.9745/GHSP-D-13-00010.

Royal Society. 2012. *People and the Planet.* London: The Royal Society.

Rutstein, S. O., K. Johnson, A. Conde-Agudelo, and A. Rosas-Bermudez. 2008. "Further Analysis of the Effects of Birth Spacing on Infant and Child Mortality: A Systematic Review and Meta-Analysis." Technical Consultation and Scientific Review of Birth Spacing, World Health Organization, Geneva, June 13–15.

Samandari, G., M. Wolf, I. Basnett, A. Hyman, and K. Andersen. 2012. "Implementation of Legal Abortion in Nepal: A Model for Rapid Scale-Up of High-Quality Care." *Reproductive Health* 9: 7.

Schutt-Aine, J., and M. Maddaleno. 2003. *Sexual Health and Development of Adolescents and Youth in the Americas: Program and Policy Implications.* Washington, DC: Pan American Health Organization.

Seamans, Y., and C. M. Harner-Jay. 2007. "Modelling Cost-Effectiveness of Different Vasectomy Methods in India, Kenya, and Mexico." *Cost Effectiveness and Resource Allocation* 5: 8.

Senderwitz, J. 1999. "Making Reproductive Health Services Youth Friendly." Research, Program and Policy Series. Pathfinder International, FOCUS on Young Adults, Washington, DC.

Seltzer, J. 2002. *The Origins and Evolution of Family Planning Programs in Developing Countries.* Santa Monica, CA: RAND.

Simmons, R., and J. Shiffman. 2007. "Scaling-up Reproductive Health Service Innovations: A Framework for Action." In *Scaling Up Health Service Delivery: From Pilot Innovations to Policies and Programmes,* edited by Ruth Simmons, Peter Fajans, and Laura Ghiron, 1–30. Geneva: World Health Organization.

Singh, J. S. 2009. *Creating a New Consensus on Population: The Politics of Reproductive Health, Reproductive Rights and Women's Empowerment.* London: Earthscan.

Sneeringer, R. K., D. L. Billings, B. Ganatra, and T. L. Baird. 2012. "Roles of Pharmacists in Expanding Access to Safe and Effective Medical Abortion in Developing Countries: A Review of the Literature." *Journal of Public Health Policy* 33 (2): 218–29.

Stephenson, R., A. O. Tsui, S. Sulzbach, P. Bardsley, G. Bekele, and others. 2004. "Franchising Reproductive Health Services." *Health Services Research* 39 (6 Pt 2): 2053–80.

Stoebenau, K., and T. W. Valente. 2003. "Using Network Analysis to Understand Community-Based Programs: A Case Study from Highland Madagascar." *International Family Planning Perspectives* 29 (4): 167–73.

Stover, J., and J. Ross. 2009. "How Increased Contraceptive Use Has Reduced Maternal Mortality." *Maternal and Child Health* 14 (5): 687–95. doi:10.1007/s10995-009-0505-y.

Sweat, M. D., J. Denison, C. Kennedy, V. Tedrow, and K. O'Reilly. 2012. "Effects of Condom Social Marketing on Condom Use in Developing Countries: A Systematic Review and Meta-Analysis, 1990–2010." *Bulletin of the World Health Organization* 90 (8): 613–22A. doi:10.2471/BLT.11.094268.

Thapa, S., S. Sharma, and N. Khatiwada. 2014. "Women's Knowledge of Abortion Law and Availability of Services in Nepal." *Journal of Biosocial Science* 46 (2): 266–77.

Todd, J. E., P. Winters, and G. Stecklov. 2010. "Evaluating the Impact of Conditional Cash Transfer Programs on Fertility: The Care of the *Red de Proteccíon Social* in Nicaragua." *Journal of Population Economics* 25 (1): 267–90. doi:10.1007/s00148-010-0337-5.

Tripney, J., I. Kwan, and K. Bird. 2013. "Postabortion Family Planning Counseling and Services for Women in Low-Income Countries: A Systematic Review." *Contraception* 87: 17–25.

Trussel, J. 2011. "Contraceptive Efficacy." In *Contraceptive Technology,* Twentieth Revised Edition, edited by R. A. Hatcher, J. Trussel, A. L. Nelson, W. Cates, D. Kowal, and M. Policar. New York: Ardent Media.

UN (United Nations). 1968. "Final Act of the International Conference on Human Rights, Teheran, April 22–May 13." UN, New York.

———. 2011. *World Population Prospects 2011.* New York: Department of Economic and Social Affairs, Population Division, UN.

UN Population Division. 2009. "What Would It Take to Accelerate Fertility Decline in the Least Developed Countries?" Policy Brief 2009/1, United Nations, New York.

———. 2013a. *World Abortion Policies 2013.* New York. http://www.un.org/en/development/desa/population/publications/policy/world-abortion-policies-2013.shtml.

———. 2013b. *World Contraceptive Patterns 2013.* New York: Department of Economic and Social Affairs, United Nations.

UNESCO (United Nations Educational, Scientific and Cultural Organization). 2009. *UNESCO's Short Guide to Essential Characteristics of Effective HIV Prevention.* Paris: UNESCO. www.unesco.org/aids

———. 2013. "Schooling for millions of Children Jeopardized by Reductions in Aid." Institute for Statistics Database, No. 25, UNESCO.

UNFPA (United Nations Population Fund). 2012. *By Choice, Not by Chance. State of World Population 2012.* New York: UNFPA.

———. 2013. *Motherhood in Childhood. Facing the Challenge of Adolescent Pregnancy.* 2013 State of the World Population Report. New York: UNFPA.

UNICEF (United Nations Children's Fund). 2005. "Progress for Children: A Report Card on Gender Parity and Primary Education." No. 2. UNICEF, New York.

———. 2011. *The State of the World's Children 2011.* New York: UNICEF.

USAID/Africa Bureau, USAID/Population and Reproductive Health, Ethiopia Federal Ministry of Health, Malawi Ministry of Health, and Rwanda Ministry of Health. 2013. *Three Successful Sub-Saharan Africa Family Planning Programs: Lessons for Meeting the MDGs.* Washington, DC: USAID.

Villarruel, A. M., Y. Zhou, E. C. Gallegos, and D. L. Ronis. 2010. "Examining Long-Term Effects of *Cuidate*—A Sexual Risk Reduction Program in Mexican

Youth." *Revista Panamericana de Salud Publica* 27 (5): 345–51.

World Bank and UNICEF. 2009. *Abolishing School Fees in Africa: Lessons from Ethiopia, Ghana, Kenya, Malawi, and Mozambique.* Washington, DC: World Bank.

WHO (World Health Organization). 1997. "Beyond Acceptability: Users' Perspectives on Contraception, Reproductive Health Matters." WHO, Geneva.

———. 2011. *Unsafe Abortion: Global and Regional Estimates of the Incidence of Unsafe Abortion and Associated Mortality in 2008,* 6th ed. Geneva: WHO.

———. 2012. *Safe Abortion: Technical and Policy Guidance for Health Systems.* Geneva: WHO.

———. 2013. *Responding to Intimate Partner Violence and Sexual Violence against Women: WHO Clinical and Policy Guidelines.* Geneva: WHO.

———. 2014a. *Global Health Estimates for Deaths by Cause, Age, and Sex for Years 2000–2012.* Geneva: WHO. http://www.who.int/healthinfo/global_burden_disease/en/.

———. 2014b. *Trends in Maternal Mortality: 1990 to 2013.* Estimates by WHO, UNFPA, World Bank, and the United Nations Population Division. Geneva: WHO.

———. 2014c. *Health Care for Women Subjected to Intimate Partner Violence or Sexual Violence. A Clinical Handbook.* Geneva: WHO

———. 2015. *Trends in Maternal Mortality: 1990 to 2015.* Estimates by WHO, UNFPA, World Bank, and the United Nations Population Division. Geneva: WHO.

Williams, T., S. Mullen, A. Karim, and J. Posner. 2007. *Evaluation of the Africa Youth Alliance Program in Ghana, Tanzania and Uganda: Impact on Sexual and Reproductive Health Behavior among Young People.* Arlington, VA: JSI Research and Training Institute.

Zuurmond, M. A., R. S. Geary, and D. A. Ross. 2012. "The Effectiveness of Youth Centers in Increasing Use of Sexual and Reproductive Health Services: A Systematic Review." *Studies in Family Planning* 43 (4): 239–54.

Chapter **7**

Interventions to Reduce Maternal and Newborn Morbidity and Mortality

A. Metin Gülmezoglu, Theresa A. Lawrie, Natasha Hezelgrave,
Olufemi T. Oladapo, João Paulo Souza, Marijke Gielen,
Joy E. Lawn, Rajiv Bahl, Fernando Althabe, Daniela Colaci,
and G. Justus Hofmeyr

INTRODUCTION

In 2015, an estimated 303,000 women died as a result of pregnancy and childbirth-related complications (WHO 2015a). Most of these deaths occurred in low- and middle-income countries (LMICs). Sub-Saharan Africa had the highest maternal mortality ratio (MMR) in 2015, an estimated 546 maternal deaths per 100,000 live births; the MMR for high-income countries (HICs) was an estimated 17 maternal deaths per 100,000 live births (map 7.1) (WHO 2015a). Although significant progress has been made since 1990 in achieving the Millennium Development Goals (MDGs), with a reduction in the global MMR from 385 to 216 maternal deaths per 100,000 live births, this reduction falls short of the 2015 MDG 5 target of a 75 percent reduction.

Similarly, mortality for children under age five years (MDG 4) declined by 49 percent, from 12.4 million in 1990 to 5.9 million in 2015, but still substantially short of the 2015 target of a reduction by two-thirds, and the decline is much slower for neonatal deaths (Liu and others 2016). Within countries, when the population is disaggregated by income, education, or place of residence, wide disparities in child mortality can be shown, even in those areas where the overall mortality

seems low. Respiratory infections, diarrhea, and malaria remain important causes of under-five mortality after the first month of life (Liu and others 2016). Neonates account for 45 percent of all deaths under age five years (Liu and others 2016); this share exceeds 50 percent in several regions (Lawn and others 2014). Of all newborn deaths, preterm birth and intrapartum-related complications account for 59 percent (Liu and others 2016), and preterm birth is now the leading direct cause of all deaths under age five years (Lawn and others 2014).

The tracking of progress does not include stillbirths. In 2009, an estimated 2.6 million stillbirths occurred in the last trimester of pregnancy, with more than 45 percent in the intrapartum period (Lawn and others 2011; Lawn and others 2016). The majority of these stillbirths (98 percent) occur in LMICs (Lawn and others 2014).

Significant proportions of these maternal, fetal, and newborn deaths are preventable. A crucial focus of recent initiatives, such as Ending Preventable Maternal Mortality, is quality of care (WHO 2015b). This chapter discusses biomedical interventions for major causes of morbidity and mortality in pregnancy and childbirth in the context of people's right to access good quality, respectful, and timely care—wherever they may live.

Corresponding author: A. Metin Gülmezoglu, Department of Reproductive Health and Research, World Health Organization, Geneva, gulmezoglum@who.int.

Map 7.1 Maternal Mortality Ratio per 100,000 Live Births, 2015

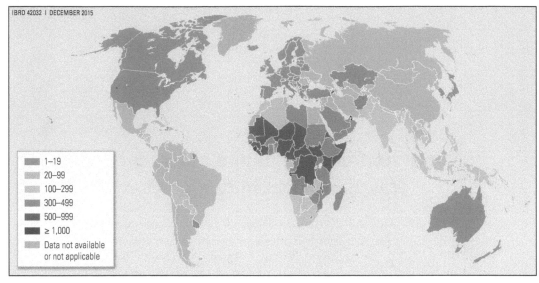

IBRD 42032 | DECEMBER 2015

- 1–19
- 20–99
- 100–299
- 300–499
- 500–999
- ≥ 1,000
- Data not available or not applicable

Source: Based on WHO 2015a; map re-created based on WHO 2015a.

INTERVENTIONS TO REDUCE MATERNAL MORTALITY AND MORBIDITY

Major obstetric causes of maternal mortality include hemorrhage (postpartum hemorrhage [PPH], and hemorrhage due to placental abruption, placenta previa, ruptured uterus, and other causes), hypertensive diseases of pregnancy (mainly preeclampsia/eclampsia), and maternal sepsis. In a study conducted across 29 countries in Asia, Latin America and the Caribbean, the Middle East and North Africa, and Sub-Saharan Africa, PPH and preeclampsia/eclampsia each accounted for more than 25 percent of maternal deaths and near-misses; maternal sepsis accounted for approximately 8 percent (Souza and others 2013). The burden of disease due to obstructed labor is difficult to estimate because these data may be coded under sepsis or hemorrhage. However, ruptured uterus, a possible consequence of obstructed labor, accounted for 4.3 percent of maternal deaths and near-miss events in the multicountry study.

Data on indirect causes of maternal deaths—those associated with conditions, such as heart disease, malaria, tuberculosis, and HIV, exacerbated by pregnancy—are also difficult to capture. However, the contribution of indirect causes of maternal deaths is estimated to be about 28 percent and seems to be increasing, particularly in Sub-Saharan Africa (Say and others 2014). In 2015, 2.0 percent of indirect maternal deaths in Sub-Saharan Africa were related to HIV, with the proportion reaching 10 percent or more in five countries (WHO 2015a). This highlights the importance of integrating service delivery during pregnancy and childbirth as recommended by the WHO

Integrated Management in Pregnancy and Childcare (IMPAC) package (WHO 2010a). Interventions to reduce indirect causes of maternal mortality and morbidity are not addressed in this chapter.

Table 7.1 provides an overview of selected medical interventions to reduce poor maternal outcomes for which there is moderate to high-quality evidence.

Postpartum Hemorrhage

Most of the evidence for PPH comes from reviews of studies in both high-income countries (HICs) and LMICs.

Preventing Postpartum Hemorrhage

The most effective intervention for preventing PPH is the use of uterotonics—drugs that contract the uterus—during the third stage of labor before the placenta is delivered. An injectable uterotonic is the drug of choice; however, oral or sublingual misoprostol may be used when injectable uterotonics are not available (table 7.2).

Oxytocin and ergot alkaloids. A Cochrane review assessed the effect of prophylactic oxytocin given during the third stage of labor on PPH (blood loss greater than 500 milliliters) (Westhoff, Cotter, and Tolosa 2013). The review included 20 randomized controlled trials (RCTs) conducted in LMICs and HICs involving 10,806 women. Prophylactic oxytocin, compared with placebo, halved the risk of PPH; when compared with ergot alkaloids, it reduced the risk of PPH by 25 percent. There was no significant difference in the risk of PPH with the combination of oxytocin and ergometrine versus ergot alkaloids alone. Oxytocin was better tolerated than ergot alkaloids.

Table 7.1 Evidence-Based Interventions that Reduce Maternal Morbidity and Mortality

Type of intervention	Main effects	Quality of evidence[a]	Source of evidence
Postpartum hemorrhage (PPH)			
Oxytocin	• Halves PPH risk when used routinely for prevention • Recommended for prevention and treatment	Moderate	Westhoff, Cotter, and Tolosa 2013; WHO 2012
Misoprostol	• Reduces PPH risk and the need for blood transfusion • Recommended for PPH prevention if oxytocin unavailable	Moderate	Tunçalp, Hofmeyr, and Gülmezoglu 2012; WHO 2012
Preeclampsia and eclampsia			
Calcium supplementation	• Halves preeclampsia risk in all women • Risk reduction is greatest in high-risk women and those with low dietary calcium intake	Moderate	Hofmeyr and others 2014; WHO 2013
Aspirin supplementation	• Reduces the risk of preeclampsia in high-risk women	Moderate	Duley and others 2007; WHO 2011b
Magnesium sulphate	• Reduces the risk of first seizure in women with preeclampsia and recurrent seizures in eclampsia, with a trend to reduced maternal mortality	High	Altman and others 2002; Duley, Gülmezoglu, and others 2010; WHO 2011b
Sepsis			
Prophylactic antibiotics at cesarean section	• Reduces risk of wound infection, endometritis, and serious maternal infectious morbidity	Moderate	Smaill and Grivell 2014

Note: This list is not comprehensive. PPH = postpartum hemorrhage.

a. Based on GRADE Working Group grades of evidence (Atkins and others 2004). The GRADE approach considers evidence from randomized trials to be high quality in the first instance, and downgrades the evidence to moderate, low, or very low if there are limitations in trial quality suggesting bias, inconsistency, imprecise or sparse data, uncertainty about directness, or high probability of publication bias. Evidence from observational studies is graded low quality in the first instance and upgraded to moderate (or high) if large effects are yielded in the absence of obvious bias.

Table 7.2 Interventions to Prevent Postpartum Hemorrhage

Evidence-based effective interventions for postpartum hemorrhage prevention
• Uterotonics used during the third stage of labor: Oxytocin (10 IU IM or IV) is the drug of choice (Westhoff, Cotter, and Tolosa 2013).
• In settings where oxytocin is unavailable, other injectable uterotonics—ergot alkaloids if appropriate, or the fixed drug combination of oxytocin and ergometrine), or oral misoprostol (600 micrograms)—are recommended (WHO 2012).

Note: IM = intramuscular; IU = international unit; IV = intravenous; μg = microgram.

Misoprostol. A Cochrane review assessed the effect of prophylactic misoprostol compared with uterotonics or no uterotonic given during the third stage of labor to women at risk of PPH (Tunçalp, Hofmeyr, and Gülmezoglu 2012). The review included 72 trials conducted in LMICs and HICs involving 52,678 women. In comparison with oxytocin, oral or sublingual misoprostol was associated with an increased risk of severe PPH (blood loss greater than 1,000 milliliters). However, misoprostol was significantly more effective than placebo in reducing PPH and blood transfusions. Misoprostol is associated with an increased risk of shivering and fever (temperature of 38°C or higher) compared with oxytocin and placebo. It does not appear to increase or decrease severe maternal morbidity or mortality (Hofmeyr and others 2013).

Misoprostol does not require refrigeration and is inexpensive and easy to administer. In settings in which skilled birth attendants are not present and oxytocin is unavailable, the World Health Organization (WHO) recommends that misoprostol (600 micrograms orally) be given to women in the third stage of labor by community health care workers and lay health workers to prevent PPH (WHO 2012). Continued vigilance for adverse effects is essential. Additional research is needed to further determine the relative effectiveness and the risks of various dosages of misoprostol and to identify the lowest effective dose.

Other Interventions

Uterine massage. Evidence on the efficacy of uterine massage for the prevention of PPH is limited and inconclusive. A Cochrane review evaluated data from two RCTs of 1,491 women that investigated the effects of uterine massage before, after, or both before and after delivery of the placenta (Hofmeyr, Abdel-Aleem, and Abdel-Aleem 2013). No significant difference was observed in uterine blood loss, irrespective of when the massage was initiated, between the intervention and control groups. The WHO does not recommend sustained uterine massage as an intervention to prevent PPH in women who have received prophylactic oxytocin. However, early postpartum identification of uterine atony—failure of the uterus to contract sufficiently—is recommended for all women.

Early versus late cord clamping. A Cochrane review assessed the effects of early cord clamping (less than one minute after birth), compared with late cord clamping after birth, on maternal and neonatal outcomes (McDonald and others 2013). The review included 15 trials conducted in LMICs and HICs involving 3,911 women and infant pairs. There was no significant difference between early versus late cord clamping groups with respect to PPH and severe PPH in the mothers. However, late cord clamping increased early hemoglobin concentrations and iron stores in infants, compared with early cord clamping, and the WHO recommends late cord clamping to improve infant outcomes (WHO 2012).

Controlled cord traction. Two large trials of controlled cord traction (CCT) have been conducted, one of 23,861 women in eight LMICs (Gülmezoglu, Lumbiganon, and others 2012) and the other of 4,013 women in France (Deneux-Tharaux and others 2013). The results of these trials suggest that CCT performed as part of the management of the third stage of labor has no clinically important effect on the incidence of PPH. The WHO weakly recommends CCT by skilled birth attendants (WHO 2012).

Treating Postpartum Hemorrhage

Evidence for the most common interventions for treating PPH due to atony is based on data extrapolated from studies of PPH prevention.

Primary interventions. Emptying the bladder and uterine massage to stimulate contractions are the first steps for the treatment of PPH. Although no high-quality evidence supports these interventions, they allow easier assessment of the uterus and its contractility. Uterine massage is strongly recommended for PPH treatment (WHO 2012). Fluid replacement is a key element in the resuscitation of women with PPH. No RCTs have assessed fluid replacement in this particular condition; the evidence in favor of crystalline fluid replacement is extrapolated from a Cochrane review of fluid replacement in critically ill patients (Perel, Roberts, and Ker 2013).

Drug interventions. The injectable uterotonic drugs oxytocin and ergometrine are both extremely effective in causing uterine contraction. Oxytocin is preferred initially, especially in women with a history of hypertension, because ergometrine can cause hypertension. The intravenous route is recommended for administration of oxytocin. Evidence suggests that administering misoprostol and injectable uterotonics together for PPH treatment does not confer additional benefits (Mousa and others 2014). However, if injectable uterotonics are not available or have been ineffective, misoprostol can be administered. Tranexamic acid may also be given (WHO 2012).

Uterine tamponade. Uterine tamponade, involving a mechanical device to exert pressure from within the uterus, has a reported success rate of between 60 percent and 100 percent (Diemert and others 2012; Georgiou 2009; Majumdar and others 2010; Porreco and Stettler 2010; Sheikh and others 2011; Thapa and others 2010; Yoong and others 2012). This evidence is indirect and comes mainly from case series. The types of devices used for uterine tamponade include urinary catheters (Sengstaken-Blakemore or Foley's), balloon catheters (Bakri and Rusch), and condoms. Although the quality of the evidence is low, the WHO considers the benefits to outweigh the disadvantages and weakly recommends this intervention (WHO 2012).

Artery embolization. Artery embolization is used to treat PPH in facilities with appropriate equipment and expertise. There are no RCTs evaluating this procedure; the evidence from case series and case reports indicates that the success rate ranges between 82 percent and 100 percent (Ganguli and others 2011; Kirby and others 2009; Lee and Shepherd 2010; Touboul and others 2008; Wang and others 2009; Zwart, Djik, and van Roosmalen 2010). The WHO weakly recommends this intervention (WHO 2012), depending on available resources.

Surgical interventions. Surgical interventions are generally used when other treatments have failed. Surgical interventions include compression sutures (for example, the B-Lynch technique); ligation of the uterine, ovarian, or iliac artery; and total or subtotal hysterectomy. The evidence supporting these procedures is limited because they are emergency, life-saving procedures. The B-Lynch technique has some advantages in that it is relatively simple to perform, preserves fertility, and has good success rates (89 percent to 100 percent) (Price and Lynch 2005). The WHO strongly recommends these life-saving procedures when indicated (WHO 2012).

Nonpneumatic antishock garment. A nonpneumatic antishock garment is a simple low-technology, first-aid device that may help stabilize women with hypovolemic shock, particularly during transport to facilities; however, high-quality research on the garment is lacking. The WHO weakly recommends this intervention, depending on available resources (WHO 2012).

Interventions in the Pipeline
Several lines of active research are underway in PPH prevention and treatment: A large RCT with a sample size of 20,000 is evaluating tranexamic acid compared with placebo in women with PPH (http://www.thewomantrial.lshtm.ac.uk/). An inhaled oxytocin development project has been awarded seed funding and is undergoing initial development research in Australia (http://www.monash.edu.au/pharm/research/iop/). The WHO is evaluating a room-temperature-stable synthetic oxytocin analogue, carbetocin. In addition, various forms of occlusive gels and foams are in development.

Preeclampsia and Eclampsia
Hypertensive disorders in pregnancy, particularly preeclampsia, complicate 2 percent to 8 percent of all pregnancies, accounting for the majority of the estimated 76,000 annual maternal deaths occurring in LMICs (Duley 2009). A WHO multicountry survey on maternal and newborn health estimates that preeclampsia is associated with more than 25 percent of severe maternal outcomes and is the direct cause of 20 percent of reported maternal deaths (Souza and others 2013). It is associated with 20 percent of infants born prematurely and 25 percent of stillbirths and neonatal deaths (Ngoc and others 2006).

The etiology of preeclampsia is unknown. It is thought to arise from the placenta and is associated with malfunction of the lining of blood vessels. The clinical spectrum of disease in preeclampsia varies, ranging from mild, asymptomatic disease, often occurring close to term, to severe, uncontrolled hypertension typically developing remote from term (less than

34 weeks). Generalized seizures (eclampsia) occur in up to 8 percent of women with preeclampsia in LMICs (Steegers and others 2010), a rate that is 10 times to 30 times more common than in HICs (Duley 2009).

Preventing Preeclampsia
The only interventions that have shown clear benefit in reducing preeclampsia risk in selected populations are low-dose aspirin (Duley and others 2007) and dietary supplementation with calcium (Hofmeyr and others 2014).

Calcium supplementation. A WHO synthesis of evidence from two Cochrane reviews (Buppasiri and others 2011; Hofmeyr and others 2014) involving 15 RCTs conducted in LMICs and HICs and 16,490 women found that calcium supplementation more than halves the incidence of preeclampsia in all women, compared with placebo, with greater reductions in high-risk women and populations with low dietary calcium intake. Calcium supplementation was associated with a 20 percent reduction in the risk of the composite outcome of maternal death or serious morbidity. The WHO strongly recommends that in areas with low dietary calcium intake, calcium supplementation commence in early pregnancy, particularly for women at high risk of preeclampsia, including those with multiple pregnancies, previous preeclampsia, preexisting hypertension, diabetes, renal or autoimmune disease, or obesity (WHO 2011a, 2013).

Low-dose aspirin. In a Cochrane review of 18 trials conducted in LMICs and HICs of prophylactic aspirin in 4,121 pregnant women, low-dose aspirin in women at high risk of preeclampsia was associated with a 25 percent risk reduction (Duley and others 2007). In addition, an 18 percent reduction in the risk of fetal or neonatal death was observed for a subgroup of trials that commenced treatment before 20 weeks' gestation. The WHO recommends low-dose aspirin (75 milligrams a day) to be prescribed and initiated before 20 weeks gestation to those women at high risk of developing preeclampsia (WHO 2011b).

Screening for preeclampsia. Early detection is vital for timely intervention and prevention of progression to severe disease. Monitoring blood pressure and performing urinalysis are the cornerstones of antenatal screening, as are asking about symptoms that may suggest preeclampsia and noting if a fetus is smaller than expected. Detection of preeclampsia should prompt referral for specialist care.

Treating Preeclampsia and Eclampsia
The only definitive cure for preeclampsia is delivery of the baby, by induction of labor or by prelabor cesarean section (CS), to prevent progression of disease and related

morbidity and mortality. The mainstays of treatment are antihypertensive drugs for blood pressure control and magnesium sulphate ($MgSO_4$) for eclampsia.

Antihypertensive therapy. Antihypertensive therapy in preeclampsia aims to reduce the risk of severe hypertension and stroke, with a steady reduction in blood pressure to safe levels, avoiding sudden drops that may compromise blood supply to the fetus. No evidence is available on the comparative efficacy of commonly used antihypertensive medications, such as labetolol, calcium channel blockers (nifedipine), hydralazine, and methyldopa, for mild to moderate or severe hypertension. All of the agents listed have been used extensively, and the WHO guidelines recognize that they are all reasonable choices for controlling hypertension. The choice of drug should be based on the prescribing clinician's experience with that particular drug, its cost, and local availability (WHO 2011b).

Anticonvulsant prophylaxis and treatment. Substantial evidence exists to demonstrate that $MgSO_4$, a low-cost intramuscular or intravenous treatment, is effective in preventing and controlling eclampsia. The Magpie study, a multicountry prospective RCT involving 33 centers and 10,141 women (two-thirds of the participating centers were in LMICs), compared $MgSO_4$ with placebo in women with preeclampsia. A reduction of more than 50 percent in preeclamptic seizures occurred in the treatment arm, with the number needed to treat of 100 women to prevent 1 case of eclampsia (Altman and others 2002); the number needed to treat fell to 63 for women with severe preeclampsia.

A Cochrane review and meta-analysis of six trials including Magpie confirmed a clinically significant reduction in risk of eclampsia of 59 percent, regardless of the route of administration of $MgSO_4$ (Duley, Gülmezoglu, and others 2010), with the risk of dying nonsignificantly reduced by 46 percent. Strong evidence indicates that $MgSO_4$ is also substantially more effective than phenytoin for the treatment of eclampsia (Duley, Henderson-Smart, and Chou 2010). The evidence regarding the effectiveness and safety of a low-dose $MgSO_4$ regimen is insufficient (Duley, Gülmezoglu, and others 2010); the WHO recommends the administration of the full intravenous or intramuscular regimen involving a loading dose followed by at least 24 hours of maintenance dosing.

Timing of delivery. For mild, moderate, and severe preeclampsia diagnosed at term, the WHO recommends a policy of early delivery by induction of labor, or cesarean section if induction is not appropriate (WHO 2011b). However, limited evidence suggests that induction at more than 36 weeks of gestation reduces poor maternal outcomes in mild preeclampsia (Koopmans and others 2009). For earlier gestations, the decision for delivery versus expectant management depends on the severity of disease and is influenced by the setting. A Cochrane review finds insufficient evidence for intervention versus expectant management for women with severe preeclampsia between 24 and 34 weeks gestation (Churchill and others 2013); however, the expectant approach is probably associated with less neonatal morbidity. No systematic reviews address the optimal timing of delivery for preeclampsia between 34 and 36 weeks gestation, and significant variation in practice exists. In the absence of robust evidence, the WHO recommends a policy of expectant management for women with severe preeclampsia, both before 34 weeks gestation and between 34 and 36 weeks gestation with a viable fetus, provided that the pregnancy can be monitored for increasing hypertension, maternal organ dysfunction, and fetal distress (WHO 2011b). Clearly, this management requires equitable access to facilities for safe delivery (including CS), skilled attendance at delivery, access to appropriate drugs, and maternal and fetal monitoring.

Technologies and Interventions in the Pipeline
Prevention and treatment. Early calcium supplementation during preconception and early pregnancy, possibly by means of food fortification, is being evaluated by the WHO/PRE-EMPT Calcium in Pre-eclampsia (CAP) study. Funded by the Bill & Melinda Gates Foundation, the trial is being conducted in centers in Argentina, South Africa, and Zimbabwe in populations with known calcium dietary deficiencies. Work is ongoing to assess whether pregnancy and pre-pregnancy supplementation with selenium, which is reduced in preeclampsia (Mistry and others 2008), will affect outcomes from preeclampsia.

The use of statins to treat early-onset preeclampsia has shown initial promise and is under investigation (Ahmed 2011).

Screening. Interest has increased in the development of a blood pressure monitor suitable for settings without medically trained health workers. Such monitors should be automated, validated for accuracy in pregnancy, affordable, and hardwearing, and should have a reliable power supply, for example, solar power or mobile phone charging technology.

Recent evidence from a diagnostic test accuracy study suggests that low plasma levels of placental growth factor can accurately predict delivery within two weeks in women with suspected preeclampsia before 35 weeks' gestation (Chappell and others 2013). In this study, normal levels of placental growth factor accurately predicted which women did not need delivery for preeclampsia within two weeks. This test, which is potentially available as a rapid bedside diagnostic tool, shows promise as an adjunct to clinical assessment of women with preeclampsia, particularly for its apparent ability to distinguish women who require intensive surveillance and delivery from those who can be managed expectantly as outpatients.

Obstructed Labor

Labor is considered obstructed when the presenting part of the fetus cannot progress through the birth canal despite strong uterine contractions. Obstruction usually occurs at the pelvic brim, but may occur in the cavity or outlet. Causes include cephalopelvic disproportion, shoulder dystocia (fetal shoulders trapped in the pelvis during delivery), and fetal malposition and malpresentation. Obstructed labor accounts for an estimated 4 percent of maternal deaths (Lozano and others 2012), which are caused by ruptured uterus, hemorrhage and puerperal sepsis. Other outcomes, such as obstetric fistulas, lead to considerable long-term maternal morbidity. In LMICs, women with obstructed labor are more likely to have stillbirths, neonatal deaths, and neonatal infections (Harrison and others 2015). Obstructed labor can only be alleviated by means of a CS or other instrumental delivery (forceps, vacuum, symphysiotomy); therefore, referral and appropriate action during labor play a crucial role in reducing the burden of disease.

Preventing Obstructed Labor

A substantial proportion of maternal deaths in LMICs due to obstructed labor occur in community settings, where women are unable to access assisted delivery at health facilities, either because they are disempowered to challenge existing social norms (for example, delivering alone or with traditional birth attendants), or because infrastructure is lacking (for example, roads, transportation, and health facilities). In addition, women may prefer to deliver in the community without skilled assistance because they are afraid of financial costs, low quality of care in health facilities, and disrespectful treatment (Stenberg and others 2013). The first priority for preventing poor outcomes related to obstructed labor is to create the demand for skilled birth assistance and to ensure that this demand can be met.

Maternity waiting homes. A maternity waiting home is a facility that is within easy reach of a hospital or health center that provides antenatal care and emergency obstetric care (van Lonkhuijzen, Stekelenburg, and van Roosmalen 2012). Women with high-risk pregnancies or those who live remotely are encouraged to stay at these facilities, if they exist, toward the end of their pregnancies. A Cochrane review conducted in 2012 sought to evaluate the role of maternity waiting homes

on reducing maternal deaths and stillbirths. However, there was insufficient evidence for robust conclusions to be drawn (van Lonkhuijzen, Stekelenburg, and van Roosmalen 2012).

External cephalic version. External cephalic version (ECV) is a method of manually encouraging a breech fetus into a cephalic presentation, through the maternal abdomen. Very low quality evidence from a Cochrane review of eight trials conducted in LMICs and HICs involving 1,308 women shows that attempting ECV from 36 weeks gestation may reduce the risk of not achieving a normal vaginal (cephalic) delivery by half, and may reduce the risk of CS by approximately 43 percent (Hofmeyr, Kulier, and West 2015). The WHO currently supports ECV in women with uncomplicated singleton breech presentations at or beyond 36 weeks, but more research is needed.

Treating Obstructed Labor

Cesarean section. CS forms the backbone of the management of obstructed labor and saves many lives. Because of the availability of operative delivery in HICs, maternal deaths there due to obstructed labor are rare; however, CS rates are often disproportionately high in these settings. Overuse of CS has important negative implications for health equity within and across countries (Gibbons and others 2010). A systematic review of ecologic studies finds that maternal, neonatal, and infant mortality decreased with increasing CS rates up to a threshold between 9 percent and 16 percent (Betran and others 2015). Above this threshold, CS rates were not associated with reductions in mortality. Therefore, increasing the availability of CS in countries that show underuse could substantially reduce maternal deaths.

Vacuum and forceps delivery. Operative vaginal delivery may be used to assist women with obstructed labor at the pelvic outlet or low or mid-cavity. Operative vaginal delivery occurs at rates of about 10 percent in HICs, in contrast with the rate of 1.6 percent reported in a large, prospective, population-based study conducted in six LMICs (Harrison and others 2015). Vacuum and forceps procedures are associated with different benefits and risks: forceps are more likely than vacuum to achieve a vaginal delivery but are associated with more vaginal trauma and newborn facial injuries (O'Mahony, Hofmeyr, and Menon 2010). Metal cups may be more effective than soft cups for vacuum delivery, but may be associated with more cephalhematomas in newborns (O'Mahony, Hofmeyr, and Menon 2010). The lack of appropriate and functional equipment, as well as the lack of knowledge, experience, and skills to perform these procedures, contributes to the low operative vaginal delivery rates in many LMICs. Operator training is vital in all facility settings to maximize benefits and reduce morbidity with vacuum and forceps deliveries.

Symphysiotomy. Symphysiotomy is an operation in which the fibers of the pubic symphysis are partially divided to allow separation of the joint and thus enlargement of the pelvic dimensions during childbirth (Hofmeyr and Shweni 2012). The procedure is performed with local analgesia and does not require an operating theater or advanced surgical skills; it may be a lifesaving procedure for the mother, the baby, or both in clinical situations in which CS is unavailable and there is failure to progress in labor, or in obstructed birth of the aftercoming head of a breech baby.

A Cochrane review found no RCTs evaluating symphysiotomy for fetopelvic disproportion (Hofmeyr and Shweni 2012). Criticism of the procedure because of potential subsequent pelvic instability and because it is considered a second-best option has resulted in its decline or disappearance from use in many countries. Proponents argue that many maternal and neonatal deaths from obstructed labor could be prevented in parts of the world without CS facilities if symphysiotomy was used. Research is needed to provide robust evidence of the relative effectiveness and safety of symphysiotomy compared with no symphysiotomy, or comparisons of alternative symphysiotomy techniques in clinical situations in which CS is not available (Hofmeyr and Shweni 2012).

Maneuvers for shoulder dystocia. A Cochrane review evaluated evidence for maneuvers to relieve shoulder dystocia by manipulating the fetal shoulders (for example, through suprapubic pressure or the corkscrew maneuver), and increasing the functional size of the maternal pelvis by utilizing an exaggerated knee-chest position (Athukorala, Middleton, and Crowther 2006). The evidence from this review of two small trials was insufficient to support or refute any benefits of these maneuvers.

Technologies and Interventions in the Pipeline

The Odon device has been developed to assist vaginal delivery. This technological innovation has the potential to facilitate assisted delivery for prolonged second stage of labor. It consists of a film-like polyethylene sleeve that is applied to the fetal head with the help of an inserter. Because the device is designed to minimize trauma to the mother and baby, it is potentially a safer alternative to forceps and vacuum delivery. A feasibility and safety study is in progress and a comparative trial is planned if it is shown to be safe (WHO Odon Device Research Group 2013).

Maternal Sepsis

Sepsis associated with pregnancy and childbirth is among the leading direct causes of maternal mortality worldwide, accounting for approximately 10 percent of the global burden of maternal deaths (Khan and others 2006). Most of these deaths occur in LMICs; in a prospective study conducted in seven LMICs, 11.6 percent of maternal deaths were due to sepsis (Saleem and others 2014). Although the reported incidence in HICs is relatively low (between 0.1 and 0.6 per 1,000 deliveries), sepsis was reported as the leading direct cause of maternal death in the United Kingdom's Confidential Enquiry into Maternal Death (2006–08 triennium).

Maternal infections occurring before or during the birth of the baby have considerable impact on newborn mortality, and an estimated 1 million newborn deaths associated with maternal infection are recorded each year. Efforts to reduce maternal sepsis have largely focused on avoiding the risk factors, with an emphasis on reducing the frequency of unsafe abortion, intrapartum vaginal examination, and prolonged or obstructed labor; providing antibiotic cover for operative delivery; and using appropriate hospital infection control.

Preventing Maternal Sepsis

The most effective intervention for preventing maternal sepsis is the use of stringent infection control measures to limit the spread of microorganisms, particularly within hospital environments. General measures, such as handwashing with soap or other cleansing agents, are widely acceptable practices for preventing hospital transmissible infections.

Antibiotic prophylaxis in operative vaginal delivery. There is a general assumption that the use of vacuum and forceps–assisted vaginal deliveries increases the incidence of postpartum infections compared with spontaneous vaginal delivery. The evidence from available Cochrane reviews is insufficient to determine whether prophylactic antibiotics given with operative delivery or following third- or fourth-degree perineal tears reduces infectious postpartum morbidities (Buppasiri and others 2010; Liabsuetrakul and others 2004). However, the use of antibiotics among women with a third- or fourth-degree perineal tear is recommended by the WHO for prevention of wound complications (WHO 2014c).

Antibiotic prophylaxis at cesarean delivery. CS is the single most important risk factor for postpartum maternal infection, and routine antibiotic prophylaxis has considerable clinical benefits. In a Cochrane review that includes 95 trials from LMICs and HICs involving more than 15,000 women (Smaill and Grivell 2014), the use of prophylactic antibiotics compared with placebo after CS was associated with substantially lower risks of endometritis (infection of the lining of the womb) (62 percent reduction), wound infection (60 percent), and serious maternal infectious complications (69 percent reduction). This evidence was considered to be moderate quality.

Preterm and term prelabor rupture of membranes. Rupture of the fetal membranes remote from term carries substantial risk of chorioamnionitis (infection of the fetal membranes) and severe maternal sepsis. Evidence on the benefits of prophylactic antibiotics with preterm rupture of membranes is demonstrated in a Cochrane review of 22 RCTs conducted in LMICs and HICs that involved 6,872 women (Kenyon, Boulvain, and Neilson 2013). Findings reveal that the use of prophylactic antibiotics was associated with a significant reduction in chorioamnionitis (moderate-quality evidence) and markers of neonatal morbidity.

There is no convincing evidence to support the use of prophylactic for prelabor rupture of membranes at term, and this practice should be avoided in its absence (Wojcieszek, Stock, and Flenady 2014).

Vaginal application of antiseptics for vaginal delivery. A Cochrane systematic review of three RCTs involving 3,012 participants assesses the effectiveness and side effects of chlorhexidine vaginal douching during labor (Lumbiganon and others 2004). The review shows no difference in the incidence of chorioamnionitis and postpartum endometritis between women who received chlorhexidine and placebo. No benefits to neonatal infection were observed.

Vaginal application of antiseptics for cesarean delivery. A Cochrane review compares the effect of vaginal cleansing with any antiseptic agent before cesarean delivery to placebo on the risk of maternal infectious morbidities (Haas, Morgan, and Contreras 2013). The review includes five trials involving 1,946 women. The risk of postoperative endometritis was reduced by 61 percent, but no clear difference was detected in postoperative fever or any wound complications. Subgroup analysis suggests that beneficial effects might be greater for women with ruptured membranes.

Treating Maternal Sepsis

Chorioamnionitis and postpartum endometritis. The mainstay of treating maternal sepsis is antibiotics. Although evidence from Cochrane reviews is limited, intrapartum treatment with potent antibiotics is clinically reasonable (Hopkins and Smaill 2002). A Cochrane review of 39 RCTs involving 4,221 women evaluates the comparative efficacy and side effects of different antibiotic regimens for postpartum endometritis (French and Smaill 2004). Wound infection was significantly reduced and treatment was less likely to fail with a combination

of an aminoglycoside (mostly gentamicin) and clindamycin compared with other regimens.

INTERVENTIONS TO REDUCE STILLBIRTHS AND NEWBORN MORTALITY AND MORBIDITY

Addressing stillbirths and neonatal mortality requires interventions across the continuum of care (preconception, antenatal, intrapartum, immediate postnatal period, and after) and interventions across the health system (family and community level, outreach, and clinical care or facility level). Most of these interventions are included in the Lives Saved Tool, developed to model the impact of the interventions at different coverage levels (Walker, Tam, and Friberg 2013), and are part of existing sets of recommended intervention packages for addressing maternal and neonatal outcomes. *The Lancet* Every Newborn Series presents Lives Saved Tool modeling with estimates of lives saved for maternal and neonatal deaths and stillbirths, showing high gains and triple return on investment, with the potential to avert 3 million deaths per year, especially with facility-based care around birth and care of small and sick newborns (Bhutta and others 2014).

RCTs for several well-established interventions that form the cornerstones of newborn care, for example, neonatal resuscitation and thermal care for term newborns, would be impossible for ethical reasons. Important interventions initiated in the antenatal or neonatal period with evidence of health benefits later in childhood, like newborn vaccination or antiretroviral therapy (ART) in babies born to HIV-positive mothers, are not included in this chapter. In addition, we have not covered preconception or adolescent care interventions, such as family planning, for which there is good evidence of a positive impact on perinatal health (Stenberg and others 2013).

Antenatal Interventions

Routine Antenatal Care Visits

A Cochrane review of antenatal care programs reveals that reduced antenatal visits may be associated with an increase in perinatal mortality, compared with standard care (Dowswell and others 2010) (table 7.3). Indirect evidence of the effectiveness of antenatal care in reducing stillbirths is available from further analysis of data from the WHO antenatal care trial, which showed that stillbirth was reduced in the standard care group for participants who received more frequent routine antenatal visits (Vogel and others 2013). This finding is consistent with those of other trials (Hofmeyr and Hodnett 2013).

Table 7.3 Evidence-Based Antenatal Interventions that Reduce Perinatal Morbidity and Mortality

Type of intervention	Main effects	Quality of evidence[a]	Source of evidence
Nutritional			
Folic acid	• Reduces the risk of neural tube defects when given periconceptually	High	De-Regil, Fernandez-Gaxiola, and others 2010
Infection prevention and treatment			
Syphilis detection and treatment	• Reduces stillbirths, neonatal deaths, and preterm birth	High	Blencowe and others 2011
IPT (malaria-endemic areas)	• Reduces neonatal mortality and low birthweight	High	Radeva-Petrova and others 2014
	• Reduces maternal anemia		
Insecticide-treated bednets (malaria)	• Reduces fetal loss and low birthweight	High	Gamble, Ekwaru, and ter Kuile 2006
Antitetanus vaccine	• Reduces neonatal mortality from tetanus	Moderate	Blencowe, Lawn, and others 2010
Intrauterine growth restriction interventions			
Antithrombotic agents in pregnancies identified as high risk	• Reduces perinatal mortality, preterm birth, and low birthweight	High	Dodd and others 2013
Doppler velocimetry in high-risk pregnancies	• Reduces perinatal mortality	Moderate	Alfirevic, Stampalija, and Gyte 2013
Other interventions			
Labor induction at 41+ weeks for postterm pregnancy	• Reduces perinatal deaths and meconium aspiration	High	Gülmezoglu, Crowther, and others 2012
Intensive management of gestational diabetes with optimal glucose control	• Reduces macrosomia, perinatal morbidity, and mortality	Moderate	Alwan, Tuffnell, and West 2009; Syed and others 2011

Note: This list is not comprehensive. IPT = intermittent preventive treatment.

a. Based on GRADE Working Group grades of evidence (Atkins and others 2004). The GRADE approach considers evidence from randomized trials to be high quality in the first instance, and downgrades the evidence to moderate, low, or very low if there are limitations in trial quality suggesting bias, inconsistency, imprecise or sparse data, uncertainty about directness, or high probability of publication bias. Evidence from observational studies is graded low quality in the first instance and upgraded to moderate (or high) if large effects are yielded in the absence of obvious bias.

Nutritional Interventions

Folic acid. Several nutritional interventions may be implemented before and during pregnancy. Supplementation of diets with folic acid and fortification of staple commodities periconceptually reduces the risk of neural tube defects that account for a small proportion of stillbirths or neonatal deaths (Blencowe, Cousens, and others 2010; De-Regil and others 2010).

Dietary advice and balanced energy supplementation. Balanced energy and protein supplementation (BES), defined as a diet that provides up to 25 percent of total energy in the form of protein, is an important intervention for the prevention of adverse perinatal outcomes in populations with high rates of food insecurity and maternal undernutrition (Imdad and Bhutta 2012). In a Cochrane review of dietary advice interventions that includes 15 trials involving 7,410 pregnant women (Ota and others 2012), the risk of stillbirth and small-for-gestational-age babies was reduced by 38 percent for women receiving BES advice, and mean birthweight was increased. Further research on the effectiveness and implementation of BES is necessary.

Maternal calcium supplementation. The WHO synthesized evidence from two systematic reviews on maternal calcium supplementation (Buppasiri and others 2011; Hofmeyr and others 2014) and found moderate-quality evidence that calcium supplementation has no effect on preterm birth overall (WHO 2013). The WHO recommends maternal calcium supplementation from 20 weeks' gestation in populations in which calcium intake is low to reduce the risk of hypertensive disorders in pregnancy (WHO 2013).

Maternal zinc supplementation. Some evidence suggests that zinc supplementation may reduce the risk of preterm birth. A Cochrane review of the intervention includes 20 RCTs involving more than 15,000 women and infants (Mori and others 2012). Zinc supplementation resulted in a small but significant reduction in preterm birth of 14 percent, without any other significant benefits compared with controls. The reviewers conclude that studies of strategies to improve the overall nutrition of populations in impoverished areas, rather than studies of micronutrient supplementation in isolation, should be a priority.

Antenatal Treatment of Maternal Infections

Maternal infections frequently have adverse effects on perinatal outcomes, and striking mortality reductions can be obtained by antenatal interventions related to malaria, HIV, syphilis, and tetanus.

Tetanus. A review of tetanus toxoid immunization concludes that there is clear evidence of the high impact of two or more doses of tetanus vaccine in pregnancy on reducing neonatal tetanus mortality (Blencowe, Lawn, and others 2010). Immunizing pregnant women or women of childbearing age with at least two doses of tetanus toxoid was estimated to reduce mortality from neonatal tetanus by 94 percent.

Syphilis. Pregnant women with untreated syphilis have a 21 percent increased risk of stillbirths (Gomez and others 2013). Evidence of the effect of antenatal syphilis detection combined with treatment with penicillin suggests a significant reduction in stillbirths, preterm births, congenital syphilis, and neonatal mortality (Blencowe and others 2011).

Malaria. Effective prevention strategies for malaria include prophylactic antimalarial drugs through intermittent preventive treatment (IPT) and insecticide-treated bednets (ITNs). IPT has been shown to improve mean birthweight and reduce the incidence of low birthweight and neonatal mortality (Radeva-Petrova and others 2014). ITNs have been shown to reduce fetal loss by 33 percent (Gamble, Ekwaru, and ter Kuile 2006). The WHO recommends the use of long-lasting ITN and IPT with sulfadoxine-pyramethamine to prevent infection during pregnancy in malaria-endemic areas in Africa (WHO 2014b).

HIV. Most children with HIV acquire it from their mothers, and ART is vital in preventing vertical (mother-to-child) transmission. Triple drug regimens commenced antenatally are most effective; however, short ART courses commencing before labor, with treatment extended to newborns during the first week of life, have been shown to significantly reduce mother-to-child HIV transmission (Siegfried and others 2011). The WHO guidelines recommend that all pregnant women who are eligible for ART (CD4 ≤ 350 cells per cubic millimeter or advanced clinical disease) should receive it (WHO 2010b). For ineligible women, combination ART should be provided during pregnancy beginning in the second trimester and should be linked with postpartum prophylaxis (WHO 2010b). Findings from the Kesho-Bora trial, in which early weaning was associated with higher HIV-related infant mortality even with maternal ART prophylaxis during breastfeeding, highlight the importance of breastfeeding in low-resource settings (Cournil and others 2015). ART prophylaxis in these settings should be provided to either the mother or infant for the duration of breastfeeding.

Other infections. There is currently no conclusive evidence of the effects on perinatal outcomes of using viral influenza, pneumococcal, and *Haemophilus influenzae* type b vaccines during pregnancy (Chaithongwongwatthana and others 2012; Salam, Das, and Bhutta 2012).

Treatment of Diabetes Mellitus and Gestational Diabetes

Complications of diabetes range from variations in birthweight to fetal malformations and potentially an excess of perinatal mortality. Any specific treatment for gestational diabetes versus routine antenatal care is associated with a reduction in perinatal mortality (Alwan, Tuffnell, and West 2009). Intensified management including dietary advice, monitoring, or pharmacotherapy for women with gestational diabetes mellitus, when compared with conventional management, resulted in a 54 percent reduction of macrosomic (> 4,000 grams) babies. It was also associated with statistically nonsignificant reductions in other outcomes, including perinatal death, stillbirths, neonatal hypoglycemia, shoulder dystocia, CS, and birthweight (Lassi and Bhutta 2013). Optimal blood glucose control in pregnancy compared with suboptimal control was associated with a 60 percent reduction in the risk of perinatal mortality but a statistically insignificant impact on stillbirths (Syed and others 2011).

Intrauterine Growth Restriction

Risk factors for stillbirths and intrauterine growth restriction (IUGR) largely overlap, and growth-restricted fetuses are at increased risk of mortality and serious morbidity. Improved detection and management of IUGR using maternal body mass index, symphysial-fundal height measurements, and targeted ultrasound could be effective in reducing IUGR-related stillbirths by 20 percent (Imdad and others 2011).

Doppler velocimetry. A Cochrane review of RCTs in HICs shows that the use of Doppler ultrasound of umbilical and fetal arteries in high-risk pregnancies was associated with a 29 percent reduction in perinatal mortality; however, the specific effect on stillbirths was not significant (Alfirevic, Stampalija, and Gyte 2013).

Antithrombotic agents. Treatment with heparin for pregnant women considered to be at high risk of complications secondary to placental insufficiency leads to a significant reduction in the risk of perinatal mortality, preterm birth, and infant birthweight below the 10th centile for gestational age when compared with no treatment (Dodd and others 2013).

Fetal movement counting. The lack of trials has resulted in insufficient evidence of any benefits of routine fetal movement counting (Mangesi, Hofmeyr, and Smith 2007). However, a reduction in fetal movements may be indicative of fetal compromise; when identified by the mother, awareness could trigger prompt care seeking and further assessment.

Postterm Pregnancy

Elective induction of labor in low-risk pregnancies at or beyond 41 weeks gestation (late term) is recommended in settings with adequate gestational age dating and appropriate facility care. In a Cochrane review of 22 RCTs involving 9,383 women of late-term labor induction, compared with expectant management, the newborns of women who were induced were 69 percent less likely to die perinatally and 50 percent less likely to aspirate meconium (Gülmezoglu, Crowther, and others 2012); there was no significant reduction in stillbirths.

Intrapartum Interventions

Labor surveillance is needed for early detection, clinical management, and referral of women for complications. Basic emergency obstetric care should be available at first-level facilities providing childbirth care. This basic emergency care includes the following:

- The capacity to perform assisted vaginal delivery (including vacuum or forceps assistance for delivery, episiotomy, advanced skills for manual delivery of the infant with shoulder dystocia, and skilled vaginal delivery of the breech infant)
- Availability of parenteral antibiotics, parenteral oxytocin, and parenteral anticonvulsants for preeclampsia or eclampsia
- Skills for manual removal of the placenta and removal of retained products.

Because stillbirths and intrapartum-related neonatal deaths are often associated with difficult and obstructed labor, assisted vaginal delivery and CS are vital to reduce perinatal morbidity and mortality.

Worldwide, an estimated 40 million births occur at home, most in LMICs and usually in the absence of skilled birth attendants. Limited evidence from two before-and-after studies of community-based skilled birth attendance shows a 23 percent significant reduction in the risk of stillbirth (Yakoob and others 2011). Although there has been an increase in the use of skilled birth attendants globally, much remains to be done for the organization and provision of services; however, this issue is beyond the scope of this chapter. An overview of selected intrapartum interventions can be found in table 7.4.

General Interventions

Hygiene. Poor hygienic conditions and poor delivery practices contribute to the burden of neonatal mortality. Pooled data from 19,754 home births at three sites in South Asia indicate that the use of clean delivery kits or clean delivery practices almost halves the risk of neonatal mortality (Seward and others 2012). The use of a plastic sheet during delivery, a boiled blade to cut the cord, a boiled thread to tie the cord, and antiseptic to clean the umbilicus were each significantly associated with reductions in mortality, independent of kit use.

The partograph. A partograph is usually a preprinted form that provides a pictorial overview of labor progress that can alert health professionals to any problems with the mother or baby (Lavender, Hart, and Smyth 2013). Although the partograph is widely used and accepted to detect abnormal labor, strong evidence to recommend its general use is lacking (Lavender, Hart, and Smyth 2013). Until stronger evidence is available, the WHO supports the use of a partograph with a four-hour action line for monitoring the progress of labor (WHO 2014a).

Fetal monitoring in labor. There is no evidence that the use of electronic fetal heart rate monitoring during labor reduces perinatal mortality. A Cochrane review of 13 RCTs involving more than 37,000 women of continuous cardiotocography compared with intermittent auscultation shows no reduction in perinatal mortality (Alfirevic, Devane, and Gyte 2013). Continuous cardiotocography halved the risk of neonatal seizures without significant reductions in cerebral palsy, infant mortality, or other standard measures of neonatal well-being and was associated with an increased risk of assisted and operative delivery.

Active management of labor. Active management refers to a package of care that includes strict diagnosis of labor, routine amniotomy, oxytocin for slow progress, and one-to-one support (Brown and others 2013). A Cochrane review of seven RCTs involving 5,390 women finds

Table 7.4 Evidence-Based Intrapartum and Neonatal Interventions that Reduce Perinatal Morbidity and Mortality

Type of intervention	Main effects	Quality of evidence[a]	Source of evidence
General			
Clean delivery kits	• Reduces neonatal mortality	Moderate	Seward and others 2012
Preterm birth and PPROM			
Antenatal Corticosteroids	• Reduces neonatal mortality • Reduces the risk of RDS and other neonatal morbidities	Moderate	Roberts and Dalziel 2006
Magnesium sulphate	• Reduces the risk of cerebral palsy in preterm infants	Moderate	Doyle and others 2009
Antibiotics (PPROM only)	• Reduces neonatal infection	High	Kenyon, Boulvain, and Neilson 2013
Surfactant	• Reduces RDS-related mortality	Moderate	Seger and Soll 2009; Soll and Özek 2010
Neonatal care			
Kangaroo mother care	• Reduces mortality in low-birthweight infants	High	Conde-Agudelo, Belizán, and Diaz-Rossello 2014
Cord cleansing (chlorhexidine)	• Reduces neonatal mortality and omphalitis in community settings	Low-Moderate	Imdad and others 2013; WHO 2014c
Hypoxic ischemic encephalopathy			
Induced hypothermia	• Reduces mortality	High	Jacobs and others 2013
Neonatal sepsis			
Community-administered antibiotics	• Reduces all-cause neonatal mortality and pneumonia-specific mortality	Moderate	Zaidi and others 2011

Note: This list is not comprehensive. PPROM = preterm premature rupture of membranes; RDS = respiratory distress syndrome.

a. Based on GRADE Working Group grades of evidence (Atkins and others 2004). The GRADE approach considers evidence from randomized trials to be high quality in the first instance, and downgrades the evidence to moderate, low, or very low if there are limitations in trial quality suggesting bias, inconsistency, imprecise or sparse data, uncertainty about directness, or high probability of publication bias. Evidence from observational studies is graded low quality in the first instance and upgraded to moderate (or high) if large effects are yielded in the absence of obvious bias.

no significant difference in poor neonatal outcomes; however, CS rates were nonsignificantly reduced in the active management group (Brown and others 2013).

Preterm Labor and Preterm Prelabor Rupture of Membranes

Antenatal corticosteroids. The administration of antenatal corticosteroids to women in preterm labor, or in whom preterm delivery is anticipated (for example, in severe preeclampsia), for the prevention of neonatal respiratory distress syndrome (RDS) has been shown to be very effective in preventing poor neonatal outcomes in well-resourced settings. A Cochrane review of 21 RCTs involving 4,269 neonates finds that a single course of steroids administered between 26 weeks and 35 weeks gestation reduced the risk of neonatal death by 31 percent and reduced neonatal morbidity including cerebroventricular hemorrhage, necrotizing enterocolitis, RDS, and systemic infections

(Roberts and Dalziel 2006). However, a large cluster randomized trial (Antenatal Corticosteroids Trial) conducted in LMICs to test provision of antenatal corticosteroids at lower levels of the health system with mainly unskilled workers and limited assessment of gestational age finds no difference in neonatal mortality with the administration of antenatal corticosteroids (Althabe and others 2015). Neonatal mortality in the intervention clusters overall was increased, which may have been due to overtreatment, as were maternal infections. This trial has important implications for the setting, implementation, and scale up of this intervention, notably that antenatal corticosteroids should be used in the context of more accurate assessment of gestational age and assessment for maternal infection; ensuring that maternal and newborn care can be provided should also be a part of this intervention. In the Antenatal Corticosteroids Trial, half of the births were at home (Althabe and others 2015).

Antibiotics. The evidence does not support the routine administration of antibiotics to women in preterm labor with intact membranes in the absence of overt signs of infection (Flenady and others 2013). However, antibiotics for preterm premature rupture of membranes are effective in reducing the risk of a number of early morbidities, including RDS and postnatal infection, without having a significant impact on mortality (Kenyon, Boulvain, and Neilson 2013).

Magnesium sulphate. A Cochrane review of five RCTs involving 6,145 babies found that $MgSO_4$ given to women considered to be at risk of preterm birth reduced the risk of cerebral palsy by 32 percent and improved long-term outcomes into childhood (Doyle and others 2009). However, evidence is insufficient to determine the existence of neuroprotective benefits for infants of women with high-risk pregnancies at term (Nguyen and others 2013), and more research is needed.

Newborn Resuscitation

Training of birth attendants. Newborn resuscitation is not available for the majority of newborns in LMICs. Limited evidence suggests that training of birth attendants improves initial resuscitation practices and reduces inappropriate and harmful practices (Carlo and others 2010; Opiyo and English 2010) but may not have a significant impact on perinatal mortality. This finding may be because advanced resuscitation, including intubation and drugs, is appropriate only in institutions that provide ventilation. A large cluster RCT of a combined community- and facility-based approach with a package of interventions including community birth attendant training, hospital transport, and facility staff training finds the intervention package to have no detectable impact on perinatal mortality (Pasha and others 2013). This finding suggests that substantially more infrastructure may be necessary, in addition to provider training and community mobilization, to have a meaningful effect on neonatal outcomes.

Essential Newborn Care

The WHO defines essential newborn care as including cleaning, drying, and warming the infant; initiating exclusive breastfeeding; and cord care (WHO 2011a). Ideally, this care should be provided by a skilled attendant; however, most of these tasks can be carried out at home by alternative attendants.

High-quality evidence shows that home visits by community health workers in the first week after birth significantly reduces neonatal mortality and are strongly recommended by the WHO (WHO 2014c).

Neonatal Interventions

The immediate cause of many of the world's 2.8 million annual neonatal deaths is an illness presenting as an emergency, either soon after birth (such as complications of preterm birth and intrapartum hypoxia) or later (due to neonatal tetanus or community-acquired infections). Other important but less prevalent conditions include jaundice and hemorrhagic disease of the newborn. These conditions all have high fatality rates, particularly tetanus and encephalopathy (Lawn and others 2014).

Preventive measures needed to adequately reduce this burden of disease include much of what has already been discussed. Other interventions include routine vitamin K administration in newborns for the prevention of vitamin K deficiency bleeding and early phototherapy for jaundice. Early phototherapy reduces both mortality and chronic disability subsequent to kernicterus and is feasible in facilities (Djik and Hulzebos 2012; Maisels and others 2012).

Postnatal Care

Kangaroo mother care. Kangaroo mother care, which is part of the extra newborn care package for small and low-birthweight infants and includes continuous skin-to-skin contact between mothers and newborns, frequent and exclusive breastfeeding, and early discharge from hospital, has been evaluated in comparison with conventional care in a Cochrane review. The review includes 18 RCTs involving 2,751 infants (Conde-Agudelo, Belizán, and Diaz-Rossello 2014). In low-birthweight infants, kangaroo mother care reduced neonatal mortality by 40 percent, hypothermia by 66 percent, and nosocomial infection by 55 percent.

Exclusive breastfeeding. The WHO recommends exclusive breastfeeding of infants until age six months (WHO 2014c). Infants who are exclusively breastfed for six months experience less gastrointestinal morbidity (Kramer and Kakuma 2012), less respiratory morbidity, and less infection-related neonatal mortality than partially breastfed neonates (WHO 2014c). A meta-analysis shows that breastfeeding education or support (or a combination of education and support) increased exclusive breastfeeding rates (Haroon and others 2013). For small or preterm babies, extra feeding support is needed (WHO 2011a).

Cord cleansing. Pooled data from three community trials involving 54,624 newborns of cord care with chlorhexidine versus dry care show a reduction in omphalitis of 27 percent to 56 percent and in neonatal mortality of 23 percent (Imdad and others 2013). Chlorhexidine cord cleansing did not have these effects when used in hospital settings

(Sinha and others 2015). The WHO recommends daily chlorhexidine application to the umbilical cord stump during the first week of life for newborns who are born at home in settings with high neonatal mortality (WHO 2014c).

Management of Neonatal Encephalopathy

Seizures are common following perinatal hypoxic ischemia. Induced hypothermia (cooling) in newborn infants who are encephalopathic because of intrapartum hypoxia reduces neonatal mortality, major neurodevelopmental disability, and cerebral palsy. This evidence is derived from a Cochrane review of 11 RCTs involving 1,505 term and late preterm infants with moderate or severe hypoxic ischemic encephalopathy (Jacobs and others 2013). Cooling reduced neonatal mortality by 25 percent and the authors conclude that induced hypothermia should be performed in term and late preterm infants with moderate or severe hypoxic ischemic encephalopathy if identified before age six hours (Jacobs and others 2013). However, most of these studies were conducted in HICs and more trials in LMICs are needed before implementing this intervention in these settings. Routine anticonvulsant prophylaxis with barbiturates for the neuroprotection of term infants with perinatal asphyxia is not recommended (Evans, Levene, and Tsakmakis 2007).

Management of Respiratory Distress Syndrome

RDS is the most important cause of mortality in preterm infants. Administration of surfactant in preterm infants significantly decreases the risk of poor neonatal outcomes, but cost is a major factor for LMICs (Seger and Soll 2009; Soll and Özek 2010). Institution of continuous positive airway pressure may bring down the requirement and cost of surfactant therapy (Rojas-Reyes, Morley, and Soll 2012).

Management of Neonatal Sepsis

Antibiotics for treatment. Over 1 million neonatal deaths annually in LMICs are attributable to infectious causes, including neonatal sepsis, meningitis, and pneumonia (Liu and others 2016). Feasible and low-cost interventions to prevent these deaths exist. Oral antibiotics administered in the community reduce all-cause mortality by 25 percent and pneumonia-specific mortality by 42 percent (Zaida and others 2011).

Presumptive antibiotics for group B streptococcus. The risk of serious infection in term newborn infants is increased if group B streptococcus (GBS) is present in the birth canal, if rupture of membranes is prolonged, and if maternal temperature is raised during labor. A Cochrane review of intrapartum antibiotic prophylaxis (IAP) for mothers colonized with GBS (three trials and 500 women) finds low-quality evidence that early neonatal GBS infection was reduced with IAP compared with no prophylaxis (Ohlsson and Shah 2014). European consensus recommends IAP based on a universal intrapartum GBS screening strategy (Di Renzo and others 2014); however, data on GBS prevalence are not routinely available to inform policies in most LMICs. In the absence of GBS screening and strong evidence to guide clinical practice regarding routine prescription of antibiotics (Ungerer and others 2004), the use of presumptive antibiotic therapy for newborns at risk of GBS and other bacterial infections is recommended (WHO 2011a).

Interventions in the Pipeline

Household air pollution is recognized as a risk factor for several health outcomes, including stillbirth, preterm birth, and low birthweight, but rigorous evidence for the impact of reducing household air pollution on these birth outcomes is lacking (Bruce and others 2013). Interventions to reduce household air pollution may reduce poor perinatal outcomes.

A habitual supine sleeping position has been associated with an increase in stillbirth (Owusu and others 2013). Whether sleeping position can be changed by advice or other interventions, and whether such a change would affect stillbirth rates, remains to be established.

COST-EFFECTIVENESS OF INTERVENTIONS

Increasing the coverage of interventions demonstrated to be effective and cost-effective is essential, but reliable data remain limited (Mangham-Jefferies and others 2014). Chapter 17 of this volume (Horton and Levin 2016) summarizes the findings of a systematic search of the cost-effectiveness literature of reproductive, maternal, newborn, and child health interventions and discusses the difficulties, including methodological gaps, multiple platforms, and outcome measures.

For the 75 high-burden Countdown countries, Bhutta and others (2014) estimate that the additional funding required to scale up effective interventions to reduce preventable maternal and newborn deaths and still births is US$5.65 billion annually, which they equate to US$1.15 per person, excluding the initial investment in new facilities. They further estimate that increased coverage and quality of care would reduce maternal and newborn deaths and prevent stillbirths at a cost of US$1,928 per life saved (or US$60 per disability adjusted life-year [DALY] averted); 82 percent of this effect would be from facility-based care.

Costs per DALY averted have been estimated for training initiatives (for example, LeFevre and others 2013), participatory women's groups (for example, Fottrell and others 2013), and safe motherhood initiatives (for example, Erim, Resch, and Goldie 2012), and range from US$150 to US$1,000. Cost estimates for CS for obstructed labor have a wider range (US$200 to US$4,000 per DALY averted, depending on the country), with a median of slightly more than US$400 (Alkire and others 2012). Other innovations with lower costs per DALY averted, in the range of US$20–US$100—for example, clean delivery kits for home births (Sabin and others 2012)—have a modest impact on DALYs averted.

CONCLUSIONS

Although evidence of effectiveness is not available for several vital interventions, these interventions save the lives of thousands of mothers and newborns every day. For other simple interventions, research has demonstrated convincingly that, if provided in the appropriate time and with the appropriate protocol, many more lives can be saved. However, effective interventions are not consistently used or available in LMICs, and accelerated investments are needed in health system infrastructure, intervention implementation, health worker training, and patient education to improve health outcomes for mothers and newborns.

Even in the poorest settings simple approaches at the family and community levels and through outreach services can save many lives now. Well-known interventions, such as neonatal resuscitation and case management of infections, can be added to existing programs, particularly Safe Motherhood and Integrated Management of Childhood Illness programs, at low marginal cost. Although community-based options are often most feasible, if the commitment to strengthen clinical care systems is lacking, the potential improvements in health outcomes from these options is limited.

Scaling-up of skilled care for pregnancy and childbirth is still required to reach the MDGs in LMICs. However, as increasing numbers of women and babies reach first-level facilities and hospitals, the quality of care challenges in these facilities need to be addressed. A shift in focus to quality of care has the potential to unlock significant returns for every mother and every newborn beyond 2015 to end preventable maternal and newborn deaths and stillbirths by 2030.

NOTE

For consistency and ease of comparison, *DCP3* is using the World Health Organization's Global Health Estimates (GHE) for data on diseases burden, except in cases where a relevant data point is not available from GHE. In those instances, an alternative data source is noted.

World Bank Income Classifications as of July 2014 are as follows, based on estimates of gross national income (GNI) per capita for 2013:

- Low-income countries (LICs) = US$1,045 or less
- Middle-income countries (MICs) are subdivided:
  a) lower-middle-income = US$1,046 to US$4,125
  b) upper-middle-income (UMICs) = US$4,126 to US$12,745
- High-income countries (HICs) = US$12,746 or more.

REFERENCES

Ahmed, A. 2011. "New Insights into the Etiology of Preeclampsia: Identification of Key Elusive Factors for the Vascular Complications." *Thrombosis Research* 127 (Suppl. 3): S72–75. doi:10.1016/S0049-3848(11)70020-2.

Alfirevic, Z., D. Devane, and G. M. L. Gyte. 2013. "Continuous Cardiotocography (CTG) as a Form of Electronic Fetal Monitoring (EFM) for Fetal Assessment during Labour." *Cochrane Database of Systematic Reviews* (5): CD006066. doi:10.1002/14651858. CD006066.pub2.

Alfirevic, Z., T. Stampalija, and G. M. L. Gyte. 2013. "Fetal and Umbilical Doppler Ultrasound in High-Risk Pregnancies." *Cochrane Database of Systematic Reviews* (11): CD007529. doi:10.1002/14651858.CD007529.pub3.

Alkire, B. C., J. R. Vincent, C. T. Burns, I. S. Metzler, P. E. Farmer, and others. 2012. "Obstructed Labor and Caesarean Delivery: The Cost and Benefit of Surgical Intervention." *PLoS One* 7 (4): e34595.

Althabe, F., J. M. Belizan, E. M. McClure, J. Hemingway-Foday, M. Berrueta, and others. 2015. "A Population-Based, Multifaceted Strategy to Implement Antenatal Corticosteroid Treatment versus Standard Care for the Reduction of Neonatal Mortality Due to Preterm Birth in Low-Income and Middle-Income Countries: The ACT Cluster-Randomised Trial." *The Lancet* 385 (9968): 629–39.

Altman, D., G. Carroli, L. Duley, B. Farrell, J. Moodley, and others. 2002. "Magpie Trial Collaboration Group. Do Women with Pre-Eclampsia, and Their Babies, Benefit from Magnesium Sulphate? The Magpie Trial: A Randomised Placebo-Controlled Trial." *The Lancet* 359 (9321): 1877–90.

Alwan, N., D. J. Tuffnell, and J. West. 2009. "Treatments for Gestational Diabetes." *Cochrane Database of Systematic Reviews* (3): CD003395. doi:10.1002/14651858.CD003395.pub2.

Athukorala, C., P. Middleton, and C. A. Crowther. 2006. "Intrapartum Interventions for Preventing Shoulder Dystocia." *Cochrane Database of Systematic Reviews* (4): CD005543. doi:10.1002/14651858.CD005543.pub2.

Atkins, D., D. Best, P. A. Briss, M. Eccles, Y. Falck-Ytter, and others. 2004. "Grading Quality of Evidence and Strength of Recommendations." *British Medical Journal* 328 (7454): 1490.

Betran, A. P., M. R. Torloni, J. Zhang, J. Ye, R. Mikolajczyk, and others. 2015. "What Is the Optimal Rate of Caesarean Section at Population Level? A Systematic Review of Ecologic Studies." *Reproductive Health* 12: 57. doi:10.1186/s12978-015-0043-6.

Bhutta, Z. A., J. K. Das, R. Bahl, J. E. Lawn, R. A. Salam, and others. 2014. "Can Available Interventions End Preventable Deaths in Mothers, Newborn Babies, and Stillbirths, and at What Cost?" *The Lancet* 384 (9940): 347–70.

Blencowe, H., S. Cousens, B. Modell, and J. Lawn. 2010. "Folic Acid to Reduce Neonatal Mortality from Neural Tube Disorders." *International Journal of Epidemiology* 39 (Suppl. 1): i110–21. doi:10.1093/ije/dyq028.

Blencowe, H., J. Lawn, J. Vandelaer, M. Roper, and S. Cousens. 2010. "Tetanus Toxoid Immunization to Reduce Mortality from Neonatal Tetanus." *International Journal of Epidemiology* 39 (Suppl. 1): i102–9. doi:10.1093/ije/dyq027.

Blencowe, H., S. Cousens, M. Kamb, S. Berman, and J. E. Lawn. 2011. "Lives Saved Tool Supplement Detection and Treatment of Syphilis in Pregnancy to Reduce Syphilis Related Stillbirths and Neonatal Mortality." *BMC Public Health* 11 (Suppl 3): S9. doi:10.1186/1471-2458-11-S3-S9.

Brown, H. C., S. Paranjothy, T. Dowswell, and J. Thomas. 2013. "Package of Care for Active Management in Labour for Reducing Caesarean Section Rates in Low-Risk Women." *Cochrane Database of Systematic Reviews* (9): CD004907. doi:10.1002/14651858.CD004907.pub3.29.

Bruce, N. G., M. K. Dherani, J. K. Das, K. Balakrishnan, H. Adair-Rohani, and others. 2013. "Control of Household Air Pollution for Child Survival: Estimates for Intervention Impacts." *BMC Public Health* 13 (Suppl. 3): S8. doi:10.1186/1471-2458-13-S3-S8.

Buppasiri, P., P. Lumbiganon, J. Thinkhamrop, and B. Thinkhamrop. 2010. "Antibiotic Prophylaxis for Third- and Fourth-Degree Perineal Tear during Vaginal Birth." *Cochrane Database of Systematic Reviews* (11): Cd005125. doi:10.1002/14651858.CD005125.pub3

Buppasiri, P., P. Lumbiganon, J. Thinkhamrop, C. Ngamjarus, and M. Laopaiboon. 2011. "Calcium Supplementation (Other than for Preventing or Treating Hypertension) for Improving Pregnancy and Infant Outcomes." *Cochrane Database of Systematic Reviews* (10): CD007079. doi:10.1002/14651858.CD007079.pub2.

Carlo, W. A., S. S. Goudar, I. Jehan, E. Chomba, A. Tshefu, and others. 2010. "Newborn-Care Training and Perinatal Mortality in Developing Countries." *New England Journal of Medicine* 362 (7): 614–23. doi:10.1056/NEJMsa0806033.

Chaithongwongwatthana, S., W. Yamasmit, S. Limpongsanurak, P. Lumbiganon, J. A. DeSimone, and others. 2012. "Pneumococcal Vaccination during Pregnancy for Preventing Infant Infection." *Cochrane Database of Systematic Reviews* (7): CD004903. doi:10.1002/14651858.CD004903.pub3.

Chappell, L. C., S. Duckworth, P. T. Seed, M. Griffin, J. Myers, and others. 2013. "Diagnostic Accuracy of Placental Growth Factor in Women with Suspected Preeclampsia: A Prospective Multicenter Study." *Circulation* 128: 2121–31. doi:10.1161/CIRCULATIONAHA.113.003215.

Churchill, D., L. Duley, J. G. Thornton, and L. Jones. 2013. "Interventionist versus Expectant Care for Severe Pre-Eclampsia between 24 and 34 Weeks' Gestation." *Cochrane Database of Systematic Reviews* (7): CD003106. doi:10.1002/14651858.CD003106.pub2.

Conde-Agudelo, A., J. M. Belizán, and J. Diaz-Rossello. 2014. "Kangaroo Mother Care to Reduce Morbidity and Mortality in Low Birthweight Infants." *Cochrane Database of Systematic Reviews* (4): CD002771. doi:10.1002/14651858.CD002771.pub3.

Cournil, A., P. Van de Perre, C. Cames, I. de Vincenzi, J. S. Read, and others. 2015. "Early Infant Feeding Patterns and HIV-Free Survival: Findings from the Kesho-Bora Trial (Burkina Faso, Kenya, South Africa)." *Pediatric Infectious Disease Journal* 34 (2): 168–74.

Deneux-Tharaux, C., L. Sentilhes, F. Maillard, E. Closset, D. Vardon, and others. 2013. "Effect of Routine Controlled Cord Traction as Part of the Active Management of the Third Stage of Labour on Postpartum Haemorrhage: Multicentre Randomised Controlled Trial (TRACOR)." *British Medical Journal* 346: f1541. doi:10.1136/bmj.f1541.

De-Regil, L. M., A. C. Fernández-Gaxiola, T. Dowswell, and J. P. Peña-Rosas. 2010. "Effects and Safety of Periconceptional Folate Supplementation for Preventing Birth Defects." *Cochrane Database of Systematic Reviews* (10): CD007950. doi: 10.1002/14651858.CD007950.pub2.

Diemert, A., G. Ortmeyer, B. Hollwitz, M. Lotz, T. Somville, and others. 2012. "The Combination of Intrauterine Balloon Tamponade and the B-Lynch Procedure for the Treatment of Severe Postpartum Hemorrhage." *American Journal of Obstetrics and Gynecology* 206 (1): 65.e1–4. doi.10.1016/j.ajog.2011.07.041.

Dijk, P. H., and C. V. Hulzebos. 2012. "An Evidence-Based View on Hyperbilirubinaemia." *Acta Paediatrica Supplement* 101 (464): 3–10. doi:10.1111/j.1651-2227.2011.02544.x.

Di Renzo, G. C., P. Melin, A. Berardi, M. Blennow, X. Carbonell-Estrany, and others. 2014. "Intrapartum GBS Screening and Antibiotic Prophylaxis: A European Consensus Conference." *Journal of Maternal, Fetal and Neonatal Medicine* 28 (7): 766–82.

Dodd, J. M., A. McLeod, R. C. Windrim, and J. Kingdom. 2013. "Antithrombotic Therapy for Improving Maternal or Infant Health Outcomes in Women Considered at Risk of Placental Dysfunction." *Cochrane Database of Systematic Reviews* (6): CD006780. doi: 10.1002/14651858.CD006780.pub3.

Dowswell, T., G. Carroli, L. Duley, S. Gates, A.M. Gülmezoglu, and others. 2010. "Alternative versus Standard Packages of Antenatal Care for Low-Risk Pregnancy." *Cochrane Database of Systematic Reviews* 10: CD000934. doi:10.1002/14651858.CD000934.pub2.

Doyle, L. W., C. A. Crowther, P. Middleton, S. Marret, and D. Rouse. 2009. "Magnesium Sulphate for Women at Risk of Preterm Birth for Neuroprotection of the Fetus."

Cochrane Database of Systematic Reviews (1): CD004661. doi:10.1002/14651858. CD004661.pub3.

Duley, L. 2009. "The Global Impact of Pre-Eclampsia and Eclampsia." *Seminars in Perinatology* 33: 130–37. doi:10.1053/j.semperi.2009.02.010.

———, A. M. Gülmezoglu, D. J. Henderson-Smart, and D. Chou. 2010. "Magnesium Sulphate and other Anticonvulsants for Women with Pre-Eclampsia." *Cochrane Database of Systematic Reviews* 11: CD000025. doi:10.1002/14651858.CD000025.pub2.

Duley, L., D. J. Henderson-Smart, D. Chou. 2010. "Magnesium Sulphate versus Phenytoin for Eclampsia." *Cochrane Database of Systematic Reviews* 10: CD000128. doi:10.1002/14651858.CD000128.pub2.

Duley, L., D. J. Henderson-Smart, S. Meher, and J. F. King. 2007. "Antiplatelet Agents for Preventing Preeclampsia and Its Complications." *Cochrane Database of Systematic Reviews* (2): CD004659. doi:10.1002/14651858.CD004659.pub2.

Duley, L., H. E. Matar, M. Q. Almerie, and D. R. Hall. 2010. "Alternative Magnesium Sulphate Regimens for Women with Pre-Eclampsia and Eclampsia." *Cochrane Database of Systematic Reviews* (8): CD007388. doi:10.1002/14651858. CD007388.pub2.

Erim, D. O., S. C. Resch, and S. J. Goldie. 2012. "Assessing Health and Economic Outcomes of Interventions to Reduce Pregnancy-Related Mortality in Nigeria." *BMC Public Health* 12: 786. doi:10.1186/1471-2458-12-786.

Evans, D. J., M. Levene, and M. Tsakmakis. 2007. "Anticonvulsants for Preventing Mortality and Morbidity in Full Term Newborns with Perinatal Asphyxia." *Cochrane Database of Systematic Reviews* (3): CD001240. doi:10.1002/14651858.CD001240.pub2.

Flenady, V., G. Hawley, O. M. Stock, S. Kenyon, and N. Badawi. 2013. "Prophylactic Antibiotics for Inhibiting Preterm Labour with Intact Membranes." *Cochrane Database of Systematic Reviews* 12: CD000246. doi:10.1002/14651858. CD000246.pub2.

Fottrell, E., K. Azad, A. Kuddus, L. Younes, S. Shaha, and others. 2013. "The Effect of Increased Coverage of Participatory Women's Groups on Neonatal Mortality in Bangladesh: A Cluster Randomized Trial." *JAMA Pediatrics* 167 (9): 816–25.

French, L., and F. M. Smaill. 2004. "Antibiotic Regimens for Endometritis after Delivery." *Cochrane Database of Systematic Reviews* (4): CD001067. doi:10.1002/14651858. CD001067.pub2.

Gamble, C. L., J. P. Ekwaru, and F. O. ter Kuile. 2006. "Insecticide-Treated Nets for Preventing Malaria in Pregnancy." *Cochrane Database of Systematic Reviews* (2): CD003755. doi:10.1002/14651858.CD003755.pub2.

Ganguli, S., M. S. Stecker, D. Pyne, R. A. Baum, and C. M. Fan. 2011. "Uterine Artery Embolization in the Treatment of Postpartum Uterine Hemorrhage." *Journal of Vascular and Interventional Radiology* 22 (2): 169–76. doi:10.1016/j.jvir.2010.09.031.

Georgiou, C. 2009. "Balloon Tamponade in the Management of Postpartum Haemorrhage: A Review." *British Journal of Obstetrics and Gynaecology* 116 (6): 748–57. doi:10.1111/j.1471-0528.2009.02113.x.

Gibbons, L., J. M. Belizán, J. A. Lauer, A. P. Betrán, M. Merialdi, and others. 2010. "The Global Numbers and Costs of Additionally Needed and Unnecessary Caesarean Sections Performed per Year: Overuse as a Barrier to Universal Coverage." World Health Report (2010), Background paper 30. http://www.who.int/healthsystems/topics/financing/healthreport/30C-sectioncosts.pdf.

Gomez, G. B., M. L. Kamb, L. M. Newman, J. Mark, N. Broutet, and S. J. Hawkes. 2013. "Untreated Maternal Syphilis and Adverse Outcomes of Pregnancy: A Systematic Review and Meta-Analysis." *Bulletin of the World Health Organization* 91 (3): 217–26. doi:10.2471/BLT.12.107623.

Gülmezoglu, A. M., C. A. Crowther, P. Middleton, and E. Heatley. 2012. "Induction of Labour for Improving Birth Outcomes for Women at or Beyond Term." *Cochrane Database of Systematic Reviews* (6): CD004945. doi:10.1002/14651858.CD004945.pub3.

Gülmezoglu, A. M., P. Lumbiganon, S. Landoulsi, M. Widmer, H. Abdel-Aleem, and others. 2012. "Active Management of the Third Stage of Labour with and without Controlled Cord Traction: A Randomised, Controlled, Non-Inferiority Trial." *The Lancet* 379 (9827): 1721–27. doi:10.1016/S0140-6736(12)60206-2.

Haas, D. M., S. Morgan, and K. Contreras. 2013. "Vaginal Preparation with Antiseptic Solution before Cesarean Section for Preventing Postoperative Infections." *Cochrane Database of Systematic Reviews* (1): CD007892. doi:10.1002/14651858.CD007892.pub3.

Haroon, S., J. K. Das, R. A. Salam, A. Imdad, and Z. A. Bhutta. 2013. "Breastfeeding Promotion Interventions and Breastfeeding Practices: A Systematic Review." *BMC Public Health* 13 (3): 1–18. doi:10.1186/1471-2458-13-S3-S20.

Harrison, M. S., A. Ali, O. Pasha, S. Saleem, F. Althabe, and others. 2015. "A Prospective Population-Based Study of Maternal, Fetal, and Neonatal Outcomes in the Setting of Prolonged Labor, Obstructed Labor and Failure to Progress in Low- and Middle-income Countries." *Reproductive Health* 12 (suppl 2): S9.

Hofmeyr, G. J., H. Abdel-Aleem, and M. A. Abdel-Aleem. 2013. "Uterine Massage for Preventing Postpartum Haemorrhage." *Cochrane Database of Systematic Reviews* (7): CD006431. doi:10.1002/14651858.CD006431.pub3.

Hofmeyr, G. J., A. M. Gülmezoglu, N. Novikova, and T. A. Lawrie. 2013. "Postpartum Misoprostol for Preventing Maternal Mortality and Morbidity." *Cochrane Database of Systematic Reviews* (7): CD008982. doi:10.1002/14651858. CD008982.pub2.

Hofmeyr, G. J., and E. D. Hodnett. 2013. "Antenatal Care Packages with Reduced Visits and Perinatal Mortality: A Secondary Analysis of the WHO Antenatal Care Trial— Commentary: Routine Antenatal Visits for Healthy Pregnant Women Do Make a Difference." *Reproductive Health* 10: 20.

Hofmeyr, G. J., R. Kulier, and H. M. West. 2015. "External Cephalic Version for Breech Presentation at Term." *Cochrane Database of Systematic Reviews* (4): CD000083.

Hofmeyr, G. J., T. A. Lawrie, Á. N. Atallah, L. Duley, and M. R. Torloni. 2014. "Calcium Supplementation during Pregnancy for Preventing Hypertensive Disorders and Related Problems." *Cochrane Database of Systematic Reviews* (8): CD001059. doi:10.1002/14651858. CD001059.pub3.

Hofmeyr, G. J., and P. M. Shweni. 2012. "Symphysiotomy for Feto-Pelvic Disproportion." *Cochrane Database of Systematic Reviews* (10): CD005299. doi:10.1002/14651858. CD005299.pub3.

Hopkins, L., and F. M. Smaill. 2002. "Antibiotic Regimens for Management of Intraamniotic Infection." *Cochrane Database of Systematic Reviews* (3): CD003254. doi:10.1002/14651858.CD003254.

Horton, S., and C. Levin. 2016. "Cost-Effectiveness of Interventions for Reproductive, Maternal, Neonatal, and Child Health." In *Disease Control Priorities* (third edition): Volume 2, *Reproductive, Maternal, Newborn, and Child Health,* edited by R. Black, R. Laxminarayan, M. Temmerman, and N. Walker. Washington, DC: World Bank.

Imdad, A., R. M. M. Bautista, K. A. A. Senen, M. E. V. Uy, J. B. Mantaring III, and others. 2013. "Umbilical Cord Antiseptics for Preventing Sepsis and Death among Newborns." *Cochrane Database of Systematic Reviews* (5): CD008635. doi:10.1002/14651858. CD008635.pub2.

Imdad, A., and Z. A. Bhutta. 2012. "Maternal Nutrition and Birth Outcomes: Effect of Balanced Protein-Energy Supplementation." *Paediatric and Perinatal Epidemiology* 26 (Suppl. 1): 178–90. doi:10.1111/j.1365-3016.2012.01308.x.

Imdad, A., M. Y. Yakoob, S. Siddiqui, and Z. A. Bhutta. 2011. "Screening and Triage of Intrauterine Growth Restriction (IUGR) in General Population and High Risk Pregnancies: A Systematic Review with a Focus on Reduction of IUGR Related Stillbirths." *BMC Public Health* 11 (Suppl. 3): S1. doi:10.1186/1471-2458-11-S3-S1.

Jacobs, S. E., M. Berg, R. Hunt, W. O. Tarnow-Mordi, T. E. Inder, and others. 2013. "Cooling for Newborns with Hypoxic Ischaemic Encephalopathy." *Cochrane Database of Systematic Reviews* (1): CD003311. doi:10.1002/14651858. CD003311.pub3.

Kenyon, S., M. Boulvain, and J. P. Neilson. 2013. "Antibiotics for Preterm Rupture of Membranes." *Cochrane Database of Systematic Reviews* (12): CD001058. doi:10.1002/14651858. CD001058.pub3.

Khan, K. S., D. Wojdyla, L. Say, A. M. Gülmezoglu, and P. F. Van Look. 2006. "WHO Analysis of Causes of Maternal Death: A Systematic Review." *The Lancet* 367 (9516): 1066–74.

Kirby, J. M., J. R. Kachura, D. K. Rajan, K. W. Sniderman, M. E. Simons, and others. 2009. "Arterial Embolization for Primary Postpartum Hemorrhage." *Journal of Vascular and Interventional Radiology* 20 (8): 1036–45. doi:10.1016/j.jvir .2009.04.070.

Koopmans, C. M., D. Bijlenga, H. Groen, S. M. Vijgen, J. G. Aarnoudse, and others. 2009. "Induction of Labour versus Expectant Monitoring for Gestational Hypertension or Mild Pre-Eclampsia after 36 Weeks' Gestation (HYPITAT): A Multicentre, Open-Label Randomised Controlled Trial." *The Lancet* 374 (9694): 979–88. doi:10.1016/S0140-6736(09)60736-4.

Kramer, M. S., and R. Kakuma. 2012. "Optimal Duration of Exclusive Breastfeeding." *Cochrane Database of Systematic Reviews* (8): CD003517. doi:10.1002/14651858. CD003517. pub2.

Lassi, Z. S., and Z. A. Bhutta. 2013. "Risk Factors and Interventions Related to Maternal and Pre-Pregnancy Obesity, Pre-Diabetes and Diabetes for Maternal, Fetal and Neonatal Outcomes: A Systematic Review." *Expert Review of Obstetrics and Gynecology* 8 (6): 639–60.

Lavender, T., A. Hart, and R. M. D. Smyth. 2013. "Effect of Partogram Use on Outcomes for Women in Spontaneous Labour at Term." *Cochrane Database of Systematic Reviews* (7): CD005461. doi:10.1002/14651858.CD005461.pub4.

Lawn, J. E., H. Blencowe, S. Oza, D. You, A. C. Lee, and others. 2014. "Every Newborn: Progress, Priorities, and Potential beyond Survival." *The Lancet* 384 (9938): 189–205.

Lawn, J. E., H. Blencowe, R. Pattinson, S. Cousens, R. Kumar, and others. 2011. "Stillbirths: Where? When? Why? How to Make the Data Count?" *The Lancet* 377 (9775): 1448–63.

Lawn, J., H. Blencowe, P. Waiswa, A. Amouzou, C. Mathers, and others. 2016. "Stillbirths: Rate, Risk Factors, and Acceleration towards 2030." *The Lancet* 387: 587–603.

Lee, J. S., and S. M. Shepherd. 2010. "Endovascular Treatment of Postpartum Hemorrhage." *Clinical Obstetrics and Gynecology* 53 (1): 209–18. doi:10.1097/GRF.0b013e3181ce09f5.

LeFevre, A. E., S. D. Shillcutt, H. R. Waters, S. Haider, S. El Arifeen, and others. 2013. "Economic Evaluation of Neonatal Care Packages in a Cluster-Randomized Controlled Trial in Sylhet, Bangladesh." *Bulletin of the World Health Organization* 91 (10): 736–45.

Liabsuetrakul, T., T. Choobun, K. Peeyananjarassri, and Q. M. Islam. 2004. "Antibiotic Prophylaxis for Operative Vaginal Delivery." *Cochrane Database of Systematic Reviews* (3): CD004455. doi:10.1002/14651858.CD004455.pub2.

Liu, L., K. Hill, S. Oza, D. Hogan, Y. Chu, and others. 2016. "Levels and Causes of Mortality under Age Five Years." In *Disease Control Priorities* (third edition): Volume 2, *Reproductive, Maternal, Newborn, and Child Health,* edited by R. Black, R. Laxminarayan, M. Temmerman, and N. Walker. Washington, DC: World Bank.

Lozano, R., M. Naghavi, K. Foreman, S. Lim, K. Shibuya, and others. 2012. "Global and Regional Mortality from 235 Causes of Death for 20 Age Groups in 1990 and 2010: A Systematic Analysis for the Global Burden of Disease Study 2010." *The Lancet* 380 (9859): 2095–128.

Lumbiganon, P., J. Thinkhamrop, B. Thinkhamrop, and J. E. Tolosa. 2004. "Vaginal Chlorhexidine during Labour for Preventing Maternal and Neonatal Infections (Excluding Group B Streptococcal and HIV)." *Cochrane Database of Systematic Reviews* (4): CD004070. doi:10.1002/14651858. CD004070.pub2.

Maisels, M. J., J. F. Watchko, V. K. Bhutani, and D. K. Stevenson. 2012. "An Approach to the Management of Hyperbilirubinaemia in the Preterm Infant Less than 35 Weeks Gestation." *Journal of Perinatology* 32 (9): 660–64. doi:10.1038/jp.2012.71.

Majumdar, A., S. Saleh, M. Davis, I. Hassan, and P. J. Thompson. 2010. "Use of Balloon Catheter Tamponade for Massive

Postpartum Haemorrhage." *Journal of Obstetrics and Gynaecology* 30 (6): 586–93. doi:10.3109/01443615.2010.494202.

Mangesi, L., G. J. Hofmeyr, and V. Smith. 2007. "Fetal Movement Counting for Assessment of Fetal Wellbeing." *Cochrane Database of Systematic Reviews* (1): CD004909. doi:10.1002/14651858.CD004909.pub2.

Mangham-Jefferies, L., C. Pitt, S. Cousens, A. Mills, and J. Schellenberg. 2014. "Cost-Effectiveness of Strategies to Improve the Utilization and Provision of Maternal and Newborn Health Care in Low-Income and Lower-Middle-Income Countries: A Systematic Review." *BMC Pregnancy Childbirth* 14: 243. doi:10.1186/1471-2393-14-243.

McDonald, S. J., P. Middleton, T. Dowswell, and P. S. Morris. 2013. "Effect of Timing of Umbilical Cord Clamping of Term Infants on Maternal and Neonatal Outcomes." *Cochrane Database of Systematic Reviews* (7): CD004074. doi:10.1002/14651858.CD004074.pub3.

Mistry, H. D., V. Wilson, M. M. Ramsay, M. E. Symonds, and F. Broughton Pipkin. 2008. "Reduced Selenium Concentrations and Glutathione Peroxidase Activity in Pre-Eclamptic Pregnancies." *Hypertension* 52 (5): 881–88. doi:10.1161/HYPERTENSIONAHA.108.116103.

Mori, R., E. Ota, P. Middleton, R. Tobe-Gai, K. Mahomed, and others. 2012. "Zinc Supplementation for Improving Pregnancy and Infant Outcome." *Cochrane Database of Systematic Reviews* (7): CD000230. doi:10.1002/14651858.CD000230.pub4.

Mousa, H. A., J. Blum, G. Abou El Senoun, H. Shakur, and Z. Alfirevic. 2014. "Treatment for Primary Postpartum Haemorrhage." *Cochrane Database of Systematic Reviews* (2): CD003249. doi:10.1002/14651858.CD003249.pub3.

Ngoc, N. T., M. Merialdi, H. Abdel-Aleem, G. Carroli, M. Purwar, and others. 2006. "Causes of Stillbirths and Early Neonatal Deaths: Data from 7993 Pregnancies in Six Developing Countries." *Bulletin of the World Health Organization* 84: 699–705.

Nguyen, T. M. N., C. A. Crowther, D. Wilkinson, and E. Bain. 2013. "Magnesium Sulphate for Women at Term for Neuroprotection of the Fetus." *Cochrane Database of Systematic Reviews* (2): CD009395. doi:10.1002/14651858.CD009395.pub2.

Ohlsson, A., and V. S. Shah. 2014. "Intrapartum Antibiotics for Known Maternal Group B Streptococcal Colonization." *Cochrane Database of Systematic Reviews* (6): CD007467. doi:10.1002/14651858.CD007467.pub4.

O'Mahony, F., G. J. Hofmeyr, and V. Menon. 2010. "Choice of Instruments for Assisted Vaginal Delivery." *Cochrane Database of Systematic Reviews* (11): CD005455. doi:10.1002/14651858.CD005455.pub2.

Opiyo, N., and M. English. 2010. "In-Service Training for Health Professionals to Improve Care of the Seriously Ill Newborn or Child in Low and Middle-Income Countries (Review)." *Cochrane Database of Systematic Reviews* (4): CD007071. doi:10.1002/14651858.CD007071.pub2.

Ota, E., R. Tobe-Gai, R. Mori, and D. Farrar. 2012. "Antenatal Dietary Advice and Supplementation to Increase Energy and Protein Intake." *Cochrane Database of*

Systematic Reviews (9): CD000032. doi:10.1002/14651858.CD000032.pub2.

Owusu, J. T., F. J. Anderson, J. Coleman, S. Oppong, J. D. Seffah, and others. 2013. "Association of Maternal Sleep Practices with Pre-Eclampsia, Low Birth Weight, and Stillbirth among Ghanaian Women." *International Journal of Gynecology and Obstetrics* 121 (3): 261–65. doi:10.1016/j.ijgo.2013.01.013.

Pasha, O., E. M. McClure, L. L. Wright, S. Saleem, S. S. Goudar, and others. 2013. "A Combined Community- and Facility-Based Approach to Improve Pregnancy Outcomes in Low-Resource Settings: A Global Network Cluster Randomized Trial." *BMC Medicine* 11: 215.

Perel, P., I. Roberts, and K. Ker. 2013. "Colloids versus Crystalloids for Fluid Resuscitation in Critically Ill Patients." *Cochrane Database of Systematic Reviews* (2): CD000567. doi:10.1002/14651858.CD000567.pub6.

Porreco, R. P., and R. W. Stettler. 2010. "Surgical Remedies for Postpartum Hemorrhage." *Clinical Obstetrics and Gynecology* 53 (1): 182–95. doi:10.1097/GRF.0b013e3181cc4139.

Price, N., and C. B. Lynch. 2005. "Technical Description of the B-Lynch Brace Suture for Treatment of Massive Postpartum Hemorrhage and Review of Published Cases." *International Journal of Fertility and Women's Medicine* 50 (4): 148–63.

Radeva-Petrova, D., K. Kayentao, F. O. ter Kuile, D. Sinclair, and P. Garner. 2014. "Drugs for Preventing Malaria in Pregnant Women in Endemic Areas: Any Drug Regimen versus Placebo or No Treatment." *Cochrane Database of Systematic Reviews* (10): CD000169.

Roberts, D., and S. R. Dalziel. 2006. "Antenatal Corticosteroids for Accelerating Fetal Lung Maturation for Women at Risk of Preterm Birth." *Cochrane Database of Systematic Reviews* (3): CD004454. doi:10.1002/14651858.CD004454.pub2.

Rojas-Reyes, M. X., C. J. Morley, and R. Soll. 2012. "Prophylactic versus Selective Use of Surfactant in Preventing Morbidity and Mortality in Preterm Infants." *Cochrane Database of Systematic Reviews* (3): CD000510. doi:10.1002/14651858.CD000510.pub2.

Sabin, L. L., A. B. Knapp, W. B. MacLeod, G. Phiri-Mazala, J. Kasimba, and others. 2012. "Costs and Cost-Effectiveness of Training Traditional Birth Attendants to Reduce Neonatal Mortality in the Lufwanyama Neonatal Survival Study (LUNESP)." *PLoS One* 7 (4): e35560.

Salam, R. A., J. K. Das, and Z. A. Bhutta. 2012. "Impact of Haemophilus Influenza Type B (Hib) and Viral Influenza Vaccinations in Pregnancy for Improving Maternal, Neonatal and Infant Health Outcomes." *Cochrane Database of Systematic Reviews* (7): CD009982. doi:10.1002/14651858.CD009982.

Saleem, S., E. M. McClure, S. S. Goudar, A. Patel, F. Esamai, and others. 2014. "A Prospective Study of Maternal, Fetal and Neonatal Deaths in Low- and Middle-Income Countries." *Bulletin of the World Health Organization* 92 (8): 605–12.

Say, L., D. Chou, A. Gemmill, Ö. Tunçalp, A. B. Moller, and others. 2014. "Global Causes of Maternal Death: A WHO Systematic Analysis." *The Lancet* 6: e323–33. doi:10.1016/S2214-109X(14)70227-X. Epub May 5.

Seger, N., and R. Soll. 2009. "Animal Derived Surfactant Extract for Treatment of Respiratory Distress Syndrome." *Cochrane Database of Systematic Reviews* (2): CD007836. doi:10.1002/14651858.CD007836.

Seward, N., D. Osrin, L. Li, A. Costello, A. M. Pulkki-Brännström, and others. 2012. "Association between Clean Delivery Kit Use, Clean Delivery Practices, and Neonatal Survival: Pooled Analysis of Data from Three Sites in South Asia." *PLoS Medicine* 9 (2): e1001180. doi:10.1371/journal.pmed.1001180.

Sheikh, L., N. Najmi, U. Khalid, and T. Saleem. 2011. "Evaluation of Compliance and Outcomes of a Management Protocol for Massive Postpartum Hemorrhage at a Tertiary Care Hospital in Pakistan." *BMC Pregnancy and Childbirth* 11: 28. doi:10.1186/1471-2393-11-28.

Siegfried, N., L. van der Merwe, P. Brocklehurst, and T. T. Sint. 2011. "Antiretrovirals for Reducing the Risk of Mother-to-Child Transmission of HIV Infection." *Cochrane Database of Systematic Reviews* (7): CD003510.

Sinha, A., S. Sazawal, A. Pradhan, S. Ramji, and N. Opiyo. 2015. "Chlorhexidine Skin or Cord Care for Prevention of Mortality and Infections in Neonates." *Cochrane Database of Systematic Reviews* (3): CD007835.

Smaill, F. M., and R. M. Grivell. 2014. "Antibiotic Prophylaxis versus no Prophylaxis for Preventing Infection after Cesarean Section." *Cochrane Database of Systematic Reviews* (10): CD007482. doi:10.1002/14651858.CD007482.pub3.

Soll, R., and E. Özek. 2010. "Prophylactic Protein Free Synthetic Surfactant for Preventing Morbidity and Mortality in Preterm Infants." *Cochrane Database of Systematic Reviews* (1): CD001079. doi:10.1002/14651858.CD001079.pub2.

Souza, J. P., A. M. Gülmezoglu, J. Vogel, G. Carroli, P. Lumbiganon, and others. 2013. "Moving beyond Essential Interventions for Reduction of Maternal Mortality (the WHO Multi-Country Survey on Maternal and Newborn Health): A Cross-Sectional Study." *The Lancet* 381 (9879): 1747–55. doi:10.1016/S0140-6736(13)60686-8.

Steegers, E. A., P. von Dadelszen, J. J. Duvekot, and R. Pijnenborg. 2010 "Preeclampsia." *The Lancet* 376 (9741): 631–44. doi:10.1016/S0140-6736(10)60279-6.

Stenberg, K., H. Axelson, P. Sheehan, I. Anderson, A. M. Gülmezoglu, and others. 2013. "Advancing Social and Economic Development by Investing in Women's and Children's Health: A New Global Investment Framework." *The Lancet* 383 (9925): 1333–54. doi:10.1016/S0140-6736(13)62231-X.

Syed, M., H. Javed, M. Y. Yakoob, and Z. A. Bhutta. 2011. "Effect of Screening and Management of Diabetes during Pregnancy on Stillbirths." *BMC Public Health* 11 (Suppl. 3): S2. doi:10.1186/1471-2458-11-S3-S2.

Thapa, K., B. Malla, S. Pandey, and S. Amatya. 2010. "Intrauterine Condom Tamponade in Management of Postpartum Haemorrhage." *Journal of Nepal Health Research Council* 8 (1): 19–22.

Touboul, C., W. Badiou, J. Saada, J. P. Pelage, D. Payen, and others. 2008. "Efficacy of Selective Arterial Embolisation for the Treatment of Life-Threatening Post-Partum Haemorrhage in a Large Population." *PLoS One* 3 (11): e3819. doi:10.1371/journal.pone.0003819.

Tunçalp, Ö., G. J. Hofmeyr, and A. M. Gülmezoglu. 2012. "Prostaglandins for Preventing Postpartum Haemorrhage." *Cochrane Database of Systematic Reviews* (8): CD000494. doi:10.1002/14651858.CD000494.pub4.

Ungerer, R. L. S., O. Lincetto, W. McGuire, H. H. Saloojee, and A. M. Gülmezoglu. 2004. "Prophylactic versus Selective Antibiotics for Term Newborn Infants of Mothers with Risk Factors for Neonatal Infection." *Cochrane Database of Systematic Reviews* (4): CD003957. doi:10.1002/14651858.CD003957.pub2.

UNICEF and WHO. 2014. "Countdown to 2015. Maternal, Newborn and Child Survival." http://www.countdown2015mnch.org/countdown-highlights.

van Lonkhuijzen, L., J. Stekelenburg, and J. van Roosmalen. 2012. "Maternity Waiting Facilities for Improving Maternal and Neonatal Outcome in Low-Resource Countries." *Cochrane Database of Systematic Reviews* (10): CD006759. doi:10.1002/14651858.CD006759.pub3.

Vogel, J. P., H. A. Ndema, J. P. Souza, M. A. Gülmezoglu, T. Dowswell, and others. 2013. "Antenatal Care Packages with Reduced Visits and Perinatal Mortality: A Secondary Analysis of the WHO Antenatal Care Trial." *Reproductive Health* 10 (1): 19.

Walker, N., Y. Tam, and I. K. Friberg. 2013. "Overview of the Lives Saved Tool (LiST)." *BMC Public Health* 13 (Suppl 3): S1. doi:10.1186/1471-2458-13-S3-S1.

Wang, M. Q., F. Y. Liu, F. Duan, Z. J. Wang, P. Song, and others. 2009. "Ovarian Artery Embolization Supplementing Hypogastric-Uterine Artery Embolization for Control of Severe Postpartum Hemorrhage: Report of Eight Cases." *Journal of Vascular and Interventional Radiology* 20 (7): 971–76.

Westhoff, G., A. M. Cotter, and J. E. Tolosa. 2013. "Prophylactic Oxytocin for the Third Stage of Labour to Prevent Postpartum Haemorrhage." *Cochrane Database of Systematic Reviews* (10): CD001808.

WHO 2010a. "Integrated Management of Pregnancy and Childbirth (IMPAC)." WHO, Geneva. http://www.who.int/maternal_child_adolescent/topics/maternal/impac/en/.

———. 2010b. "PMTCT Strategic Vision 2010–2015." WHO, Geneva. http://whqlibdoc.who.int/publications/2010/9789241599030_eng.pdf?ua=1.

———. 2011a. "Essential Interventions, Commodities and Guidelines for Reproductive Maternal, Newborn, and Child Health." WHO, Geneva. http://www.who.int/pmnch/topics/part_publications/essential_interventions_18_01_2012.pdf.

———. 2011b. *Recommendations for Prevention and Treatment of Pre-Eclampsia and Eclampsia*. Geneva: WHO.

———. 2012. "WHO Recommendations for the Prevention and Treatment of Postpartum Haemorrhage." WHO, Geneva. http://www.who.int/reproductivehealth/publications/maternal_perinatal_health/9789241548502/en/.

———. 2013. *Guideline: Calcium Supplementation in Pregnant Women*. Geneva: WHO.

———. 2014a. "Effect of Partogram Use on Outcomes for Women in Spontaneous Labour at Term." The WHO Reproductive Health Library. http://apps.who.int/rhl/pregnancy_childbirth/childbirth/routine_care/cd005461/en/.

———. 2014b. "WHO Policy Brief for the Implementation of Intermittent Preventive Treatment of Malaria in Pregnancy Using Sulfadoxine-Pyrimethamine (IPTp-SP)." WHO, Geneva.

———. 2014c. *WHO Recommendations on Postnatal Care of the Mother and Newborn.* Geneva: WHO.

———. 2015a. *Trends in Maternal Mortality: 1990 to 2015: Estimates by WHO, UNICEF, UNFPA, World Bank, and the United Nations Population Division.* Geneva: WHO.

———. 2015b. "Strategies toward Ending Preventable Maternal Mortality (EPMM)." Geneva, WHO.

WHO Odon Device Research Group. 2013. "Feasibility and Safety Study of a New Device (Odon device) for Assisted Vaginal Deliveries: Study Protocol." *Reproductive Health* 10: 33. doi:10.1186/1742-4755-10-33.

Wojcieszek, A. M., O. M. Stock, and V. Flenady. 2014. "Antibiotics for Prelabour Rupture of Membranes at or Near Term." *Cochrane Database of Systematic Reviews* (10): CD001807.

Yakoob, M. Y., M. A. Ali, M. U. Ali, A. Imdad, J. E. Lawn, and others. 2011. "The Effect of Providing Skilled Birth Attendance and Emergency Obstetric Care in Preventing Stillbirths." *BMC Public Health* 11 (Suppl. 3): S7. doi:10.1186/1471-2458-11-S3-S7.

Yoong, W., A. Ridout, M. Memtsa, A. Stavroulis, M. Aref-Adib, and others. 2012. "Application of Uterine Compression Suture in Association with Intrauterine Balloon Tamponade ('Uterine Sandwich') for Postpartum Hemorrhage." *Acta Obstetricia et Gynecologica Scandinavica* 91 (1): 147–51. doi:10.1111/j.1600-0412.2011.01153.x.

Zaidi, A. K., H. A. Ganatra, S. Syed, S. Cousens, A. C. Lee, and others. 2011. "Effect of Case Management on Neonatal Mortality Due to Sepsis and Pneumonia." *BMC Public Health* 11 (Suppl. 3): S13. doi:10.1186/1471-2458-11-S3-S13.

Zwart, J. J., P. D. Dijk, and J. van Roosmalen. 2010. "Peripartum Hysterectomy and Arterial Embolization for Major Obstetric Hemorrhage: A 2-Year Nationwide Cohort Study in the Netherlands." *American Journal of Obstetrics and Gynecology* 202 (2): 150. e1–7. doi:10.1016/j.ajog.2009.09.003.

Chapter 8

Diagnosis and Treatment of the Febrile Child

Julie M. Herlihy, Valérie D'Acremont, Deborah C. Hay Burgess, and Davidson H. Hamer

INTRODUCTION

Fever is one of the most common presenting symptoms of pediatric illnesses. Fever in children under age five years signifies systemic inflammation, typically in response to a viral, bacterial, parasitic, or less commonly, a noninfectious etiology. Patients' ages and geographic settings can help direct the appropriate diagnostic approach and treatment, if local epidemiology is well understood.

The combined proportion of deaths due to AIDS, diarrheal diseases, pertussis, tetanus, measles, meningitis/encephalitis, malaria, pneumonia and sepsis was 58.5 percent for children ages 1–59 months in 2015; it was 23.4 percent for neonates (Liu and others 2016, chapter 4 of this volume). Evidence regarding fever incidence is variable, with country-specific reports from cross-sectional surveys or weekly active case detection ranging from two to nine febrile episodes per child under age five years per year, a mean of 5.88 fever episodes per child under age five years per year (Gething and others 2010). National survey data from 42 Sub-Saharan African countries (excluding Botswana, Cabo Verde, Eritrea, and South Africa) were collected and analyzed for an estimated 655.6 million under-five fever episodes in 2007; 32 percent of these episodes occurred in 11 outpatient units in the Democratic Republic of Congo, Ethiopia, and Nigeria (Gething and others 2010). At the health facility and community levels, fever is by far the most common pediatric presenting symptom.

Multiple studies summarized in table 8.1 highlight the most common presenting symptoms at the facility and community levels.

Before the availability of affordable and accurate malaria rapid diagnostic tests (RDTs), most health care providers in malaria-endemic countries presumed that malaria was the cause of fever; the proportion of fevers due to malaria was very high in the early 1990s, and the priority was to reduce malaria mortality by any means.

The 1997 World Health Organization's (WHO's) initial Integrated Management of Childhood Illness (IMCI) guidelines recommended the use of injectable antimalarials and antibiotics in children in malaria-endemic areas who were suspected of having severe disease with the presence of danger signs (Gove 1997; Communicable Disease Surveillance and Response Vaccines and Biologicals 1997). Until 2010, the first edition of the WHO guidelines for the treatment of malaria recommended empiric, oral, antimalarial therapy for fever without other source in children under age five years living in malaria-endemic areas (WHO 2006). The decline of malaria incidence; rise of antimicrobial resistance; and availability of accurate, low-cost, point-of-care diagnostics have challenged the effectiveness of the presumptive treatment of febrile illnesses and reopened the discussion of the most accurate and cost-effective approaches for fever diagnosis and treatment. There are settings with very high malaria transmission and limited availability of diagnostic test where presumptive treatment would

Corresponding author: Julie M. Herlihy, MD, MPH, Director of Pediatric Global Health, Department of Pediatrics, University of California Davis, Sacramento, California; herlihyj@gmail.com.

Table 8.1 Clinical Findings and Final Classification in Studies on Integrated Management of Fevers

	Level of health care										
	Health facilities (outpatients)							Community health workers (children <5 years)			
Reference	Gouws and others 2004	Gouws and others 2004	Gouws and others 2004	D'Acremont and others 2011	D'Acremont and others 2011	D'Acremont and others 2014	Shao and others 2011	Rowe and others 2001	Mukanga, Tiono, and Anyorigiya 2012	Mukanga, Tiono, and Anyorigiya 2012	Mukanga, Tiono, and Anyorigiya 2012
Year(s) of study	2000	2000	2002	2007–08	2007–08	2008	2011	1997–2002	2009	2009	2009
Country	Tanzania	Uganda	Brazil	Tanzania	Tanzania	Tanzania	Tanzania	Kenya	Uganda	Burkina Faso	Ghana
Algorithm used	Original IMCI	Original IMCI	Original IMCI	Usual care	Usual care	Modified IMCI	Modified IMCI	Original IMCI	iCCM	iCCM	iCCM
Age group (years)	<5	<5	<5	<5	>5	<10	<5	<5	<5	<5	<5
Total number of patients	419	516	653	1,270	1,254	1,005	842	7,151	182	525	584
% with one or more danger signs	—	—	—	—	—	5	—	10	—	—	—
% who required referral	—	—	—	—	—	8	—	17	—	—	—
% with fever	76	81	29	84	74	100	73	88	—	—	—
% positive RDT results among febrile patients	—	—	—	—	—	10	3	—	78	74	84
% with cough	35	33	52	46	24	46	53	44	—	48	21
% with difficult breathing	—	—	—	2	1	2	—	—	—	—	—

table continues next page

Table 8.1 Clinical Findings and Final Classification in Studies on Integrated Management of Fevers (continued)

	Level of health care										
	Health facilities (outpatients)							Community health workers (children < 5 years)			
Reference	Gouws and others 2004	Gouws and others 2004	Gouws and others 2004	D'Acremont and others 2011	D'Acremont and others 2011	D'Acremont and others 2014	Shao and others 2011	Rowe and others 2001	Mukanga, Tiono, and Anyorigiya 2012	Mukanga, Tiono, and Anyorigiya 2012	Mukanga, Tiono, and Anyorigiya 2012
Year(s) of study	2000	2000	2002	2007–08	2007–08	2008	2011	1997–2002	2009	2009	2009
% with fast breathing among those with cough	—	—	—	—	—	40	22	—	—	44	24
% with chest indrawing among those with cough	—	—	—	—	—	2	—	—	—	—	—
% with pneumonia	28	31	3	—	—	18	12	—	35	—	—
% with diarrhea	24	34	17	17	6	10	18	22	—	26	36
% with blood in stools among those with diarrhea	—	—	—	—	—	5	1	—	—	—	—
% with ear pain	—	—	—	2	1	1	1	—	—	—	—
% with measles	—	—	—	—	0.1	0	0.8	—	—	—	—
% with skin problems	—	—	—	7	3	8	10	—	—	—	—
% with more than one diagnostic classification	—	—	—	—	—	—	—	36	29	33	22

Source: WHO 2013a. Reproduced with permission.

Note: — = not available; iCCM = Integrated Community Case Management; IMCI = Integrated Management of Childhood Illness; RDT = rapid diagnostic test.

be most practical and cost-effective (*DCP3* volume 6, Babigumira, forthcoming). In 2009, experts debated whether sufficient information was available to abandon presumptive treatment guidelines and move to an emphasis on diagnosis before treatment (D'Acremont, Lengeler, and Genton 2007; D'Acremont and others 2009; English and others 2009).

Mounting evidence demonstrated the decline of *Plasmodium falciparum* infections in response to intense national and multinational initiatives to control malaria. In 2012 more than US$2.5 billion was invested from global partners, including the Global Fund to Fight AIDS, Tuberculosis and Malaria; the World Bank Malaria Booster Program; the U.S. President's Malaria Initiative; the Bill & Melinda Gates Foundation's Malaria Control and Evaluation Partnership in Africa; and the Roll Back Malaria Partnership (D'Acremont, Lengeler, and Genton 2010; Feachem and others 2010; Leslie and others 2012; WHO 2013a). Countries with previously defined high-transmission regions are reporting decreasing malaria incidence, making the management of nonmalarial fevers critically important (Feachem and others 2010; WHO 2013a; Hertz and others 2013; Ishengoma and others 2011).

In 2010, the WHO revised its fever treatment guidelines to recommend antimalarial treatment only for those with a positive malaria test result, either point-of-care or microscopy (WHO 2010a). This new strategy is being implemented in the public sector in most Sub-Saharan African countries (Bastiaens and others 2011). However, many patients first present for care in the informal private sector, and more research is needed to better understand treatment decision making in this context and how to reduce overuse of antimicrobials and ensure appropriate care. The epidemiology of pediatric febrile illness is undoubtedly shifting; understanding the etiology of nonmalarial fevers in each context is the logical next step to improve pediatric clinical outcomes of other treatable serious febrile illnesses, such as pneumonia, sepsis, bacterial meningitis, enteric fever, rickettsioses, and influenza. Given rampant and expanding antimicrobial drug resistance globally, care must be taken to use antibiotics only when indicated and to develop careful guidelines when resources are limited. Present guidelines are based on clinical features that are unfortunately poorly predictive of the diseases causing fever. Low-cost, accurate, point-of-care diagnostics are needed to determine which children can benefit from antibacterial therapies to guide the most effective use of antibiotics.

This chapter discusses the evidence that informs current etiologies of fever, stratified by regional geography. It presents the clinical presentation, diagnosis, and treatment of the most common diseases, with special considerations for certain age groups, the burden of disease for different conditions, classification and treatment strategies, and a review of available diagnostic tests. In addition, different health systems approaches to diagnosis and treatment of the febrile child at the community and health-facility levels are discussed, as is the evidence base for WHO-sponsored approaches such as IMCI and Integrated Community Case Management (iCCM). Fever in adults and RDT use for malaria are discussed further in volume 6 (Holmes, Bertozzi, Bloom, Jha, and Nugent, forthcoming).

ETIOLOGY OF FEVER IN CHILDREN UNDER AGE FIVE YEARS

Infectious etiologies of fever differ according to age and geographic region. Recent evidence from multiple health care and low- and middle-income country (LMIC) settings confirms that viral infections are predominantly responsible for fever within all age groups (Animut and others 2009; Crump and others 2013; D'Acremont and others 2014; Kasper and others 2012; Mayxay and others 2013). The studies described in table 8.2 used different study designs with significant variation in study population, case definitions, and available diagnostics. Although these studies are informative, they need to be interpreted in the context of the individual study design and context. Following are common themes across the available research:

- Predominance of acute respiratory infections (ARIs) in outpatient visits for fever
- Identification of multiple pathogens after molecular laboratory investigations, making it difficult to declare a specific diagnosis
- High proportion of fever etiologies due to viral pathogens when appropriate viral diagnostic tests are available; studies without viral diagnostics reveal a high proportion of undiagnosed febrile illnesses
- Clinically overestimated malaria, compared with RDT or microscopy-confirmed diagnosis.

Although the available evidence suggests that most viral and some specific bacterial diseases, such as rickettsiosis and leptospirosis, are likely to be underdiagnosed, data are either not available or are limited from several countries where the fever burden is highest, such as the Democratic Republic of Congo, India, and Nigeria. Ongoing surveillance of fever etiology in multiple representative geographies to establish trends in predominant pathogens and to identify emerging infections early would be ideal. Additionally, little research is available on fever etiology of young infants (age 0–2 months); a concerted research effort is underway to better understand the distribution

Table 8.2 Summary of Evidence for Etiology of Fever Studies

	World Bank region									
	Sub-Saharan Africa					South Asia				
Study	D'Acremont and others (2014)	Crump and others (2013)	Animut and others (2009)	WHO 2013a	Njama-Meya and others (2007)	Mayxay and others (2013)	WHO 2013a	WHO 2013a	WHO 2013a	Kasper and others (2012)
Study setting	Tanzania: One urban and one rural outpatient clinic	Tanzania, hospitalized patients	Four outpatient clinics in Gojjam zone in northwest Ethiopia	Zanzibar, Tanzania	Uganda, study clinic within a referral third-level hospital	Lao PDR, two province-level hospitals	Pakistan, small peripheral clinic	Cambodia, setting unknown	Cambodia, nine outpatient clinics in south central region	
Study design	N = 1,005 (younger than age 10 years with fever) Computer-algorithm-generated diagnosis using history, physical, and wide array of lab investigations	N = 467 (ages 2 months to 13 years) Diagnoses by case definitions and convalescent serum at four to six weeks post discharge	N = 653 (ages 3–17 years)	N = 677 cases, 200 controls (ages 2–59 months) Diagnoses by IMCI classifications plus laboratory investigations	N =1,602 (less than age 10 years with fever in last 24 hours) Clinical diagnoses for RDT or microscopy negative for malaria per local clinical guidelines	N = 1,938 (ages 5 months to 49 years) with fever	N = 1,248 febrile episodes, all ages Case definition plus laboratory investigations	N = 1,193 febrile patients, all ages, 282 controls Tested for malaria, leptospirosis, rickettsial diseases, scrub typhus, dengue, influenza, and bacteremia	N = 9,997 patients with fever, all ages, median 13 years Lab investigations of respiratory secretions, blood, serum	
Most common diagnoses	62 percent ARI (5 percent chest X-ray-confirmed pneumonia); 11.9 percent nasopharyngeal viral infection; 10.5 percent malaria; 10.3 percent gastroenteritis; 5.9 percent UTI	1.3 percent malaria; 3.4 percent bacteremia; 0.9 percent fungemia; **Zoonotic:**; 2 percent brucellosis; 7.7 percent leptospirosis; 2.6 percent Q fever	62 percent malaria; 7 percent clinical pneumonia; **Serologically diagnosed:**; 5.8 percent typhoid; 5.1 percent typhus; 2.6 percent brucellosis	25 percent watery diarrhea; 2 percent bloody diarrhea; 5 percent skin infections; 0.2 percent malaria; **65 percent ARIs:**; 57 percent pneumonia; 9 percent tonsillitis	10 percent diarrhea; **93 percent ARIs:**; 47 percent URI; 29 percent common cold; 12 percent pharyngitis; 4 percent pneumonia; 1 percent otitis media	8 percent dengue; 7 percent scrub typhus; 6 percent Japanese encephalitis virus; 6 percent leptospirosis; 2 percent bacteremia; less than 3 percent malaria confirmed by microscopy or RDT	47 percent ARI; 23 percent diarrhea or dysentery; 17 percent enteric fever; 2 percent bacteremia other than S. typhi; 0.5 percent UTI; 0.4 percent malaria	32 percent RDT-confirmed malaria; 68 percent RDT-negative:; 76 percent URI; 0.6 percent LRI; 17 percent enteric fever	19.9 percent PCR-confirmed influenza; 7.2 percent microscopy-confirmed malaria; 6.3 percent bacteremia	

table continues next page

Table 8.2 Summary of Evidence for Etiology of Fever Studies (continued)

	World Bank region						
	Sub-Saharan Africa				South Asia		
	3.7 percent typhoid fever; 1.5 percent skin/mucosal infections; 0.2 percent meningitis	7.4 percent spotted fever rickettsial disease; 10 percent chikungunya virus	4 percent otitis; 31 percent other ARI; (54 percent viral, 12 percent bacterial, 18 percent unknown)	2 percent UTIs; 8 percent skin infections	Six-month testing for influenza: 32 percent influenza-positive		
Undiagnosed (percent)	3.2	64	Unknown	15	59	Unknown	62
Multiple diagnoses (percent)	22.6	Unknown	Unknown	Unknown	Unknown		3.5 more than one pathogen identified
Notes	Availability of extensive viral diagnostics correlated with clinical diagnoses	Limited viral testing. High prevalence of zoonoses; consider different empiric antibiotic regimens	Of the viral ARIs most common PCR results: 16 percent RSV; 9 percent influenza (A/B); 9 percent rhinovirus	Limited testing for bacterial illnesses such as typhoid	Role of influenza during outbreak	High proportion of enteric disease	Clinical presentation and lab diagnoses did not always correlate; many pathogens found in similar rates in controls

Note: ARI = acute respiratory infection; IMCI = Integrated Management of Childhood Illness; LRI = lower respiratory tract infection; PCR = polymerase chain reaction; RDT = rapid diagnostic test; RSV = respiratory syncytial virus; URI = upper respiratory tract infection; UTI = urinary tract infection.

of infections in young infants via the Aetiology of Neonatal Infection in South Asia research group, which is building on results from the WHO Young Infants Study Group and the WHO Young Infants Clinical Signs Study Group (YICSSG) (WHO Young Infants Study Group 1999; YICSSG 2008). Infection-related neonatal deaths contributed at least 10 percent to overall mortality in children under age five years in 2013 (Liu and others 2015).

DIAGNOSIS AND TREATMENT OF COMMON CHILDHOOD FEBRILE ILLNESSES

Febrile Illnesses in Young Infants

Infection-related mortality and morbidity for young infants from birth to age 59 days is one of the most challenging health issues to address; signs and symptoms are often nonspecific, and illnesses can rapidly progress to severe disease. Care seeking for young infant illness often occurs too late or not at all, making community-based efforts critical to increasing access to early treatment and addressing this disproportionate morbidity and mortality. Using the CHERG estimates, sepsis (15 percent) and pneumonia (6 percent) are the highest infection-related contributors to neonatal death, with tetanus and diarrheal disease both contributing approximately 1 percent (chapter 4 in this volume, Liu and others 2016). None of the etiology studies discussed in table 8.2 captures the causes of fever in the young infant age group.

Sepsis

Sepsis in young infants presents in two varieties: early onset (fewer than seven days after birth) and late onset (seven days or more). Early-onset neonatal sepsis is thought to be the result of exposure to pathogens in the maternal birth canal; late-onset sepsis is thought to be secondary to environmental exposures. Symptoms of bacteremia and related sepsis in young infants are often vague and may include fever, hypothermia, poor tone, jaundice, or inability to suck. A decrease in urine production, poor perfusion, bulging fontanelle, excessive sleepiness, or alternatively, excessive irritability are signs of more serious disease. Without antibiotic treatment, many young infants will rapidly progress to severe bacterial sepsis, which may prove fatal.

A review by Ganatra and Zaidi (2010) of five neonatal sepsis studies reports incidences of blood culture–confirmed early-onset sepsis ranging from 2.2 to 9.8 per 1,000 live births, and clinical sepsis incidence ranging from 20.7 to 50 per 1,000 live births. Two of these studies report case fatality rates (CFRs) of 18 percent and 19 percent (Ganatra and Zaidi 2010). A systematic review that included 27 hospital-based studies of the etiology of neonatal sepsis reports CFRs in children younger than 60 days as low as 3 percent in Europe and as high as 70 percent in South-East Asia (Waters and others 2011).

Although a positive blood culture is the gold standard for diagnosing bacteremia, cultures are known to lack sensitivity, especially in children, and may take several hours to days before results are available; cultures require significant laboratory infrastructure, which is a challenge in low-resource settings. Total leukocyte count, leukocyte differential, levels of acute phase reactants (for example, C-reactive protein), and screening panels using a variety of cytokine markers may provide supportive evidence of infection when abnormal, but these measures have been shown to have limited value in diagnosing bacteremia (Remington and others 2006).

According to a systematic review of 27 studies performed by Waters and others (2011), the most common documented pathogens for early-onset sepsis (N = 282 isolates) include *Escherichia coli* (16.3 percent), *Staphylococcus aureus* (11.7 percent), nonpneumococcal streptococcal species (8.5 percent), *Klebsiella* species (7.8 percent), *Pseudomonas* species (7.8 percent), Group B streptococcus (GBS; 6.7 percent), *Acinetobacter* species (6.7 percent), and *Streptococcus pneumoniae* (4.6 percent). The distribution of pathogens for late-onset sepsis (N = 1,784) was similar to early onset but with notably less GBS (1.7 percent) and a higher proportion of *Serratia* species (2.2 percent), *Salmonella* species (1.5 percent), *H. influenzae* (1.7 percent), and *Neisseria meningitidis* (0.7 percent). Overall, there was a similar proportion of gram-positive isolates (34.4 percent early onset, 34.6 percent late onset) compared with gram-negative isolates (63.8 percent early onset, 60.5 percent late-onset) (Waters and others 2011). These results suggest that empiric antibiotic regimens for both early- and late-onset sepsis should be broad spectrum to treat both gram-positive and -negative infections.

Meningitis, Herpes Simplex Virus, and Urinary Tract Infections

In addition to bacteremia, a young infant presenting with a nonfocal fever should be evaluated for meningitis and urinary tract infections (UTIs). A lumbar puncture to check for pleocytosis (an elevated number of white blood cells in cerebral spinal fluid), elevated protein, or low glucose levels can indicate whether infection is present in the central nervous system.

Herpes simplex virus-2 (HSV-2) may cause encephalitis, an infection more common in the first three weeks of life secondary to exposure via the birth canal. HSV-2 is responsible for genital herpes, the prevalence of which is rising globally; it is of particular concern in HIV-endemic countries where genital ulcers increase risk of human immunodeficiency virus (HIV) transmission. HSV-2 seroprevalence has been measured at roughly 50 percent in many LMICs (WHO, UNAIDS, and LSHTM 2001). Many newborns are exposed to HSV-2 in asymptomatic mothers, making surveillance for neonatal HSV-2 a challenge. Further research is needed to determine whether HSV-2 is a major contributor to neonatal morbidity and mortality in LMICs.

UTIs are best evaluated by urine culture; in low-resource settings, point-of-care urinalysis can provide potentially valuable information. The presence of leukocyte esterase, blood, or nitrates may suggest a bacterial urinary infection, however, only if the urine sample is not contaminated. The difficulty of obtaining a sterile sample from a young infant has made implementation of this test less feasible in the community setting. UTIs are the most common reason for nonfocal fever in young infants; urinary vesicoureteral reflux is associated with higher risk (Byington and others 2003; Greenhow and others 2014).

Group B Streptococcus Disease

GBS *(Streptococcus agalactiae)* is a bacterium that can cause bacteremia, sepsis, pneumonia, and meningitis in newborns. GBS may present as early-onset disease, which is usually due to transmission from a colonized mother immediately before or during delivery, and late-onset disease (later than seven days of age), at which time infection may be acquired from the mother or environmental sources. Overall, the CFR tends to be high (9.6 percent), with a higher case fatality in early-onset infections (Edmond and others 2012).

Although GBS is a common cause of neonatal sepsis in high-income countries (HICs), the global burden in LMICs is less established. Variable incidence levels have been reported, with Sub-Saharan Africa reporting rates almost threefold higher than North and South America. In contrast, South-East Asian studies have reported a low incidence and even no cases of GBS. This disparity may be due to differences in study design, previous antibiotic use, and the severity of illness, with young infants dying before they can be fully evaluated. In HICs, the standard of care is to conduct surveillance cultures for GBS at 36 weeks gestation. Pregnant women colonized with GBS receive intrapartum antibiotics at least four hours before delivery to reduce the incidence of GBS neonatal illness. In the meta-analysis (Edmond and others 2012), studies that report intrapartum prophylaxis were associated with lower incidence of early-onset GBS (0.23 per 1,000 live births [95 percent confidence interval 0.13–0.59]) compared with those with no prophylaxis (0.75 per 1,000 live births [95 percent confidence interval 0.58–0.89]). Whether this practice would be beneficial in low-resource countries is difficult to determine because of insufficient data on the burden of GBS disease in these contexts.

Acute Respiratory Infections

ARIs in young infants (age 0–59 days) are particularly dangerous because immature immune systems increase vulnerability for systemic spread, and the fatigue from the increased work of breathing is a major clinical concern. Liu and others (chapter 4 in this volume, 2016) estimate that ARIs contribute 6 percent to total all-cause neonatal mortality (0–28 days), and the WHO repository suggests 4 percent of children age 0–59 days die from ARI (WHO-CHERG 2011). It is difficult to disentangle primary respiratory infections from sepsis and other pulmonary conditions related to premature lungs and congenital anomalies. Viral respiratory infections often infect the smallest of airways—bronchioles—causing inflammation, bronchospasm, and difficulty breathing.

Febrile Illnesses in Older Infants and Young Children

Acute Respiratory Infections

ARIs became the second largest killer of children under age five years. Recent WHO-CHERG data describe ARIs as responsible for approximately 15 percent of all under-five deaths and 24 percent of mortality for ages 1–59 months (chapter 4 in this volume, Liu and others 2016). Estimates vary depending on the sources and modeling approach, with ARI-related deaths among children under five years of age ranging from 890,000 (GBD 2013 Collaborators 2015) in 2013 to approximately 922,000 in 2015 (chapter 4 in this volume, Liu and others 2016). ARIs include upper respiratory tract infections, such as the common cold, otitis media, sinusitis, and pharyngitis, as well as lower respiratory tract infections (LRIs), such as laryngitis, tracheitis, bronchitis, bronchiolitis, and pneumonia. Bronchiolitis and pneumonia are the largest contributors to child ARI deaths through progressive respiratory failure or systemic infection, inflammation, or toxins spread from the lungs.

Acute lower respiratory tract infections (ALRIs) in older infants and children under age five years are the most common reason for hospitalization. An assessment of the global burden of severe pneumonia estimated that in 2010, 11.9 million (95 percent confidence interval 10.3 million to 13.9 million) episodes of severe and 3.0 million (95 percent confidence interval 2.1 million to 4.2 million) episodes of very severe LRI resulted in hospital admissions in young children worldwide (Nair and others 2013). This analysis uses data from 37 hospital studies reporting CFRs for severe ALRI to estimate that approximately 265,000 (95 percent confidence interval 160,000–450,000) in hospital deaths occurred in young children; 99 percent of these deaths occurred in developing countries. These data capture the inpatient CFR; however, the at-home CFR is likely higher in areas with poor access to care. Although many children with ARI are diagnosed and treated in the private sector, data on these ARI episodes and their outcome is sorely lacking; investment to better understand the role of the informal sector in disease diagnosis and treatment is paramount.

In 2009, the WHO and UNICEF released a Global Action Plan for Prevention and Control of Pneumonia (WHO and UNICEF 2009a). In 2013, this plan was updated to include diarrheal disease control and renamed the Integrated Global Action Plan for Prevention and Control of Pneumonia and Diarrhoea (WHO and UNICEF 2013). These calls to action outlined the research and programming priorities for ARIs to include the following:

- Etiology research to better direct antimicrobial therapy
- Vaccine development
- Scale-up of community-based programming to recognize and treat cases of severe ARI before disease progression.

The Pneumonia Etiology Research for Child Health project was designed in response to the call for enhanced understanding of the etiology of pneumonia. This multicountry case-control study of hospitalized pediatric patients in Bangladesh, The Gambia, Kenya, Mali, South Africa, Thailand, and Zambia will reflect the changes in severe pneumonia etiology resulting from wider vaccine availability, the HIV/AIDS epidemic and resulting opportunistic infections, and increasing antimicrobial resistance. Results are expected in 2016–17. Annex 8A provides a summary of the current understanding of pneumonia etiology.

Respiratory viruses play a major role in infants of all ages presenting with severe ALRI, clinically known as bronchiolitis. Although these viruses exist in older children with ARIs, the clinical presentation in infants is associated with higher morbidity and mortality. Common viral etiologies of bronchiolitis include respiratory syncytial virus, influenza (types A and B), parainfluenza, human metapneumovirus, rhinovirus, adenovirus, coronaviruses, and human bocavirus (García and others 2010).

In 2012, the WHO updated the technical guidelines for treatment of pneumonia, based on available evidence from studies reviewed by an expert panel. On the basis of recent studies, the 2014 version of the IMCI guidelines (table 8.3) recommends that pneumonia with fast breathing or chest indrawing but no other danger signs be managed at the outpatient level, potentially reducing the number of children needing referral (WHO 2012b, 2014a).

Pulse oximetry, which measures a patient's oxygen saturation, can provide important triage information—peripheral oxygen saturation of less than 90 percent predicts clinical severity and need for supplemental oxygen (WHO 2013a). To reduce mortality from ARIs, clear community-based algorithms to identify and refer children with severe pneumonia are needed, and referral-level facilities need to deliver supplemental oxygen. The cost-effectiveness of an oxygen systems strategy compares favorably with other higher-profile child survival interventions, such as new vaccines (Duke and others 2008). Although most portable oxygen systems lack sufficient oxygen flow rates to provide adequate respite for increased work of breathing in infants with bronchiolitis, oxygen concentrators provide the most consistent and least expensive source of oxygen in health facilities with reliable power supplies. Future research efforts that focus on reducing the power needs of or using alternative energy sources for oxygen concentrators will facilitate their introduction to lower levels of the health care system. The capacity to perform routine maintenance and to source necessary replacement parts locally needs to be addressed if this technology is to be sustainable at the community or facility level.

Viral Exanthems

A discussion of febrile illnesses in children is incomplete without the mention of the myriad viruses that present nonfocally and ultimately declare themselves clinically with a characteristic exanthema or rash. For example, the clinical syndromes of roseola (HHV-6), varicella, measles, parvovirus B19, and coxsackievirus may initially present with fever before erupting into a rash. Of these conditions, only measles is incorporated into the IMCI algorithms, which recommend treatment with vitamin A for uncomplicated infections, or urgent referral, a first dose of an antibiotic, and vitamin A for severe complicated measles (Gove 1997). Many other classic

Table 8.3 WHO IMCI Respiratory Illness Clinical Guidelines

IMCI classification for children age 2–59 months	Treatment	Strength of recommendation
Nonsevere pneumonia (fast breathing[a] or chest indrawing without danger signs)	Without chest indrawing and HIV-negative: Amoxicillin 40 mg/kg twice daily for three days	Weak recommendation, moderate quality of evidence
	Without chest indrawing and HIV-positive: Amoxicillin 40 mg/kg twice daily for five days	
	With chest indrawing: Amoxicillin 40 mg/kg twice daily for five days	Strong recommendation, moderate quality of evidence
Severe pneumonia (fast breathing with danger signs, with or without chest indrawing)	Children age 2–59 months: Ampicillin 50 mg/kg IV every six hours for five days OR Benzyl penicillin 50,000 IU/kg every six hours for five days AND gentamicin 7.5 mg/kg IV daily for five days Third-generation cephalosporin as second-line therapy[b]	Strong recommendation, moderate quality of evidence
Wheezing	Inhaled salbutamol delivered via metered dose inhaler with spacer devices for up to three times 15–20 minutes apart, to relieve bronchoconstriction and to assess the respiratory rate again and classify accordingly	Strong recommendation, low quality of evidence
	Oral salbutamol should not be used for treatment of acute or persistent wheezing, except where inhaled salbutamol is not available[b]	

Source: WHO IMCI Chart Booklet 2014 (http://www.who.int/maternal_child_adolescent/documents/IMCI_chartbooklet/en/).
Note: IMCI = Integrated Management of Childhood Illness; IU = international unit; IV = intravenous; mg/kg = milligrams per kilogram.
a. Fast breathing is defined as respiratory rate ≥ 50 breaths per minute in infants age 2–12 months, and ≥ 40 breaths per minute in infants age 12–59 months.
b. Expert consensus.

viral exanthema are difficult to diagnose on darker skin, are typically self limited, and do not require treatment. Measles and, to a lesser extent, varicella are highly contagious viruses and have the potential for serious sequelae. Parvovirus B19 is an important condition to consider in patients with sickle-cell disease because infection can lead to aplastic anemia. An emphasis on identifying these syndromes and prophylactic vaccination for measles is warranted in refugee or displaced populations, and in HIV-endemic areas where outbreaks could spread rapidly.

Enteric Fever

Enteric fever is an all-encompassing term for the disease caused by several serovars of *Salmonella enterica* including *S. typhi* and *S. paratyphi A*. The clinical picture of typhoid is nonspecific with symptoms of severe headache, nausea, and loss of appetite associated with sustained, high fever and few other specific signs. The Institute for Health Metrics and Evaluation (IHME)

reports a mortality burden of 190,000 for enteric fever in the 2010 Global Burden of Diseases (Lozano and others 2012). In 2015, the IHME released updated mortality estimates with disaggregated cause of death; they report an estimated 54,262 paratyphoid-caused deaths and 160,645 typhoid-caused deaths worldwide annually (GBD 2013 Collaborators 2015). These data come from 73 Gavi, the Vaccine Alliance, countries within which more than 70 percent of mortality burden comes from Asia and more than 50 percent comes from South Asia (Lozano and others 2012; GBD 2013 Collaborators 2015). CFRs, ranging from 10 percent to 30 percent without antibiotic treatment, drop to less than 1 percent to 4 percent in the antibiotic-treated patient. As part of Millennium Development Goal (MDG) 7, improvements in water, sanitation, and hygiene have reduced environmental contamination exposure to typhoid. However, treatment with antibiotics and prevention through vaccination are ultimately needed to reduce typhoid mortality and morbidity (United Nations 2013).

Malaria

Despite substantial control efforts since 2000, malaria remains responsible for substantial morbidity and mortality worldwide; in 2015, there were an estimated 214 million cases and at least 438,000 deaths (WHO 2015). Four species of *Plasmodium* are responsible for most human cases (*P. falciparum, P. vivax, P. ovale,* and *P. malariae*), although *P. knowlesi,* a cause of primate malaria, has been identified as a cause of human infections in Malaysia and other parts of South-East Asia. Clinically, malaria ranges from asymptomatic parasitemia to uncomplicated malaria to severe malaria (typically manifested as cerebral malaria, severe anemia, hypoglycemia, and potentially multisystem organ failure). Further detail on etiology and control strategies for malaria can be found in volume 6 (Holmes, Bertozzi, Bloom, Jha, and Nugent, forthcoming).

A paradigm shift has occurred in recent years, away from the presumption that all fevers in endemic areas should be treated as malaria toward the recommendation that laboratory testing should occur before treatment. Although thick and thin blood smears have been the mainstay of diagnosis, since 2005 the use of antigen-based RDTs with high sensitivity and specificity has increased. This recommendation has not been implemented in all regions given lack of resources to acquire RDTs or provider preference for relying on clinical diagnosis or blood smears, despite a convincing body of research to support RDTs as reliable and cost-effective diagnostic tools. Artemisinin-based combination therapy (ACT) is the preferred treatment modality for uncomplicated and severe disease caused by *P. falciparum*; chloroquine remains the treatment of choice for the other three species in most regions.

Dengue and Chikungunya Virus

Dengue fever, a mosquito-borne arbovirus of the genus *Flavivirus,* has become one of the most common and rapidly spreading vector-borne diseases after malaria and is a major international public health concern. Dengue is responsible for an estimated 50 million to 100 million illnesses annually, including 250,000 to 500,000 cases of dengue hemorrhagic fever—a severe manifestation of dengue—and approximately 29,000 deaths (Lozano and others 2012; CDC 2012). Approximately 95 percent of cases occur in children younger than age 15 years; infants constitute 5 percent of all cases. Dengue has mainly been documented in Asia; data from Sub-Saharan Africa are lacking, although reports from Gabon and elsewhere are creating concern that it is an emerging disease or has been previously not recognized because of a lack of diagnostic testing (Caron and others 2013).

The grading of the severity of dengue can be based on a WHO classification system, updated in 2009 (WHO and Special Programme for Research and Training in Tropical Diseases 2009). No specific therapeutic agents exist for dengue fever apart from analgesics and medications to reduce fever. Treatment is supportive; steroids, antivirals, or carbazochrome, which decreases capillary permeability, have no proven role. Mild or classic dengue is treated with antipyretic agents such as acetaminophen, bed rest, and fluid replacement; most cases can be managed on an outpatient basis. The management of dengue hemorrhagic fever and dengue shock syndrome is purely supportive. Aspirin and other nonsteroidal anti-inflammatory drugs should be avoided, owing to the increased risk for Reye's syndrome and hemorrhage (Simmons and others 2012).

Chikungunya, an alpha virus transmitted by mosquitoes of the *Aedes* genus, is responsible for a clinical syndrome characterized by fever, rash, headache, myalgias, and arthralgias (Thiboutot and others 2010). It can affect all ages, including young children; transplacental transmission with congenital infection has been described (Gérardin and others 2008). Although past outbreaks of chikungunya have primarily occurred in Sub-Saharan Africa and regions of South Asia and East Asia and Pacific, this vector-borne viral infection has emerged in Latin America and the Caribbean, where it spread rapidly from island to island. No specific antiviral therapy is available, and treatment is largely supportive.

DIAGNOSTIC TOOLS AVAILABLE OR UNDER DEVELOPMENT

Malaria

In many endemic areas, malaria accounts for a minority of fever episodes and is clinically indistinguishable from other common illnesses, including pneumonia, meningitis, typhoid, sepsis, and viral infections such as dengue and chikungunya. The WHO recommends that malaria case management be based on parasitological diagnosis of malaria infections before treatment (WHO 2010a, 2012a); the use of antigen-detecting RDTs is supportive of this strategy, particularly in areas where good quality microscopy cannot be maintained. The number of commercially available malaria RDTs that detect one or more of the three parasite antigens—histidine rich protein-2 (HRP-2), parasite lactate dehydrogenase (pLDH), or aldolase—have increased substantially since their introduction in the late 1990s (table 8.4). RDTs can play a key role in febrile illness management, providing they are sensitive enough to detect nearly all clinically significant cases of malaria and have a high specificity to rule out nonmalarial causes of febrile illness. Multiple rounds of laboratory-based evaluations have identified those RDTs that consistently detect malaria at low parasite densities (WHO 2012c).

Table 8.4 Average Sensitivity and Specificity of Malarial Tests

Test type	Species detected	Sensitivity (95% CI)	Specificity (95% CI)
Type 1 Pf HRP-2	*Plasmodium falciparum* only	94.8% (93.1%–96.1%)	95.2% (93.2%–96.7%)
Type 2 Pf HRP-2 and pan aldolase	*Plasmodium falciparum, Plasmodium vivax, Plasmodium malariae* and *Plasmodium ovale*	96.0% (94.0%–97.3%)	95.3% (87.3%–98.3%)
Type 3 Pf HRP-2 and pan pLDH	*Plasmodium falciparum, Plasmodium vivax, Plasmodium malariae* and *Plasmodium ovale*	99.5% (71.0%–100%)	90.6% (80.5%–95.7%)

Sources: Baiden and others 2012; Abba and others 2011.
Note: CI = confidence interval; Pf HRP2 = histidine rich protein-2; pLDH = parasite lactate dehydrogenase.

However, the declining malaria burden in many endemic regions and an increasing programmatic focus on malaria elimination mean that novel target antigens, use of gold nanoparticles, or other diagnostic approaches may be needed to create point-of-care tests with increased sensitivity. Several diagnostic approaches are based on selective microscopic detection of infected blood cells by methods such as third-harmonic generation imaging (Bélisle and others 2008), photoacoustic flowmetry (Samson and others 2012), and more recently, magneto-optical detection of the malaria pigment (Mens and others 2010) hemozoin using hand-held devices with polarized light and laser pulse detection of vapor nanobubbles generated by the parasite (Lukianova-Hleb and others 2014).

Respiratory and Other Bacterial Illnesses

A detailed discussion of diagnostic tools available and under development for ARI or other serious bacterial illnesses can be found in annex 8B (available online).

HEALTH SYSTEMS APPROACHES TO CHILDREN WITH FEBRILE ILLNESSES

Children with fever present to all levels and sectors of the health system. Trials of algorithmic approaches have been undertaken at the community and facility levels to identify seriously ill children to indicate referral to a higher level of care. Two WHO-supported platforms to identify and treat children with fever and common pediatric illnesses are IMCI for the facility level and iCCM for the community level. Further research is needed to identify best practice models for the formal and informal private sector to create a synergistic approach to providing appropriate treatment and referral to more advanced care, when needed.

Integrated Management of Childhood Illness

The WHO developed the IMCI strategy in the 1990s to improve the quality of disease management and to reduce mortality of children under age five years (Gove 1997). Using a series of algorithms and flow charts, IMCI gives health care providers a systematic way to assess children for danger signs that trigger immediate referral or hospitalization; to classify the illness based on the level of severity for pneumonia, diarrhea, measles, fever, otitis media, and malnutrition (Tulloch 1999); and to identify those requiring antibiotic treatment. The classifications are color coded, with pink calling for hospital referral or admission, yellow for treatment at home, and green for children with mild illness who require only supportive care at home and can be counseled with return precautions (figure 8.1). IMCI has been adapted at the national level with increasing attention to HIV screening and management of illness in infants under age two months.

Several assessments of the quality of care delivered by IMCI have been performed since the early 2000s. In Bangladesh, a systematic evaluation of 669 sick children age 2–59 months, using a gold-standard physician diagnosis and treatment decision, found a sensitivity of 78 percent and specificity of 47 percent for identifying children with probable bacterial infections requiring antibiotics (Factor and others 2001). In this low malaria prevalence site, the majority of children with meningitis, pneumonia, otitis media, and UTIs fulfilled IMCI criteria for at least one classification that would have resulted in antibiotic initiation. However, many children with bacteremia, skin infections, and dysentery would not have received antibiotics. This evaluation was based on a comparison with an expert diagnosis that is subject to clinical subjectivity and the limited accuracy of available diagnostic tools. A study assessing the safety of using a slightly modified version of IMCI showed that the rate

Figure 8.1 Sample Fever Algorithm from 2014 IMCI

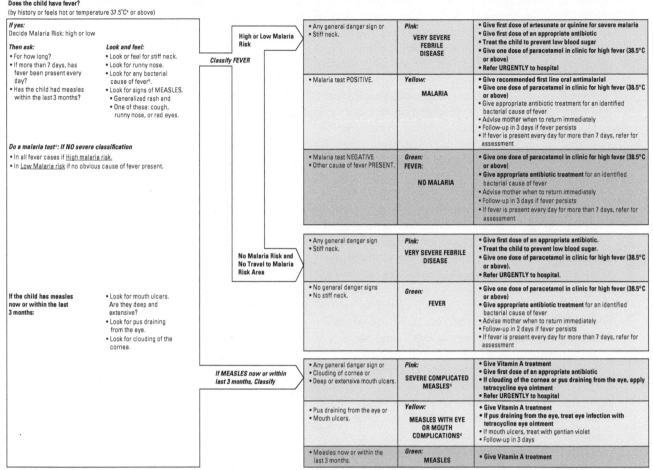

Does the child have fever?
(by history or feels hot or temperature 37.5°C[a] or above)

If yes:
Decide Malaria Risk: high or low

Then ask:
• For how long?
• If more than 7 days, has fever been present every day?
• Has the child had measles within the last 3 months?

Look and feel:
• Look or feel for stiff neck.
• Look for runny nose.
• Look for any bacterial cause of fever[b].
• Look for signs of MEASLES.
  • Generalized rash and
  • One of these: cough, runny nose, or red eyes.

Do a malaria test[c]: If NO severe classification
• In all fever cases if High malaria risk.
• In Low Malaria risk if no obvious cause of fever present.

If the child has measles now or within the last 3 months:
• Look for mouth ulcers. Are they deep and extensive?
• Look for pus draining from the eye.
• Look for clouding of the cornea.

Classify FEVER

High or Low Malaria Risk

Signs	Classify as	Treatment
• Any general danger sign or • Stiff neck.	**Pink: VERY SEVERE FEBRILE DISEASE**	• Give first dose of artesunate or quinine for severe malaria • Give first dose of an appropriate antibiotic • Treat the child to prevent low blood sugar • Give one dose of paracetamol in clinic for high fever (38.5°C or above) • Refer URGENTLY to hospital
• Malaria test POSITIVE.	**Yellow: MALARIA**	• Give recommended first line oral antimalarial • Give one dose of paracetamol in clinic for high fever (38.5°C or above) • Give appropriate antibiotic treatment for an identified bacterial cause of fever • Advise mother when to return immediately • Follow-up in 3 days if fever persists • If fever is present every day for more than 7 days, refer for assessment
• Malaria test NEGATIVE • Other cause of fever PRESENT.	**Green: FEVER: NO MALARIA**	• Give one dose of paracetamol in clinic for high fever (38.5°C or above) • Give appropriate antibiotic treatment for an identified bacterial cause of fever • Advise mother when to return immediately • Follow-up in 3 days if fever persists • If fever is present every day for more than 7 days, refer for assessment

No Malaria Risk and No Travel to Malaria Risk Area

Signs	Classify as	Treatment
• Any general danger sign • Stiff neck.	**Pink: VERY SEVERE FEBRILE DISEASE**	• Give first dose of an appropriate antibiotic. • Treat the child to prevent low blood sugar. • Give one dose of paracetamol in clinic for high fever (38.5°C or above). • Refer URGENTLY to hospital.
• No general danger signs • No stiff neck.	**Green: FEVER**	• Give one dose of paracetamol in clinic for high fever (38.5°C or above) • Give appropriate antibiotic treatment for an identified bacterial cause of fever • Advise mother when to return immediately • Follow-up in 2 days if fever persists • If fever is present every day for more than 7 days, refer for assessment

If MEASLES now or within last 3 months, Classify

Signs	Classify as	Treatment
• Any general danger sign or • Clouding of cornea or • Deep or extensive mouth ulcers.	**Pink: SEVERE COMPLICATED MEASLES[d]**	• Give Vitamin A treatment • Give first dose of an appropriate antibiotic • If clouding of the cornea or pus draining from the eye, apply tetracycline eye ointment • Refer URGENTLY to hospital
• Pus draining from the eye or • Mouth ulcers.	**Yellow: MEASLES WITH EYE OR MOUTH COMPLICATIONS[d]**	• Give Vitamin A treatment • If pus draining from the eye, treat eye infection with tetracycline eye ointment • If mouth ulcers, treat with gentian violet • Follow-up in 3 days
• Measles now or within the last 3 months.	**Green: MEASLES**	• Give Vitamin A treatment

a. These temperatures are based on axillary temperature. Rectal temperature readings are approximately 0.5°C higher.

b. Look for local tenderness; oral sores; refusal to use a limb; hot tender swelling; red tender skin or boils; lower abdominal pain or pain on passing urine in older children.

c. If no malaria test available: High malaria risk - classify as MALARIA; Low malaria risk AND NO obvious cause of fever - classify as MALARIA.

d. Other important complications of measles - pneumonia, stridor, diarrhoea, ear infection, and acute malnutrition - are classified in other tables.

Source: IMCI Chart Booklet 2014 (http://www.who.int/maternal_child_adolescent/documents/IMCI_chartbooklet/en/).

of clinical failure at day seven was very low (2.7 percent), and lower than in the control group (8.0 percent) in which routine care was used; only 15 percent received an antibiotic compared with 84 percent in the control group (Shao and others 2015).

A multicountry evaluation of IMCI effectiveness, cost, and impact was conducted in Bangladesh, Brazil, Peru, Tanzania, and Uganda (Bryce and others 2005). In Tanzania, the survey results demonstrate that children in IMCI districts received higher-quality care, including more thorough evaluations, a greater likelihood of being properly diagnosed and correctly treated, and better counseling and knowledge of caretakers of children in IMCI districts relative to comparison districts (Armstrong Schellenberg and others 2004). Several other studies also show that IMCI case management training resulted in improved quality of care, especially when there were minimum standards of training quality and sufficient coverage of trained health workers (Arifeen and others 2005; Gouws and others 2004; Pariyo and others 2005; Nguyen and others 2013). The multicountry evaluation also reveals that the IMCI approach provided many benefits in addition to improved quality of care, including better record keeping and strengthened supervision. However, four of the five countries encountered challenges in expanding the IMCI strategy at the national level (Bryce and others 2005).

A multicountry study finds that the quality of child health care associated with IMCI training was similar across different cadres of health workers and that the duration and level of preservice training did not appear to influence the quality of care (Huicho and others 2008). A cluster randomized controlled trial in Bangladesh demonstrates that IMCI implementation resulted in improved health worker skills, increased oral rehydration solution (ORS) utilization, and exclusive breastfeeding, and it reduced stunting prevalence in intervention areas relative to comparison areas (Arifeen and others 2009). IMCI implementation was also associated with a nonsignificant 13 percent reduction in mortality in children under age five years. Mortality impact is examined in two other studies. In the first, a cluster randomized controlled trial in India that used Integrated Management of Neonatal and Childhood Illness (IMNCI) and community workers to conduct postnatal home visits, the infant mortality rate was 15 percent lower (adjusted hazard ratio 0.85, 95 percent confidence interval 0.77–0.94), and the neonatal mortality rate after the first 24 hours was 14 percent lower (adjusted hazard ratio 0.86, 95 percent confidence interval 0.79–0.95) in intervention, relative to control clusters (Bhandari and others 2012). In the second, a retrospective pre/post analysis of IMCI implementation in the Arab Republic of Egypt found a nearly twofold reduction in under-five mortality (3.3 percent versus 6.3 percent) in one year (Rakha and others 2013). These three studies provide evidence to suggest that effective scale-up and implementation of IMCI can help reduce infant and under-five all-cause mortality.

In HIV-endemic countries such as South Africa, local adaptations of the IMCI algorithm have been created to identify and manage HIV-infected children using a set of common signs and symptoms that are predictive of HIV infection, for example, recurrent or persistent diarrhea, persistent fever, or history of tuberculosis (Horwood and others 2003). The presence of three signs or a maternal report of HIV infection prompts testing for HIV in children. An evaluation of the IMCI HIV guidelines in South Africa finds that the algorithm correctly classified 71 percent of 76 HIV-infected children as suspected symptomatic HIV; approximately 20 percent were identified as HIV-exposed (Horwood and others 2009). This approach missed only 9 percent of HIV-infected children. Unfortunately, the study also finds that this approach is not being used consistently in routine clinical practice.

Although the IMCI strategy has the potential to increase the quality of care in health facilities, absolute levels of performance often are low, and adherence to the guidelines has been unsatisfactory. An assessment of health worker practices in Benin in 2000 revealed multiple problems with local adaptation of the IMCI guidelines. Problems included the failure to treat children in accordance with the guideline (incorrect choice of drug, dosage, and duration); missed opportunities for vaccination; treatment with unnecessary and occasionally dangerous medications; prescription of a large number of drugs for some children; and failure to perform counseling tasks, including how to administer medications (Rowe and others 2001). In Uganda, even after IMCI training, only about 50 percent of the children classified as having malaria or pneumonia received complete and appropriate treatment (Pariyo and others 2005). New training strategies are necessary, especially for respiratory rate measurement and identification of danger signs.

In addition, the IMCI clinical algorithms have the advantage of being highly sensitive but the drawback of having inadequate specificity. A prospective hospital-based study in Mozambique finds substantial symptom overlap between malaria and severe pneumonia among hospitalized children (Bassat and others 2011). Some 24 percent of children were classified using IMCI as having both malaria and severe pneumonia; however, when using stricter criteria based on radiological confirmation of pneumonia and *P. falciparum* parasitemia, the authors find that fewer than 1 percent had both malaria and severe pneumonia. Similar to other studies, there was a significant association between underlying HIV infection and prevalence of severe pneumonia, duration of hospitalization, and CFRs (Lanata 2004).

For implementation of the IMCI guidelines, the WHO recommends an 11-day in-service training course for first-level (that is, primary care) health facilities, job aids, and a follow-up visit to the facility at four to six weeks to reinforce IMCI practices. As of 2009, 76 countries had scaled up IMCI beyond a few pilot districts; many countries have adapted the IMCI algorithm to their local contexts. Some countries have started to use an electronic version of IMCI called ICATT that allows easy and rapid country adaptation of the algorithm and computer-based self training (http://www.icatt-impactt .org). Distance learning for IMCI has been developed as a strategy to increase IMCI training coverage (WHO 2014b). Other research into IMCI implementation highlights challenges related to care seeking, resources and supply chain, training, and supervision requirements to ensure implementation at large scale. Frequent staff rotation and attrition require that countries revise preservice curricula to include training on the WHO algorithms (WHO 2001, 2010b).

Management of Sick Young Infants: IMNCI and Beyond

Given the need to strengthen the capacity of health workers to identify young infants age 0–59 days with possible serious bacterial infections, two multicountry studies were performed to provide evidence to strengthen the IMCI algorithm to include newborns and young infants. To obtain information on clinical signs of sepsis in young infants age 0–59 days, the WHO conducted a large study of the clinical features and etiologies of serious bacterial disease from 1990 to 1992 in the Philippines (Gatchalian and others 1999), The Gambia (Mulholland and others 1999), Ethiopia (Muhe and others 1999), and Papua New Guinea (Lehmann and others 1999). This information contributed to the development of the IMCI algorithms during the mid-1990s, which standardized the management of sick young infants at first-level health facilities (Gove 1997; Tulloch 1999; Weber and others 2003).

Neonates in the first week of life were still not included. Accordingly, the YICSSG designed a multicenter study to analyze recognition of young infants, including neonates younger than seven days, requiring referral to higher levels of the health system. The YICSSG found that 12 symptoms or signs showed statistical evidence of independent predictive value for severe illness requiring hospital admission in the first week of life. A decision rule requiring the presence of any of these 12 signs had high sensitivity (87 percent) and specificity (74 percent). However, a simplified algorithm that required only seven signs—history of difficulty feeding, history of convulsions, movement only when stimulated, respiratory rate ≥ 60 breaths per minute, temperature ≥ 37.5°C or < 35.5°C, and severe chest indrawing—had a similar sensitivity (85 percent) and specificity (75 percent). This seven-sign algorithm also performed well in infants age 7–59 days (sensitivity 74 percent, specificity 79 percent) (WHO Young Infants Study Group 1999; Weber and others 2003). This clinical algorithm was validated at the community level during routine household visits in rural Bangladesh (Darmstadt and others 2011). A simplified six-sign algorithm had a sensitivity of 81 percent and specificity of 96 percent for screening neonates requiring referral, and sensitivity of 58 percent and specificity of 94 percent for identifying newborns at risk of dying.

The WHO IMCI guidelines recommend that any young infant presenting with danger signs should be referred to an appropriate level facility and treated with injectable gentamicin and ampicillin. Although data are limited, multiple reviews cite widespread resistance to ampicillin and gentamicin among sepsis-causing common pathogens *E. coli*, *S. aureus*, and *Klebsiella* species (Thaver, Ali, and Zaidi 2009; Waters and others 2011). Similarly, data from the YICSSG, which represent community-acquired bacteremia in young infants, reveals the wide distribution of multi-drug-resistant gram-negative rods, and 11 percent of *S. aureus* isolates were methicillin resistant (Hamer and others 2015). Although broad-spectrum cephalosporins show better sensitivities to most pathogens, they are expensive and their use will increase drug pressure. Recommended antimicrobial therapies need to be regionally specific, and considerations to empirically cover for HSV-2 infections must be considered in the youngest infants. The Aetiology of Neonatal Infection in South Asia study will provide even more current data for LMICs that reflect current epidemiology and antimicrobial susceptibilities (WHO Young Infants Study Group 1999; YICSSG 2008).

A seminal study in India demonstrates a 16 percent reduction in neonatal sepsis case fatality and a 62 percent reduction in overall neonatal mortality by instituting a package of home-based newborn care services by trained community health workers (CHWs); the services included an assessment for sepsis and prereferral administration of injectable gentamicin if indicated (Bang and others 1999). A more detailed discussion of this study is provided in chapter 18 in this volume (Ashok, Nandi, and Laxminarayan 2016). In Zambia, a cluster randomized controlled trial assessed the impact of training birth attendants to perform a modified neonatal resuscitation protocol for newborns with respiratory distress and to recognize a set of cardinal symptoms and signs of possible neonatal infection. If any signs of possible serious bacterial infection were observed in the first four weeks of life, intervention-trained birth assistants were to administer a 500 milligram dose of oral amoxicillin and facilitate referral to the nearest rural health center. This combination of interventions resulted in a 45 percent reduction in neonatal mortality for all live births in intervention as compared with controls (Gill and others 2011).

Several studies from India, Nepal, and Pakistan evaluate a variety of community-based perinatal packages that deploy newborn home visitation; each trial has shown significant impact on neonatal mortality (Baqui and others 2008; Bhutta and others 2008; Kumar and others 2008). As a result of this growing body of evidence, the WHO and UNICEF released a joint statement on home visits in 2009 (WHO and UNICEF 2009b). Several countries have developed adaptations of IMNCI. The Indian IMNCI program, which integrates home visits for newborn care with improved treatment of illness, evaluated the effectiveness of this strategy in a cluster randomized controlled trial. This study demonstrated more optimal newborn care practices in intervention clusters and a significant reduction of neonatal mortality only among babies born at home receiving intervention (hazard ratio intervention/control 0.80 for home births [95 percent confidence interval 0.68–0.93] versus 1.06 for facility births [95 percent confidence interval 0.91–1.23]) (Bhandari and others 2012).

Integrated Community Case Management

In many resource-limited countries, access to health facilities for prompt, appropriate management of common childhood illnesses is limited and often complicated by shortages of essential medicines and insufficient human resources. Children in the lowest wealth quintile are less likely to receive early and appropriate treatment for malaria, pneumonia, and diarrhea (Young and Wolfheim 2012). To address this access gap and provide early access to treatment, many countries have been testing and scaling up community-based programs for the treatment of common childhood infectious diseases. iCCM provides an integrated algorithmic approach to identifying and treating ill children with limited access to health facilities. These algorithms alert CHWs to signs and symptoms of severe disease to indicate referral into the formal health system while treating minor illness in the community, serving as an extension of the formal health care system. This approach has several potential benefits, including improving the rational use of drugs

by deploying diagnostics-guided, evidence-based pediatric treatment algorithms and improving early access to effective treatment, thereby decreasing the risk that a child's illness will progress to severe disease. The WHO and UNICEF released a joint statement justifying the need for iCCM and making recommendations on its implementation in 2012 (WHO and UNICEF 2012).

The effectiveness and feasibility of community-based management of individual disease conditions have been demonstrated for pneumonia, diarrheal disease, and malaria (Mubi and others 2011; Mukanga, Tiono, and Anyorigiya 2012; Theodoratou 2010; Yeboah-Antwi and others 2010). Home-based management of diarrhea has been practiced for decades; the WHO's Special Programme for Research and Training in Tropical Diseases and others have extensively tested approaches to community-level management of malaria (Ajayi and others 2008; Pagnoni 2009). Studies have been conducted to assess effectiveness of the full iCCM package for management of malaria, pneumonia, and diarrhea, which is often coupled with screening for acute malnutrition. This package generally consists of training either volunteer or paid cadres of community-based health workers to follow a simple algorithm (figure 8.2) to classify and

Figure 8.2 Sample Integrated Community Case Management Algorithm

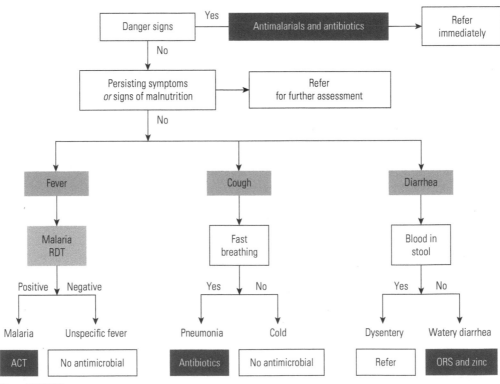

Source: WHO 2009.

Note: ACT = artemisinin-based combination therapy; ORS = oral rehydration solution; RDT = rapid diagnostic test.

treat children under age five years who present with fever, cough, difficulty breathing, or diarrhea. Necessary equipment includes a timer for counting respiratory rates and a tape for measuring mid-upper arm circumference if screening for acute malnutrition is performed; supplies include malaria RDTs, weight- and age-appropriate dose packs of an ACT, dispersible amoxicillin tablets (or cotrimoxazole because supply of amoxicillin is a frequent challenge), zinc, and low osmolarity ORS.

Quality and Safety of iCCM delivery

Several studies show that CHWs can appropriately classify and treat malaria, pneumonia, and diarrhea in children. Studies in Cambodia, Sudan, and Zambia show that with minimal training and job aids, CHWs can perform and interpret RDTs (Elmardi and others 2009; Harvey and others 2008; Mayxay and others 2004). In contrast with some studies of health workers in first-level health centers that demonstrate a tendency to ignore malaria diagnostic test results and to overprescribe ACT, several other studies clearly highlight the ability of CHWs to correctly perform RDTs and appropriately not prescribe antimalarials for RDT-negative patients (Bisoffi and others 2009; Hamer and others 2007; Harvey and others 2008; Reyburn and others 2007; Yasuoka and others 2010). Exceptions have been noted: Sudanese community volunteers have prescribed ACT in 30 percent of subjects with fever but a negative RDT result (Elmardi and others 2009), indicating that the inappropriate prescription of ACT may be an issue in some settings at the community level; lack of or inappropriate CHW training and supervision is one of several possible reasons.

A study in Zambia that evaluated two models of integrated delivery of treatment for malaria and pneumonia demonstrates that CHWs correctly classified 1,017 children who presented with fever or fast or difficult breathing as having malaria and pneumonia 94 percent to 100 percent of the time. Appropriate treatment based on disease classification was correct in 94 percent to 100 percent of episodes (Hamer and others 2012). In Uganda, a study that compared CHWs trained in integrated malaria and pneumonia management to those only trained in malaria case management demonstrated that CHWs with high illness knowledge scores used correct doses of medications for malaria and pneumonia, and correctly classified 75 percent of children with pneumonia (Kalyango, Rutebemberwa, and Alfven 2012). However, the CHWs did not count respiratory rate accurately—only 49 percent measured respiratory rates within the bounds of the gold-standard criteria of five breaths per minute of the physician. This study

and an earlier evaluation in Kenya (Kelly and others 2001) suggest problems with pneumonia evaluation, emphasizing the need for ongoing supervision, training, and quality measurement of CHWs. This issue is further discussed in a systematic review of pneumonia community case management (CCM), which suggests that evidence on the efficacy and effectiveness of this approach in Sub-Saharan Africa is still lacking (Druetz and others 2013).

Several studies conducted in Benin, Tanzania, Uganda, and Zambia demonstrate that febrile RDT-negative children can be managed safely without antimalarial therapy (D'Acremont and others 2010; Faucher and others 2010; Msellem and others 2009; Njama-Meya and others 2007; Yeboah-Antwi and others 2010). In the Zambian study, children were evaluated five to seven days after their visit to the CHW; treatment failure at this point occurred in 9.3 percent of children (N = 1,017) in the study arm that implemented an iCCM package of malaria RDTs, ACTs, and amoxicillin. Notably, only 0.4 percent of children were hospitalized and 0.2 percent died. These findings provide additional confirmation that the WHO's guidelines for malaria treatment (WHO 2010a), which recommend treatment based on a positive diagnostic test for all patients, including children under age five years, can also be safely implemented at the community level in malaria-endemic areas of Sub-Saharan Africa.

All of the studies discussed focus on the management of children with nonsevere pneumonia at the community level. However, substantial evidence indicates that children with the former WHO-defined severe pneumonia (pneumonia with chest indrawing but no danger signs) can be managed with oral amoxicillin at the community level. In Pakistan, a five-day course of high-dose amoxicillin was shown to be equivalent to parenteral ampicillin for 48 hours, followed by a three-day course of oral amoxicillin for children with severe pneumonia (Hazir and others 2008). Subsequently, a multicountry observational study conducted in Bangladesh, Egypt, Ghana, and Vietnam demonstrated the safety and efficacy of home-based management of severe pneumonia with oral high-dose amoxicillin (Addo-Yobo and others 2011). An average of 9.2 percent of children met a rigorous definition of treatment failure at day 6 and 2.7 percent relapsed by day 14, but all children survived; only one adverse drug reaction (among 823 children) was documented. Two parallel community-based studies in rural Pakistan provide further evidence of the effectiveness and safety of the home-based management of chest indrawing pneumonia with oral amoxicillin by female health workers (Bari and others 2011; Soofi and others 2012).

Impact of iCCM

iCCM has several benefits, including early care seeking for illness; early access to appropriate treatment for children; reduced use of expensive antimalarial drugs when RDTs are used; reductions in health center attendance, which helps reduce the workload at primary health care centers; and probably decreased all-cause mortality for children under age five years.

Given the substantial workload at rural health centers, which are often understaffed, iCCM offers a potential opportunity to increase access to effective therapy at the community level (Guenther and others 2012) while decreasing the volume of health facility visits. In the Zambian study (Yeboah-Antwi and others 2010), cross-sectional household surveys on health care–seeking practices were performed before and immediately after the 12-month integrated malaria and pneumonia intervention period. A significant increase was observed in the proportion of mothers who sought care from CHWs between baseline and poststudy in both groups (empiric ACT for fever plus referral of children with pneumonia versus RDT-based ACT for malaria and amoxicillin for nonsevere pneumonia). Care seeking from CHWs increased for all types of illness, and use of health facilities and traditional healers decreased (Seidenberg and others 2012). This pattern was noted in both groups for children presenting with fever, cough, and diarrhea; however, there was a trend toward greater use of the CHWs that could provide amoxicillin for children with fast breathing or difficulty breathing relative to those CHWs who were trained to refer children with signs of pneumonia.

Limited data are available on the impact of iCCM on child mortality under age five years. Some earlier studies of the home management of malaria, based on maternal recall of a history of fever, found that home management of malaria is associated with a reduction in the development of severe malaria by more than 50 percent and all-cause mortality by 40 percent (Kidane and Morrow 2000; Sirima and others 2003). More recently, a study in Ghana that used a stepped-wedge cluster-randomized design evaluated the impact of adding amoxicillin to an antimalarial (artesunate-amodiaquine) for treating fever among children age 2–59 months on all-cause mortality. In clusters in which artesunate-amodiaquine alone was used for fever treatment, mortality decreased by 30 percent (rate ratio = 0.70, 95 percent confidence interval 0.53–0.92, P = 0.011) and in clusters that used both an ACT and amoxicillin, mortality was reduced by 44 percent (rate ratio = 0.56, 95 percent confidence interval 0.41–0.76, P = 0.011) when compared with control clusters. A 21 percent mortality reduction was observed with the addition of amoxicillin to the ACT;

however, this difference was not statistically significant (rate ratio = 0.79, 95 percent confidence interval 0.56–1.12, P = 0.195). This study also showed reductions in anemia, severe anemia, and severe disease among children in both study arms (Chinbuah and others 2013). Although this trial suggests a mortality benefit of both an ACT alone and the combination of an ACT with an antibiotic, its design has several limitations, including the lack of use of malaria RDTs and the empiric use of antibiotics for all children with fever, regardless of the respiratory rate in the combined arm (Chinbuah and others 2012).

A limited number of studies have evaluated the cost-effectiveness of iCCM. An economic analysis of the study in Ghana that compared an ACT to ACT plus amoxicillin (Chinbuah and others 2012) finds that the cost per DALY averted was US$90.25 for artesunate-amodiaquine and US$114.21 for this ACT plus amoxicillin (Nonvignon and others 2012). The authors conclude that both approaches were cost-effective. However, the diagnosis of malaria did not involve the use of RDTs; all children in the ACT plus amoxicillin arm with fever were given antibiotics, an approach that carries a high risk of antimicrobial resistance and potential adverse events among children who do not require antibiotics. A cost-effectiveness analysis of malaria case management using RDTs and artemether-lumefantrine in Zambia reveals that home-based management was more cost-effective than facility-based management (US$4.22 per case at the home versus US$6.12 at the facility) (Chanda and others 2011). A cost analysis from Pakistan that focuses on household costs of illness finds that home management of pneumonia by women health workers was associated with a substantially lower cost to the household than for children who were referred for treatment (Sadruddin and others 2012).

CHALLENGES AND FUTURE DIRECTIONS

The Catalytic Initiative, an evaluation in six Sub-Saharan African countries—Ethiopia, Ghana, Malawi, Mali, Mozambique, and Niger—provides a useful summary of challenges and lessons learned during the scale-up of iCCM. Some of the major challenges to delivery of iCCM include the deployment, supervision, motivation, and retention of CHWs; maintenance of reliable supply chains; demand-side barriers to utilization; inadequate monitoring and evaluation systems; and a need for supportive government policies and engagement to achieve sustainable progress (UNICEF 2012).

In 2009–10, a survey of 68 countries in the Countdown to 2015 initiative was conducted to assess CCM of childhood illnesses (de Sousa and others 2012).

Most (81 percent) of the 59 countries that responded had policies for CCM of diarrhea and malaria (75 percent); only 54 percent had CCM policies for pneumonia. Only 17 (32 percent) of the 53 malaria-endemic countries providing responses had policies for all three of these conditions. According to the survey, CHWs administered the recommended treatments for diarrhea, malaria, or pneumonia in 34 percent (17 of 50), 100 percent (41 of 41), and 100 percent (34 of 34) of the countries implementing CCM of these conditions, respectively. Many programs identified similar implementation-related concerns, including problems with drug supplies; quality of care; and CHW incentives, training, and supervision. Implementation issues around supervision, quality control, supply chain, and remuneration of CHWs are important areas of research for iCCM because best practices will inform approaches to the scale-up of iCCM.

Economic studies confirm that international guidelines for treatment of fever in children are also cost-effective. Community use of rectal artesunate for children with severe malaria during their referral to higher-level care has been shown to be cost-effective. Similarly, RDTs for malaria are cost-effective if used appropriately (where *P. falciparum* is dominant and ACTs are the appropriate therapy, and where care providers abide by test results in their prescribing behavior). Finally, IMCI was shown in one study to be cost-effective (Armstrong Schellenberg and others 2004); however, precisely because it is effective, it can increase costs to the health service as patients shift from using private clinics (needs Prinja and others 2013).

Future research needs for diagnosis and treatment approaches for the febrile child are plentiful. Box 8.1 highlights considerations for future research, policy, and programming.

Box 8.1

Future Research Needs

Epidemiology
- Ongoing surveillance of febrile illness etiology, with particular emphasis on high burden countries, such as the Democratic Republic of Congo, Ethiopia, India, and Nigeria; on regions at high risk of zoonotic illness; on regions in conflict; and on neonatal infections
- Role of HSV-2 and GBS in neonatal illness, as well as impact of HSV-2 and GBS prophylaxis on neonatal outcomes
- Patterns of antimicrobial resistance to direct empiric therapies for pediatric serious bacterial infections

Implementation
- Field evaluation of commercially available diagnostic point-of-care tools to determine feasibility, cost-effectiveness, and level of health system; various tools should be introduced
- Creation and evaluation of innovative solutions to reduce power needs or use of alternative energy sources (for example, solar power, battery operated) for oxygen concentrators, pulse oximeters, and other tools that require power
- Operational research to determine best practices for supply chain management, training, and supervision for IMCI and iCCM when scaled up
- Qualitative and quantitative research to better understand the role of the private sector in influencing care-seeking behaviors, diagnosis, and treatment

Economics
- Cost analysis of diagnostic tools versus empiric therapy for common pediatric illnesses in newborn period, and for pneumonia, diarrheal disease, and nonfocal fevers
- Cost comparisons of investments in preventive interventions (for example, vaccines, malnutrition treatment, exclusive breastfeeding) compared with diagnosis and treatment for common pediatric illnesses

Note: GBS = Group B streptococcus; HSV-2 = herpes simplex virus-2; iCCM = integrated community case management; IMCI = Integrated Management of Childhood Illness.

CONCLUSIONS

Ample evidence suggests a shift in the etiology of pediatric febrile illnesses, especially in countries with declining rates of malaria transmission. More etiology studies are needed in LMICs with high disease burdens (for example, Democratic Republic of Congo, Ethiopia, India, Nigeria, Pakistan), particularly for young infants. Ongoing surveillance is required to track epidemiological shifts given that drug pressure and policies influence which diseases are prominent in each region. The research evidence is concentrated in a few regions of the world; thus, advocacy for research in high burden countries, regions at high risk of zoonotic illness, regions in conflict, and neonatal infections is paramount to shaping global, national, and region-specific policy. Many diagnostic tools are commercially available or are in the development pipeline, tools that could aid in narrowing differential diagnoses and that could help providers determine whether antimicrobials are indicated. However, these tools need to be evaluated in the field to assess the cost-effectiveness and utility in the clinical context.

Finally, although both WHO-sponsored IMCI and iCCM offer promising health facility and community platforms for integrated service delivery, challenges including adherence to guidelines, supply chain, supervision, and scale up while maintaining quality are barriers to successful implementation. Adaptation of these models to reflect local epidemiology and available resources is paramount. In areas without CHWs or regions with prominent informal private sectors, work needs to be done to determine how to align approaches to children with fever to ensure appropriate treatment and decrease antibiotic overuse. The role of the private informal sector has been underestimated, and careful thought is needed about how to motivate and partner with private sector drug providers.

Because febrile illnesses are still the predominant disease presentation of most pediatric illnesses, high-quality impact and process research that can inform which models work best in which contexts is needed. This research, along with expanded fever etiology surveillance and innovative technologies for low-resource diagnostics and treatment delivery, is critical for further reductions in child mortality and morbidity. A unified call for an organized agenda and framework that unites the pneumonia, malaria, measles, other febrile illnesses, and neonatal illness agendas would benefit the global child survival agenda. MDG 4 has motivated numerous national-level planning efforts and now there is substantial country-specific programming. A forum to discuss evidence for best practices would further benefit this unmet need.

ANNEXES

The annexes to this chapter are as follows. They are available at http://www.dcp-3.org/RMNCH.

- Annex 8A. Common Etiologies of Childhood Pneumonia in Low- and Middle-Income Countries
- Annex 8B. Diagnostic Tools Available and Under Development for ARI or Other Serious Bacterial Illnesses

NOTE

For consistency and ease of comparison, *DCP3* is using the World Health Organization's Global Health Estimates (GHE) for data on diseases burden, except in cases where a relevant data point is not available from GHE. In those instances, an alternative data source is noted.

World Bank Income Classifications as of July 2014 are as follows, based on estimates of gross national income (GNI) per capita for 2013:

- Low-income countries (LICs) = US$1,045 or less
- Middle-income countries (MICs) are subdivided:
  a) lower-middle-income = US$1,046–US$4,125
  b) upper-middle-income (UMICs) = US$4,126–US$12,745
- High-income countries (HICs) = US$12,746 or more.

REFERENCES

Abba, K., J. J. Deeks, P. L. Olliaro, C.-M. Naing, S. M. Jackson, and others. 2011. "Rapid Diagnostic Tests for Diagnosing Uncomplicated *P. falciparum* Malaria in Endemic Countries." *Cochrane Database of Systematic Reviews* (7): CD008122.

Addo-Yobo, E., D. D. Anh, H. El-Sayed, L. M. Fox, M. P. Fox, and others. 2011. "Outpatient Treatment of Children with Severe Pneumonia with Oral Amoxicillin in Four Countries: The MASS Study." *Tropical Medicine and International Health* 16 (8): 995–1006.

Ajayi, I. O., E. N. Browne, F. Bateganya, D. Yar, C. Happi, and others. 2008. "Effectiveness of Artemisinin-Based Combination Therapy Used in the Context of Home Management of Malaria: A Report from Three Study Sites in Sub-Saharan Africa." *Malaria Journal* 7: 190.

Animut, A., Y. Mekonnen, D. Shimelis, and E. Ephraim. 2009. "Febrile Illnesses of Different Etiology among Outpatients in Four Health Centers in Northwestern Ethiopia." *Japanese Journal of Infectious Disease* 62 (2): 107–10.

Arifeen, S. E., J. Bryce, E. Gouws, A. Baqui, R. E. Black, and others. 2005. "Quality of Care for Under-Fives in First-Level Health Facilities in One District of Bangladesh." *Bulletin of the World Health Organization* 83 (4): 260–67.

Arifeen, S. E., D. M. E. Hoque, T. Akter, M. Rahman, M. E. Hoque, and others. 2009. "Effect of the Integrated Management of Childhood Illness Strategy on Childhood Mortality and Nutrition in a Rural Area in Bangladesh: A Cluster Randomised Trial." *The Lancet* 374 (9687): 393–403.

Armstrong Schellenberg, J., J. Bryce, D. de Savigny, T. Lambrechts, C. Mbuya, and others. 2004. "The Effect of Integrated Management of Childhood Illness on Observed Quality of Care of Under-Fives in Rural Tanzania." *Health Policy Planning* 19 (1): 1–10.

Ashok, A., A. Nandi, and R. Laxminarayan. 2016. "The Benefits of a Universal Home-Based Neonatal Care Package in Rural India: An Extended Cost-effectiveness Analysis." In *Disease Control Priorities* (third edition): Volume 2, *Reproductive, Maternal, Newborn, and Child Health*, edited by R. Black, R. Laxminarayan, M. Temmerman, and N. Walker. Washington, DC: World Bank.

Baiden, F., J. Webster, M. Tivura, R. Delimini, Y. Berko, and others. 2012. "Accuracy of Rapid Tests for Malaria and Treatment Outcomes for Malaria and Non-Malaria Cases among Under-Five Children in Rural Ghana." *PLoS One* 7 (4): e34073.

Bang, A. T., R. A. Bang, S. B. Baitule, M. H. Reddy, and M. D. Deshmukh. 1999. "Effect of Home-Based Neonatal Care and Management of Sepsis on Neonatal Mortality: Field Trial in Rural India." *The Lancet* 354 (9194): 1955–61.

Baqui, A. H., S. El-Arifeen, G. L. Darmstadt, S. Ahmed, E. K. Williams, and others. 2008. "Effect of Community-Based Newborn-Care Intervention Package Implemented through Two Service-Delivery Strategies in Sylhet District, Bangladesh: A Cluster-Randomised Controlled Trial." *The Lancet* 371 (9628): 1936–44.

Bari, A., S. Sadruddin, A. Khan, Iu Khan, A. Khan, and others. 2011. "Community Case Management of Severe Pneumonia with Oral Amoxicillin in Children Aged 2–59 Months in Haripur District, Pakistan: A Cluster Randomised Trial." *The Lancet* 378 (9805): 1796–803.

Bassat, Q., S. Machevo, C. O'Callaghan-Gordo, B. Siga úque, L. Morais, and others. 2011. "Distinguishing Malaria from Severe Pneumonia among Hospitalized Children Who Fulfilled Integrated Management of Childhood Illness Criteria for Both Diseases: A Hospital-Based Study in Mozambique." *American Journal of Tropical Medicine and Hygiene* 85 (4): 626–34.

Bastiaens, G. J. H., E. Schaftenaar, A. Ndaro, M. Keuter, T. Bousema, and others. 2011. "Malaria Diagnostic Testing and Treatment Practices in Three Different *Plasmodium falciparum* Transmission Settings in Tanzania: Before and after a Government Policy Change." *Malaria Journal* 10: 76.

Bélisle, J. M., S. Costantino, M. L. Leimanis, M.-J. Bellemare, D. S. Bohle, and others. 2008. "Sensitive Detection of Malaria Infection by Third Harmonic Generation Imaging." *Biophysical Journal* 94 (4): L26–28.

Bhandari, N., S. Mazumder, S. Taneja, H. Sommerfelt, and T. A. Strand. 2012. "Effect of Implementation of Integrated Management of Neonatal and Childhood Illness (IMNCI) Programme on Neonatal and Infant Mortality: Cluster Randomised Controlled Trial." *British Medical Journal* 344: e1634.

Bhutta, Z. A., Z. A. Memon, S. Soofi, M. S. Salat, S. Cousens, and others. 2008. "Implementing Community-Based Perinatal Care: Results from a Pilot Study in Rural Pakistan." *Bulletin of the World Health Organization* 86 (6): 452–59.

Bisoffi, Z., B. S. Sirima, A. Angheben, C. Lodesani, F. Gobbi, and others. 2009. "Rapid Malaria Diagnostic Tests vs. Clinical Management of Malaria in Rural Burkina Faso: Safety and Effect on Clinical Decisions: A Randomized Trial." *Tropical Medicine and International Health* 14 (5): 491–98.

Bryce, J., C. G. Victora, J.-P. Habicht, R. E. Black, and R. W. Scherpbier. 2005. "Programmatic Pathways to Child Survival: Results of a Multi-Country Evaluation of Integrated Management of Childhood Illness." *Health Policy Planning* 20 (Suppl 1): i5–17.

Byington, C. L., K. K. Rittichier, K. E. Bassett, H. Castillo, T. S. Glasgow, and others. 2003. "Serious Bacterial Infections in Febrile Infants Younger Than 90 Days of Age: The Importance of Ampicillin-Resistant Pathogens." *Pediatrics* 111 (5): 964–68.

Caron, M., G. Grard, C. Paupy, and I. Mombo. 2013. "First Evidence of Simultaneous Circulation of Three Different Dengue Virus Serotypes in Africa." *PLoS One* 8 (10): e78030.

CDC (Centers for Disease Control and Prevention). 2012. "Fact Sheet: Dengue." CDC, Atlanta, GA. www.cdc.gov/Dengue/faqFacts/fact.html.

Chanda, P., B. Hamainza, H. Moonga, V. Chalwe, P. Banda, and F. Pagnoni. 2011. "Relative Costs and Effectiveness of Treating Uncomplicated Malaria in Two Rural Districts in Zambia: Implications for Nationwide Scale-Up of Home-Based Management." *Malaria Journal* 10: 159.

Chinbuah, M., M. Adjuik, F. Cobelens, K. A. Koram, M. Abbey, and others. 2013. "Impact of Treating Young Children with Antimalarials with or without Antibiotics on Morbidity: A Cluster-Randomized Controlled Trial in Ghana." *International Health* 5 (3): 228–35.

Chinbuah, M., P. Kager, M. Abbey, M. Gyapong, E. Awini, and others. 2012. "Impact of Community Management of Fever (Using Antimalarials with or without Antibiotics) on Childhood Mortality: A Cluster-Randomized Controlled Trial in Ghana." *American Journal of Tropical Medicine and Hygiene* 87 (5 Suppl): 11–20.

Communicable Disease Surveillance and Response Vaccines and Biologicals. 1997. "The Diagnosis, Treatment and Prevention of Typhoid Fever." World Health Organization, Geneva.

Crump, J. A., A. B. Morrissey, W. L. Nicholson, R. F. Massung, R. A. Stoddard, and others. 2013. "Etiology of Severe Non-Malaria Febrile Illness in Northern Tanzania: A Prospective Cohort Study." *PLoS Neglected Tropical Diseases* 7 (7): e2324.

D'Acremont, V., J. Kahama-Maro, N. Swai, D. Mtasiwa, B. Genton, and C. Lengeler. 2011. "Reduction of Anti-Malarial Consumption after Rapid Diagnostic Tests implementation in Dar es Salaam: A Before-After and Cluster Randomized Controlled Study." *Malaria Journal* 10: 107.

D'Acremont, V., M. Kilowoko, E. Kyungu, S. Philipina, W. Sangu, and others. 2014. "Beyond Malaria: Causes of Fever in Outpatient Tanzanian Children." *New England Journal of Medicine* 370: 809–17.

D'Acremont, V., C. Lengeler, and B. Genton. 2007. "Stop Ambiguous Messages on Malaria Diagnosis." *British Medical Journal* 334: 489.

———. 2010. "Reduction in the Proportion of Fevers Associated with *Plasmodium falciparum* Parasitaemia in Africa: A Systematic Review." *Malaria Journal* 9: 240.

D'Acremont, V., C. Lengeler, H. Mshinda, D. Mtasiwa, M. Tanner, and others. 2009. "Time to Move from Presumptive Malaria Treatment to Laboratory-Confirmed Diagnosis and Treatment in African Children with Fever." *PLoS Medicine* 6 (1): e252.

D'Acremont, V., A. Malila, N. Swai, R. Tillya, J. Kahama-Maro, and others. 2010. "Withholding Antimalarials in Febrile Children Who Have a Negative Result for a Rapid Diagnostic Test." *Clinical Infectious Disease* 51 (5): 506–11.

Darmstadt, G. L., A. H. Baqui, Y. Choi, S. Bari, S. M. Rahman, and others. 2011. "Validation of a Clinical Algorithm to Identify Neonates with Severe Illness during Routine Household Visits in Rural Bangladesh." *Archive of Disease in Childhood* 96 (12): 1140–46.

de Sousa, A., K. E. Tiedje, J. Recht, I. Bjelic, and D. H. Hamer. 2012. "Community Case Management of Childhood Illnesses: Policy and Implementation in Countdown to 2015 Countries." *Bulletin of the World Health Organization* 90: 183–90.

Druetz, T., K. Siekmans, S. Goossens, V. Ridde, and S. Haddad. 2013. "The Community Case Management of Pneumonia in Africa: A Review of the Evidence." *Health Policy Planning* 30 (2): 253–66.

Duke, T., W. Francis, J. Merilyn, M. Sens, K. Magdalene, and others. 2008. "Improved Oxygen Systems for Childhood Pneumonia: A Multihospital Effectiveness Study in Papua New Guinea." *The Lancet* 372 (9646): 1328–33.

Edmond, K. M., C. Kortsalioudaki, S. Scott, S. J. Schrag, A. K. M. Zaidi, and others. 2012. "Group B Streptococcal Disease in Infants Aged Younger Than 3 Months: Systematic Review and Meta-Analysis." *The Lancet* 379 (9815): 547–56.

Elmardi, K. A., E. M. Malik, T. Abdelgadir, S. H. Ali, A. H. Elsyed, and others. 2009. "Feasibility and Acceptability of Home-Based Management of Malaria Strategy Adapted to Sudan's Conditions Using Artemisinin-Based Combination Therapy and Rapid Diagnostic Test." *Malaria Journal* 8: 39.

English, M., H. Reyburn, C. Goodman, and R. W. Snow. 2009. "Abandoning Presumptive Antimalarial Treatment for Febrile Children Aged Less Than Five Years—A Case of Running before We Can Walk?" *PLoS Medicine* 6 (1): e1000015.

Factor, S. H., J. A. Schillinger, H. D. Kalter, S. Saha, H. Begum, and others. 2001. "Diagnosis and Management of Febrile Children Using the WHO/UNICEF Guidelines for IMCI in Dhaka, Bangladesh." *Bulletin of the World Health Organization* 79 (12): 1096–105.

Faucher, J., P. Makoutode, G. Abiou, T. Beheton, P. Houze, and others. 2010. "Can Treatment of Malaria Be Restricted to Parasitologically Confirmed Malaria? A School-Based Study in Benin in Children with and without Fever." *Malaria Journal* 9: 104.

Feachem, R. G., A. A. Phillips, J. Hwang, C. Cotter, B. Wielgosz, and others. 2010. "Shrinking the Malaria Map: Progress and Prospects." *The Lancet* 376 (9752): 1566–78.

Ganatra, H. A., and A. K. M. Zaidi. 2010. "Neonatal Infections in the Developing World." *Seminars in Perinatology* 34 (6): 416–25.

García, C. G., R. Bhore, A. Soriano-Fallas, M. Trost, R. Chason, and others. 2010. "Risk Factors in Children Hospitalized with RSV Bronchiolitis versus Non-RSV Bronchiolitis." *Pediatrics* 126 (6): e1453–60.

Gatchalian, S., B. Quiambao, A. Morelos, L. Abraham, C. Gepanayao, and others. 1999. "Bacterial and Viral Etiology of Serious Infections in Very Young Filipino Infants." *Pediatric Infectious Disease Journal* 18 (10 Suppl): S50–55.

GBD (Global Burden of Disease) 2013 Mortality and Causes of Death Collaborators. 2015. "Global, Regional, and National Age-Specific All-Cause and Cause-Specific Mortality for 240 Causes of Death, 1999–2013: A Systematic Analysis for the Global Burden of Disease Study 2013." *The Lancet* 385: 117–71. Epub December 17.

Gérardin, P., G. Barau, A. Michault, M. Bintner, H. Randrianaivo, and others. 2008. "Multidisciplinary Prospective Study of Mother-to-Child Chikungunya Virus Infections on the Island of La Réunion." *PLoS Medicine* 5 (3): e60.

Gething, P. W., V. C. Kirui, V. A. Alegana, E. A. Okiro, A. M. Noor, and R. W. Snow. 2010. "Estimating the Number of Paediatric Fevers Associated with Malaria Infection Presenting to Africa's Public Health Sector in 2007." *PLoS Medicine* 7 (7): e1000301.

Gill, C. J., G. Phiri-Mazala, N. G. Guerina, J. Kasimba, C. Mulenga, and others. 2011. "Effect of Training Traditional Birth Attendants on Neonatal Mortality (Lufwanyama Neonatal Survival Project): Randomised Controlled Study." *British Medical Journal* 342: d346.

Gouws, E., J. Bryce, J.-P. Habicht, J. Amaral, G. Pariyo, and others. 2004. "Improving Antimicrobial Use among Health Workers in First-Level Facilities: Results from the Multi-Country Evaluation of the Integrated Management of Childhood Illness Strategy." *Bulletin of the World Health Organization* 82 (7): 509–15.

Gove, S. 1997. "Integrated Management of Childhood Illness by Outpatient Health Workers: Technical Basis and Overview. The WHO Working Group on Guidelines for Integrated Management of the Sick Child." *Bulletin of the World Health Organization* 75 (Suppl 1): 7–24.

Greenhow, T. L., Y.-Y. Hung, A. M. Herz, E. Losada, and R. H. Pantell. 2014. "The Changing Epidemiology of Serious Bacterial Infections in Young Infants." *Pediatric Infectious Disease Journal* 33 (6): 595–99.

Guenther, T., S. Sadruddin, T. Chimuna, B. Sichamba, K. Yeboah-Antwi, and others. 2012. "Beyond Distance: An Approach to Measure Effective Access to Case Management for Sick Children in Africa." *American Journal of Tropical Medicine and Hygiene* 87 (5 Suppl): 77–84.

Hamer, D. H., E. Brooks, K. Semrau, P. Pilingana, W. MacLeod, and others. 2012. "Quality and Safety of Integrated Community Case Management of Malaria Using Rapid

Diagnostic Tests and Pneumonia by Community Health Workers." *Pathology in Global Health* 106 (1): 32–39.

Hamer, D. H., G. L. Darmstadt, J. B. Carlin, A. K. M. Zaidi, K. Yeboah-Antwi, and others. 2015. "Etiology of Bacteremia in Young Infants in Six Countries." *Pediatric Infectious Disease Journal* 34 (1): e1–8.

Hamer, D. H., M. Ndhlovu, D. Zurovac, M. Fox, K. Yeboah-Antwi, and others. 2007. "Does Improving Coverage of Parasitological Diagnostic Tests Change Malaria Treatment Practices? An Operational Cross-Sectional Study in Zambia." *Journal of American Medicine* 297: 2227–31.

Harvey, S. A., L. Jennings, M. Chinyama, F. Masaninga, K. Mulholland, and others. 2008. "Improving Community Health Worker Use of Malaria Rapid Diagnostic Tests in Zambia: Package Instructions, Job Aid and Job Aid-Plus-Training." *Malaria Journal* 7: 160.

Hazir, T., L. M. Fox, Y. B. Nisar, M. P. Fox, Y. P. Ashraf, and others. 2008. "Ambulatory Short-Course High-Dose Oral Amoxicillin for Treatment of Severe Pneumonia in Children: A Randomised Equivalency Trial." *The Lancet* 371 (9606): 49–56.

Hertz, J. T., O. M. Munishi, J. P. Sharp, E. A. Reddy, and J. A. Crump. 2013. "Comparing Actual and Perceived Causes of Fever among Community Members in a Low Malaria Transmission Setting in Northern Tanzania." *Tropical Medicine and International Health* 18 (11): 1406–15.

Holmes, K. K., S. Bertozzi, B. Bloom, P. Jha, and R. Nugent, editors. Forthcoming. *Disease Control Priorities* (third edition): Volume 6, *HIV/AIDS, STIs, Tuberculosis, and Malaria*. Washington, DC: World Bank.

Horwood, C., S. Liebeschuetz, D. Blaauw, S. Cassol, and S. Qazi. 2003. "Diagnosis of Paediatric HIV Infection in a Primary Health Care Setting with a Clinical Algorithm." *Bulletin of the World Health Organization* 81 (12): 858–66.

Horwood, C., K. Vermaak, N. Rollins, L. Haskins, P. Nkosi, and others. 2009. "Paediatric HIV Management at Primary Care Level: An Evaluation of the Integrated Management of Childhood Illness (IMCI) Guidelines for HIV." *BioMed Central Pediatrics* 9: 59.

Huicho, L., R. W. Scherpbier, A. M. Nkowane, and C. G. Victora. 2008. "How Much Does Quality of Child Care Vary between Health Workers with Differing Durations of Training? An Observational Multicountry Study." *The Lancet* 372 (9642): 910–16.

Ishengoma, D. S., F. Francis, B. P. Mmbando, J. P. A. Lusingu, P. Magistrado, and others. 2011. "Accuracy of Malaria Rapid Diagnostic Tests in Community Studies and their Impact on Treatment of Malaria in an Area with Declining Malaria Burden in North-Eastern Tanzania." *Malaria Journal* 10: 176.

Kalyango, J., E. Rutebemberwa, and T. Alfven. 2012. "Performance of Community Health Workers under Integrated Community Case Management of Childhood Illnesses in Eastern Uganda." *Malaria Journal* 11: 282.

Kasper, M. R., P. J. Blair, S. Touch, B. Sokhal, C. Y. Yasuda, and others. 2012. "Infectious Etiologies of Acute Febrile Illness among Patients Seeking Health Care in South-Central Cambodia." *American Journal of Tropical Medicine and Hygiene* 86 (2): 246–53.

Kelly, J. M., B. Osamba, R. M. Garg, J. M. Hamel, J. J. Lewis, and others. 2001. "Community Health Worker Performance in the Management of Multiple Childhood Illnesses: Siaya District, Kenya, 1997–2001." *American Journal of Public Health* 91 (10): 1617–24.

Kidane, G., and R. H. Morrow. 2000. "Teaching Mothers to Provide Home Treatment of Malaria in Tigray, Ethiopia: A Randomised Trial." *The Lancet* 356 (9229): 550–55.

Kumar, V., S. Mohanty, A. Kumar, R. P. Misra, M. Santosham, and others. 2008. "Effect of Community-Based Behaviour Change Management on Neonatal Mortality in Shivgarh, Uttar Pradesh, India: A Cluster-Randomised Controlled Trial." *The Lancet* 372 (9644): 1151–62.

Lanata, C. F., I. Rudan, C. Boschi-Pinto, L. Tomaskovic, T. Cherian, and others. 2004. "Methodological and Quality Issues in Epidemiological Studies of Acute Lower Respiratory Infections in Children in Developing Countries." *International Journal of Epidemiology* 33 (6): 1362–72.

Lehmann, D., A. Michael, M. Omena, A. Clegg, T. Lupiwa, and others. 1999. "Bacterial and Viral Etiology of Severe Infection in Children Less Than Three Months Old in the Highlands of Papua New Guinea." *Pediatric Infectious Disease Journal* 18 (10 Suppl): S42–49.

Leslie, T., A. Mikhail, I. Mayan, S. Anwar, S. Bakhtash, and others. 2012. "Overdiagnosis and Mistreatment of Malaria among Febrile Patients at Primary Healthcare Level in Afghanistan: Observational Study." *British Medical Journal* 345: e4389.

Liu, L., K. Hill, S. Oza, D. Hogan, Y. Chu, and others. 2016. "Levels and Causes of Mortality under Age Five Years." In *Disease Control Priorities* (third edition): Volume 2, *Reproductive, Maternal, Newborn, and Child Health*, edited by R. Black, R. Laxminarayan, M. Temmerman, and N. Walker. Washington, DC: World Bank.

Liu, L., H. L. Johnson, S. Cousens, J. Perin, S. Scott, and others. 2012. "Global, Regional, and National Causes of Child Mortality: An Updated Systematic Analysis for 2010 with Time Trends since 2000." *The Lancet* 379 (9832): 2151–61.

Liu, L., S. Oza, D. Hogan, J. Perin, I. Rudan, and others. 2015. "Global, Regional, and National Causes of Child Mortality in 2000–13, with Projections to Inform Post-2015 Priorities: An Updated Systematic Analysis." *The Lancet* 385 (9966): 430–40.

Lozano, R., M. Naghavi, K. Foreman, S. Lim, K. Shibuya, and others. 2012. "Global and Regional Mortality from 235 Causes of Death for 20 Age Groups in 1990 and 2010: A Systematic Analysis for the Global Burden of Disease Study 2010." *The Lancet* 380 (9859): 2095–128.

Lukianova-Hleb, E. Y., K. M. Campbell, P. E. Constantinou, J. Braam, J. S. Olson, and others. 2014. "Hemozoin-Generated Vapor Nanobubbles for Transdermal Reagent- and Needle-Free Detection of Malaria." *Proceedings of the National Academy of Sciences of the United States* 111 (9859): 900–95.

Mayxay, M., J. Castonguay-Vanier, V. Chansamouth, A. Dubot-Pérès, D. H. Paris, and others. 2013. "Causes of Non-Malarial Fever in Laos: A Prospective Study." *The Lancet Global Health* 1 (3): e46–54.

Mayxay, M., P. N. Newton, S. Yeung, T. Pongvongsa, S. Phompida, and others. 2004. "Short Communication: An Assessment of the Use of Malaria Rapid Tests by Village Health Volunteers in Rural Laos." *Tropical Medicine and International Health* 9 (3): 325–29.

Mens, P. F., R. J. Matelon, B. Y. M. Nour, D. M. Newman, and H. D. Schallig. 2010. "Laboratory Evaluation on the Sensitivity and Specificity of a Novel and Rapid Detection Method for Malaria Diagnosis Based on Magneto-Optical Technology (MOT)." *Malaria Journal* 9: 207.

Msellem, M. I., A. Mårtensson, G. Rotllant, A. Bhattarai, J. Strömberg, and others. 2009. "Influence of Rapid Malaria Diagnostic Tests on Treatment and Health Outcome in Fever Patients, Zanzibar: A Crossover Validation Study." *PLoS Medicine* 6: e1000070.

Mubi, M., A. Janson, M. Warsame, A. Mårtensson, K. Källander, and others. 2011. "Malaria Rapid Testing by Community Health Workers Is Effective and Safe for Targeting Malaria Treatment: Randomised Cross-Over Trial in Tanzania." *PLoS One* 6: e19753.

Muhe, L., M. Tilahun, S. Lulseged, S. Kebede, D. Enaro, and others. 1999. "Etiology of Pneumonia, Sepsis and Meningitis in Infants Younger Than Three Months of Age in Ethiopia." *Pediatric Infectious Disease Journal* 18 (10 Suppl): S56–61.

Mukanga, D., A. Tiono, and T. Anyorigiya. 2012. "Community Case Management of Fever in Children Under Five Using Rapid Diagnostic Tests and Respiratory Rate Counting: A Multi-Country Cluster Randomized Trial." *American Journal of Tropical Medicine and Hygiene* 87 (5 Suppl): 21–29.

Mulholland, E. K., O. O. Ogunlesi, R. A. Adegbola, M. W. Weber, A. Palmer, and others. 1999. "The Aetiology of Serious Infections in Young Gambian Infants." *Pediatric Infectious Disease Journal* 18 (10 Suppl): S35–42.

Nair, H., E. A. F. Simões, I. Rudan, B. D. Gessner, E. Azziz-Baumgartner, and others. 2013. "Global and Regional Burden of Hospital Admissions for Severe Acute Lower Respiratory Infections in Young Children in 2010: A Systematic Analysis." *The Lancet* 381 (9875): 1380–90.

Nguyen, D. T. K., K. K. Leung, L. McIntyre, W. A. Ghali, and R. Sauve. 2013. "Does Integrated Management of Childhood Illness (IMCI) Training Improve the Skills of Health Workers? A Systematic Review and Meta-Analysis." *PLoS One* 8 (6): e66030.

Njama-Meya, D., T. D. Clark, B. Nzarubara, S. Staedke, M. R. Kamya, and others. 2007. "Treatment of Malaria Restricted to Laboratory-Confirmed Cases: A Prospective Cohort Study in Ugandan Children." *Malaria Journal* 6: 7.

Nonvignon, J., M. A. Chinbuah, M. Gyapong, M. Abbey, E. Awini, and others. 2012. "Is Home Management of Fevers a Cost-Effective Way of Reducing Under-Five Mortality in Africa? The Case of a Rural Ghanaian District." *Tropical Medicine and International Health* 17 (8): 951–57.

Pagnoni, F. 2009. "Malaria Treatment: No Place Like Home." *Trends in Parasitology* 25 (3): 115–19.

Pariyo, G. W., E. Gouws, J. Bryce, and G. Burnham. 2005. "Improving Facility-Based Care for Sick Children in Uganda: Training Is Not Enough." *Health Policy and Planning* 20 (Suppl 1): i58–68.

Prinja, S., S. Mazumder, S. Taneja, P. Bahuguna, N. Bhandari, and others. 2013. "Cost of Delivering Child Health Care through Community Level Health Workers: How Much Extra Does IMNCI Program Cost?" *Journal of Tropical Pediatrics* 59 (6): 489–95.

Rakha, M. A., A.-N. Abdelmoneim, S. Farhoud, S. Pieche, S. Cousens, and others. 2013. "Does Implementation of the IMCI Strategy Have an Impact on Child Mortality? A Retrospective Analysis of Routine Data from Egypt." *British Medical Journal* 3 (1): e001852.

Remington, J., J. O. Klein, C. B. Wilson, V. Nizet, and Y. Maldonado. 2006. *Infectious Diseases of the Fetus and Newborn Infant*, 6th edition. Philadelphia, PA: Elsevier Saunders.

Reyburn, H., H. Mbakilwa, R. Mwangi, O. Mwerinde, R. Olomi, and others. 2007. "Rapid Diagnostic Tests Compared with Malaria Microscopy for Guiding Outpatient Treatment of Febrile Illness in Tanzania: Randomised Trial." *British Medical Journal* 334 (7590): 403.

Rowe, A. K., F. Onikpo, M. Lama, F. Cokou, and M. S. Deming. 2001. "Management of Childhood Illness at Health Facilities in Benin: Problems and Their Causes." *American Journal of Public Health* 91 (10): 1625–35.

Sadruddin, S., S. Shehzad, A. Bari, A. Khan, Ibad-ul-Haque, and others. 2012. "Household Costs for Treatment of Severe Pneumonia in Pakistan." *American Journal of Tropical Medicine and Hygiene* 87 (5 Suppl): 137–43.

Samson, E. B., B. S. Goldschmidt, P. J. D. Whiteside, A. S. M. Sudduth, J. R. Custer, and others. 2012. "Photoacoustic Spectroscopy of β-Hematin." *Journal of Optics* 14 (6): 065302.

Seidenberg, P., D. H. Hamer, H. Iyer, P. Pilingana, K. Siazeele, and others. 2012. "Impact of Integrated Community Case Management on Health-Seeking Behavior in Rural Zambia." *American Journal of Tropical Medicine and Hygiene* 87 (5 Suppl): 105–10.

Shao, A., C. Rambaud-Althaus, S. Perri, N. Swai, J. Kahama-Maro, and others. 2011. "Safety of a New Algorithm for the Management of Childhood Illness (ALMANACH) to Improve Quality of Care and Rational Use of Drugs." In Abstracts of the 7th European Congress on Tropical Medicine and International Health, October 3–6, 2011, Barcelona, Spain.

Shao, A., C. Rambaud-Althaus, J. Samaka, A. F. Faustine, S. Perri-Moore, and others. 2015. "Clinical Outcome and Antibiotic Prescription Rate Using a New Algorithm for the Management of Childhood Illnesses (ALMANACH) in Tanzania." *PLoS One* 10 (7): e0132316.

Simmons, C., J. Farrar, N. van Vinh Chau, and B. Wills. 2012. "Dengue." *New England Journal of Medicine* 15: 1423–32.

Sirima, S. B., A. Konaté, A. B. Tiono, N. Convelbo, S. Cousens, and F. Pagnoni. 2003. "Early Treatment of Childhood Fevers with Pre-Packaged Antimalarial Drugs in the Home Reduces Severe Malaria Morbidity in Burkina Faso." *Tropical Medicine and International Health* 8 (2): 133–39.

Soofi, S., S. Ahmed, M. P. Fox, W. B. MacLeod, D. M. Thea, and others. 2012. "Effectiveness of Community Case Management of Severe Pneumonia with Oral Amoxicillin in Children Aged 2–59 Months in Matiari District, Rural

Pakistan: A Cluster-Randomised Controlled Trial." *The Lancet* 379 (9817): 729–37.

Thaver, D., S. Ali, and A. Zaidi. 2009. "Antimicrobial Resistance among Neonatal Pathogens in Developing Countries." *Pediatric Infectious Disease Journal* 29 (1 Suppl): S19–21.

Theodoratou, E., S. Al-Jilaihawi, F. Woodward, J. Ferguson, A. Jhass, and others. 2010. "The Effect of Case Management on Childhood Pneumonia Mortality in Developing Countries." *International Journal of Epidemiology* 39 (Suppl. 1): i155–71.

Thiboutot, M. M., S. Kannan, O. U. Kawalekar, D. J. Shedlock, A. S. Khan, and others. 2010. "Chikungunya: A Potentially Emerging Epidemic?" *PLoS Neglected Tropical Diseases* 4 (4): e623.

Tulloch, J. 1999. "Integrated Approach to Child Health in Developing Countries." *The Lancet* 354 (Suppl 2): 16–20.

UNICEF (United Nations Children's Fund). 2012. *Review of Systematic Challenges to the Scale-Up of Integrated Community Case Management. Emerging Lessons & Recommendations from the Catalytic Initiative (CI/IHSS).* New York: UNICEF.

United Nations. 2013. *The Millennium Development Goals Report 2013.* New York: United Nations.

Waters, D., I. Jawad, A. Ahmad, I. Lukšic, H. Nair, and others. 2011. "Aetiology of Community-Acquired Neonatal Sepsis in Low and Middle Income Countries." *Journal of Global Health* 1 (2): 154–70.

Weber, M., J. Carlin, S. Gatchalian, D. Lehmann, L. Muhe, and others. 2003. "Predictors of Neonatal Sepsis in Developing Countries." *Pediatric Infectious Disease Journal* 22 (8): 711–27.

WHO (World Health Organization). 2001. *Integrated Management of Child Health: Guide to Planning for Implementation of IMCI at District Level.* Cairo: World Health Organization, Regional Office for the Eastern Mediterranean.

———. 2006. *Guidelines for the Treatment of Malaria.* 1st edition. Geneva: WHO.

———. 2009. *Integrated Management of Adolescent and Adult Illness: Interim Guidelines for First-Level Facility Health Workers at Health Centre and District Outpatient Clinic: Acute Care.* Geneva: WHO.

———. 2010a. *Guidelines for the Treatment of Malaria.* 2nd edition. Geneva: WHO.

———. 2010b. *IMCI Pre-Service Education: Guide to Evaluation.* Geneva: WHO.

———. 2012a. *Recommendations for Management of Common Childhood Conditions.* Geneva: WHO.

———. 2012b. *Malaria Rapid Diagnostic Test Performance: Results of WHO Product Testing of Malaria RDTs—Rounds 1–4.* Geneva: WHO.

———. 2013a. *WHO Informal Consultation on Fever Management in Peripheral Health Care Settings: A Global Review of Evidence and Practice.* Geneva: WHO.

———. 2013b. *World Malaria Report 2013.* Geneva: WHO.

———. 2014a. *Integrated Management of Childhood Illnesses (IMCI) Chart Booklet.* Geneva: WHO.

———. 2014b. *Integrated Management of Childhood Illness Distance Learning Modules.* Geneva: WHO.

———. 2015. *World Malaria Report: 2015.* Geneva: WHO.

WHO-CHERG (Child Health Epidemiology Reference Group). 2011. "Global Health Observatory Data Depository." Geneva: WHO.

WHO Division of Child Health and Development. 1997. "Integrated Management of Childhood Illness: Conclusions." *Bulletin of the World Health Organization* 75 (Suppl 1): 119–28.

WHO and Special Programme for Research and Training in Tropical Diseases. 2009. *Dengue Guidelines for Diagnosis, Treatment, Prevention and Control: New Edition.* Geneva: WHO.

WHO, UNAIDS, and LSHTM (London School of Hygiene and Tropical Medicine). 2001. *Herpes Simplex Virus Type 2: Programmatic and Research Priorities of Developing Countries.* Geneva: WHO, UNAIDS, and LSHTM.

WHO and UNICEF. 2009a. *Global Action Plan for Prevention and Control of Pneumonia.* Geneva: WHO and UNICEF.

———. 2009b. "Joint Statement: Home Visits for the Newborn Child: A Strategy to Improve Survival." Geneva: WHO and UNICEF.

———. 2012. "Integrated Community Case Management: An Equity-Focused Strategy to Improve Access to Essential Treatment Services for Children." Joint Statement, WHO and UNICEF, Geneva and New York.

———. 2013. *Ending Preventable Child Deaths from Pneumonia and Diarrhoea by 2025: The Integrated Global Action Plan for Pneumonia and Diarrhoea.* Geneva: WHO.

WHO Young Infants Study Group. 1999. "Clinical Prediction of Serious Bacterial Infections in Young Infants in Developing Countries." *Pediatric Infectious Disease Journal* 18 (10 Suppl): S23–31.

Yasuoka, J., K. Poudel, K. Poudel-Tandukar, C. Nguon, P. Ly, and others. 2010. "Assessing the Quality of Service of Village Malaria Workers to Strengthen Community-Based Malaria Control in Cambodia." *Malaria Journal* 9: 109.

Yeboah-Antwi, K., P. Pilingana, W. B. Macleod, K. Semrau, K. Siazeele, and others. 2010. "Community Case Management of Fever Due to Malaria and Pneumonia in Children Under Five in Zambia: A Cluster Randomized Controlled Trial." *PLoS Medicine* 7 (9): e1000340.

YICSSG (Young Infants Clinical Signs Study Group). 2008. "Clinical Signs That Predict Severe Illness in Children Under Age 2 Months: A Multicentre Study." *The Lancet* 371 (9607): 135–42.

Young, M., and C. Wolfheim. 2012. "World Health Organization/United Nations Children's Fund Joint Statement on Integrated Community Case Management: An Equity-Focused Strategy to Improve." *American Journal of Tropical Medicine and Hygiene* 87 (5 Suppl): 6–10.

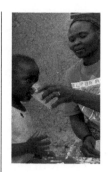

Chapter **9**

Diarrheal Diseases

Gerald T. Keusch, Christa Fischer Walker, Jai K. Das,
Susan Horton, and Demissie Habte

INTRODUCTION

The annual number of deaths from diarrheal diseases among the 0–4 year age group in low- and middle-income countries (LMICs) has dropped by 89 percent, from 4.6 million in 1980 to 526,000 in 2015 (Liu, Hill and others 2016). This striking improvement occurred without vaccines against the major pathogens, except for rotavirus, which is now being scaled-up in LMICs. The incidence of diarrhea has not significantly diminished, especially in young infants (Fischer Walker and others 2012). Therefore, success in reducing mortality appears to be driven largely by improved management rather than prevention (box 9.1). Each day, 4.7 million episodes of diarrheal disease occur, including 100,000 cases of severe diarrhea, along with nearly 1,600 deaths, approximately 9 percent of the mortality in children under age five years (chapter 4 in this volume, Liu, Oza, and others 2016).

Increasing awareness of the adverse effects of nonfatal episodes of diarrhea on infant and childhood growth and development, particularly the role of repeated illness and the potential impact of frequent subclinical infections with the same pathogens, presents a new challenge. Interventions will depend on enhanced understanding of causal pathways, pathogenesis, and sequelae of these infections, with or without symptomatic diarrhea.

Diarrheal diseases are good indicators of the stage of development of communities in LMICs because of the impact of proximal and distal determinants of diarrheal morbidity and mortality, including the availability of safe drinking water; sanitation; level of education, particularly of mothers; income; food security; nutrition; and access to health care, both preventive and therapeutic. Continued progress depends on recognition that intersectoral interventions are integral to required measures to reduce or eliminate diarrheal diseases as a public health concern.

This chapter explores the still-limited evidence on subclinical infections due to known microbial causes of diarrhea, and impacts on intestinal physiology, nutrient absorption, and nutritional status as plausible mechanisms underlying growth stunting and developmental delays. The potential interventions for clinical and subclinical intestinal infections are not necessarily identical, although they undoubtedly overlap. Accordingly, we consider epidemiology, transmission, and mechanisms of disease, as well as social and cultural factors instrumental in determining outcomes. Nutritional needs of infants and young children, breastfeeding practices, use of complementary foods, and management of nutritional rehabilitation of acute malnutrition are covered in greater depth in Das and others (2016, chapter 12 of this volume).

DIARRHEAL DISEASES

Definitions and Classification

Diarrheal diseases are most prevalent in and cause greater morbidity and mortality in children younger than age five years in low-income countries (LICs). The term covers a

Corresponding author: Gerald T. Keusch, Boston University School of Medicine, Boston, Massachusetts, United States, keusch@bu.edu.

Major Interventions in Diarrheal Disease

- Early use of oral rehydration solutions
- Appropriate use of antibiotics for bloody diarrhea and dysentery
- Continued breastfeeding
- Nutritional interventions for persistent diarrhea
- Rapid restoration of nutritional status in all diarrhea patients

Figure 9.1 Regional Burden of Diarrhea, Ages 0–4 Years, 2010

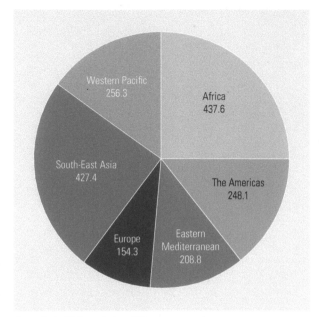

Source: Fischer Walker and others 2013.

multitude of infectious causes, ranging from viruses and bacteria to protozoa and occasionally worms, each with distinctive effects. There are three discernable epidemiological and clinical presentations with vastly different consequences for the individuals affected:

- Acute dehydrating watery diarrhea
- Acute inflammatory (bloody) diarrhea and dysentery
- Persistent diarrhea lasting 14 days or more.

Burden of Infection

Children younger than age five years in LMICs in South Asia and Sub-Saharan Africa experience an average of 2.7 (uncertainty range: 2.1–3.2) episodes of diarrhea per year (Fischer Walker and others 2012). Most are mild and self-limited, lasting an average of 4.3 days. From 0.5 percent to 2 percent are severe, and last an average of 8.4 days (Lamberti, Fischer Walker, and Black 2012). Incidence rates vary but are higher in children in LICs and lower-middle-income countries, and highest in Sub-Saharan Africa (3.3 episodes per child per year) (Fischer Walker and others 2013) (figure 9.1).

Incidence

Despite targeted investments, estimated global diarrhea incidence rates have not changed significantly since 1980 (Bern and others 1992; Fischer Walker and others 2013; Kosek, Bern, and Guerrant 2003; Snyder and Merson 1982). Incidence consistently varies by age, peaking between 6 and 11 months, as immunity transferred from the mother in utero and via breastfeeding wanes; potentially contaminated complementary foods are introduced; and infant mobility increases, allowing for greater contact with sources of pathogens (Fischer Walker and others 2012). The consequences are also determined by

disease severity, although few studies separately analyze severe episodes or identify bloody diarrhea or dysentery or episodes that become persistent. One systematic review of the limited data available suggests that 5 percent to 15 percent of watery diarrhea cases progress to persistent diarrhea (Lamberti, Fischer Walker, and Black 2012). More than 50 percent of severe episodes occur in Sub-Saharan Africa and South-East Asia (figure 9.2).

Mortality

The 2015 estimated number of deaths due to diarrhea—526,000 under age five years—represents an 89 percent decline from 1980 and a striking 58 percent reduction from 2000 to 2015 (Liu, Oza, and others 2016, chapter 4 in this volume), even though the total population in this age group increased by approximately 11 percent (figure 9.3). Because 72 percent of diarrhea deaths occur in the first two years of life, targeting this age group will yield the greatest future impact on mortality (Fischer Walker and others 2013). A thorough discussion of the cause-of-death structure and mortality decline is presented in Liu, Hill, and others (2016, chapter 4 in this volume); Sub-Saharan Africa and South Asia account for 90 percent of the total.

Etiologies

Although many agents cause diarrheal disease, a few account for a major portion of the burden. In one study, almost 40 percent of cause-specific attributable

Figure 9.2 Regional Burden of Severe Diarrhea Episodes, Ages 0–4 Years, 2010

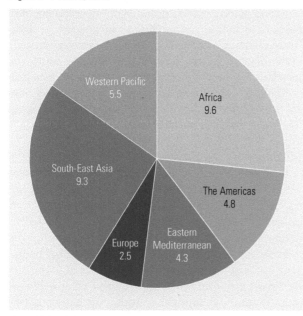

Source: Fischer Walker and others 2013.

Figure 9.3 Regional Burden of Diarrhea Mortality, Ages 0–4 Years, 2015

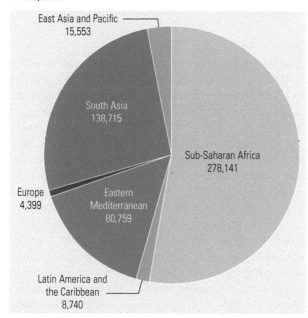

Source: Liu, Hill, and others 2016.

diarrhea mortality was due to two organisms: rotavirus (27.8 percent) and enteropathogenic *Escherichia coli* (11.1 percent) (Lanata and others 2013). Another large, multisite, clinic-based prospective case-control study of children under age five years with moderate

to severe illness identified four pathogens—rotavirus, *Cryptosporidium,* enterotoxigenic *E. coli,* and *Shigella*—responsible for most attributable episodes of moderate to severe diarrhea (Kotloff and others 2013).

Rotavirus was the leading cause during the first year of life, followed by *Cryptosporidium.* Rotavirus remained first in the age 12–23 month cohort, followed by *Shigella;* among children ages 24–59 months, that ranking reversed. The odds of dying for children with moderate to severe diarrhea were 8.5 times higher (95 percent confidence interval 5.8–12.5, $p < 0.0001$) than for control subjects, with 33 percent of deaths occurring 21 days to 90 days following enrollment in the study. Most deaths were in infants (56 percent) and toddlers (32 percent); 55 percent of the deaths occurred at home or outside a medical facility. Certain pathogens, such as rotavirus, *Shigella, Vibrio cholerae,* and adenovirus serotypes 40/41, were more commonly isolated in children with moderate to severe illness. Almost three-quarters (72 percent) of controls without diarrhea also harbored one or more putative pathogens, and 31 percent had two or more, reflecting the fecally contaminated environment in which they live (Kotloff and others 2013). Future studies that include diagnostic capacity for noroviruses and other emerging pathogens may change these rankings.

Transmission and Epidemiology

Understanding transmission routes and epidemiology is critical for effective prevention and mitigation. Although transmission is fundamentally the same for all agents (fecal-oral transmission), there are diverse pathways and routes involved, including direct person-to-person transmission mediated through feces-contaminated fingers or inanimate objects (fomites); and indirect transmission via contaminated food or water in or outside the home, including agricultural fields or seafood sources irrigated or contaminated with pathogen-laden sewage. Microbial characteristics determine the number of organisms required to cause illness (the inoculum size); small inoculum pathogens are readily transmitted directly from person to person, whereas high inoculum pathogens first need to multiply in food or water. Host characteristics, such as immunity, often interplay with microbial characteristics. Pathogens also must survive diverse nonspecific host defenses, such as stomach acid. Some pathogens, for example, *Shigella,* are inherently acid resistant, so small inocula survive into the duodenum; others, like *V. cholerae,* are acid sensitive, and large inocula are essential to survive passage through the stomach.

Reduced gastric acidity significantly reduces the required inoculum size for acid-sensitive pathogens, for example, in individuals with peptic ulcer disease treated by gastric surgery or drugs to reduce acid secretion. Infants, including preterm, produce acid, but the amounts and response to stimuli are diminished compared with older children, potentially increasing their susceptibility. Malnutrition (Gilman and others 1988) and *Helicobacter pylori* infection of the stomach (Windle, Kelleher, and Crabtree 2007) also impair gastric acid production in young children. Sustained early infection with *H. pylori* in Gambian infants under age one year was associated with subsequent growth faltering, even though they had access to good primary health care, treatment of acute childhood illness, and nutritional supplements (Thomas and others 2004).

Other factors include lack of refrigeration for food, or flies that can transfer pathogens from feces in the environment to unprotected food or water in households (Farag and others 2013; Lindsay and others 2012). A risk factor study for *Shigella* infection in Thailand identified poor breastfeeding practices; poor water supply; unsafe sanitation; lack of fly control; and inadequate personal hygiene, in particular handwashing, as major targets for interventions (Chompook and others 2006). Multiple routes of transmission exist; hence any single intervention may have limited impact.

Natural History

Exposure to pathogens does not necessarily lead to infection, and infection does not necessarily result in clinical illness. Several factors explain the differences:

- The inoculum size and the biology of the pathogen, in particular, its virulence attributes
- The susceptibility of the host, including previous exposure and preexisting immunity, including passively acquired immunity in utero or from breast milk consumption
- The health and nutritional status of the individual at the time of exposure.

As a result, natural history following infection can vary from no symptoms, to mild-moderate self-limited illness, to severe life-threatening disease. Individuals who are healthier and better nourished at exposure are less likely to develop severe illness after a given inoculum of a specific pathogen. Early and appropriate management of clinical manifestations improves outcomes and can be effectively promoted at the community level.

Watery Diarrhea

Watery diarrhea is classified according to stool volume: mild when less than 5 percent of body weight, moderate between 5 percent and 10 percent, and severe and potentially life-threatening when in excess of 10 percent. With increasing fluid losses, intravascular volume diminishes and blood pressure drops. Without replacement of fluids (rehydration), hypotension can progress to circulatory failure, dysfunction of critical organs, and death. Early initiation of rehydration, for example, using oral rehydration solutions (ORS), can mitigate or prevent progression to more severe dehydration. Such interventions are not only life saving; they can also reduce duration of illness and extent of nutrient losses.

Inflammatory Diarrhea and Dysentery

Some pathogens cause inflammation of the bowel wall, with leukocyte (white blood cell) infiltration and damage resulting in mucosal ulcers; bleeding; leukocyte exudates; production of peptide cytokines that mediate dramatic, often prolonged, changes in appetite and metabolism; and direct nutrient losses. Bacterial pathogens causing inflammatory diarrhea and dysentery (a clinical syndrome of frequent small-volume bloody mucoid stools, abdominal cramps, and tenesmus [the urgency to pass stool]) generally require antibiotics to treat the infection, resolve inflammation, allow the mucosa to heal, and reverse nutritional deterioration. Early effective antibiotic treatment shortens duration of these illnesses, limits acute complications, and reduces longer-term impacts.

Persistent Diarrhea

Diarrhea episodes lasting from 7 days to 13 days, termed *prolonged,* impair growth and increase the risk of progression to *persistent diarrhea* (Moore and others 2010). Moore and others (2010) find that prolonged diarrhea accounted for only 11.7 percent of episodes but 25.2 percent of all days of diarrhea; persistent diarrhea accounted for only 4.7 percent of episodes but 24.5 percent of days with diarrhea. Progression from acute to prolonged diarrhea increased the overall risk of persistent diarrhea from 4.8 percent to 29.0 percent (relative risk 6.09, 95 percent confidence interval 4.96–7.45). Once diarrhea is persistent, mortality rates increase sharply (Grimwood and Forbes 2009), in some settings accounting for as much as 50 percent of overall diarrhea mortality. Continuing reductions in acute diarrhea deaths has increased attention to mortality associated with persistent diarrhea, which is relatively heightened as a consequence.

A few pathogens have been particularly associated with persistence or are preferentially identified when an episode becomes persistent, including a subgroup of diarrhea-causing *E. coli* designated enteroaggregative, *Cryptosporidium parvum, S. flexneri, S. dysenteriae* type 1, and *Giardia intestinalis (lamblia).* Serial exposure to these or other pathogens may also be involved. As the duration of illness extends, malnutrition becomes increasingly prominent because of ongoing mucosal injury, anorexia, malabsorption, and nutrient losses (Newman and others 2000). *Shigella* infection, characterized by intense tissue catabolism and nutrient losses, almost doubles the risk of persistent diarrhea (Ahmed and others 2001). As the frequency of *Shigella* infection dropped from 1991 to 2010 in Bangladesh, the frequency of persistent diarrhea diminished as well (Das and others 2012). Mucosal injury also explains why the manifestations of persistent diarrhea are primarily those of malabsorption and malnutrition, and why careful dietary and nutritional management is needed until mucosal damage is reversed and new, normally functioning epithelial cells are regenerated.

NEW FRONTIERS: SUBCLINICAL INFECTIONS AND ENVIRONMENTAL ENTERIC DYSFUNCTION

Subclinical Infections

Mounting and diverse evidence suggests that subclinical infections with diarrhea pathogens can cause physiological and structural alterations of the gut with adverse consequences on child nutrition and growth. For example, a handwashing intervention not only reduced the number of diarrhea episodes by 31 percent (4.3 versus 3.0 episodes, $p < 0.05$) and days of diarrhea by 41 percent (9.67 versus 16.33, $p = 0.023$) (Langford, Lunn, and Panter-Brick 2011) but also showed that, *independent of clinical diarrhea*, infants with the highest values of a biomarker of mucosal damage (lactose-to-creatinine ratio) indicative of abnormal mucosal permeability had significantly lower height-for-age z-scores ($p = 0.01$), weight-for-age z-scores ($p < 0.001$), and weight-for-height z-scores ($p = 0.034$) (Langford, Lunn, and Panter-Brick 2011). This finding suggests that subclinical infections may reduce nutrient absorption and impair growth by many of the same mechanisms present during clinical episodes. Although the malabsorption may be limited, chronicity may be sufficient to produce overt malnutrition over time, especially when dietary nutrient intake is marginal.

Subclinical infections with intestinal pathogens have been shown to underlie growth faltering (Guerrant and others 1999). *Giardia intestinalis*, which causes diarrhea associated with growth retardation in infants (Newman and others 2001), is often identified in the stools of asymptomatic children in endemic areas, and a correlation between asymptomatic *Giardia* infection and growth faltering has been reported (Prado and others 2005). Asymptomatic first *Cryptosporidium* infections

in Peruvian infants are also associated with slower weight gain compared with uninfected infants, albeit to a lesser extent than infants with symptomatic infections (Checkley and others 1997). However, because asymptomatic infections were twice as common as diarrhea, their ultimate effects might exceed those of clinical diarrhea. Moreover, infants infected with *Cryptosporidium* during the first six months of life remained stunted at age one year, despite some interval catch-up growth (Bushen and others 2007; Checkley and others 1998). Early colonization with *H. pylori* has also been identified as a precursor of growth faltering in children under age five years in The Gambia (Thomas and others 2004).

Environmental Enteric Dysfunction

Intestinal biopsy studies of the upper small intestine from asymptomatic adults in tropical countries reported 30 years to 40 years ago documented structural differences compared with healthy adults from temperate countries, including shorter blunted villi, which reduced the surface area covered by epithelial cells, and increased inflammatory cells, accompanied by diminished ability to absorb test sugars, fat, or vitamin B12 (Baker 1976). Limited biopsies from infants and young children revealed normal, slender finger-like villi at birth, but jejunum of older infants and children resembled the adult gut, suggesting these changes were acquired after birth (Baker 1976). Similar changes occurred over one to two years in healthy young adult expatriates living in Bangladesh (Lindenbaum, Kent, and Sprinz 1966) and Thailand (Keusch, Plaut, and Troncale 1972), with few or no symptoms other than soft stools and mild weight loss. This constellation of findings was called *tropical* or *subclinical enteropathy/jejunitis/malabsorption*, and normalized after the subjects returned home (Lindenbaum, Gerson, and Kent 1971). The same resolution was observed in healthy South Asians living in the United States or the United Kingdom the longer they resided outside their home countries (Gerson and others 1971; Wood, Gearty, and Cooper 1991). However, the significance of enteropathy remained unclear, and interest waned because no relationship to pathogenesis of tropical sprue, a real disease, was apparent.

In retrospect, the extent of the weight loss associated with enteropathy in adults was dismissed too quickly; the same decrement occurring in young infants would raise concerns about incipient malnutrition. Recently, investigators in Sub-Saharan Africa, using newer assessments of intestinal permeability, identified alterations in young infants associated with altered gut histology and poor growth in early childhood (Campbell, Lunn, and Elia 2002; Campbell and others 2004). Inflammatory cells present in the intestinal mucosa were identified as immunoreactive T cells (Veitch and others 1991), linked to strong pro-inflammatory local cytokine responses (Campbell and others 2003). These findings have rekindled interest in their physiological significance, analogous to inflammatory bowel disease. Although the mechanisms have remained uncertain, a nexus of microbial exposure, mucosal pathology, increased permeability and malabsorption, immune activation leading to poor response to mucosal vaccines, and growth stunting has been postulated (Prendergast and Kelly 2012). Inadequacy of dietary intake, especially when diet quality is also marginal, would likely exacerbate the impact of any level of malabsorption.

In parallel, growth stunting, a marker of chronic undernutrition that is common among infants and children living in poverty in LMICs, is associated with increased childhood morbidity and mortality and poor longer-term functional outcomes, including cognitive development; reduced years of schooling; and diminished productivity in adulthood, measured by income attained and other economic productivity markers (Dewey and Begum 2011). If changes in intestinal structure and function develop in young infants in impoverished communities early in life, presumably due to environmental exposure to still-unknown inciting factors, the consequence may be initial malabsorption leading to early malnutrition, growth faltering, and increased susceptibility to diarrheal disease (Keusch and others 2013). This has been termed *environmental enteric dysfunction* (EED) to stress the importance of the functional alterations.

Although systematic serial observations of intestinal structure in these young infants remains limited, a number of surrogate biomarkers of gut inflammation or immune activation have been identified (Kosek and others 2013). A composite activity score of three stool biomarkers of intestinal inflammation (neopterin, alpha1-antitrypsin, and myeloperoxidase) during periods without diarrhea is inversely correlated with linear growth. Children with the highest score grew 1.08 centimeters less than children with the lowest score during the subsequent six months, even controlling for the incidence of diarrheal disease. Similarly, fecal levels of REG1B protein, which plays a role in cell differentiation and proliferation in the intestinal tract and is reported to be increased in other gut inflammatory conditions, was predictive of linear growth in three-month-old birth cohorts in Bangladesh and Peru, independent of their length-for-age z-score at the time the sample was taken (Peterson and others 2013). If confirmed, such assessments of intestinal health may become important biomarkers of EED and a predictor of growth (box 9.2).

If EED leads to malnutrition, impaired immune function, and increased susceptibility to and severity of subsequent diarrheal episodes in early infancy, it may be a major force for stunting, particularly when recurrent episodes restrict the capacity for catch-up growth (Salomon, Mata, and Gordon 1968). The effects of diarrheal diseases can be both short term and long term. In the short term, patients experience adverse systemic impacts on appetite, metabolism, and nutrition due to the infection. In the longer term, mucosal changes can alter digestion, absorption, and assimilation of nutrients from food. In bloody diarrhea and dysentery, structural mucosal damage leads to protein-losing enteropathy as blood proteins leak into the gut lumen (Bennish, Salam, and Wahed 1993). These effects can continue for weeks after shigellosis (Alam and others 1994; Raqib and others 1995), resulting

---

Box 9.2

Biomarkers to Assess Environmental Enteric Dysfunction

Category	Potential biomarkers
Intestinal absorption and mucosal permeability	D-Xylose, mannitol, or rhamnose absorption; lactulose paracellular uptake; α1-antitrypsin leakage into gut lumen
Enterocyte mass and function border	Plasma citrulline, conversion of alanyl-glutamine to citrulline, or both; lactose tolerance test (as a marker of microvillus damage)
Inflammation	Plasma cytokines, stool calprotectin, myeloperoxidase, or lactoferrin
Microbial translocation and immune activation	Stool neopterin; plasma lipopolysaccharide (LPS) core antibody, LPS binding protein, or both; circulating soluble CD14

in progressive malnutrition rather than convalescence and repair. As a consequence, mortality over the three months following successful discharge from an expert treatment center in Bangladesh almost doubled (2.8 percent versus 4.9 percent) in children with documented shigellosis compared with watery diarrhea without evidence of *Shigella* (Bennish and Wojtyniak 1991).

The early effects of EED can lead to repeated infection because of similar risk factors, including increased exposure to enteric pathogens, limited and poor quality water, lack of sanitary facilities, poor household hygiene, and poor diets. Understanding the pathogenesis of EED is a prerequisite to the selection of optimal interventions.

INTERVENTIONS FOR DIARRHEAL DISEASES

Interventions for diarrheal diseases can be divided into therapeutic and preventive (box 9.3). Some interventions, such as nutritional support and zinc supplementation, can be beneficial for both purposes. Interventions can also be classified by scale: individuals, households, or communities. Some depend on infrastructure; others are behavioral, determined by understanding and compliance at the level of the household, community, or health care system. Although most interventions are not new, innovations to make them more accessible or effective can have adverse unintended consequences, such as increased and inappropriate use of antibiotics.

Therapeutic Interventions

Treatment with therapeutic interventions focuses on reversing dehydration, providing antibiotics for inflammatory bacterial diarrhea and dysentery, and special nutritional interventions to overcome malabsorption associated with persistent diarrhea, although general dietary interventions to mitigate nutritional deterioration during and after diarrhea are relevant to all diarrheal diseases. Two analyses of a package of interventions individually shown to have an impact on mortality (ORS; zinc; antibiotics for dysentery; rotavirus vaccination; vitamin A supplementation; improved access to safe water, sanitation, and hygiene; and breastfeeding) estimate a reduction in mortality of 54 percent to 78 percent if implemented to a feasible level, and by 92 percent to 95 percent if universally applied (Bhutta and others 2013; Fischer Walker and others 2011).

Other strategies, including pre- and probiotics to counter adverse changes in intestinal microecology, or fecal transplants to reconstitute a healthy microbiota after illness or antibiotic treatment, are not discussed further because available efficacy data are limited, often

---

Box 9.3

Interventions for Diarrheal Diseases

Category	Options
Therapeutic	Oral rehydration solutions
	Antimicrobials for bloody diarrhea or dysentery
	Nutritional treatment of persistent diarrhea
	Zinc supplementation
Preventive	Protected safe water
	Handwashing Sanitary disposal of fecal waste
	Vaccines
	Improved nutrition: vitamin A, zinc

---

contradictory, of poor reliability, or difficult to interpret. Similarly, the use of drugs to restore physiological functions of the intestine is not considered because of limited reliable data in target human populations.

Oral Rehydration Solutions

ORS may prevent as many as 93 percent of diarrheal deaths (Munos, Fischer Walker, and Black 2010). The therapy works because the co-absorption of glucose and sodium is preserved during watery diarrheas; hence, ORS containing optimal concentrations of glucose and salt results in net uptake of sodium and chloride, effectively expanding the intravascular compartment regardless of age, and significantly reduces the need for intravenous fluids for all but the most severely dehydrated patients or those with intractable vomiting. New formulations with lower concentrations of glucose and sodium reduce the likelihood of hypernatremia during treatment of noncholera dehydration, reduce total stool output and vomiting, and reduce the need for supplementary intravenous fluids (Hahn, Kim, and Garner 2002); the World Health Organization (WHO) now recommends such formulations (WHO and UNICEF 2004).

Further modifications have been proposed, for example, rice-based formulations or the addition of certain amino acids (glycine, alanine, or glutamine) to further increase sodium absorption and hasten intestinal repair (Atia and Buchman 2009), or supplementation with zinc to improve outcomes (Awasthi and IC-ZED Group 2006;

Lazzerini and Ronfani 2013). However, the primary goal of ORS remains enhancing salt and water absorption. Although simple home-prepared ORS may be sufficient in mild diarrhea, the WHO formulation is preferred for more severely dehydrated patients.

Cholera and cholera-like enterotoxigenic *E. coli* infections raise additional issues because of prodigious volume losses; vomiting; and comorbidities, such as pneumonia, that affect outcomes. When intravenous rehydration is required because of shock, switching to maintenance ORS when clinical status improves is effective. Interest in antiemetic drugs, for example, ondansetron, is limited because safety and efficacy data in poorly nourished children under age five years are not available, and because of the added cost (Ciccarelli, Stolfi, and Caramia 2013).

Unfortunately, use of ORS for clinic- and home-based treatment has stagnated in most countries reaching, on average, 30 percent to 38 percent of the children who should receive it (Santosham and others 2010; WHO and UNICEF 2009). This absence of use is due in part to a lack of parental understanding of the benefit of ORS, because stool volumes may remain high even as hydration improves. Parental expectations of treatment are also influenced by previous experience. For example, Brazilian physicians recommend intravenous fluids for most children with moderate dehydration, which sends the wrong message to caregivers about professionals' trust in the efficacy of ORS (Costa and Silva 2011). Community-based initiatives, such as home visits by community health workers, and community-based delivery mechanisms have increased the use of ORS by an average of 160 percent, with an 80 percent increase in the use of zinc-ORS, as well as a 75 percent reduction in antibiotic use (Das, Lassi, and others 2013). Limited information precludes rigorous assessment of the impact of community case management on mortality, but trends suggest a decrease of 63 percent among children ages 0–4 years (95 percent confidence interval 7–85 percent) and 92 percent (95 percent confidence interval 13–100 percent) among children age 0–1 year.

Antibiotics

The pervasive, indiscriminate overuse of antibiotics is dangerous because it promotes emergence of drug resistance. Overuse is fostered by multiple causes: caregiver expectations; lack of knowledge; prescriber behavior; lack of etiology-specific point-of-care diagnostics; failure of regulation and its enforcement to control quality of and access to medicines; and availability without prescription in pharmacies, shops, and markets even when prescriptions are required (Adriaenssens and others 2011). Improved practitioner and parent knowledge and attitudes reduce inappropriate use (Clavenna and Bonati 2011).

Despite repeated pleas for more evidence-based use of antibiotics, better education of practitioners and the public, and systematic surveillance of antibiotic use and resistance, more than 50 percent of all medicines are still inappropriately prescribed, dispensed, or sold, and 50 percent of patients use them incorrectly (WHO 2010). Examples abound. Government health centers in The Gambia ordered antibiotics for 45 percent of young children with simple diarrhea without dehydration (Risk and others 2013). In the Democratic Republic of Congo, more practitioners relied on pharmaceutical companies for prescribing recommendations (73.9 percent) than on professional guidelines (66.3 percent) or university training (63.6 percent), and more practitioners used the Internet for guidance (45.7 percent) than used WHO publications (26.6 percent) (Thriemer and others 2013). Although 85 percent of caregivers in a peri-urban slum in Lima, Peru, expressed confidence in decisions made by physicians, even withholding antibiotics when advised, 65 percent of caregivers still believed antibiotics were necessary for acute diarrhea, and nearly 25 percent reporting leftover antibiotics at home said they would use them for a future illness (Ecker and others 2013). In Nigeria, 47 percent of young children with diarrhea seen at a third-level hospital had already received antibiotics without a clinician's recommendation (Ekwochi and others 2013). Caregivers in India and Kenya ranked antibiotics higher than ORS for diarrhea by more than two to one, partially explaining the low use of ORS and the high use of antibiotics (Zwisler, Simpson, and Moodley 2013).

Inappropriate use of antibiotics. Experts agree that antibiotics are usually unnecessary for acute watery diarrhea; most episodes are mild and self-limited, and many are due to viruses, especially among young children (Kotloff and others 2013). It is time to abandon routine use of antibiotics to shorten duration of illness in moderate to severe dehydration. Although *V. cholerae* has remained sensitive to most antibiotics, the long-term tradeoff of antibiotic use is selection for drug resistance, which is now increasing among *V. cholerae* strains (Ghosh and Ramamurthy 2011) and is potentially transferable to other enteric pathogens as well (Kruse and others 1995). The emergence of resistance in *V. cholerae* to quinolone (Kim and others 2010), the most useful antibiotic for grossly bloody diarrhea and dysentery, further raises the level of concern about routine inclusion of antibiotics for cholera. Routine use of quinolone may be appropriate in certain circumstances. These include treatment of the most severely purging cases (Harris and others 2012), during epidemics that overwhelm clinical capacity (Ernst and others 2011), or when elimination of viable *V. cholerae* in stool would diminish the potential for spread within or between countries (MacPherson and others 2009; Tatem, Rogers, and Hay 2006).

Appropriate use of antibiotics. Morbidity and mortality due to inflammatory diarrheas, most often caused by *Shigella* invading the intestinal mucosa, are not caused by dehydration but rather by tissue damage. Large numbers of leukocytes are recruited to the invasion site, leading to epithelial cell death and ulceration, with release of cytokine mediators of metabolism that result in nutritional deterioration. These metabolic responses persist for weeks after acute infection, and drive continuing malnutrition (Raqib and others 1995), a major reason why post-shigellosis mortality remains high for months after bloody diarrhea or dysentery ceases. The clinical hallmarks of inflammatory diarrhea for which antibiotics are indicated include grossly bloody stools or dysentery, usually with accompanying fever. Most episodes are bacterial in etiology, and *Shigella* or sometimes-related enteroinvasive *E. coli* serotypes are most common.

Without point-of-care diagnostics to identify specific causes, the pragmatic assumption is that bloody diarrhea is bacterial in origin and antibiotics appropriate for shigellosis should be initiated. This regimen will likely be adequate for other possible bacterial etiologies. However, resistance of *Shigella* species to some, or multiple, antibiotics is increasing (Bhattacharya and others 2011; Mota and others 2010), but the pattern is locale specific and dynamic (Das, Ahmed, and others 2013). Ongoing drug sensitivity surveillance is essential to guide therapeutic decisions (O'Ryan, Prado, and Pickering 2005). Because such surveillance is not yet feasible in most LMICs, empiric treatment decisions remain the norm. Ciprofloxacin, azithromycin, or pivmecillinam, where available, are reasonable initial choices, reserving ceftriaxone for treatment failures, defined as lack of clinical improvement within 48 hours to 72 hours (Erdman, Buckner, and Hindler 2008; Traa and others 2010).

ORS may be useful but insufficient, because dehydration is minor and, unlike inflammation, does not drive severity or mortality. Mild shigellosis, typically associated with *S. sonnei* infection, without grossly bloody stools is generally self-limited and can be treated like other watery diarrheas with ORS alone, even if stool microscopy reveals some red or white blood cells. The challenge is to increase adherence to current principles and guidelines to limit the use of antibiotics unless clinical criteria are met.

Preventive Interventions

Preventive measures to reduce exposure to enteric pathogens involve improving the quality of water for drinking and cooking; the quantity of water available for personal and household hygiene; safe storage of food; handwashing; and sanitary disposal of fecal waste, including treatment of sewage to inactivate microbial pathogens. Vaccines to improve immunity are presently limited to rotavirus, the only vaccine approved and increasingly available to prevent moderate to severe rotavirus diarrhea. Improving health and immune function by improving nutritional status is another effective measure.

Vaccines

For public health, prevention is always preferable to treatment, but effective treatment is necessary when prevention fails. Immunization is among the more cost-effective public health tools when deployed at scale (WHO, UNICEF, and World Bank 2009). The complexity for diarrheal disease is that vaccines are pathogen specific and often serotype or serogroup specific. For example, different formulations would be necessary for *V. cholerae* O1 and O139; even if combined in the final product, a vaccine for each would be required. Unfortunately, vaccines for diarrheal diseases have met with developmental challenges, in part because the basis of effective immunity is poorly understood, and because diarrheal disease is most problematic in LICs where resources to purchase vaccines is limited, thereby reducing incentives for research and development.

Rotavirus. Two vaccines produced by Merck and GlaxoSmithKline are widely used in high-income countries and many middle-income countries but are only beginning to be introduced in LICs. Other rotavirus vaccines have been licensed in China or Vietnam for local use only. A less expensive Indian-manufactured vaccine named ROTAVAC® (Bharat Biotech) has been prequalified by the WHO and is approved for use in India. In efficacy trials, it reduced severe episodes by more than 56 percent in the first year of life, by nearly 49 percent in the second year of life, and overall by 55 percent (Bhandari and others 2014). It was also safe. The most important adverse event associated with rotavirus vaccines, intussusception, was assessed through active surveillance. Eight events occurred in India between 112 days and 587 days after vaccination, well beyond the known timing of vaccine-related intussusception, and so were unlikely to be vaccine related. Continued monitoring subsequent to introduction is necessary and is planned (Bhandari and others 2014).

Delayed introduction of rotavirus vaccines in LICs, where the vast majority of severe rotavirus infection and most mortality occurs, is a consequence of several factors:

• Price
• Lower reported efficacy than in high-income countries
• Uncertainty about the risk of complications, such as intussusception
• National policy failures to prioritize national childhood vaccine programs.

Gavi, the Vaccine Alliance has added rotavirus to its support program, and 19 of the 35 Gavi-eligible countries now include rotavirus vaccine in their routine immunization programs; this number is expected to increase to 30 during 2015 (Gavi Alliance 2014). ROTAVAC may ultimately be marketed outside of India in LICs. Universal implementation of rotavirus vaccine could prevent many episodes of severe diarrhea (Fischer Walker and Black 2011) and reduce the number of diarrhea deaths under age five years by 70,000–85,000 per year, and reduce hospitalizations and associated costs by an average of 94 percent (Munos, Fischer Walker, and Black 2010). The cost of hospital admission for rotavirus diarrhea in India may be as much as 5.8 percent of annual household income (Mendelsohn and others 2008), or about US$66 per hospitalization (Sowmyanarayanan and others 2012).

Cholera. The global burden of morbidity and mortality of cholera is high; an estimated 2.8 million cases and 91,000 deaths occur annually in endemic countries (Ali and others 2012). Incidence is highest in children under age five years, who may account for as much as 50 percent of cholera mortality. It is notable that 67 percent of inpatient cholera deaths in Bangladesh were actually associated with pneumonia rather than dehydration (Ryan and others 2000), increasing to 80 percent in children under age one year. Identification and appropriate treatment of these patients will reduce mortality.

Inexpensive oral killed whole bacteria cholera vaccines developed in India and Vietnam are effective (Clemens 2011); the former is WHO prequalified. Production and use of these vaccines remains limited, even for domestic needs, although widespread introduction could reduce incidence by as much as 52 percent (Das, Tripathi, and others 2013). Modeling based on clinical trials in Bangladesh suggests a herd immunity effect with as high as a 93 percent reduction in incidence if only 50 percent of the population is immunized (Longini and others 2007). Reduced incidence would also reduce the use of antibiotics (Okeke 2009).

In contrast to endemic cholera, the experience in Haiti following the introduction of cholera in 2010 is enlightening. In the first two years, 604,634 cases—with 329,697 hospitalizations and 7,436 deaths—were reported to the Ministry of Health (Barzilay and others 2013). With international support to improve case management, the case fatality rate rapidly decreased; within three months it was approximately 1 percent, a threshold indicator of effective case management for cholera (WHO 2012).

Mass immunization was under consideration as a way to prevent cholera from becoming endemic in Haiti. However, analyses concluded it should not be deployed because of serious obstacles, including limited vaccine availability, complex logistics, operational challenges of a multidose regimen, and population displacement and potential civil unrest (Kashmira and others 2011). Cholera has indeed become endemic in Haiti and is the leading etiology of diarrhea in hospitalized patients (Steenland and others 2013). A subsequent vaccine demonstration trial in Haiti showed that high coverage with two doses of vaccine was, in fact, feasible (Rouzier and others 2013). This paved the way for an ambitious immunization program, justified by the dreadful state of water and sanitation facilities in the country. The potential of vaccines to mitigate the extent of epidemic cholera and improve the impact of effective case management for dehydration has led to a proposal for an oral cholera vaccine stockpile that would be available for use in future emergency and humanitarian disaster settings (Waldor, Hotez, and Clemens 2010); this plan is being implemented through the WHO and the International Coordinating Group (WHO 2013).

Other pathogens. Vaccines for other enteric pathogens remain under research and development; no licensed products are available, particularly for agents highly associated with moderate to severe diarrhea, including enterotoxigenic *E. coli*, *Shigella*, and *Cryptosporidium*. More recently, norovirus has been identified as a potential significant cause of global diarrhea morbidity and mortality and a target for vaccine development (Patel and others 2008). Vaccines for these infections are a high priority, but it will be many years before licensed products become available for scale up in LICs.

It has long been recognized that measles immunization also reduces incidence and mortality from diarrheal disease (Feachem and Koblinsky 1983), presumably because measles is immunosuppressive and exacerbates malnutrition. The current campaign for measles elimination through universal immunization not only addresses measles, but has additional beneficial effects on diarrheal disease mortality and morbidity.

Nutrition

General Nutritional Support

Nutritional support is both a therapeutic and a preventive intervention. Malnutrition is a consequence of and a risk factor for diarrheal disease (Mondal and others 2012). Nutritional support during diarrhea and nutritional rehabilitation during convalescence reduce the severity of associated nutritional deficits and improves resistance to and recovery from future diarrheal episodes. Improving nutrition enhances the ability to respond to future exposure to diarrhea pathogens and mitigates the severity of nutritional losses when diarrhea occurs. Dietary management of acute diarrhea with locally available age-appropriate foods is effective for the majority of acute diarrhea episodes, even in the presence of lactose malabsorption; commercial preparations or specialized diets are not necessary (Gaffey and others 2013). Recent studies of community management of severe or moderate acute malnutrition using commercial ready-to-use therapeutic foods (RUTFs), which are energy dense, solid or semisolid, low-moisture-content preparations of peanut butter enriched with dried skimmed milk, sugar, vegetable oil, vitamins, and minerals that can be eaten direct from the package, have had positive effects (Santini and others 2013). Such products can also be locally made and will facilitate community management of malnutrition (Choudhury and others 2014; Schoonees and others 2013). Local production has certain benefits over imported commercially produced RUTF, which are more costly, can exert adverse impacts on breastfeeding, may medicalize and commercialize malnutrition treatment, and may be difficult to scale up to meet global needs (Latham and others 2010).

Exclusive breastfeeding is another fundamental nutritional support modality for very young infants, with many health impacts beyond improved nutrition and reduced susceptibility to diarrheal disease and other infections (Bhutta and others 2013; Dey and others 2013; Strand and others 2012). Alternating breastfeeding and ORS during acute watery diarrhea in infants combines the nutrient and resistance factors in breast milk with the impact of ORS on dehydration, but faces common cultural biases against feeding during diarrhea (Chouraqui and Michard-Lenoir 2007; King and others 2003). Strand and others (2012) conclude that breastfeeding is the most important modifiable risk factor to reduce the frequency of prolonged diarrhea.

Zinc Supplementation

Zinc deficiency is associated with increased risk of diarrhea, adversely affects intestinal structure and function, and impairs immune function (Bhan and Bhandari 1998; Gebhard and others 1983). Zinc administration may curtail the severity of diarrheal episodes (Haider and Bhutta 2009) and prevent future episodes because it is vital for protein synthesis, cell growth and differentiation, and immune function, and promotes intestinal transport of water and electrolytes (Castillo-Duran and others 1987; Shankar and Prasad 1998). A systematic review of 13 studies from LMICs of zinc supplementation in diarrhea finds a significant 46 percent (relative risk 0.64, 95 percent confidence interval 0.32–0.88) reduction in all-cause mortality and 23 percent (relative risk 0.77, 95 percent confidence interval 0.69–0.85) reduction in diarrhea-related hospital admissions (Fischer Walker and Black 2010). No statistically significant impact on diarrhea-related mortality and subsequent prevalence was found; however, it was not possible to completely separate the effect of zinc from that of ORS in large-scale effectiveness trials, because introduction of zinc also increased ORS use rates. Zinc supplementation for more than three months was associated with a 13 percent (relative risk 0.87, 95 percent confidence interval 0.81–0.94) reduction in incidence of diarrhea in children under age five years in LMICs (Yakoob and others 2011). Efficacy has also been documented in children younger than age six months (Mazumder and others 2010). There have been no reports of severe adverse reactions from any form of zinc supplementation used in the treatment of diarrhea, and the WHO recommends therapeutic zinc supplementation for children with acute diarrhea for 10 days to 14 days.

Zinc supplementation may also be useful in the treatment of persistent diarrhea. A randomized controlled trial in children ages 6–18 months showed that persistent diarrhea led to depletion of zinc whereas oral zinc administration improved zinc status (Sachdev, Mittal, and Yadav 1990). A pooled analysis of the effect of supplementary oral zinc in children under age five years with persistent diarrhea reduced the probability of continuing diarrhea by 24 percent (relative risk 0.76, 95 percent confidence interval 0.63–0.91) and decreased the rate of treatment failure or death by 42 percent (relative risk 0.58, 95 percent confidence interval 0.37–0.90) (Bhutta and others 2000).

Zinc also plays a vital role in normal growth and development of children, with or without diarrhea. Preventive zinc supplementation at a dose of 10 milligrams per day for 24 weeks leads to a net gain of 0.19 (±0.08) centimeters in height in children under age five years (Imdad and Bhutta 2011). Zinc sulfate is low cost, safe, and efficacious, and tablets can be crushed and fed to children or dispersed in breast milk, ORS, or water. Baby zinc sulfate tablets and formulations in syrup form are also available.

Although many countries have changed diarrhea management policies by adding zinc to ORS, a gap remains between policy change and effective program implementation (Bhutta and others 2013). Bottlenecks include limited knowledge among care providers and parents, price, and availability. Scaling-up use of zinc, including promotion and distribution through community programs, can increase use by 80 percent (Das, Lassi, and others 2013). Free distribution, social marketing, education of caregivers, and provision of zinc through both government and private providers at the community level, and copackaging of zinc and ORS are additional strategies to increase coverage.

Water, Sanitation, and Hygiene

Because diarrhea is ultimately transmitted from infected stools, clean water and safe disposal of feces have major impacts on diarrhea incidence. If, as suspected, EED is also a consequence of continuing ingestion of fecal microorganisms, water and sanitation improvements should also reduce EED as a cause of early malnutrition. Reductions in diarrhea risk of 17 percent and 36 percent have been shown for improved water quality and excreta disposal, respectively (Cairncross and others 2010). Demographic and Health Surveys between 1986 and 2007 also suggest that access to improved water reduces risk of diarrhea (odds ratio 0.91, 95 percent confidence interval 0.88–0.94) and mild or severe stunting (odds ratio 0.92, 95 percent confidence interval 0.89–0.94), while improved sanitation reduces diarrhea mortality (odds ratio 0.77, 95 percent confidence interval 0.68–0.86), incidence (odds ratio 0.87, 95 percent confidence interval 0.85–0.90), and risk of mild to moderate stunting (odds ratio 0.73, 95 percent confidence interval 0.71–0.75) (Fink, Günther, and Hill 2011).

Water, sanitation, and hygiene interventions are collectively known as *WASH*. Somewhat surprisingly, a 2005 meta-analysis of WASH interventions failed to document greater effectiveness of combinations over single interventions (Fewtrell and others 2005). Current assessments are not sufficiently robust to influence investment decisions in one strategy over another, although all make sense and improve quality of life (Arnold and others 2013).

As infrastructure projects, water and sanitation improvements can be built at the community, neighborhood, or individual household levels; may be more or less technically complex; and may be more or less expensive. Unfortunately, the majority of sanitation systems fail to treat sewage to render it safe; as a result, irrigation water or seafood sources may become contaminated (Hutton and Chase, forthcoming, volume 7). In 2008, the World Bank

and the WHO estimated that the global cost of water and sanitation projects to meet Millennium Development Goal (MDG) targets would be US$42 billion and US$142 billion in 2005 dollars through 2014 for water and sanitation, respectively, exclusive of programmatic costs beyond the intervention delivery point (Hutton and Bartram 2008). This investment equates to US$4 billion and US$14 billion per year for water and sanitation projects, respectively, or US$8 and US$28 per capita, respectively. When maintenance, the cost of replacing existing infrastructure and facilities, and the extension of coverage to include future population growth are added, expenditures increase to US$360 billion for each intervention. Once built, however, water and sanitation infrastructure need to be maintained; this ongoing requirement leads to substantial additional financial as well as human capacity investments, without which infrastructure deteriorates and the initial investment can be lost. Further economic analysis of WASH interventions is provided in Hutton and Chase (forthcoming).

Limited evidence suggests that combining development and health interventions results in facilities that are better built and maintained, and used more effectively. Six years after completion of a project in Bolivia, the use of facilities in intervention communities was 44 percent higher than in control communities; from 66 percent to 86 percent of intervention households continued to practice four promoted maternal and child health behaviors compared with 14 percent to 30 percent of households in control communities (Eder and others 2012). Unfortunately, current assessments indicate that the 2015 MDG 7 for water and sanitation targets will not be met in five of nine regions (WHO and UNICEF 2013).

Behavioral Interventions

Many actions or decisions by caregivers, health care providers, and public health officials require behavior changes and the decision to act. If improved practices became the norm, risk of diarrhea and morbidity and mortality rates would diminish. Each of these behaviors may be difficult to sustain, but each would have a major impact.

Handwashing

The transfer of infectious agents via the hands directly between individuals or indirectly through contamination of inanimate objects (fomites), such as dishes, utensils, and other objects (Abad and others 2001), is a common route for the transmission of low inoculum diarrhea pathogens (as well as respiratory infections). Contaminated hands readily inoculate food or water, allowing high inoculum pathogens to multiply. Simple handwashing procedures significantly reduce transmission rates in health care facilities (Bolon 2011); households (Bloomfield 2003); schools (Lee and Greig 2010); and even day care and pre-school settings, which are notoriously difficult environments in which to enforce good hygiene (Churchill and Pickering 1997). Handwashing has an additional benefit in also reducing transmission of respiratory infections (Luby and others 2005).

Provision of soap to an urban squatter community in Karachi, Pakistan, supported by weekly meetings with trained health care workers from the same communities to reinforce the behavior, reduced days with diarrhea by 39 percent (95 percent confidence interval −61 percent to −16 percent) among infants compared with controls over one year (Luby and others 2004). Even severely malnourished children (weight-for-age z-score < −3.0) had 42 percent (95 percent confidence interval −69 percent to −16 percent) fewer days of diarrhea, compared with equally malnourished children in the control group. An additional benefit was a 50 percent reduction in the incidence of pneumonia (95 percent confidence interval −65 percent to −34 percent).

Handwashing with water alone is also worthwhile. In Bangladesh, the risk of diarrhea diminished when caregivers washed both hands with water before preparing food (odds ratio 0.67, 95 percent confidence interval 0.51–0.89); the effect was greater if one or both hands were washed with soap (odds ratio 0.30, 95 percent confidence interval 0.19–0.47) (Luby and others 2011). Risk was also reduced when caregivers washed hands with soap after defecation, but not with water alone (odds ratio 0.45, 95 percent confidence interval 0.26–0.77). Five key times for handwashing were identified: after defecation, after handling children's feces or cleaning the anus, before preparing food, before feeding children, and before eating. Direct observations identified more than 20 opportunities per day for handwashing, a frequency considered impossible to achieve, especially when the added cost of soap is considered. Handwashing after contact with feces is poorly practiced globally (Freeman and others 2014), and Luby and others (2011) recommended prioritizing handwashing before food preparation because it was the single most effective opportunity to reduce diarrhea risk.

How feasible is it to embed handwashing in daily behavior? A randomized intervention in Pakistan compared provision of soap for handwashing with a method to disinfect water or no intervention, including weekly visits over nine months to encourage either practice (Luby and others 2006). The study documented a 55 percent reduction in diarrhea (95 percent confidence interval 17 percent to 80 percent) compared with control neighborhoods, but no difference between the soap or water disinfection groups. When reenrolled in a follow-up surveillance 18 months later, handwashing intervention households were still 1.5 times more likely to wash with soap and water (79 percent versus 53 percent, $p = 0.001$) and 2.2 times (50 percent versus 23 percent, $p = 0.002$) more likely to rub their hands together compared with controls (Bowen and others 2013). During weekly follow-up throughout the 14 months without active educational intervention there was no difference between the groups in the proportion of person-days with diarrhea (1.59 percent versus 1.88 percent, $p = 0.66$) or the amount of soap purchased. Three years later, however, the investigators reengaged 461 original households (69 percent) and found the original intervention households were 3.4 times more likely than controls to have soap available (97 percent versus 28 percent, $p < 0.0001$), more commonly reported handwashing before cooking (relative risk 1.2, 95 percent confidence interval 1.0–1.4) and before meals (relative risk 1.7, 95 percent confidence interval 1.3–2.1), and purchased more soap per person per month (0.91–1.1 bars versus 0.65 for controls, $p < 0.0001$).

The critical question is not whether improving handwashing practices is effective, but rather how to best promote consistent behavior. The behavior requires availability of water and household handwashing stations designed and located to facilitate rather than inhibit the practice (Hulland and others 2013). Educational support from health care workers is useful, but how much is feasible and affordable remains in question. Increasingly, integrated behavioral models will be needed to improve the outcome of WASH interventions (Dreibelbis and others 2013).

Health Care Seeking

To ensure optimal care of infants and children with diarrheal disease, caregivers must recognize there is a problem, know what to do and do it, be alert to signs of clinical deterioration needing professional care, and know how to access such care without delay. Knowledge and experience are necessary but not sufficient; caregivers must also have the authority to act promptly. Initiatives to scale up prompt decision making and action generally focus on technical details and acquisition of practical skills, but frequently overlook social and cultural dimensions. These factors may influence whether a caregiver recognizes that fluid losses are beyond normal limits, are becoming dangerous, and require professional intervention (Larrea-Killinger and Muñoz 2013).

Higher levels of education promote quicker care-seeking action; however, cultural influences, for example, gender discrimination, can delay action for female infants (Malhotra and Upadhyay 2013). In rural Burkina Faso caregivers failed to recognize mild diarrhea, especially among infants, and made intervention choices that were not clinically based and recommended (Wilson and others 2012). Only 55 percent of caregivers sought care outside of the household, and 22 percent of these were with traditional healers or drug vendors, only 12 percent of whom recommended ORS. In rural Kenya, where caregivers understood the significance of diarrhea and dehydration, their primary concern was stopping the diarrhea, preferring antibiotics or antidiarrheals over ORS (Blum and others 2011). Cost of treatment is the major pragmatic impediment to care seeking outside of the home (Nasrin and others 2013). Anthropological and ethnographic approaches may help improve educational messaging and responses, but cost, travel and access to facilities, and wait times are likely to be critical determinants of behavior, and these require very different inputs to address.

Community-Based Interventions

Limited access to health facilities with trained primary care workers means that many children fail to receive simple but effective early interventions when diarrhea develops. However, a systematic review (Das, Lassi, and others 2013) concludes that community-based interventions improve care seeking by 9 percent (relative risk 1.09, 95 percent confidence interval 1.06–1.11), increase ORS use by 160 percent (relative risk 2.6, 95 percent confidence interval 1.59–4.27), produce a 29-fold increase in use of zinc supplements (relative risk 29.8, 95 percent confidence interval 12.33–71.97), and reduce antibiotic use by 75 percent (relative risk 0.25, 95 percent confidence interval 0.12–0.51).

Because diarrheal disease risk not only depends on the behavior of individuals and households but also on the practices of neighbors and communities, a systems approach to increase "attention to multiple transmission pathways, and highlight the need to widen the causal lens and pay more conceptual attention to socioeconomic status, gender, remoteness, and ecosystem changes" (Eisenberg and others 2012, 242) can improve outcomes. However, measuring these effects will require innovative study designs that reveal social patterns of interaction and the movement of pathogens through the environment.

Community-Led Total Sanitation

Interventions to improve the safe disposal of human excreta can be difficult to implement and maintain, and documenting a positive result is challenging, especially in rural settings in LMICs (Clasen and others 2010). For full impact, children and adults must learn to consistently use improved sanitation, and stools from infants and toddlers must be handled safely as well. Because water and sanitation improvements are often implemented together, separating the influence of each, and under which circumstances, can be difficult. Community-Led Total Sanitation (CLTS) is a participatory approach to improving sanitation in communities, in which communities mobilize to achieve total abandonment of open defecation and replace it with subsidized construction of facilities, household by household. The goal is to generate social pressure on all members of a community to understand the health implications of open defecation, and convince the community to join together, without external resources except guidance and facilitation, to agree on and act to completely eliminate open defecation and build a community sanitary infrastructure (Kar 2003). Its relevance is suggested by an analysis of Demographic and Health Survey data indicating that open defecation explains almost twice as much (54 versus 29 percent) of the international variation in child height compared with gross domestic product (Spears 2013). A 20 percent reduction in open defecation predicted a 0.1 standard deviation increase in child height.

CLTS begins with a facilitator engaging a community or village to promote understanding of the link between open defecation and illness. Initial engagement is followed by a survey and mapping of actual practices, often led by motivated school-age children. Finally, community deliberations lead to communal decisions to make the necessary changes. In the process, the facilitator may "provoke people through... tactics that trigger powerful emotions such as disgust, shame and fear... [to] enable local people to confront an unpleasant reality, and in doing this deliberately shocks, provokes, jokes and teases. Sparking these emotions and affects is key to triggering CLTS" (Deak 2008, 11). Although some have criticized the use of shame or social stigma to promote compliance (Bartram and others 2012), others have noted that shame, social pressure, and peer monitoring with government subsidies to build latrines markedly increases the adoption of improved sanitation (Pattanayak and others 2009).

Many tensions continue to surround the CLTS movement because organizations, government ministries, and development funders may be committed to different models of improving sanitation infrastructure; yet many examples of success and the spread of CLTS exist. This juxtaposition of tensions and successes indicates the need for careful analysis of the role of CLTS and how and where to introduce it most effectively. A number of issues must be considered, such as how to promote learning by doing; careful training of facilitators; cultural changes in institutional environments to a more participatory, responsive, transparent, and downward-accountability approach; and changing from a top-down to a bottom-up development model that is sensitive to local context and the longer time horizon required (Deak 2008).

COST AND COST-EFFECTIVENESS OF INTERVENTIONS

Several cost-effective and low-cost interventions are available to help prevent and treat diarrhea (table 9.1). Since the analysis of cost-effectiveness of interventions for diarrhea in LMICs in the second edition of *Disease Control Priorities in Developing Countries* (Keusch and others 2006), the ranking of various modalities has changed because of new evidence on the benefits of zinc as adjunct therapy for diarrhea (optimally in combination with ORS), substantial decreases in the cost of rotavirus vaccine, and additional research separating the cost-effectiveness of water supply from that of sanitation. The large gains in measles immunization have stopped additional work on its cost-effectiveness for diarrhea because it has become standard care. Although it is self evident that breastfeeding promotion reduces diarrhea, this practice has not been as high on the research and policy agenda.

The following is a brief discussion of the cost-effectiveness of selected diarrhea interventions. Details are presented in table 10.1 (Feikin and others 2016, chapter 10 in this volume). Das and others (2016, chapters 10 and 12 in this volume), and Stenberg and others (2016, chapter 16 in this volume) provide relevant information on vaccines and nutrition.

The most cost-effective interventions currently available for diarrhea (as measured in 2012 U.S. dollars per disability adjusted life year [DALY] averted) are prophylactic zinc supplementation (alone and as an adjunct to ORS), ORS, rotavirus vaccine, and household-level water treatment (primarily in rural areas using chlorination or solar disinfection) (see table 10.1). The second most cost-effective group includes rural sanitation, piped water, and in selected countries, cholera vaccine. Nutrition interventions are the least cost-effective for diarrhea; however, they have other major benefits, and cost-effectiveness of community management of severe acute malnutrition is addressed in Lenters, Wazny, and Bhutta (2016, chapter 11 in this volume).

Table 9.1 includes just one study of behavior change, identified through a focused search in PubMed. Such interventions tend to have very heterogeneous results; the one reviewed here (see table 10.1 for further details), a handwashing education intervention in Burkina Faso

Table 9.1 Cost-Effectiveness and Unit Cost of Interventions for Diarrheal Diseases

Intervention	Region	Cost-effectiveness (US$/DALY averted)	Unit cost (US$)
Oral rehydration solution (versus no ORS)	AFR-E	< 200	2.20/diarrhea episode
Prophylactic zinc with ORS (versus ORS alone)	AFR-E and SEA-D	< 100	0.61/diarrhea episode
Rotavirus vaccine (versus no vaccine)	Low-income countries	< 200 at 5/dose (less at 0.20/dose)	5/dose for two doses (Gavi price); Gavi-eligible countries pay 0.20/dose for two doses
Clean water (at household: chlorination or solar disinfection versus untreated water)	AFR-E and SEA-D	< 200	0.07/person/year SEA-D 0.13/person/year AFR-E (in 2000 U.S. dollars)
Improved rural water and sanitation (versus unimproved)	AFR-E and SEA-D	< 2,000	28/household (well); 52/household (latrine)
Piped water and sewer connection (versus no connections)	AFR-E	< 2,000	136/household (water); 160/household (sewer)
	SEA-D	< 3,000	
Cholera vaccine (versus no vaccine)	High-endemicity countries	2,000–10,000	1.33/person
Behavior change	Low-income countries	Large variation	Large variation
RUTF added to standard rations (versus standard rations)	AFR-E	> 10,000 considering only benefits for diarrhea	527/child/year

Source: See Horton and Levin 2016, chapter 17, on cost-effectiveness in this volume.
Note: AFR-E = high-mortality Africa (WHO subregion); DALY = disability adjusted life year; Gavi, the Vaccine Alliance; ORS = oral rehydration solution; RUTF = ready-to-use therapeutic foods; SEA-D = high-mortality South-East Asia (WHO subregion). Costs and cost per DALY averted are higher in other regions. Interventions costing less than US$240 per DALY in 2012 would be very cost-effective even in the poorest low-income country; those costing less than US$720 would be cost-effective even in the poorest low-income country (Burundi's per capita gross national income was US$240 in 2012) (World Bank 2014). All costs converted to 2012 U.S. dollars (except as noted otherwise).

(Borghi and others 2002), falls into the most cost-effective group. Well-designed behavior change interventions to increase use of clean water, latrines, ORS, prophylactic zinc, and vaccines could all be cost-effective. Neither table 9.1 nor table 10.1 contains cost-effectiveness results for drug treatment of dysentery because focused searches in PubMed returned no relevant citations. Typically, cost-effectiveness studies are performed when a drug is new or is being tested for a new use, which is not the case here. Drug treatment for dysentery is known to be highly effective if the pathogens are sensitive; the high case fatality rates for dysentery indicate that drug treatment is extremely likely to be cost-effective.

It is not sufficient for an intervention to be cost-effective to be adopted. Cost or affordability in relation to health expenditures also matters. One major advance has been the addition of zinc as a complementary therapy to ORS; as an adjunct to an existing treatment, it appears to be particularly cost-effective and affordable. Robberstad and others (2004) estimate that zinc tablets cost approximately US$0.61 for a three-week course of treatment, in addition to the US$2.20 in recurrent costs per course of treatment with ORS, excluding personnel costs in delivering the intervention.

Introduction of rotavirus vaccine is progressing as a result of Gavi interventions, although the negotiated price for the vaccine at US$5 per dose for the two-dose course remains a substantial addition to current costs of the WHO's Expanded Program on Immunization. Gavi provides the vaccine at a highly subsidized price to eligible countries (US$0.40 for two doses); countries that graduate from eligibility are required to pay 20 percent of the Gavi cost in the first year, increasing by US$1 per year until the full price of US$5 per dose is paid (Verguet and others 2016, chapter 19 in this volume). Given that diarrhea rates and mortality rates are higher in LICs, the vaccine is particularly cost-effective in these countries.

Sanitation and, to a lesser extent, water supply interventions, are subject to affordability considerations. Initial investment costs per household for standard urban requirements—water piped to the house and a sewer connection—are US$136 and US$160, respectively. The lowest-cost clean water interventions in rural areas are still substantial at US$28 per household for a dug well, US$31 per household for a borehole, and US$52 per household for a pit latrine (Haller, Hutton, and Bartram 2007). Household point-of-use disinfection of water (using chlorine or solar disinfection) costs pennies per capita per year in recurrent costs, but requires behavior change. Although improved water supply and sanitation are essential in the long term to decrease diarrhea, intestinal parasites, and stunting, the investment costs mean the transition is likely to be slow.

Most of the results in tables 9.1 and 10.1 describe the cost-effectiveness of implementing a single intervention. If interventions are combined, the incremental cost-effectiveness of each additional intervention can decline. Fischer Walker and others (2011) estimate the combined effect of 10 interventions designed to reduce diarrhea in 68 countries with high child mortality, using the Lives Saved Tool. Two scenarios were modeled: an ambitious strategy designed to reach MDG 4 goals (to reduce child mortality) in a realizable way; and a universal strategy designed to bring coverage of many interventions to 90 percent or more of the target population, and water, sanitation, and handwashing interventions to 55 percent or more. Both strategies were scaled up from current coverage to the target over five years. The ambitious strategy saved 3.8 million lives during a five-year period, at a cost of US$52.5 billion, or US$13,700 per death averted, approximately US$432/DALY averted assuming one life saved in infancy or early childhood is about 32 DALYs averted. The universal strategy saved 5 million lives at a cost of US$20,752 per death averted, or US$648 per DALY averted. Although these rates would be considered cost-effective or very cost-effective for most countries, affordability is still an obstacle. The main issue is the water and sanitation components, which account for 84 percent of the cost of the ambitious package and 87 percent of the universal strategy.

Extended cost-effectiveness analysis provides further insight. Chapters 18 and 19 in this volume (Ashok, Nandi, and Laxminarayan 2016; Verguet and others 2016) present extended cost-effectiveness analyses of the introduction of rotavirus vaccine in India and water and sanitation improvements in Ethiopia. These interventions are pro-poor—the poor benefit disproportionately from reduced child mortality and from out-of-pocket savings on treatment costs, because they bear a disproportionately higher burden of ill health from diarrhea. They have less access to clean water and improved sanitation, and therefore their children have poorer nutritional status and are at higher risk of mortality from diarrhea-related illness.

CONCLUSIONS

The burden of diarrheal diseases in children under age five years in LMICs has been reduced dramatically. These reductions are the result of focused attention and resources applied, originally through vertical programs and advocacy through the WHO and international donor agencies, and more recently through more integrated programs for primary care and community-based programming. Although there are no magic bullets to control the incidence of diarrheal diseases, the following are highly effective: improved nutrition of young children to increase their ability to respond to infection; water and sanitation improvements to reduce the number of microorganisms in the environment; handwashing; and implementation of simple but highly effective interventions, such as ORS, that have enabled early treatment and mitigation of dehydration due to watery diarrhea.

When antibiotics are used appropriately for inflammatory diarrheas, survival is enhanced; however, targeting only those individuals who truly need antibiotic treatment remains problematic. Most uses of antibiotics are not only ineffective, for example, in the treatment of viral infections, but counterproductive, due to selective pressure for drug resistance. Indeed, many important diarrheal disease agents now exhibit serious resistance to multiple medications. Improved understanding of the pathogenesis of persistent diarrhea has helped the development of nutritional interventions to address the malabsorption and malnutrition that characterize persistent diarrhea and lead to serious morbidity and increased mortality.

This chapter reviews interventions and policy strategies that are effective, can often be packaged together, and can be delivered at the community level. Many of these interventions have impacts far beyond diarrheal disease, and these additional rationales for implementation enhance their cost-effectiveness. Some are both effective and highly inexpensive, for example, the early use of ORS, so there is no reason not to promote them. Continued attention to delivering an appropriate package of interventions, coupled with monitoring and continuous quality improvement of health care delivery services, can be expected to continue to drive down the mortality and sequelae of diarrheal diseases in the coming decade. In addition to the development of point-of-care diagnostics, medications, and vaccines, many issues need continuing study, including better water and safe sanitation methods, food and water safety behavior within households and along the food chain, and the cause and role of EED and asymptomatic infection on intestinal function and nutrition.

NOTE

World Bank Income Classifications as of July 2014 are as follows, based on estimates of gross national income (GNI) per capita for 2013:

- Low-income countries (LICs) = US$1,045 or less
- Middle-income countries (MICs) are subdivided:
  a) lower-middle-income = US$1,046–US$4,125
- b) upper-middle-income (UMICs) = US$4,126–US$12,745
- High-income countries (HICs) = US$12,746 or more.

REFERENCES

Abad, F. X., C. Villena, S. Guix, S. Caballero, R. M. Pintó, and others. 2001. "Potential Role of Fomites in the Vehicular Transmission of Human Astroviruses." *Applied Environmental Microbiology* 67 (9): 3904–07.

Adriaenssens, N., S. Coenen, A. Versporten, A. Muller, G. Minalu, and others. 2011. "European Surveillance of Antimicrobial Consumption (ESAC): Outpatient Antibiotic Use in Europe (1997–2009)." *Journal of Antimicrobial Chemotherapy* 66 (Suppl 6): vi3–12. doi:10.1093/jac/dkr453.

Ahmed, R., M. Ansaruzzaman, E. Haque, M. R. Rao, and J. D. Clemens. 2001. "Epidemiology of Postshigellosis Persistent Diarrhea in Young Children." *Pediatric Infectious Diseases Journal* 20 (5): 525–30.

Alam, A. N., S. A. Sarker, K. A. Wahed, M. Khatun, and M. M. Rahaman. 1994. "Enteric Protein Loss and Intestinal Permeability Changes in Children during Acute Shigellosis and after Recovery: Effect of Zinc Supplementation." *Gut* 35 (12): 1707–11.

Ali, M., A. L. Lopez, Y. A. You, Y. E. Kim, B. Sah, and others. 2012. "The Global Burden of Cholera." *Bulletin of the World Health Organization* 90: 209–18.

Arnold, B. F., C. Null, S. P. Luby, L. Unicomb, C. P. Stewart, and others. 2013. "Cluster-Randomised Controlled Trials of Individual and Combined Water, Sanitation, Hygiene and Nutritional Interventions in Rural Bangladesh and Kenya: The WASH Benefits Study Design and Rationale." *BMJ Open* 3: e003476. doi:10.1136/bmjopen-2013-003476.

Ashok, A., A. Nandi, and R. Laxminarayan. 2016. "The Benefits of a Universal Home-Based Neonatal Care Package in Rural India: An Extended Cost-Effectiveness Analysis." In *Disease Control Priorities* (third edition): Volume 2, *Reproductive, Maternal, Newborn, and Child Health*, edited by R. Black, R. Laxminarayan, M. Temmerman, and N. Walker. Washington, DC: World Bank.

Atia, A. N., and A. L. Buchman. 2009. "Oral Rehydration Solutions in Non-Cholera Diarrhea: A Review." *American Journal of Gastroenterology* 104 (10): 2596–04.

Awasthi, S., and IC-ZED (INCLEN Childnet Zinc Effectiveness for Diarrhea) Group. 2006. "Zinc Supplementation in Acute Diarrhea Is Acceptable, Does Not Interfere with Oral Rehydration, and Reduces the Use of Other Medications: A Randomized Trial in Five Countries." *Journal of Pediatric Gastroenterology and Nutrition* 42 (3): 300–05.

Baker, S. J. 1976. "Subclinical Intestinal Malabsorption in Developing Countries." *Bulletin of the World Health Organization* 54 (5): 485–94.

Bartram, J., K. Charles, B. Evans, L. O'Hanlon, and S. Pedley. 2012. "Commentary on Community-Led Total Sanitation and Human Rights: Should the Right to Community-Wide Health Be Won at the Cost of Individual Rights?" *Journal of Water and Health* 10 (4): 499–503.

Barzilay, E. J., N. Schaad, R. Magloire, K. S. Mung, J. Boncy, and others. 2013. "Cholera Surveillance during the Haiti Epidemic—The First 2 Years." *New England Journal of Medicine* 368: 599–609.

Bennish, M. L., M. A. Salam, and M. A. Wahed. 1993. "Enteric Protein Loss during Shigellosis." *American Journal of Gastroenterology* 88 (1): 53–57.

Bennish, M. L., and B. J. Wojtyniak. 1991. "Mortality Due to Shigellosis: Community and Hospital Data." *Reviews of Infectious Diseases* 13 (Suppl 4): S245–51.

Bern, C., J. Martines, I. de Zoysa, and R. I. Glass. 1992. "The Magnitude of the Global Problem of Diarrhoeal Disease: A Ten-Year Update." *Bulletin of the World Health Organization* 70: 705–14.

Bhan, M. K., and N. Bhandari. 1998. "The Role of Zinc and Vitamin A in Persistent Diarrhea among Infants and Young Children." *Journal of Pediatric Gastroenterology and Nutrition* 26 (4): 446–53.

Bhandari, N., T. Rongsen-Chandola, A. Bavdekar, J. John, K. Antony, and others. 2014. "Efficacy of a Monovalent Human-Bovine (116E) Rotavirus Vaccine in Indian Children in the Second Year of Life." *Vaccine* 32 (Suppl 1): A110–16. doi:10.1016/j.vaccine.2014.04.079.

Bhattacharya, D., S. A. Purushottaman, H. Bhattacharjee, R. Thamizhmani, S. D. Sudharama, and others. 2011. "Rapid Emergence of Third-Generation Cephalosporin Resistance in Shigella sp. Isolated in Andaman and Nicobar Islands, India." *Microbial Drug Resistance* 17 (2): 329–32.

Bhutta, Z. A., S. M. Bird, R. E. Black, K. H. Brown, J. M. Gardner, and others. 2000. "Therapeutic Effects of Oral Zinc in Acute and Persistent Diarrhea in Children in Developing Countries: Pooled Analysis of Randomized Controlled Trials." *American Journal of Clinical Nutrition* 72 (6): 1516–22.

Bhutta, Z. A., J. K. Das, N. Walker, A. Rizvi, H. Campbell, and others. 2013. "Interventions to Address Deaths from Childhood Pneumonia and Diarrhoea Equitably: What Works and at What Cost?" *The Lancet* 381 (9875): 1417–29.

Bloomfield, S. F. 2003. "Home Hygiene: A Risk Approach." *International Journal of Hygiene and Environmental Health* 206 (1): 1–8.

Blum, L. S., P. A. Oria, C. K. Olson, R. F. Breiman, and P. K. Ram. 2011. "Examining the Use of Oral Rehydration Salts and Other Oral Rehydration Therapy for Childhood Diarrhea in Kenya." *American Journal of Tropical Medicine and Hygiene* 85 (6): 1126–33.

Bolon, M. 2011. "Hand Hygiene." *Infectious Disease Clinics of North America* 25: 21–43.

Borghi, J., L. Guinness, J. Ouedraogo, and V. Curtis. 2002. "Is Hygiene Promotion Cost-Effective? A Case Study in Burkina Faso." *Tropical Medicine and International Health* 7 (11): 960–69.

Bowen, A., M. Agboatwalla, T. Ayers, T. Tobery, M. Tariq, and others. 2013. "Sustained Improvements in Handwashing Indicators More Than 5 Years after a Cluster-Randomised, Community-Based Trial of Handwashing Promotion in Karachi, Pakistan." *Tropical Medicine and International Health* 18 (3): 259–67.

Bushen, O. Y., A. Kohli, R. C. Pinkerton, K. Dupnik, R. D. Newman, and others. 2007. "Heavy Cryptosporidial Infections in Children in Northeast Brazil: Comparison of *Cryptosporidium hominis* and *Cryptosporidium parvum*."

Transactions of the Royal Society of Tropical Medicine and Hygiene 101 (4): 378–84.

Cairncross, S., C. Hunt, S. Boisson, K. Bostoen, V. Curtis, and others. 2010. "Water, Sanitation and Hygiene for the Prevention of Diarrhoea." *International Journal of Epidemiology* 39 (Suppl 1): i193–205.

Campbell, D. I., P. G. Lunn, and M. Elia. 2002. "Age-Related Association of Small Intestinal Ucosal Enteropathy with Nutritional Status in Rural Gambian Children." *British Journal of Nutrition* 88 (5): 499–505.

Campbell, D. I., G. McPhail, P. G. Lunn, M. Elia, and D. J. Jeffries. 2004. "Intestinal Inflammation Measured by Fecal Neopterin in Gambian Children with Enteropathy: Association with Growth Failure, *Giardia lamblia*, and Intestinal Permeability." *Journal of Pediatric Gastroenterology and Nutrition* 39 (2): 153–57.

Campbell, D. I., S. H. Murch, M. Elia, P. B. Sullivan, M. S. Sanyang, and others. 2003. "Chronic T Cell-Mediated Enteropathy in Rural West African Children: Relationship with Nutritional Status and Small Bowel Function." *Pediatric Research* 54 (3): 306–11.

Castillo-Duran, C., G. Heresi, M. Fisberg, and R. Uauy. 1987. "Controlled Trial of Zinc Supplementation during Recovery from Malnutrition: Effects on Growth and Immune Function." *American Journal of Clinical Nutrition* 45 (3): 602–8.

Checkley, W., L. D. Epstein, R. H. Gilman, R. E. Black, L. Cabrera, and others. 1998. "Effects of *Cryptosporidium parvum* Infection in Peruvian Children: Growth Faltering and Subsequent Catch-Up Growth." *American Journal of Epidemiology* 148 (5): 497–506.

Checkley, W., R. H. Gilman, L. D. Epstein, M. Suarez, J. F. Diaz, and others. 1997. "Asymptomatic and Symptomatic Cryptosporidiosis: Their Acute Effect on Weight Gain in Peruvian Children." *American Journal of Epidemiology* 145 (2): 156–63.

Chompook, P., J. Todd, J. G. Wheeler, L. von Seidlein, J. Clemens, and others. 2006. "Risk Factors for Shigellosis in Thailand." *International Journal of Infectious Diseases* 10 (6): 425–33.

Choudhury, N., T. Ahmed, M. I. Hossain, B. N. Mandal, M. Golam, and others. 2014. "Community-Based Management of Acute Malnutrition in Bangladesh: Feasibility and Constraints." *Food and Nutrition Bulletin* 35 (2): 277–85.

Chouraqui, J. P., and A. P. Michard-Lenoir. 2007. "Feeding Infants and Young Children with Acute Diarrhea." *Archives of Pediatrics* 14 (Suppl 3): S176–80.

Churchill, R. B., and L. K. Pickering. 1997. "Infection Control Challenges in Child-Care Centers." *Infectious Disease Clinics of North America* 11 (2): 347–65.

Ciccarelli, S., I. Stolfi, and G. Caramia. 2013. "Management Strategies in the Treatment of Neonatal and Pediatric Gastroenteritis." *Infection and Drug Resistance* 6: 133–61.

Clasen, T. F., K. Bostoen, W. P. Schmidt, S. Boisson, I. C. Fung, and others. 2010. "Interventions to Improve Disposal of Human Excreta for Preventing Diarrhoea." *Cochrane Database of Systematic Reviews* Jun 16: (6): CD007180. doi:10.1002/14651858.CD007180.pub2.

Clavenna, A., and M. Bonati. 2011. "Differences in Antibiotic Prescribing in Paediatric Outpatients." *Archives of Disease in Childhood* 96 (6): 590–95.

Clemens, J. 2011. "(1579)." *Philosophical Transactions of the Royal Society B* 366: 2799–805.

Costa, A. D., and G. A. Silva. 2011. "Oral Rehydration Therapy in Emergency Departments." *Jornal de Pediatria* 87 (2): 175–79.

Das, J. K., Z. S. Lassi, R. A. Salam, and Z. A. Bhutta. 2013. "Effect of Community Based Interventions on Childhood Diarrhea and Pneumonia: Uptake of Treatment Modalities and Impact on Mortality." *BMC Public Health* 13 (Suppl 3): S29. doi:10.1186/1471-2458-13-S3-S29.

Das, J. K., R. A. Salam, A. Imdad, and Z. A. Bhutta. 2016. "Infant and Young Child Growth." In *Disease Control Priorities* (third edition): Volume 2, *Reproductive, Maternal, Newborn, and Child Health*, edited by R. Black, R. Laxminarayan, M. Temmerman, and N. Walker. Washington, DC: World Bank.

Das, J. K., A. Tripathi, A. Ali, A. Hassan, C. Dojosoeandy, and others. 2013. "Vaccines for the Prevention of Diarrhea Due to Cholera, *Shigella*, ETEC and Rotavirus." *BMC Public Health* 13 (Suppl 3): 511. https://www.biomedcentral.com/1471-2458/13/S3/S11.

Das, S. K., S. Ahmed, F. Ferdous, F. D. Farzana, M. J. Chisti, and others. 2013. "Etiological Diversity of Diarrhoeal Disease in Bangladesh." *Journal of Infection in Developing Countries* 7 (12): 900–9.

Das, S. K., A. S. Faruque, M. J. Chisti, M. A. Malek, M. A. Salam, and others. 2012. "Changing Trend of Persistent Diarrhoea in Young Children over Two Decades: Observations from a Large Diarrhoeal Disease Hospital in Bangladesh." *Acta Paediatrica* 101 (10): e452–57. doi:10.1111/j.1651-2227.2012.02761.x.

Deak, A. 2008. "Taking Community-Led Total Sanitation to Scale: Movement, Spread and Adaptation." Working Paper 298, Institute of Development Studies at the University of Sussex, Brighton, UK.

Dewey, K. G., and K. Begum. 2011. "Long-Term Consequences of Stunting in Early Life." *Maternal and Child Nutrition* 7 (Suppl 3): 5–18.

Dey, S. K., M. J. Chisti, S. K. Das, C. K. Shaha, F. Ferdous, and others. 2013. "Characteristics of Diarrheal Illnesses in Non-Breast Fed Infants Attending a Large Urban Diarrheal Disease Hospital in Bangladesh." *PLoS One* 8 (3): e58228. doi:10.1371/journal.pone.0058228.

Dreibelbis, R., P. J. Winch, E. Leontsini, K. R. Hulland, P. K. Ram, and others. 2013. "The Integrated Behavioural Model for Water, Sanitation, and Hygiene: A Systematic Review of Behavioural Models and a Framework for Designing and Evaluating Behaviour Change Interventions in Infrastructure-Restricted Settings." *BMC Public Health* 13: 1015. doi:10.1186/1471-2458-13-1015.48.

Ecker, L., T. J. Ochoa, M. Vargas, L. J. Del Valle, and J. Ruiz. 2013. "Factors Affecting Caregivers' Use of Antibiotics Available without a Prescription in Peru." *Pediatrics* 131 (6): e1771–79. doi:10.1542/peds.2012-1970.

Eder, C., J. Schooley, J. Fullerton, and J. Murguia. 2012. "Assessing Impact and Sustainability of Health, Water, and Sanitation Interventions in Bolivia Six Years Post-Project." *Revista Panamericana de Salud Pública* 32: 43–48.

Eisenberg, J. N., J. Trostle, R. J. Sorensen, and K. F. Shields. 2012. "Toward a Systems Approach to Enteric Pathogen Transmission: From Individual Independence to Community Interdependence." *Annual Review of Public Health* 33: 239–57.

Ekwochi, U., J. M. Chinawa, I. Obi, H. A. Obu, and S. Agwu. 2013. "Use and/or Misuse of Antibiotics in Management of Diarrhea among Children in Enugu, Southeast Nigeria." *Journal of Tropical Pediatrics* 59 (4): 314–16.

Erdman, S. M., E. E. Buckner, and J. F. Hindler. 2008. "Options for Treating Resistant *Shigella* Species Infections in Children." *Journal of Pediatric Pharmacology and Therapeutics* 13: 29–43.

Ernst, S., C. Weinrobe, C. Bien-Aime, and I. Rawson. 2011. "Cholera Management and Prevention at Hôpital Albert Schweitzer, Haiti." *Emerging Infectious Diseases* 17: 2155–57.

Farag, T. H., A. S. Faruque, Y. Wu, S. K. Das, A. S. Hossain, and others. 2013. "Housefly Population Density Correlates with Shigellosis among Children in Mirzapur, Bangladesh: A Time Series Analysis." *PLoS Neglected Tropical Diseases* 7: e2280. doi:10.1371/journal.pntd.0002280.

Feachem, R. G., and M. A. Koblinsky. 1983. "Interventions for the Control of Diarrhoeal Diseases among Young Children: Measles Immunization." *Bulletin of the World Health Organization* 61 (4): 641–52.

Feikin, D. R., B. M. J. Flannery Hamel, M. Stack, and P. Hansen. 2016. "Vaccines for Children in Low- and Middle-Income Countries." In *Disease Control Priorities* (third edition): Volume 2, *Reproductive, Maternal, Newborn, and Child Health*, edited by R. Black, R. Laxminarayan, M. Temmerman, and N. Walker. Washington, DC: World Bank.

Fewtrell, L., R. B. Kaufmann, D. Kay, W. Enanoria, L. Haller, and others. 2005. "Water, Sanitation, and Hygiene Interventions to Reduce Diarrhoea in Less Developed Countries: A Systematic Review and Meta-Analysis." *The Lancet Infectious Diseases* 5 (1): 42–52.

Fink, G., I. Günther, and K. Hill. 2011. "The Effect of Water and Sanitation on Child Health: Evidence from the Demographic and Health Surveys 1986–2007." *International Journal of Epidemiology* 40 (5): 1196–204.

Fischer Walker, C.L., and R. E. Black. 2010. "Zinc for the Treatment of Diarrhoea: Effect on Diarrhoea Morbidity, Mortality and Incidence of Future Episodes." *International Journal of Epidemiology* 39 (Suppl 1): i63–69.

Fischer Walker, C. L., and R. E. Black. 2011. "Rotavirus Vaccine and Diarrhea Mortality: Quantifying Regional Variation in Effect Size." *BMC Public Health* 11 (Suppl 3): S16. doi:10.1186/1471-2458-11-S3-S16.

Fischer Walker, C. L., I. K. Friberg, N. Binkin, M. Young, N. Walker, and others. 2011. "Scaling Up Diarrhea Prevention and Treatment Interventions: A Lives Saved Tool Analysis." *PLoS Medicine* 8: e1000428. doi:10.1371/journal.pmed.1000428.

Fischer Walker, C. L., J. Perin, M. J. Aryee, C. Boschi-Pinto, and R. E. Black. 2012. "Diarrhea Incidence in Low- and Middle-Income Countries in 1990 and 2010: A Systematic Review." *BMC Public Health* 12: 220. doi:10.1186/1471-2458-12-220.

Fischer Walker, C. L., I. Rudan, L. Liu, H. Nair, E. Theodoratou, and others. 2013. "Global Burden of Childhood Pneumonia and Diarrhoea." *The Lancet* 381 (9875): 1405–16.

Freeman, M. C., M. E. Stocks, O. Cumming, A. Jeandron, J. P. Higgins, and others. 2014. "Hygiene and Health: Systematic Review of Handwashing Practices Worldwide and Update of Health Effects." *Tropical Medicine and International Health* 19 (8): 906–16.

Gaffey, M. F., K. Wazny, D. G. Bassani, and Z. A. Bhutta. 2013. "Dietary Management of Childhood Diarrhea in Low- and Middle-Income Countries: A Systematic Review." *BMC Public Health* 13 (Suppl 3): S17. doi:10.1186/1471-2458-13-S3-S17.

Gavi Alliance. 2014. "Rotavirus Vaccine Support." http://www .gavialliance.org/support/nvs/rotavirus/.

Gebhard, R. L., R. Karouani, W. F. Prigge, and C. J. McClain. 1983. "The Effect of Severe Zinc Deficiency on Activity of Intestinal Disaccharidases and 3-Hydroxy-3-Methylglutaryl Coenzyme A Reductase in the Rat." *Journal of Nutrition* 113 (4): 855–89.

Gerson, C. D., T. H. Kent, J. R. Saha, N. Siddiqi, and J. Lindenbaum. 1971. "Recovery of Small-Intestinal Structure and Function after Residence in the Tropics. II. Studies in Indians and Pakistanis Living in New York City." *Annals of Internal Medicine* 75 (1): 41–48.

Ghosh, A., and T. Ramamurthy. 2011. "Antimicrobials and Cholera: Are We Stranded?" *Indian Journal of Medical Research* 133: 225–31.

Gilman, R. H., R. Partanen, K. H. Brown, W. M. Spira, S. Khanam, and others. 1988. "Decreased Gastric Acid Secretion and Bacterial Colonization of the Stomach in Severely Malnourished Bangladeshi Children." *Gastroenterology* 94 (6): 1308–14.

Grimwood, K., and D. A. Forbes. 2009. "Acute and Persistent Diarrhea." *Pediatric Clinics of North America* 56 (6): 1343–61.

Guerrant, R. L., A. A. Lima, M. Barboza, S. Young, T. Silva, and others. 1999. "Mechanisms and Impact of Enteric Infections." *Advances in Experimental Medicine and Biology* 473: 103–12.

Hahn, S., S. Kim, and P. Garner. 2002. "Reduced Osmolarity Oral Rehydration Solution for Treating Dehydration Caused by Acute Diarrhoea in Children." *Cochrane Database of Systematic Reviews* 1: CD002847.

Haider, B. A., and Z. A. Bhutta. 2009. "The Effect of Therapeutic Zinc Supplementation among Young Children with Selected Infections: A Review of the Evidence." *Food and Nutrition Bulletin* 30 (Suppl 1): S41–59.

Haller, L., G. Hutton, and J. Bartram. 2007. "Estimating the Costs and Health Benefits of Water and Sanitation Improvements at Global Level." *Journal of Water and Health* 5 (4): 467–80.

Harris, J. B., R. C. LaRocque, F. Qadri, E. T. Ryan, and S. B. Calderwood. 2012. "Cholera." *The Lancet* 379 (9835): 2466–76.

Horton, S., and C. Levin. 2016. "Cost-Effectiveness of Interventions for Reproductive, Maternal, Neonatal, and Child Health." In *Disease Control Priorities* (third edition): Volume 2, *Reproductive, Maternal, Newborn, and Child Health,* edited by R. Black, R. Laxminarayan, M. Temmerman, and N. Walker. Washington, DC: World Bank.

Hulland, K. R., E. Leontsini, R. Dreibelbis, L. Unicomb, A. Afroz, and others. 2013. "Designing a Handwashing Station for Infrastructure-Restricted Communities in Bangladesh Using the Integrated Behavioural Model for Water, Sanitation and Hygiene Interventions (IBM-WASH)." *BMC Public Health* 13: 877. doi:10.1186/1471-2458-13-877.

Hutton, G., and J. Bartram. 2008. "Global Costs of Attaining the Millennium Development Goal for Water Supply and Sanitation." *Bulletin of the World Health Organization* 86: 13–19.

Hutton, G., and C. Chase. "Water Supply, Sanitation, and Hygiene." Forthcoming. In *Disease Control Priorities* (third edition): Volume 7, *Injury Prevention and Environmental Health,* edited by C. N. Mock, O. Kobusingye, and R. Nugent. Washington, DC: World Bank.

Imdad, A., and Z. A. Bhutta. 2011. "Effect of Preventive Zinc Supplementation on Linear Growth in Children under 5 Years of Age in Developing Countries: A Meta-Analysis of Studies for Input to the Lives Saved Tool." *BMC Public Health* 11(Suppl 3): S22. doi:10.1186/ 1471-2458-11-S3-S22.

Kar, K. 2003. "Subsidy or Self-Respect? Participatory Total Community Sanitation in Bangladesh." Working Paper 184, Institute for Development Studies, Brighton, UK.

Kashmira, A., K. A. Date, A. Vicari, T. B. Hyde, E. Mintz, and others. 2011. "Considerations for Oral Cholera Vaccine Use during Outbreak after Earthquake in Haiti, 2010–2011." *Emerging Infectious Diseases* 17 (11): 2105–12.

Keusch, G. T., O. Fontaine, A. Bhargava, C. Boschi-Pinto, A. A. Bhutta, and others. 2006. "Diarrheal Diseases." In *Disease Control Priorities in Developing Countries*, 2nd ed., edited by D. T. Jamison, J. G. Breman, A. R. Measham, G. Alleyene, M. Claeson, D. B. Evans, P. Jha, A. Mills, and P. Musgrove, 371–88. Washington, DC: World Bank and Oxford University Press.

Keusch, G. T., A. G. Plaut, and F. J. Troncale. 1972. "Subclinical Malabsorption in Thailand: II. Intestinal Absorption in American Military and Peace Corps Personnel." *American Journal of Clinical Nutrition* 25 (10): 1067–73.

Keusch, G. T., I. H. Rosenberg, D. M. Denno, C. Duggan, R. L. Guerrant, and others. 2013. "Implications of Acquired Environmental Enteric Dysfunction for Growth and Stunting in Infants and Children Living in Low- and Middle-Income Countries." *Food and Nutrition Bulletin* 34 (3): 357–64.

Kim, H. B., M. Wang, S. Ahmed, C. H. Park, R. C. LaRocque, and others. 2010. "Transferable Quinolone Resistance in *Vibrio cholerae.*" *Antimicrobial Agents and Chemotherapy* 54 (2): 799–803.

King, C. K., R. Glass, J. S. Bresee, and C. Duggan. 2003. "Managing Acute Gastroenteritis among Children: Oral Rehydration, Maintenance, and Nutritional Therapy." *Morbidity and Mortality Weekly Reports. Recommendations and Reports* 52 (RR16): 1–16. http://www.cdc.gov/mmwr /preview/mmwrhtml/rr5216a1.htm.

Kosek, M., C. Bern, and R. L. Guerrant. 2003. "The Global Burden of Diarrhoeal Disease, as Estimated from Studies Published between 1992 and 2000." *Bulletin of the World Health Organization* 81 (3): 197–204.

Kosek, M., R. Haque, A. Lima, S. Babji, S. Shrestha, and others. 2013. "Fecal Markers of Intestinal Inflammation and Permeability Associated with the Subsequent Acquisition of Linear Growth Deficits in Infants." *American Journal of Tropical Medicine and Hygiene* 88 (2): 390–96.

Kotloff, K. L., J. P. Nataro, W. C. Blackwelder, D. Nasrin, T. H. Farag, and others. 2013. "Burden and Aetiology of Diarrhoeal Disease in Infants and Young Children in Developing Countries (the Global Enteric Multicenter Study, GEMS): A Prospective, Case-Control Study." *The Lancet* 382 (9888): 209–22.

Kruse, H., H. Sørum, F. C. Tenover, and O. Olsvik. 1995. "A Transferable Multiple Drug Resistance Plasmid from *Vibrio cholerae* O1." *Microbial Drug Resistance* 1 (3): 203–10.

Lamberti, L. M., C. L. Fischer Walker, and R. E. Black. 2012. "Systematic Review of Diarrhea Duration and Severity in Children and Adults in Low- and Middle-Income Countries." *BMC Public Health* 12: 276. doi:10.1186/1471-2458-12-276.

Lanata, C. F., C. L. Fischer Walker, A. C. Olascoaga, C. X. Torres, M. J. Aryee, and others. 2013. "Child Health Epidemiology Reference Group of the World Health Organization and UNICEF. Global Causes of Diarrheal Disease Mortality in Children <5 Years of Age: A Systematic Review." *PLoS One* September 4: 8:e72788. doi:10.1371/journal.pone.0072788.

Langford, R., P. Lunn, and C. Panter-Brick. 2011. "Hand-Washing, Subclinical Infections, and Growth: A Longitudinal Evaluation of an Intervention in Nepali Slums." *American Journal of Human Biology* 23 (5): 621–29.

Larrea-Killinger, C., and A. Muñoz. 2013. "The Child's Body without Fluid: Mother's Knowledge and Practices about Hydration and Rehydration in Salvador, Bahia, Brazil." *Journal of Epidemiology and Community Health* 67 (6): 498–507.

Latham, M. C., U. Jonsson, E. Sterken, and G. Kent. 2010. "RUTF Stuff: Can the Children Be Saved with Fortified Peanut Paste?" *World Nutrition* 2 (2): 62–85.

Lazzerini, M., and L. Ronfani. 2013. "Oral Zinc for Treating Diarrhoea in Children." *Cochrane Database of Systematic Reviews* 1: CD005436. doi:10.1002/14651858.CD005436.pub4.

Lee, M. B., and J. D. Greig. 2010. "A Review of Gastrointestinal Outbreaks in Schools: Effective Infection Control Interventions." *Journal of School Health* 80 (12): 588–98.

Lenters, L., K. Wazny, and Z. A. Bhutta. 2016. "Management of Severe and Moderate Acute Malnutrition in Children." In *Disease Control Priorities* (third edition): Volume 2, *Reproductive, Maternal, Newborn, and Child Health*, edited by R. Black, R. Laxminarayan, M. Temmerman, and N. Walker. Washington, DC: World Bank.

Lindenbaum, J., C. D. Gerson, and T. H. Kent. 1971. "Recovery of Small Intestinal Structure and Function after Residence in the Tropics: I. Studies in Peace Corps Volunteers." *Annals of Internal Medicine* 74 (2): 218–22.

Lindenbaum, J., T. H. Kent, and H. Sprinz. 1966. "Malabsorption and Jejunitis in American Peace Corps Volunteers in Pakistan." *Annals of Internal Medicine* 65 (6): 1201–09.

Lindsay, S. W., T. C. Lindsay, J. Duprez, M. J. Hall, B. A. Kwambana, and others. 2012. "Chrysomya Putoria, a Putative Vector of Diarrheal Diseases." *PLoS Neglected Tropical Diseases* 6: e1895. doi:10.1371/journal.pntd.0001895.

Liu, L., K. Hill, S. Oza, D. Hogan, S. Cousens, and others. 2016. "Levels and Causes of Mortality under Age Five Years." In *Disease Control Priorities* (third edition): Volume 2, *Reproductive, Maternal, Newborn, and Child Health*, edited by R. Black, R. Laxminarayan, M. Temmerman, and N. Walker. Washington, DC: World Bank.

Liu, L., S. Oza, D. Hogan, J. Perin, I. Rudan, and others. 2015. "Global, Regional, and National Causes of Child Mortality in 2000–13, with Projections to Inform Post-2015 Priorities: An Updated Systematic Analysis." *The Lancet* 385 (9832): 430–40.

Longini, I. M. Jr, A. Nizam, M. Ali, M. Yunus, N. Shenvi, and J. D. Clemens. 2007. "Controlling Endemic Cholera with Oral Vaccines." *PLoS Medicine* 4: e336.

Luby, S. P., M. Agboatwalla, D. R. Feikin, J. Painter, W. Billhimer, and others. 2005. "Effect of Handwashing on Child Health: A Randomised Controlled Trial." *The Lancet* 366 (9481): 225–33.

Luby, S. P., M. Agboatwalla, J. Painter, A. Altaf, W. Billhimer, and others. 2006. "Combining Drinking Water Treatment and Hand Washing for Diarrhoea Prevention: A Cluster Randomised Controlled Trial." *Tropical Medicine and International Health* 11 (4): 479–89.

Luby, S. P., M. Agboatwalla, J. Painter, A. Altaf, W. L. Billhimer, and R. M. Hoekstra. 2004. "Effect of Intensive Handwashing Promotion on Childhood Diarrhea in High-Risk Communities in Pakistan: A Randomized Controlled Trial." *Journal of the American Medical Association* 291 (21): 2547–54.

Luby, S. P., A. K. Halder, T. Huda, L. Unicomb, and R. B. Johnston. 2011. "The Effect of Handwashing at Recommended Times with Water Alone and with Soap on Child Diarrhea in Rural Bangladesh: An Observational Study." *PLoS Med* 8: e1001052. doi:10.1371/journal.pmed.1001052.

MacPherson, D. W., B. D. Gushulak, W. B. Baine, S. Bala, P. O. Gubbins, and others. 2009. "Population Mobility, Globalization, and Antimicrobial Drug Resistance." *Emerging Infectious Diseases* 15 (11): 1727–32.

Malhotra, N., and R. P. Upadhyay. 2013. "Why Are There Delays in Seeking Treatment for Childhood Diarrhoea in India?" *Acta Paediatrica* 102 (9): e413–18. doi:10.1111/apa.12304.

Mazumder, S., S. Taneja, N. Bhandari, B. Dube, R. C. Agarwal, and others. 2010. "Effectiveness of Zinc Supplementation Plus Oral Rehydration Salts for Diarrhoea in Infants Aged Less than 6 Months in Haryana State, India." *Bulletin of the World Health Organization* 88: 754–60.

Mendelsohn, A. S., J. R. Asirvatham, D. Mkaya Mwamburi, T. V. Sowmynarayanan, and others. 2008. "Estimates of the Economic Burden of Rotavirus-Associated and All-Cause Diarrhoea in Vellore, India." *Tropical Medicine and International Health* 13 (7): 934–42.

Mondal, D., J. Minak, M. Alam, Y. Liu, J. Dai, and others. 2012. "Contribution of Enteric Infection, Altered Intestinal Barrier Function, and Maternal Malnutrition to Infant Malnutrition in Bangladesh." *Clinical Infectious Diseases* 54 (2): 185–92.

Moore, S. R., N. L. Lima, A. M. Soares, R. B. Oriá, R. C. Pinkerton, and others. 2010. "Prolonged Episodes of Acute Diarrhea Reduce Growth and Increase Risk of Persistent Diarrhea in Children." *Gastroenterology* 139 (4): 1156–64.

Mota, M. I., M. P. Gadea, S. González, G. González, L. Pardo, and others. 2010. "Bacterial Pathogens Associated with Bloody Diarrhea in Uruguayan Children." *Revista Argentina de Microbiologia* 42 (2): 114–17.

Munos, M. K., C. L. Fischer Walker, and R. E. Black. 2010. "The Effect of Oral Rehydration Solution and Recommended Home Fluids on Diarrhoea Mortality." *International Journal of Epidemiology* 39 (Suppl 1): 175–87.

Nasrin, D., Y. Wu, W. C. Blackwelder, T. H. Farag, D. Saha, and others. 2013. "Health Care Seeking for Childhood Diarrhea in Developing Countries: Evidence from Seven Sites in Africa and Asia." *American Journal of Tropical Medicine and Hygiene* 89 (Suppl 1): 3–12.

Newman, R. D., S. R. Moore, A. A. Lima, J. P. Nataro, R. L. Guerrant, and others. 2001. "A Longitudinal Study of *Giardia lamblia* Infection in North-East Brazilian Children." *Tropical Medicine and International Health* 6 (8): 624–34.

Newman, R. D., C. L. Sears, J. P. Nataro, D. P. Fedorko, T. Wuhib, and others. 2000. "Persistent Diarrhea Signals a Critical Period of Increased Diarrhea Burdens and Nutritional Shortfalls: A Prospective Cohort Study among Children in Northeastern Brazil." *Journal of Infectious Diseases* 181 (5): 1643–51.

O'Ryan, M., V. Prado, and L. K. Pickering. 2005. "A Millennium Update on Pediatric Diarrheal Illness in the Developing World." *Seminars in Pediatric Infectious Diseases* 16 (2): 125–36.

Okeke, I. N. 2009. "Cholera Vaccine Will Reduce Antibiotic Use." *Science* 325 (5941): 326.

Patel, M. M., M. A. Widdowson, R. I. Glass, K. Akazawa, J. Vinjé, and others. 2008. "Systematic Literature Review of Role of Noroviruses in Sporadic Gastroenteritis." *Emerging Infectious Diseases* 14 (8): 1224–31.

Pattanayak, S. K., J. C. Yang, K. L. Dickinson, C. Poulos, S. R. Patil, and others. 2009. "Shame or Subsidy Revisited: Social Mobilization for Sanitation in Orissa, India." *Bulletin of the World Health Organization* 87 (8): 580–87.

Peterson, K. M., J. Buss, R. Easley, Z. Yang, P. S. Korpe, and others. 2013. "REG1B as a Predictor of Childhood Stunting in Bangladesh and Peru." *American Journal of Clinical Nutrition* 97 (5): 1129–33.

Prado, M. S., S. Cairncross, A. Strina, M. L. Barreto, A. M. Oliveira-Assis, and others. 2005. "Asymptomatic Giardiasis and Growth in Young Children: A Longitudinal Study in Salvador, Brazil." *Parasitology* 131 (Pt 1): 51–56.

Prendergast, A., and P. Kelly. 2012. "Review: Enteropathies in the Developing World: Neglected Effects on Global Health." *American Journal of Tropical Medicine and Hygiene* 86 (5): 756–63.

Raqib, R., A. A. Lindberg, B. Wrwetlind, P. K. Bardhan, U. Andersson, and others. 1995. "Persistence of Local Cytokine Production in Shigellosis in Acute and Convalescent Stages." *Infection and Immunity* 63 (1): 289–96.

Risk, R., H. Naismith, A. Burnett, S. E. Moore, M. Cham, and S. Unger. 2013. "Rational Prescribing in Paediatrics in a Resource-Limited Setting." *Archives of Disease in Childhood* 98 (7): 503–9.

Robberstad, B., T. Strand, R. E. Black, and H. Sommerfelt. 2004. "Cost-Effectiveness of Zinc as Adjunct Therapy for Acute Childhood Diarrhoea in Developing Countries." *Bulletin of the World Health Organization* 82 (7): 523–31.

Rouzier, V., K. Severe, M. A. Juste, M. Peck, C. Perodin, and others. 2013. "Cholera Vaccination in Urban Haiti." *American Journal of Tropical Medicine and Hygiene* 89 (4): 671–81.

Ryan, E. T., U. Dhar, W. A. Khan, M. A. Salam, A. S. Faruque, and others. 2000. "Mortality, Morbidity, and Microbiology of Endemic Cholera among Hospitalized Patients in Dhaka, Bangladesh." *American Journal of Tropical Medicine and Hygiene* 63 (1–2): 12–20.

Sachdev, H. P., N. K. Mittal, and H. S. Yadav. 1990. "Oral Zinc Supplementation in Persistent Diarrhea in Infants." *Annals of Tropical Paediatrics* 10 (1): 63–69.

Salomon, J. B., L. J. Mata, and J. E. Gordon. 1968. "Malnutrition and the Common Communicable Diseases of Childhood in Rural Guatemala." *American Journal of Public Health* 58 (3): 505–16.

Santini, A., E. Novellino, V. Armini, and A. Ritieni. 2013. "State of the Art of Ready-to-Use Therapeutic Food: A Tool for Nutraceuticals Addition to Foodstuff." *Food Chemistry* 140 (4): 843–49. doi:10.1016/j.foodchem.2012.10.098.

Santosham, M., A. Chandran, S. Fitzwater, C. Fischer Walker, A. H. Baqui, and others. 2010. "Progress and Barriers for the Control of Diarrhoeal Disease." *The Lancet* 376 (9734): 63–67.

Schoonees, A., M. Lombard, A. Musekiwa, E. Nel, and J. Volmink. 2013. "Ready-to-Use Therapeutic Food for Home-Based Treatment of Severe Acute Malnutrition in Children from Six Months to Five Years of Age." *Cochrane Database of Systematic Reviews* 6: CD009000. doi:10.1002/14651858.CD009000.pub2.

Shankar, A. H., and A. S. Prasad. 1998. "Zinc and Immune Function: The Biological Basis of Altered Resistance to Infection." *American Journal of Clinical Nutrition* 68 (Suppl 2): 447S–63S.

Snyder, J. D., and M. E. Merson. 1982. "The Magnitude of the Global Problem of Acute Diarrhoeal Disease: A Review of Active Surveillance Data." *Bulletin of the World Health Organization* 60 (4): 605–13.

Sowmyanarayanan, T. V., T. Patel, R. Sarkar, S. Broor, S. D. Chitambar, and others. 2012. "Direct Costs of Hospitalization for Rotavirus Gastroenteritis in Different Health Facilities in India." *Indian Journal of Medical Research* 136 (1): 68–73.

Spears, D. 2013. "How Much International Variation in Child Height Can Sanitation Explain?" Policy Research Working Paper WPS 6351, World Bank, Washington, DC. http://go.worldbank.org/SZE5WUJBI0.

Steenland, M. W., G. A. Joseph, M. A. Lucien, N. Freeman, M. Hast, and others. 2013. "Laboratory-Confirmed Cholera and Rotavirus among Patients with Acute Diarrhea in Four Hospitals in Haiti, 2012–2013." *American Journal of Tropical Medicine and Hygiene* 89 (4): 641–46.

Stenberg, K., K. Sweeny, H. Axelson, and P. Sheehan. 2016. "Returns on Investment in the Continuum of Care for Reproductive, Maternal, Newborn, and Child Health." In *Disease Control Priorities* (third edition): Volume 2, *Reproductive, Maternal, Newborn, and Child Health,* edited by R. Black, R. Laxminarayan, M. Temmerman, and N. Walker. Washington, DC: World Bank.

Strand, T. A., P. R. Sharma, H. K. Gjessing, M. Ulak, R. K. Chandyo, and others. 2012. "Risk Factors for Extended Duration of Acute Diarrhea in Young Children." *PLoS One* 7: e36436. doi:10.1371/journal.pone.0036436.

Tatem, A. J., D. J. Rogers, and S. I. Hay. 2006. "Global Transport Networks and Infectious Disease Spread." *Advances in Parasitology* 62: 293–343.

Thomas, J. E., A. Dale, J. E. Bunn, M. Harding, W. A. Coward, and others. 2004. "Early *Helicobacter pylori* Colonisation: The Association with Growth Faltering in The Gambia." *Archives of Disease in Childhood* 89 (12): 1149–54.

Thriemer, K., Y. Katuala, B. Batoko, J. P. Alworonga, H. Devlieger, and others. 2013. "Antibiotic Prescribing in DR Congo: A Knowledge, Attitude and Practice Survey among Medical Doctors and Students." *PLoS One* 8: e55495. doi:10.1371 /journal.pone.0055495.

Traa, B. S., C. L. Fischer Walker, M. Munos, and R. E. Black. 2010. "Antibiotics for the Treatment of Dysentery in Children." *International Journal of Epidemiology* 39 (Suppl 1): i70–74.

Veitch, A. M., P. Kelly, I. S. Zulu, I. Segal, and M. J. Farthing. 1991. "Tropical Enteropathy: A T-Cell-Mediated Crypt Hyperplastic Enteropathy." *European Journal of Gastroenterology and Hepatology* 13 (10): 1175–81.

Verguet, S., C. Pecenka, K. A. Johansson, S. T. Memirie, I. K. Friberg, and others. 2016. "Health Gains and Financial Risk Protection Afforded by Treatment and Prevention of Diarrhea and Pneumonia in Ethiopia: An Extended Cost-Effectiveness Analysis." In *Disease Control Priorities* (third edition): Volume 2, *Reproductive, Maternal, Newborn, and Child Health,* edited by R. Black, R. Laxminarayan, M. Temmerman, and N. Walker. Washington, DC: World Bank.

Waldor, M. K., P. J. Hotez, and J. D. Clemens. 2010. "A National Cholera Vaccine Stockpile—A New Humanitarian and Diplomatic Resource." *New England Journal of Medicine* 363 (24): 2279–82.

WHO (World Health Organization). 2010. "Medicines: Rational Use of Medicines." Fact Sheet 338. http://www .wiredhealthresources.net/WHO-FS_MedicinesRational Use.pdf.

———. 2012. "Cholera." Fact Sheet 107. http://www.who.int /mediacentre/factsheets/fs107/en.

———. 2013. "Oral Cholera Vaccine Stockpile." http://www .who.int/cholera/vaccines/ocv_stockpile_2013/en/index .html.

WHO and UNICEF (United Nations Children's Fund). 2004. *Clinical Management of Acute Diarrhoea.* New York: WHO and UNICEF.

———. 2009. *Diarrhoea: Why Children Are Still Dying and What Can Be Done.* Geneva: WHO and UNICEF.

———. 2013. *Progress on Sanitation and Drinking-Water, 2013 Update: Joint Monitoring Programme for Water Supply and Sanitation.* Geneva: WHO and UNICEF. http://www .who.int/water_sanitation_health/publications/2013/jmp _report/en/index.html.

WHO, UNICEF, and World Bank. 2009. *State of the World's Vaccines and Immunization.* 3rd ed. Geneva: WHO.

Wilson, S. E., C. T. Ouédraogo, L. Prince, A. Ouédraogo, S. Y. Hess, and others. 2012. "Caregiver Recognition of Childhood Diarrhea, Care Seeking Behaviors and Home Treatment Practices in Rural Burkina Faso: A Cross-Sectional Survey." *PLoS One* 7: e33273. doi:10.1371/journal .pone.0033273.

Windle, H. J., D. Kelleher, and J. E. Crabtree. 2007. "Childhood *Helicobacter pylori* Infection and Growth Impairment in Developing Countries: A Vicious Cycle?" *Pediatrics* 119 (3): e754–59.

Wood, G. M., J. C. Gearty, and B. T. Cooper. 1991. "Small Bowel Morphology in British Indian and Afro-Caribbean Subjects: Evidence of Tropical Enteropathy." *Gut* 32 (3): 256–59.

Yakoob, M. Y., E. Theodoratou, A. Jabeen, A. Imdad, T. P. Eisele, and others. 2011. "Preventive Zinc Supplementation in Developing Countries: Impact on Mortality and Morbidity Due to Diarrhea, Pneumonia and Malaria." *BMC Public Health* 11 (Suppl 3): S23. doi:10.1186/1471-2458-11-S3-S23.

Zwisler, G., E. Simpson, and M. Moodley. 2013. "Treatment of Diarrhea in Young Children: Results from Surveys on the Perception and Use of Oral Rehydration Solutions, Antibiotics, and Other Therapies in India and Kenya." *Journal of Global Health* 3 (1): 010403. doi:10.7189/jogh.03.010403.

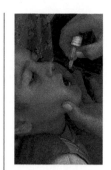

Chapter **10**

Vaccines for Children in Low- and Middle-Income Countries

Daniel R. Feikin, Brendan Flannery, Mary J. Hamel,
Meghan Stack, and Peter M. Hansen

INTRODUCTION

Vaccination is the centerpiece of preventive care of the well child. Vaccination has been one of the singular public health successes of the past half century, and its full potential remains unrealized. Pneumonia and diarrhea, two of the leading causes of child mortality, account for approximately 1.4 million deaths annually (Liu and others 2016); vaccination with currently available vaccines has the potential to prevent 59 percent of pneumonia-related deaths and 29 percent of diarrhea-related deaths (Fischer Walker, Munos, and Black 2013). Other leading causes of childhood deaths are already preventable through available and effective vaccines, such as measles and meningitis, and other diseases, such as malaria, may become vaccine preventable in the near future (Agnandji and others 2011; Liu and others 2012). Forecasts for vaccine use in the 73 countries supported by Gavi, the Vaccine Alliance, project that 17.7 million deaths will be averted in children under age five years as a result of vaccinations administered from 2011 to 2020 (Lee and others 2013). Childhood vaccination contributed greatly to progress made toward achieving the fourth United Nations Millennium Development Goal, a two-thirds reduction in childhood mortality between 1990 and 2015 (UN 2015), and the centerpiece of several other major global initiatives (PHR 2014; WHO 2012a). Vaccination is central to the health goal included in the post-2015 Sustainable Development Goals, which is on a critical pathway to delivering on its targets.

In addition to the clear health benefits, vaccination has been one of the most cost-effective public health interventions (Brenzel and others 2006; WHO, UNICEF, and World Bank 2002). Based on 2001 data, the cost per death averted through routine vaccination with the six original antigens in the Expanded Program on Immunization (EPI) was US$205 in South Asia and Sub-Saharan Africa; estimated cost per disability-adjusted life year (DALY) averted was US$7 to US$16 (Brenzel and others 2006). New vaccines, although more expensive, have also been determined to be cost-effective in Gavi-eligible countries (Atherly and others 2012; Sinha and others 2007) (see box 10.1).

This chapter describes the epidemiology and burden of vaccine-preventable diseases and provides estimates of the value of vaccines in health impact as well as broader economic benefits. The focus is on vaccination of infants during routine well-child visits and not on other important vaccines for older children and young adults, such as human papillomavirus vaccine, typhoid vaccine, and dengue vaccines.

Corresponding author: Daniel R. Feikin, Chief, Epidemiology Branch/Division of Viral Diseases, Centers for Disease Control and Prevention, Atlanta, Georgia, United States; drf0@cdc.gov.

Gavi, The Vaccine Alliance

Disparities exist in vaccination status between countries and within the same country, where some regions or sectors of society remain substantially undervaccinated. For example, in Nigeria's 2008 Demographic and Health Survey, the coverage of the third dose of the diphtheria-tetanus-pertussis vaccine varied from 67 percent in the southeast to 9 percent in the northwest (NPC and ICF Macro 2009). Disparities are largely driven by socioeconomic status; the poorest children, with the highest disease burden, are the least vaccinated (Cutts, Izurieta, and Rhoda 2013).

To address low coverage and inequitable access to life-saving vaccines, Gavi, the Vaccine Alliance was launched in 2000 to increase access to immunization in poor countries. Gavi is a public-private partnership involving the World Health Organization (WHO), the United Nations Children's Fund, and the World Bank; civil society organizations; public health institutes; donors and implementing country governments; major private philanthropists, such as the Bill & Melinda Gates Foundation; vaccine manufacturers; and the financial community (Gavi 2013). Gavi's support for 2011–15 has focused on 73 countries based on eligibility criteria determined through per capita gross national income.

Gavi has expanded its initial support for hepatitis B, pentavalent, and yellow fever vaccines to include measles vaccine second dose and those against pneumococcus, rotavirus, meningococcus serogroup A, measles-rubella, human papillomavirus, Japanese encephalitis, and inactivated polio vaccine. Gavi has approved a contribution to the global cholera stockpile for use in epidemic and endemic settings. From its inception through 2014, Gavi has committed US$8.8 billion in program support to eligible countries; 75 percent of the total commitment is for the purchase of vaccines. From 2000 through early 2015, Gavi-supported vaccines have helped countries vaccinate approximately 500 million children through routine programs. Annex table 10A.3 shows the vaccine introduction status in 73 Gavi-eligible countries.

Advanced Market Commitment

An innovative financing mechanism called the Advanced Market Commitment was established to accelerate the introduction of and scale up the pneumococcal conjugate vaccine through Gavi (Cernuschi and others 2011). The Advanced Market Commitment secured US$1.5 billion from six donor countries and the Bill & Melinda Gates Foundation, which provided a financial commitment to purchase pneumococcal conjugate vaccine for introduction and scale-up in Gavi-supported countries at predetermined terms.

Eligibility and Transition to Self-Financing

As of January 2014, per capita gross national income in 17 of 73 Gavi-supported countries had risen above the eligibility threshold, resulting in a five-year transition period during which such countries finance an increasingly larger share of their vaccines each year. These countries need to mobilize domestic resources to sustainably finance their vaccines when they complete the transition to self-financing.

Vaccine Investment Strategy

Gavi uses a vaccine investment strategy to determine which vaccines to add to its portfolio of support to countries every five years, taking into account the selection criteria and the date when different vaccines will be available. The Gavi Board decided in 2014 that Gavi will undertake the following:

- *Yellow fever.* Increase support for additional yellow fever campaigns.
- *Cholera.* Contribute to a global vaccine stockpile from 2014 to 2018 to increase access in outbreak situations and further a learning agenda on its use in endemic settings.
- *Malaria.* Consider supporting the vaccine that is now in development when it is licensed, WHO-prequalified, and recommended for use by the joint meeting of the WHO Strategic Advisory Group of Experts on Immunization and the Malaria Policy Advisory Committee.

box continues next page

Box 10.1 (continued)

- *Rabies and influenza.* Recommend further assessment of the impact and operational feasibility of supporting rabies and influenza vaccines for pregnant women, fund an observational study to address critical knowledge gaps around access to rabies vaccine, and monitor the evolving evidence base for maternal influenza vaccination.

By forecasting and pooling demand from eligible countries and purchasing large volumes of vaccines, Gavi has created a reliable market for vaccines in these settings. Gavi's market-shaping strategy aims to ensure adequate supply to meet demand,

minimize the cost of vaccines, and ensure the availability of quality and innovative products.

Improved vaccine delivery strategies are needed to ensure that immunization programs and health systems are able to implement programs of increasing size and complexity at high levels of coverage and equity. It will be necessary to build on the unprecedented momentum achieved in new vaccine introduction and market shaping to take to scale innovative approaches to generating demand for immunization; upgrading country supply chain management systems; strengthening country health information systems; and enhancing political will and country capacity related to leadership, management, and coordination.

METHODS

We describe vaccines in three categories:

- Vaccines among the six original EPI antigens: Bacille Calmette-Guérin (BCG); diphtheria, tetanus, and pertussis (DTP); and measles and polio
- Vaccines classified as new or underutilized and supported by Gavi since its inception in 2000
- New vaccines that might be introduced into routine immunization for infants at the well-child visit in the next decade.

For the epidemiology and vaccine characteristics, we used a nonsystematic review of the published literature, recommendations of the World Health Organization (WHO), and a search of relevant updated websites on vaccines. For the impact of vaccination using the original EPI vaccines, we referenced existing models. For the new vaccines, we used a methodology adopted through an expert process, with leading modeling groups co-convened by Gavi and the Bill & Melinda Gates Foundation, to estimate the number of future deaths and DALYs averted attributable to vaccinations administered in the 73 Gavi-supported countries (annex 10A and table 10A.1).

EXPANDED PROGRAM ON IMMUNIZATIONS

The EPI program was created in 1974 to improve vaccine availability globally (WHO 1974). Global policies and recommended schedules based on immunologic data

were codified in 1984, with the goal of reaching every child with vaccines against six diseases: diphtheria, pertussis, tetanus, measles, poliomyelitis, and tuberculosis (Hadler and others 2004; Mitchell and others 2013). The fulcrum of the EPI program is the fixed health facility, where parents bring their children to be immunized.

The immunization visit has been expanded into the well-child visit, where the contact with the health system is used to add other preventive interventions (for example, vitamin A and growth monitoring). Vaccination is also delivered in many low- and middle-income countries (LMICs) through modes and mechanisms outside the well-child visit, such as mobile outreach clinics, supplemental immunization activities as part of eradication and elimination campaigns, and mass vaccination for control of outbreaks.

VACCINE-PREVENTABLE DISEASES: EPIDEMIOLOGY, BURDEN, AND VACCINES

This section describes the epidemiology, burden, and vaccines available for vaccine-preventable diseases among children in LMICs. The section is divided into the six original EPI vaccines, new and underutilized vaccines introduced since 2000, and vaccines that might become more widely used in young children during the next decade (summarized in annex table 10A.2).

Original EPI Vaccines

Bacille Calmette-Guérin Vaccine
Tuberculosis is caused by the bacterium *Mycobacterium tuberculosis* and is spread from person to person through

the air; it primarily causes disease in the lung, although it can spread to many parts of the body. Infection with *M. tuberculosis* may lie dormant for years. In 2012, the WHO estimated a global burden of 8.6 million cases and 1.3 million deaths due to tuberculosis; 55,000 of these were in children under age five years, 95 percent of which occurred in LMICs. Co-infection with human immunodeficiency virus (HIV) greatly increases the risk of developing active tuberculosis. The treatment of tuberculosis worldwide is becoming more complicated because of the rise of multidrug-resistant strains (Bloom and others, forthcoming; Connelly Smith, Orme, and Starke 2013; WHO 2015a).

BCG vaccine is a live-attenuated strain of a related mycobacterium, *Mycobacterium bovis*, originally isolated from an infected cow and attenuated through repeated passage. BCG is most effective against tuberculous meningitis and disseminated (miliary) tuberculosis. However, BCG vaccination does not prevent *M. tuberculosis* infection in childhood, when most infections occur, or reactivation of latent infection and pulmonary tuberculosis later in life, which is the principal source of community transmission (WHO 2004). In 2012, BCG was included in routine infant immunization schedules in 159 of 194 WHO member states; worldwide coverage was estimated to be 90 percent in 2012 (WHO, UNICEF, and World Bank 2002). Approximately 100 million infants receive BCG annually; more than 4 billion people have been vaccinated (Connelly Smith, Orme, and Starke 2013). The 100 million BCG vaccinations given worldwide to infants in 2002 prevented approximately 30,000 cases of tuberculous meningitis and 11,000 cases of miliary tuberculosis (Trunz, Fine, and Dye 2006).

Vaccination is recommended for all infants in countries with high tuberculosis disease burden and infants at high risk of exposure in low-burden countries. Because it is a live-attenuated vaccine, BCG is not recommended for immunocompromised children, including those with congenital severe combined immunodeficiency syndrome and those with symptomatic HIV infection.

Tuberculosis will not be eliminated without new, more effective tuberculosis vaccines (Connelly Smith, Orme, and Starke 2013). For the prevention of severe childhood diseases, a single BCG dose is recommended as soon as possible after birth (WHO 2004). BCG is the only vaccine in the EPI program routinely administered by intradermal injection, which requires specific injection supplies and health care worker training. BCG is produced by a large number of countries using different vaccine seed strains, which may contribute to the variability in effectiveness observed in different studies.

Diphtheria, Tetanus, and Pertussis Vaccine

Despite progress, these three bacterial diseases of infancy and early childhood remain endemic in some countries. Diphtheria is a respiratory illness characterized by membranous inflammation of the upper respiratory tract caused by toxin-producing *Corynebacterium diphtheriae* and is transmitted through respiratory droplets and coughing. Before vaccination, an estimated 1 million cases and 50,000–60,000 deaths occurred annually (Walsh and Warren 1979). In 2008, only 7,000 cases of diphtheria were reported; more than 85 percent of these occurred in India (WHO and UNICEF 2014). Tetanus is caused by a toxin produced by *Clostridium tetani*, a ubiquitous organism found in the soil and transmitted through contamination of wounds or unsterile procedures, including care of the umbilical cord. Neonatal tetanus is mostly present in LMICs, resulting in an estimated 34,481 deaths in 2015 in children in LMICs, which account for 99 percent of all under-five tetanus deaths worldwide (Liu and others 2016). Pertussis, or whooping cough, is a highly communicable respiratory illness caused by *Bordetella pertussis* and characterized by paroxysmal cough that may last for many weeks. Estimates from the WHO suggest that about 63,000 children died from this disease in 2008, 95 percent of them in LMICs (Black and others 2010).

DTP vaccines are composed of inactivated diphtheria and tetanus toxins (referred to as toxoids) and pertussis antigens, either killed, whole-cell *Bordetella pertussis* or purified antigens (acellular pertussis [aP] vaccine). Whole-cell pertussis acts as a potent adjuvant that improves the immune response to diphtheria and tetanus toxoids, but periodic boosting is required because of waning immune responses; waning may occur more quickly with aP vaccines (Edwards and Decker 2013). DTP vaccines combined with hepatitis B and *Haemophilus influenzae* type b (Hib) antigens are widely used in LMICs, while combination vaccines with aP are common in upper-middle- and high-income countries. Because the risk of pertussis complications is highest in infants too young to be vaccinated, maternal vaccination is a strategy that could protect young infants (CDC 2011).

DTP vaccine coverage is an important indicator of immunization program performance. Initiatives to strengthen routine immunization services often monitor progress as measured by coverage with the third DTP dose (DTP3) in infancy, which requires multiple immunization visits in the first year of life. The difference between coverage with the first versus the third DTP dose, often called *dropout*, measures loss to follow-up and challenges to completion of infant vaccinations. Many newer vaccines, including pneumococcal, meningococcal, and rotavirus vaccines, have adapted to DTP immunization schedules to reach the maximum number of children during scheduled immunization visits.

DTP vaccines are included in routine childhood immunization programs in all 194 WHO member states. Global DTP3 coverage rose from 20 percent in 1980 to 84 percent in 2013 (WHO and UNICEF 2014), preventing 76,000 deaths from diphtheria and 1.6 million deaths from pertussis annually. In conjunction with improved maternal immunization against tetanus, the vaccines prevented approximately 408,000 deaths from tetanus (WHO 2013a). Despite increased coverage, more than 20 million infants remained unvaccinated in 2013 (WHO and UNICEF 2014). More than 80 percent of these children live in Gavi-eligible countries. If these countries achieved and maintained their DTP3 coverage at 90 percent between 2015 and 2020, 439,000 deaths and 16 million cases of pertussis could be averted during the 10 years from the scale-up (Stack and others 2011).

Polio Vaccine

The goal of universal polio vaccination is eradication. In 1988, when the Global Polio Eradication Initiative was established, poliomyelitis crippled more than 350,000 children each year, with transmission of wild poliovirus serotypes (1, 2, and 3) reported from 125 countries (WHO 2014c). From January to December 2015, only 66 cases of wild poliovirus type 1 were reported worldwide, compared with 359 cases in January to December 2014, and no cases of wild poliovirus had been reported on the African continent for 12 months; wild type 2 polioviruses have not been identified since 1999; and the last case of wild type 3 poliovirus occurred in 2012 (Global Polio Eradication Initiative 2013; WHO 2014b).

Implementation of routine childhood immunization and supplemental immunization activities with oral polio vaccine (OPV) containing attenuated polioviruses of all three types substantially decreased cases in LMICs and eliminated poliovirus circulation in the WHO regions of the Americas, Europe, Western Pacific, and South-East Asia. Clinical trials showed that three doses of OPV were needed for greater than 90 percent protection against paralytic poliomyelitis. However, the immune response was lower among children in LMICs, requiring more vaccine doses to achieve the high levels of population immunity necessary for elimination (Estívariz and others 2012; Grassly and others 2007). In 2014, the WHO recommended that all countries using OPV include at least one dose of inactivated polio vaccine (IPV) in their routine immunization schedule (WHO 2014c). Most immunization schedules in LMICs include a three-dose primary polio immunization schedule, and many include booster doses in the second year of life. For high-risk countries, the WHO recommends four doses beginning as soon as possible after birth, with at least one dose of IPV at age 14 weeks if only one IPV dose is given.

There are several steps to the Polio Eradication and Endgame Strategic Plan 2013–2018, and this transition in polio vaccination strategy has several phases. First, all OPV-using countries should introduce at least one dose of IPV (containing inactivated polioviruses of all three types) to boost immunity to poliovirus type 2 (WHO 2014b). Then, trivalent OPV will be replaced with more immunogenic bivalent OPV containing type 1 and 3 viruses. IPV introduction will pave the way for future total cessation of all OPV use after eradication has been achieved. Most high-income countries adopted routine childhood immunization with IPV to prevent rare cases of paralytic polio caused by OPV. However, achieving high coverage with IPV will require strengthening of routine immunization services.

Measles Vaccine

Measles is one of the most contagious diseases of humans (Fine and Mulholland 2013). It is caused by a paramyxovirus, manifesting as a febrile rash illness, which can result in multiple life-threatening complications, including pneumonia, diarrhea, and encephalitis. In 2000, measles was the leading vaccine-preventable cause of childhood deaths and the fifth leading cause of under-five mortality; that year, measles alone accounted for 5 percent of the estimated 10.9 million deaths among children under age five years (Strebel and others 2012). By 2010, measles-related deaths had declined by 75 percent following accelerated measles control activities in Sub-Saharan Africa and other regions (Simons and others 2012); declines in measles-related deaths accounted for almost 10.1 percent of overall declines in childhood mortality from 2000 to 2015 (Liu and others 2016). Further progress is expected as countries implement measles elimination strategies; as of 2014, all six WHO regions had established target dates for measles elimination.

Measles vaccination can prevent illness and death directly among vaccinated persons and indirectly among unvaccinated persons as a result of decreased transmission. In countries with ongoing transmission of measles and high risk of measles among infants, the WHO recommends vaccination at age nine months when protection provided by maternal antibody wanes and seroconversion rates improve among infants. In countries with low rates of measles transmission, the WHO recommends the first dose of vaccine at age 12 months to take advantage of higher seroconversion rates achieved at this age (Strebel and others 2012).

Between 1980 and 2011, global measles vaccination coverage rose from 18 percent to 84 percent globally (WHO 2013d; WHO, UNICEF, and World Bank 2002).

In one analysis, a projected 624 million children in Gavi-eligible countries would be vaccinated with one dose of measles-containing vaccine between 2011 and 2020, averting 10.3 million deaths relative to a hypothetical scenario in which countries were not administering measles vaccine (Lee and others 2013).

Because of its high risk of contagion, high levels of immunity are needed to interrupt measles transmission. A two-dose strategy is deemed essential for measles elimination, to immunize children who missed the first dose and protect up to 15 percent of children who do not seroconvert after primary immunization (WHO 2013d). Childhood immunization schedules in many countries include two doses. In countries with poor access to preventive services, the second opportunity for measles vaccination is most often provided through nationwide supplementary immunization activities or mass campaigns.

New and Underutilized Vaccines or Vaccine Strategies Supported by Gavi

Table 10.1 summarizes the large impact of vaccination for averting death and reducing disease burden in 73

countries receiving support from Gavi, with a focus on 10 new and previously underutilized vaccines. Expected impact is shown separately for vaccinations administered from 2001 to 2012 and vaccinations forecasted to be administered from 2013 to 2020. The total expected impact is shown as estimated numbers of persons immunized, as well as future deaths and DALYs averted. Estimates of future deaths and DALYs averted are based on a comparison of the number of deaths and DALYs expected over the lifetime of vaccinated cohorts relative to a hypothetical scenario in which the cohorts do not receive the vaccinations in question.

Hepatitis B Vaccine

Hepatitis B vaccine is included in routine infant immunization schedules to prevent serious disease and death later in life caused by chronic infection with hepatitis B virus, a member of the hepadnavirus family. Hepatitis B virus is a blood-borne pathogen that may also be transmitted sexually. Hepatitis B, one of five viruses known to cause hepatitis in humans, is responsible for most of the worldwide hepatitis burden: more than 2 billion people have been infected with hepatitis B virus, and 360 million have become chronically infected (WHO 2010b).

Table 10.1 Impact of Vaccination: Children Immunized and Deaths Averted in 73 Gavi-Supported Countries, Based on Strategic Demand Forecast Version 9

	Estimates for 2001–12			Projections for 2013–20		
	Children immunized	Deaths averted	DALYs averted	Children immunized	Future deaths averted	Future DALYs averted
Hepatitis B	377,000,000	3,400,000	99,000,000	480,000,000	3,700,000	109,000,000
Haemophilus influenzae type B	160,000,000	830,000	52,000,000	440,000,000	1,800,000	126,000,000
Japanese encephalitis (campaign)	83,000,000	19,000	1,000,000	71,000,000	9,000	1,100,000
Japanese encephalitis (routine)	21,000,000	6,000	840,000	93,000,000	20,000	3,300,000
Measles (routine 2nd dose)	71,000,000	90,000	6,000,000	350,000,000	220,000	14,000,000
Measles (campaign)	1,000,000,000	2,800,000	167,000,000	800,000,000	1,900,000	117,000,000
Meningitis A (campaign)	103,000,000	140,000	7,700,000	215,000,000	310,000	14,000,000
Meningitis A (routine)	n.a.	n.a.	n.a.	70,000,000	6,000	430,000
Pneumococcus	11,000,000	70,000	4,900,000	260,000,000	1,500,000	105,000,000
Rotavirus	4,000,000	4,000	320,000	230,000,000	380,000	24,000,000
Rubella (campaign)	105,000,000	20,000	1,800,000	650,000,000	190,000	18,000,000
Rubella (routine)	21,000,000	5,000	500,000	210,000,000	50,000	5,300,000
Yellow fever (campaign)	70,000,000	260,000	8,000,000	140,000,000	170,000	4,400,000
Yellow fever (routine)	84,000,000	540,000	21,000,000	120,000,000	570,000	23,000,000

Sources: Children immunized derived from the World Health Organization–United Nations Children's Fund Estimates of National Immunization Coverage and United Nations Population Division; vaccine introduction and scale-up scenario based on Gavi Strategic Demand Forecast Version 9; future deaths averted derived from Lee and others (2013); future DALYs averted derived from personal communication with S. Ozawa.
Note: Gavi = Gavi, the Vaccine Alliance; n.a. = not applicable; DALY = disability-adjusted life year.

Chronic hepatitis B virus infection is the leading cause of cirrhosis and cancer of the liver, which result in approximately 600,000 deaths annually (Goldstein and others 2005). Hepatitis B virus transmission may occur prenatally and during early childhood, adolescence, and adulthood. Vaccination is more than 95 percent effective in infants and more than 72 percent effective in preventing perinatal transmission. Vaccination must be part of a comprehensive prevention strategy. Humans are the only reservoir of hepatitis B virus, making disease elimination possible (WHO 2010b).

Modern hepatitis B vaccines containing recombinant hepatitis B virus surface antigen (HBsAg) were introduced in 1986 (Van Damme and others 2013). The WHO has recommended routine infant vaccination against hepatitis B since 1992. In 2013, hepatitis B vaccine was included in routine infant immunization schedules in 94 percent of 194 WHO member states. Infant immunization schedules include at least three doses of hepatitis B vaccine, which may be combined with other antigens, such as DTP and *Haemophilus influenzae* type b. In 2013, worldwide coverage with three doses of hepatitis B vaccine was estimated to be 81 percent. In countries with a high prevalence of hepatitis B virus infection, the WHO recommends administering the first dose within 24 hours of birth to prevent perinatal transmission. In 2013, 93 countries included hepatitis B birth dose in their routine immunization schedules, with global coverage estimated to be 38 percent. Better birth dose coverage and monitoring are needed; timely delivery of birth dose should be a performance measure of immunization programs (WHO 2013h).

Haemophilus influenzae Type b Vaccine

Haemophilus influenzae is a Gram-negative bacterium surrounded by a polysaccharide capsule, which is a major virulence factor. While six serotypes (a, b, c, d, e, f) and unencapsulated strains cause disease—including meningitis, pneumonia, septicemia, epiglottitis, cellulitis, septic arthritis, osteomyelitis, and otitis media (mainly due to unencapsulated *H. influenzae*)—Hib was the leading cause of meningitis in children under age five years in most countries before widespread vaccination (Bennett and others 2002). The mean case fatality rate (CFR) of Hib meningitis was 67 percent (44 percent to 75 percent) in Sub-Saharan Africa and 43 percent (23 percent to 55 percent) globally. In 2000, before widespread Hib vaccination, Hib caused an estimated 371,000 deaths (Watt and others 2009). By 2008, Hib vaccines were used in 136 countries, and estimated deaths had fallen to 203,000 (Black and others 2010; WHO 2013b).

Evidence from several clinical trials of Hib conjugate vaccine demonstrated the importance of Hib in causing severe pneumonia; Hib accounted for 25 percent of severe pneumonia in The Gambia and 22 percent in Chile (Levine and others 1999; Mulholland and others 1997). Hib pneumonia rates are higher than Hib meningitis rates; consequently, pneumonia accounted for the majority (79 percent) of the approximately 200,000 Hib-related deaths worldwide in children ages 1–59 months in 2010 (WHO 2013h).

The multiple formulations of Hib conjugate vaccines include several different conjugated proteins and combination vaccines, such as the most widely used pentavalent vaccine (DTP–Hepatitis B–Hib). Hib conjugate vaccines are more than 80 percent effective against Hib meningitis, sepsis, and bacteremic pneumonia; in most Sub-Saharan African countries that have introduced Hib vaccine into the national program, Hib disease has virtually disappeared (Adegbola and others 2005; Cowgill and others 2006; WHO 2006b). However, Hib vaccines likely have reduced efficacy in HIV-infected children, and evidence from South Africa suggests a booster dose might be required (Mangtani and others 2010). In many settings, three doses of Hib vaccine in infancy may control the disease and do not appear to increase rates of *H. influenzae* disease caused by serotypes other than type b (Ribeiro and others 2007; Zanella and others 2011). By 2013, 186 countries had introduced Hib vaccines, and as of 2014, all 73 Gavi countries vaccinated against Hib alongside hepatitis B, diphtheria, tetanus, and pertussis through the pentavalent vaccine as part of their routine infant immunization programs.

Future needs include introduction of Hib vaccine into countries that have not yet introduced it, particularly in Asia.

Pneumococcal Conjugate Vaccine

Streptococcus pneumoniae, the pneumococcus, is a Gram-positive encapsulated bacterium commonly found in the respiratory tract. Pneumococci are surrounded by polysaccharide capsules that confer serotype; more than 90 pneumococcal serotypes have been identified, although a limited number cause most disease. Pneumococcal disease is the leading bacterial cause of pneumonia in children and also causes meningitis and septicemia. The CFR of pneumococcal disease worldwide is approximately 5 percent (range 4 percent to 9 percent), but it is more than double that rate in Sub-Saharan Africa (CFR 11 percent; range 7 percent to 18 percent) (O'Brien and others 2009). About 90 percent of pneumococcal deaths are due to pneumonia. Pneumococcal meningitis, though rare, has a higher CFR of 59 percent (range 27 percent to 80 percent); it can be as high as 73 percent in Sub-Saharan Africa. Before widespread pneumococcal conjugate vaccination, pneumococcus caused an estimated 826,000 deaths (O'Brien and others 2009) in 2000, and 541,000 deaths among children younger than age five years worldwide in 2008 (WHO 2013b).

Pneumococcal conjugate vaccines are at least 80 percent effective against meningitis, septicemia, and bacteremic pneumonia (Lucero and others 2009); like Hib vaccines, pneumococcal conjugates likely have reduced efficacy in HIV-infected children (Klugman and others 2003). Two pneumococcal conjugate vaccines are currently commercially available; one contains the conjugated polysaccharides of 10 serotypes, and the other contains 13 serotypes. Evidence suggests that declines in disease caused by vaccine serotypes with pneumococcal conjugate vaccine use may be partially offset by increased disease due to nonvaccine serotypes (referred to as *serotype replacement*); however, according to one meta-analysis of invasive pneumococcal disease in high-income countries, childhood vaccination resulted in 50 percent reductions in pneumococcal disease overall, despite some serotype replacement (Feikin and others 2013). Introduction of pneumococcal conjugate vaccine into Asian countries has lagged Gavi-supported introduction into Africa.

Rotavirus Vaccine

Rotavirus, a member of the reovirus family, causes watery diarrhea that can lead to dehydration and death. It is the leading cause of childhood diarrhea-related mortality worldwide (Parashar and others 2003), responsible for an estimated 453,000 deaths in 2008 (Tate and others 2012). Rotavirus accounts for 35 percent to 50 percent of acute severe diarrhea in children, varying by region (Mwenda and others 2010), with the highest proportions in children younger than age one year (Kotloff and others 2013). Unlike bacterial and parasitic causes of diarrhea, the occurrence of rotavirus diarrhea is not higher in settings with poor water, sanitation, and hygiene. A recent study of moderate-to-severe diarrhea in seven low-income settings found a CFR from rotavirus presenting to a health facility of 2.5 percent (Kotloff and others 2013). This figure is higher in areas without good access to health care (Feikin and others 2012) (see Keusch and others 2016, chapter 9 in this volume).

Two rotavirus vaccines are commercially available (WHO 2009). Both have been efficacious in randomized controlled trials in low-income settings, with efficacies generally ranging from 50 percent to 80 percent against rotavirus diarrhea; the lowest efficacy was seen in lower-socioeconomic, higher-mortality countries (Armah and others 2010; Madhi and others 2010). Nonetheless, because of higher rates of disease in these countries, the number of serious rotavirus infections prevented is likely to be higher, and the WHO strongly recommends rotavirus vaccine use in these countries

(WHO 2009). Lower-cost rotavirus vaccines are still needed (Bharat Biotech 2011). Infants who receive rotavirus vaccines have a slightly elevated risk of a rare but serious condition called *intussusception*, which can result in potentially fatal bowel obstruction, although increased incidence of intussusception is small relative to the overall impact of the vaccine (Patel and others 2012; Patel and others 2011). Future needs include development of vaccines with improved efficacy in high-burden countries and introduction of rotavirus vaccine into high-burden Asian countries.

Rubella Vaccine

The rubella virus, a member of the togavirus family, is one of the most teratogenic viruses known. In the absence of vaccination, rubella is a common cause of febrile rash illness in children, often misdiagnosed as measles. Infection of susceptible women early in pregnancy can result in miscarriage, fetal death, or a constellation of congenital defects known as congenital rubella syndrome (CRS) in up to 90 percent of infected infants. The incidence of rubella and CRS has been reduced in many high-burden countries following implementation of rubella vaccination strategies.

The goal of rubella vaccination in high-burden countries is to prevent the substantial disease burden associated with CRS. It is estimated that more than 100,000 CRS cases occur worldwide each year (Vynnycky, Gay, and Cutts 2003). Through 2013, 137 countries have included rubella-containing vaccines in national immunization schedules; the introduction of rubella vaccination in Asia and Sub-Saharan Africa lags other regions (WHO 2011b). Live-attenuated rubella virus vaccines were first licensed in 1970, but they were not included in EPI programs because of concerns that suboptimal vaccine coverage could delay age at natural rubella virus infection and result in higher incidence among women of childbearing age, paradoxically increasing the risk of CRS. Since 2011, the WHO has recommended introduction of rubella vaccination strategies as part of measles control and elimination activities, taking advantage of the availability of combined measles-rubella (MR) and measles-mumps-rubella (MMR) vaccines (WHO 2011b).

The preferred strategy for the introduction of rubella vaccination is to begin with MR/MMR vaccine in a campaign targeting a wide range of ages, in combination with universal childhood vaccination (Reef and Plotkin 2013). The first dose of combined MR vaccine can be delivered at age 9 months or 12 months, depending on the level of measles virus transmission (WHO 2011b). The effectiveness is at least 95 percent, even at age 9 months; only one dose of rubella vaccine is required to achieve rubella elimination if high coverage is achieved (WHO 2011b).

Meningococcal Meningitis Serogroup A Conjugate Vaccine

Neisseria meningitidis, also referred to as the meningococcus, is a Gram-negative encapsulated bacterium transmitted by respiratory droplets that can cause severe bloodstream infections and meningitis; it is the leading cause of bacterial meningitis in many LMICs. Explosive outbreaks of meningococcal meningitis occur with high attack rates and case fatality across broad age ranges. Six *N. meningitidis* serogroups (A, B, C, W, X, Y) cause almost all cases, although prevalence varies temporally and geographically. Sub-Saharan African countries from Senegal to Ethiopia in a zone referred to as *the meningitis belt* have experienced frequent and devastating epidemics of meningococcal meningitis, most often caused by serogroup A meningococcal strains. From 1993 to 2012, countries in the meningitis belt reported nearly 1 million meningitis cases, including 100,000 deaths (WHO 2013f).

Meningococcal vaccines prevent diseases caused by specific serogroups: vaccines against serogroups A, C, W, and Y contain purified polysaccharide alone or conjugated to carrier proteins (based on diphtheria or tetanus toxoids), while serogroup B vaccines contain outer membrane vesicles extracted from outbreak strains with the addition of recombinant proteins. Conjugate vaccines provide better long-lasting immunity, particularly in children younger than age two years, and indirect protection of unvaccinated groups through the reduction of disease transmission. Meningococcal conjugate vaccines have been introduced into routine immunization programs in many high-burden countries. In 2010, a serogroup A meningococcal conjugate vaccine developed by the Meningitis Vaccine Project, with funding from the Bill & Melinda Gates Foundation, was licensed for use in countries in the meningitis belt (LaForce and Okwo-Bele 2011). In the Sub-Saharan African meningitis belt, the WHO recommends mass vaccination of the population ages 1–29 years (WHO 2011a), a highly effective strategy for prevention of serogroup A meningococcal disease (Novak and others 2012), followed by routine childhood vaccination with a single dose at age 9–18 months (WHO 2015b).

Yellow Fever Vaccine

Yellow fever is a viral hemorrhagic fever that was one of the most feared epidemic diseases in the world before vaccination. Despite the availability of an effective vaccine, yellow fever continues to cause an estimated 84,000 to 170,000 severe cases annually, with 29,000 to 60,000 deaths (WHO 2013e). Most reported cases and deaths occur in 31 endemic Sub-Saharan African countries with a total population of 610 million, more than 33 percent of whom live in urban settings. Since the 1980s, yellow fever has reemerged in some areas or appeared for the first time in others.

Yellow fever vaccines contain live-attenuated virus and have been used since the 1930s (Monath and others 2013). Routine infant immunization against yellow fever is only recommended in 44 at-risk countries and territories, of which 35 included yellow fever vaccine in their routine infant immunization schedules in 2013. A single dose of yellow fever vaccine at age nine months or later is assumed to provide lifelong immunity.

Japanese Encephalitis Vaccine

Japanese encephalitis (JE) is the most common cause of viral encephalitis in Asia (WHO 2013c). JE virus, a flavivirus, is transmitted by mosquitoes in natural cycles involving domestic pigs or water birds; human disease is common in areas with rice cultivation and pig farming. Of the estimated 67,900 annual cases in the 24 endemic countries, 51,000 (75 percent) occur in children ages 0–14 years, resulting in about 10,000 deaths and 15,000 cases of long-term neuropsychiatric sequelae (Campbell and others 2011). Reported cases underestimate geographic distribution of risk because of underreporting and occurrence of disease in less than 1 percent of human infections (Halstead, Jacobson, and Dubischar-Kastner 2013). In recent decades, outbreaks have occurred in several previously nonendemic areas.

The WHO recommends the introduction of JE immunization through EPI programs in areas where JE constitutes a public health problem (WHO 2006a). In 2012, JE vaccines were used in immunization programs in 11 (46 percent) of 24 at-risk countries (WHO 2013c). The most effective strategy for controlling JE has been to conduct wide age-range (catch-up) vaccination followed by routine infant immunization. In upper-middle- and high-income economies—including Japan; the Republic of Korea; and Taiwan, China—routine immunization since 1965 using inactivated, mouse-brain-derived vaccine has successfully controlled the disease (Halstead, Jacobson, and Dubischar-Kastner 2013). However, disadvantages of the mouse-brain vaccine include the need for multiple doses, frequent boosting, and high prices (WHO 2006a). In 2013, the WHO and the United Nations Children's Fund approved a live-attenuated JE vaccine from a Chinese manufacturer based on the SA 14-14-2 strain, which induces protection for several years after one or two doses (WHO 2013g). Approval of the live-attenuated JE vaccine should increase access in endemic countries.

Additional and Future Vaccines with Potential Public Health Impacts in Young Children

Malaria Vaccine

Approximately 198 million malaria cases and 584,000 malaria deaths occurred globally in 2013; most deaths were in young children living in Sub-Saharan Africa (WHO 2015c). *Plasmodium falciparum* is the most virulent of the five *Plasmodium* species that cause human malaria. The RTS,S/AS01 candidate malaria vaccine is a partially effective vaccine that targets the pre-erythrocytic stage of the *P. falciparum* parasite resulting in a reduction in the number of clinical malaria episodes experienced. RTS,S/AS01 recently underwent testing in a large phase 3 clinical trial, the final stage before licensure. In total, 15,460 children and young infants participated in the trial, which was conducted at 11 sites in seven Sub-Saharan African countries across a wide range of malaria transmission levels (RTS,S Clinical Trials Partnership 2015). Among children ages 5–17 months at first vaccination followed for a median of 48 months, RTS,S/AS01 vaccine efficacy against clinical malaria was 37 percent (95 percent confidence interval 32–41) when the primary vaccination series of three doses administered monthly was followed by a booster given 18 months after the primary vaccination series, and 28 percent (95 percent confidence interval 23–33) when no booster was given. Vaccine efficacy was lower in young infants who received the primary vaccination series coadministered with EPI vaccines beginning at ages 6–12 weeks: 26 percent (95 percent confidence interval 20–32) with a booster and 18 percent (95 percent confidence interval 12–24) without. Despite modest efficacy estimates, the impact was substantial: 1,774 cases of clinical malaria were averted per 1,000 children vaccinated when a booster was administered; 1,363 cases were averted without a booster. The number of cases averted per 1,000 young infants was 983 in those who received a booster and 558 in those who did not. Meningitis and febrile seizures were reported more frequently in those who received the RTS,S/AS01 primary vaccination series than in those in the comparator group.

In July 2015, the European Medicines Agency issued a positive scientific opinion on RTS,S/AS01 for the prevention of malaria in children in Sub-Saharan Africa. Subsequently, the WHO's Strategic Advisory Group of Experts on Immunization and the Malaria Policy Advisory Committee reviewed the evidence on RTS,S/AS01 efficacy and safety as well as other relevant information surrounding vaccine implementation. In October 2015, the WHO advisory groups recommended the implementation of the vaccine through pilot projects designed to better understand how well the vaccine can be implemented and to further assess the relationship of safety signals to the vaccine (WHO 2015d). The WHO is considering these recommendations and was expected to provide guidance in early 2016. RTS,S/AS01 may become the first malaria vaccine licensed for use in children in Sub-Saharan African countries (RTS,S Clinical Trials Partnership 2015).

Influenza Vaccine

Influenza viruses are orthomyxoviruses that cause respiratory illness, ranging from mild febrile illness to severe pneumonia. Because influenza viruses change rapidly, vaccines are reformulated and delivered annually through routine immunization or seasonal campaigns. Influenza viruses infecting humans are transmitted person to person, mostly by droplets and aerosols from the respiratory secretions of infected people. Influenza viruses cause seasonal influenza epidemics, mostly in the winter months in temperate climates, with less distinct seasonality in the tropics. Influenza has an annual attack rate of 5 percent to 10 percent in adults and 20 percent to 30 percent in children. When complicated by subsequent bacterial pneumonia, influenza infections can have high mortality rates. In general, the role of influenza in LMICs has been underestimated. A review suggests that 6.5 percent of hospital admissions for respiratory illness among Sub-Saharan African children were due to influenza (Gessner, Shindo, and Briand 2011). Another meta-analysis estimates that 28,000 to 111,500 influenza-associated deaths occur annually in children, with 99 percent occurring in LMICs (Nair and others 2013).

Licensed influenza vaccines include inactivated or live-attenuated influenza type A and B viruses. Inactivated influenza vaccines (IIVs) are administered by injection; live-attenuated virus vaccines are delivered as nasal spray. Only IIV is licensed for children younger than age two years. Two doses of influenza vaccine given four weeks apart are recommended during the first season a child is vaccinated. Vaccine effectiveness varies annually according to protection provided against circulating influenza viruses, but in general, vaccination has provided significant protection in children (Jefferson and others 2012), although few studies of vaccine effectiveness have been conducted among children in LMICs (WHO 2012b). Maternal influenza immunization has gained support as a way of protecting infants too young to be vaccinated against influenza disease. A study in Bangladesh shows that giving influenza vaccine to pregnant women led to an efficacy of 63 percent against lab-confirmed influenza and 29 percent against febrile respiratory illness in their infants' first six months of life (Zaman and others 2008). Maternal influenza vaccination with IIV is now recommended in some countries and is being studied in LMICs as a method for preventing influenza in young infants (CDC 2013;

WHO 2012a). No cost-effectiveness data on the use of influenza vaccine in LMICs are available. The WHO suggests that countries make their respective decisions on influenza vaccines based on local disease burden, resources, capacity, and other health priorities (WHO 2012a).

Oral Cholera Vaccine

Cholera is caused by ingestion of toxigenic serogroups (O1 and O139) of *Vibrio cholerae* bacteria, leading to diarrhea, dehydration, and rapid death. Periodically, new strains of *V. cholerae* emerge to cause pandemics. In 1970, the seventh pandemic strain appeared in Sub-Saharan Africa, where it is now endemic and accounts for the majority of cholera mortality (Mintz and Guerrant 2009). Cholera incidence and mortality is greatest in children (Ali and others 2012; Deen and others 2008), who account for 50 percent of all cholera deaths. Globally, cholera kills at least 45,000 children under age five years annually; this number is likely to be twice as high when considering out-of-hospital mortality (Ali and others 2012; Sack 2014). In 2010, cholera was introduced into Haiti following a massive earthquake, causing more than 500,000 cases (Barzilay and others 2013). Although the cholera CFR can be less than 1 percent in settings with good access to health care and proper treatment, these conditions rarely exist in most LMICs, where CFRs often exceed 5 percent and can be as high as 50 percent during outbreaks (Gaffga, Tauxe, and Mintz 2007; WHO 2010a).

There are two WHO-approved oral cholera vaccines, which contain formalin-inactivated or heat-killed whole-cell *V. cholerae*. One vaccine showed greater than 80 percent effectiveness against cholera for at least the first six months after administration (Clemens, Sack, and Ivanoff 2001; van Loon and others 1996); the second showed 67 percent effectiveness against cholera during the first two years of follow-up among children vaccinated at ages 1–4 years (Sur and others 2011).

These vaccines were cost-effective in a crowded city like Kolkata, India, at US$1 per dose; they would likely be cost-effective in other settings, such as Sub-Saharan Africa, if significant herd protection occurs with the vaccine, as has been hypothesized. In 2010, the WHO recommended use of oral cholera vaccines in addition to other preventive strategies, such as provision of safe water, in cholera-endemic countries or areas likely to experience outbreaks, with priority for vaccination given to children in settings of limited vaccine supply (Jeuland and others 2009; Longini and others 2007; WHO 2010a). For vaccination during large outbreaks like those in Haiti and Zimbabwe (Ahmed and others 2011; Barzilay and others 2013), the WHO plans to create an emergency stockpile of 2 million doses of cholera vaccine (Martin, Costa, and Perea 2012).

COST AND COST-EFFECTIVENESS OF VACCINATIONS

Cost

Despite the relatively low cost of traditional EPI vaccines, more than 20 million infants did not receive the third dose of DTP-containing vaccine in 2013; the majority of these children lived in five countries: the Democratic Republic of Congo, Ethiopia, India, Nigeria, and Pakistan. National EPI programs have evolved in the past 15 years; the WHO universally recommends vaccines against 11 different diseases for infants—tuberculosis, hepatitis B, polio, diphtheria, tetanus, pertussis, Hib, pneumococcus, rotavirus, measles, and rubella. As more countries increase coverage of new and underutilized vaccines, the cost of fully immunizing a child increases.

The costs of delivering existing and new vaccines to beneficiary populations can be challenging to quantify, especially over time with the introduction of new vaccines. Early studies of the principal EPI vaccines estimated the cost of fully immunizing a child to range from US$10 to $US20, depending on the region and place of vaccine delivery (Brenzel and Claquin 1994). Using more recent immunization financing data after the advent of Gavi (from Financial Sustainability Plans), the cost of fully immunizing a child in 50 of the poorest Gavi-eligible countries was estimated to increase from US$6.00 to US$17.50 per infant with the addition of hepatitis B and Hib vaccines and increased coverage (Lydon and others 2008). An updated estimate in Gavi-eligible countries based on financial data from the WHO (Comprehensive Multi-Year Plans) increased the cost to US$23 per infant for 2008–11, increasing to a projected cost of US$42 per infant in 2016 (Brenzel, Young, and Walker 2015). There was substantial variability by WHO region, with Europe having the highest costs and South-East Asia and the Western Pacific regions the lowest; more than one-third of the total projected cost of vaccination from 2011 to 2020 (US$57.5 billion) is expected to be spent in India, Nigeria, and Pakistan (Gandhi and others 2013). Non-vaccine delivery costs can account for nearly half of the total costs of vaccination (Brenzel 2015; Gandhi and others 2013; Lydon and others 2008).

As highly effective yet more expensive vaccines become available, many countries with already-strained resources will have to find the right balance between increasing coverage with available vaccines in often hard-to-reach areas or introducing new vaccines into the national immunization schedule.

A systematic review of cost-effectiveness analyses from 44 published articles of 23 vaccines in 51 countries finds that vaccines cost less than US$100 per DALY averted in more than half of the articles, and less than

US$1,000 per DALY averted in nearly 90 percent of the articles (Horton, Wu, and Brouwer 2015).

Table 10.2 shows the relative cost-effectiveness of different vaccines using the accepted metric of cost per DALY averted. For comparison, if the cost per DALY averted for an intervention is less than per capita gross national income (GNI), it is very cost-effective; if less than three times per capita GNI, it is cost-effective (WHO 2001). Those vaccines in the third column are very cost-effective in upper-middle-income countries, as long as cost per DALY does not exceed US$4,087, the cutoff in 2012 between lower-middle- and upper-middle-income countries, per the World Bank. A more detailed analysis of cost-effectiveness of vaccines is presented in chapter 17 in this volume (Horton and Levin 2016).

Direct Social and Economic Benefits

Immunization coverage has traditionally been monitored using DTP3 coverage or measles vaccine coverage as indicators. Most countries now deliver DTP through newer combination vaccines—for example, as of 2014, all 73 Gavi countries were using the pentavalent vaccine that combines Hib and hepatitis B with DTP. However, even though DTP3 coverage in 2013 was high—84 percent globally and 76 percent in the 73 Gavi countries—fewer than 5 percent of children received all 11 WHO-recommended immunizations. Clearly, immunization platforms are effective in reaching many children with some vaccines, but large gaps in protection remain.

The timeliness of vaccination is critical, particularly for diseases for which most mortality occurs in the first six months of life, for example, pertussis and Hib. Additionally, timely vaccination ensures maximal herd immunity and protects those who are too young to be fully vaccinated (Akmatov and others 2008; Clark and Sanderson 2009; Patel and others 2011). A review of immunization timeliness in 45 countries found a median delay of six weeks for receipt of DTP3; in countries with the greatest delays, 25 percent of children received DTP3 at least 19 weeks late (Clark and Sanderson 2009).

Fully immunized children who receive on-time vaccinations obtain the greatest protection and greatest reduction of the risk of mortality in the first six months of life from preventable childhood diseases. Such immunization also conveys broader direct social and economic benefits, leading to greater adult productivity and contributing to economic development. Directly averting illness through immunization can lead to lower medical costs and missed wages by caretakers. Vaccines that prevent diseases that cause disabilities have improved school enrollment and attainment rates (Simmerman and others 2006) and cognitive ability linked to test scores (Bloom, Canning, and Seiguer 2011), thereby increasing a population's human capital in the long term (Bloom, Canning, and Jamison 2004). Ozawa and others (2012) quantify the impact of vaccination on health care cost saving, care-related productivity gains, and outcome-related productivity gains.

Most of the evidence on the economic benefit of vaccines has been for health care savings and care-related productivity gains that directly affect the finances of

Table 10.2 Approximate Range of Cost-Effectiveness of Various Childhood Vaccines, Various Contexts (2012 U.S. dollars per DALY averted)

< US$100/DALYª	US$100 to <US$1,036/DALYᵇ	Over US$1,036/DALYᶜ
Original EPI-6: BCG, DTP, measles, polio	*Haemophilus influenzae* type B	Cholera (final price point pending)
Hepatitis B	Yellow fever, where endemic	Pneumococcus, low-child-mortality countries
Pneumoccocus, high-child-mortality countries	Japanese encephalitis, where endemic	Rotavirus, low-child-mortality countries
Rotavirus, high-child-mortality countries	Pneumococcus, medium-child-mortality countries	
	Rotavirus, medium-child-mortality countries	
	Meningitis A, where endemic	

Source: For details on sources and references, see table 17.1 of chapter 17 of this volume (Horton and Levin 2016).
Note: EPI = Expanded Program on Immunization; BCG = Bacille Calmette-Guérin; DALY = disability-adjusted life year; DTP = diphtheria, tetanus, and pertussis. For vaccines, cost-effectiveness is sensitive to vaccine price as well as variability in underlying disease burden by country.
a. Vaccines in the first column are very cost-effective in all low-income countries because cost per DALY averted is less than per capita gross national income (GNI) of even the poorest low-income country (World Bank definition of "low-income country" is per capita GNI of less than US$1,035 in 2012 and in 2012 the per capita income of the poorest low-income country was approximately US$250).
b. Vaccines in the second column are very cost-effective in all lower-middle-income countries (World Bank definition of "lower-middle-income country" is per capita GNI in 2012 ranging between US$1,036 and US$4,085).
c. Vaccines in the third column may be very cost-effective in upper-middle-income countries (World Bank definition of "upper-middle-income country" is per capita GNI in 2012 ranging between US$4,086 and US$12,615).

the vaccinated child's household. These savings can greatly affect household economies and health system expenditures in resource-strained settings. Scaling up coverage with vaccines against pneumococcal disease, Hib, rotavirus, pertussis, measles, and malaria to 90 percent over 10 years could save US$6.2 billion in treatment costs and avert US$1.2 million in caretaker lost wages in 73 Gavi-supported countries (Stack and others 2011).

Indirect Social and Economic Benefits

The wider indirect economic impact of vaccines on societies lies beyond vaccinated households. Many childhood vaccines have proven to have additional value by protecting persons who are still susceptible to infection, including those who are too young and too old to be vaccinated, through a mechanism referred to as herd protection, herd immunity, or community immunity. This indirect impact of vaccination has been shown for many vaccines, including those against measles, Hib, influenza, meningococcus, and pneumococcus (Fine, Eames, and Heymann 2011; Fine and Mulholland 2013). When the disease burden is large in adults, more disease is possibly prevented among unvaccinated adults than among vaccinated children, as has been shown in the United States with pneumococcal conjugate vaccine (CDC 2005).

- Between 1995 and 2001, the seven routine vaccines in the United States resulted in an estimated savings of US$10 billion in direct costs and US$43 billion in societal costs (Zhou and others 2005).
- Averting morbidity and mortality by scaling up the six original EPI vaccines to 90 percent over 10 years could increase productivity in 73 Gavi-eligible countries by US$145 billion over the lifetime of vaccinated children (Stack and others 2011).
- Behavior-related productivity gains due to vaccination include the effects of longer life expectancies (Bloom, Canning, and Weston 2005; Meij and others 2009) and alleviated poverty (Bawah and others 2010) on societal productivity. By 2020, the investments by Gavi could result in internal rates of return of 18 percent (Bloom, Canning, and Weston 2005).
- Finally, preventing outbreaks through immunization saves societies the opportunity cost of reacting to outbreaks after they have occurred. For example, modeling (Khan 2008) shows that introducing IPV in the 148 countries using OPV would save US$163 million in poliomyelitis outbreak containment costs per year over 10 years.

CONCLUSION

Vaccines have been one of the most important forces in reducing childhood mortality during the past 40 years. With the advent of new vaccines and the promise of others, immunizations have the potential to further drive down childhood mortality and deliver broader health and economic benefits. Remaining challenges need to be addressed in the coming decade:

- Progress in controlling and eliminating many diseases—including polio, measles, rubella, meningococcal meningitis, yellow fever, and JE—will increasingly depend on coordination between routine immunization services and supplementary immunization activities, including mass vaccination. It is important to ensure that supplementary immunization activities are planned and implemented in such a manner that they strengthen routine immunization programs, wherever possible.
- Immunization programs need to reduce disparities in levels of effective vaccination coverage and to monitor progress in fully immunizing children.
- Additional resources are required for immunization programs as new vaccines become available and national governments assume greater shares of program costs.
- The number of immunization visits required to ensure full immunization coverage of all recommended vaccines has increased relative to the original EPI schedule, which served as the foundation for delivering many interventions. These schedule changes lead to logistical and programmatic challenges and require enhancements to health workforce and program capacities. They also present opportunities to strengthen the delivery of other services in coordination with vaccination.
- Innovations are needed to make vaccine delivery easier, such as heat-stable vaccines that do not require cold chain, and to provide alternate delivery mechanisms, such as microneedle patches.
- Programs need to work to improve immunization timeliness and take advantage of opportunities to provide multiple interventions.
- Newer vaccines (for example, rotavirus vaccine and malaria vaccine) may be less effective than traditional EPI vaccines but may prevent a substantial burden of disease, given the high incidence of these diseases (Gessner and Feikin 2014). The evaluation process for vaccines will likely need to shift from an exclusive focus on vaccine efficacy to a focus on the vaccine-preventable disease burden.

Despite these challenges, immunization will remain central to childhood disease prevention, and the well-child visit will continue to serve as the axis upon which preventive activities evolve. The unprecedented momentum in global immunizations during the past decade must be sustained. To maximize the health and economic well-being of populations, it is especially important to fully immunize children with all recommended vaccines and to effectively use immunization as a platform to deliver other cost-effective and life-saving services as part of a comprehensive well-child approach.

ACKNOWLEDGMENTS

The authors recognize and thank the following individuals for their contributions to the impact estimates described in this chapter: Andrew Clark, Matthew Ferrari, Heather Franklin, Ingrid K. Friberg, Tini Garske, Sue Goldie, Gavin Grant, Hope Johnson, Lisa Lee, Michelle Li, Andrew Mirelman, Susan Reef, Sachiko Ozawa, Anushua Sinha, Chutima Suraratdecha, Steven Sweet, Yvonne Tam, Emilia Vynnycky, Damian Walker, and Neff Walker.

REFERENCES

Adegbola, R. A., O. Secka, G. Lahai, N. Lloyd-Evans, S. Ussen, and others. 2005. "Elimination of *Haemophilus influenzae* Type B (Hib) Disease from The Gambia after the Introduction of Routine Immunisation with a Hib Conjugate Vaccine: A Prospective Study." *The Lancet* 366 (9480): 144–50.

Agnandji, S. T., B. Lell, S. S. Soulanoudjingar, J. F. Fernandes, B. P. Abossolo, and others. 2011. "First Results of Phase 3 Trial of RTS,S/AS01 Malaria Vaccine in African Children." *New England Journal of Medicine* 365 (20): 1863–75.

Ahmed, S., P. K. Bardhan, A. Iqbal, R. N. Mazumder, A. I. Khan, and others. 2011. "The 2008 Cholera Epidemic in Zimbabwe: Experience of the Icddr,B Team in the Field." *Journal of Health, Population and Nutrition* 9 (5): 541–46.

Akmatov, M. K., M. Kretzschmar, A. Kramer, and R. T. Mikolajczyk. 2008. "Timeliness of Vaccination and Its Effects on Fraction of Vaccinated Population." *Vaccine* 26 (31): 3805–11.

Ali, M., A. L. Lopez, Y. A. You, Y. E. Kim, B. Sah, and others. 2012. "The Global Burden of Cholera." *Bulletin of the World Health Organization* 90: 209–18A.

Armah, G. E., S. O. Sow, R. F. Breiman, M. J. Dallas, M. D. Tapia, and others. 2010. "Efficacy of Pentavalent Rotavirus Vaccine against Severe Rotavirus Gastroenteritis in Infants in Developing Countries in Sub-Saharan Africa: A Randomised, Double-Blind, Placebo-Controlled Trial." *The Lancet* 376 (9741): 606–14.

Atherly, D. E., K. D. Lewis, J. Tate, U. D. Parashar, and R. D. Rheingans. 2012. "Projected Health and Economic Impact of Rotavirus Vaccination in GAVI-Eligible Countries: 2011–2030." *Vaccine* 30 (1): A7–14.

Barzilay, E. J., N. Schaad, R. Magloire, K. S. Mung, J. Boncy, and others. 2013. "Cholera Surveillance during the Haiti Epidemic: The First 2 Years." *New England Journal of Medicine* 368 (7): 599–609.

Bawah, A. A., J. F. Phillips, M. Adjuik, M. Vaughan-Smith, B. Macleod, and F. N. Binka. 2010. "The Impact of Immunization on the Association between Poverty and Child Survival: Evidence from Kassena-Nankana District of Northern Ghana." *Scandinavian Journal of Public Health* 38 (1): 95–103.

Bennett, J. V., A. E. Platonov, M. P. E. Slack, and P. Mala. 2002. Haemophilus influenzae *Type B (Hib) Meningitis in the Pre-Vaccine Era: A Global Review of Incidence, Age Distributions, and Case-Fatality Rates*. Geneva: World Health Organization.

Bharat Biotech. 2011. "Affordable Vaccines." http://www.bharatbiotech.com/affordable-vaccines.

Black, R. E., S. Cousens, H. L. Johnson, J. E. Lawn, I. Rudan, and others. 2010. "Global, Regional, and National Causes of Child Mortality in 2008: A Systematic Analysis." *The Lancet* 375 (9730): 1969–87.

Bloom, D. E., D. Canning, and D. T. Jamison. 2004. "Health, Wealth, and Welfare." *Finance and Development* 41: 10–15.

Bloom, D. E., D. Canning, and M. Weston. 2005. "The Value of Vaccination." *World Economics* 6 (3): 15.

Bloom, D. E., D. Canning, and E. Seiguer. 2011. "The Effect of Vaccination on Children's Physical and Cognitive Development in the Philippines." Working Paper 69, Program on the Global Demography of Aging, Harvard School of Public Health, Cambridge, MA.

Bloom, B., and others. Forthcoming. In *Disease Control Priorities* (third edition): Volume 6, *HIV/AIDS, STIs, Tuberculosis, and Malaria*, edited by K. K. Holmes, S. Bertozzi, B. Bloom, P. Jha, and R. Nugent. Washington, DC: World Bank.

Brenzel, L. 2015. "What Have We Learned on Costs and Financing of Routine Immunization from the Comprehensive Multi-Year Plans in Gavi-Eligible Countries?" *Vaccine* 33: A93–98.

Brenzel, L., and P. Claquin. 1994. "Immunization Programs and Their Costs." *Social Science and Medicine* 39 (4): 527–36.

Brenzel, L., L. J. Wolfson, J. Fox-Rushby, M. Miller, and N. A. Halsey. 2006. "Vaccine-Preventable Diseases." In *Disease Control Priorities in Developing Countries*, 2nd ed., edited by D. T. Jamison, J. G. Bremen, A. R. Measham, G. Alleyne, M. Claeson, D. B. Evans, A. Mills, and P. Musgrove, 389–411. Washington, DC: World Bank and Oxford University Press.

Brenzel, L., D. Young, and D. G. Walker. 2015. "Costs and Financing of Routine Immunization: Approach and Selected Findings of a Multi-Country Study (EPIC)." *Vaccine* 33: A13–20.

Campbell, G. L., S. L. Hills, M. Fischer, J. A. Jacobson, C. H. Hoke, and others. 2011. "Estimated Global Incidence of Japanese Encephalitis: A Systematic Review." *Bulletin of the World Health Organization* 89 (10): 766–74.

CDC (Centers for Disease Control and Prevention). 2005. "Direct and Indirect Effects of Routine Vaccination of

Children with 7-Valent Pneumococcal Conjugate Vaccine on Incidence of Invasive Pneumococcal Disease: United States, 1998–2003." *Morbidity and Mortality Weekly Report* 54 (36): 893–97.

———. 2011. "Updated Recommendations for Use of Tetanus Toxoid, Reduced Diphtheria Toxoid and Acellular Pertussis Vaccine (Tdap) in Pregnant Women and Persons Who Have or Anticipate Having Close Contact with an Infant Aged < 12 Months—Advisory Committee on Immunization Practices (ACIP), 2011." *Morbidity and Mortality Weekly Report* 60 (41): 1424–26. http://www.cdc.gov/mmwr/preview/mmwrhtml/mm6041a4.htm.

———. 2013. "Prevention and Control of Seasonal Influenza with Vaccines: Recommendations of the Advisory Committee on Immunization Practices—United States, 2013–2014." *MMWR Recommendations and Reports* 62 (RR07): 1–43.

Cernuschi, T., E. Furrer, S. McAdams, A. Jones, J. Fihman, and N. Schwalbe. 2011. "Pneumococcal Advance Market Commitment: Lessons Learnt on Disease and Design Choices and Processes." Gavi Alliance White Paper, Gavi, the Vaccine Alliance, Geneva.

Clark, A., and C. Sanderson 2009. "Timing of Children's Vaccinations in 45 Low-Income and Middle-Income Countries: An Analysis of Survey Data." *The Lancet* 373 (9674): 1543–49.

Clemens, J. D., D. A. Sack, and B. Ivanoff. 2001. "Misleading Negative Findings in a Field Trial of Killed, Oral Cholera Vaccine in Peru." *Journal of Infectious Diseases* 183 (8): 1306–8.

Connelly Smith, K., I. M. Orme, and J. R. Starke. 2013. "Tuberculosis Vaccines." In *Vaccines,* 6th ed., edited by S. A. Plotkin, W. A. Orenstein, and P. A. Offit, 789–811. Philadelphia, PA: Saunders.

Cowgill, K. D., M. Ndiritu, J. Nyiro, M. P. Slack, S. Chiphatsi, and others. 2006. "Effectiveness of *Haemophilus influenzae* Type B Conjugate Vaccine Introduction into Routine Childhood Immunization in Kenya." *Journal of the American Medical Association* 296 (6): 671–78.

Cutts, F. T., H. S. Izurieta, and D. A. Rhoda. 2013. "Measuring Coverage in MNCH: Design, Implementation, and Interpretation Challenges Associated with Tracking Vaccination Coverage Using Household Surveys." *PLoS Medicine* 10 (5): E1001404.

Deen, J. L., L. von Seidlein, D. Sur, M. Agtini, M. Lucas, and others. 2008. "The High Burden of Cholera in Children: Comparison of Incidence from Endemic Areas in Asia and Africa." *PLoS Neglected Tropical Diseases* 2 (2): E173.

Edwards, K. M., and M. D. Decker. 2013. "Pertussis Vaccines." In *Vaccines,* 6th ed., edited by S. A. Plotkin, W. A. Orenstein, and P. A. Offit, 447–92. Philadelphia, PA: Saunders.

Estívariz, C. F., H. Jafari, R. W. Sutter, T. J. John, V. Jain, and others. 2012. "Immunogenicity of Poliovirus Vaccines Administered at Age 6–9 Months in Moradabad District, India: A Randomized Controlled Phase 3 Trial." *The Lancet Infectious Diseases* 12 (2): 128–35.

Feikin, D. R., E. W. Kagucia, J. D. Loo, R. Link-Gelles, M. A. Puhan, and others. 2013. "Serotype-Specific Changes in Invasive Pneumococcal Disease after Pneumococcal

Conjugate Vaccine Introduction: A Pooled Analysis of Multiple Surveillance Sites." *PLoS Medicine* 10 (9): E1001517.

Feikin, D. R., K. F. Laserson, J. Ojwando, G. Nyambane, V. Ssempiija, and others. 2012. "Efficacy of Pentavalent Rotavirus Vaccine in a High HIV Prevalence Population in Kenya." *Vaccine* 30 (Suppl 1): A52–60.

Fine, P. E. M., K. Eames, and D. L. Heymann. 2011. "Herd Immunity: A Rough Guide." *Clinical Infectious Diseases* 52 (7): 911–16.

Fine, P. E. M., and E. K. Mulholland. 2013. "Community Immunity." In *Vaccines,* 6th ed., edited by S. A. Plotkin, W. A. Orenstein, and P. A. Offit, 1395–1412. Philadelphia, PA: Saunders.

Fischer Walker, C. L., M. K. Munos, and R. E. Black. 2013. "Quantifying the Indirect Effects of Key Child Survival Interventions for Pneumonia, Diarrhoea, and Measles." *Epidemiology and Infection* 141 (1): 115–31.

Gaffga, N. H., R. V. Tauxe, and E. D. Mintz. 2007. "Cholera: A New Homeland in Africa?" *American Journal of Tropical Medicine and Hygiene* 77 (4): 705–13.

Gandhi, G., P. Lydon, S. Cornejo, L. Brenzel, S. Wrobel, and H. Chang. 2013. "Projections of Costs, Financing, and Additional Resource Requirements for Low- and Middle-Income Country Immunization Programs over the Decade, 2011–2020." *Vaccine* 31 (Suppl 2): B137–48.

Gavi, the Vaccine Alliance. 2013. "Innovative Financing Mechanism Accelerates Global Roll Out of Vaccine against World's Leading Cause of Child Deaths." Pneumococcal AMC. http://www.gavialliance.org/funding/pneumococcal-amc/.

Gessner, B. D., and D. R. Feikin. 2014. "Vaccine Preventable Disease Incidence as a Complement to Vaccine Efficacy for Setting Vaccine Policy." *Vaccine* 32 (26): 3133–38.

Gessner, B. D., N. Shindo, and S. Briand. 2011. "Seasonal Influenza Epidemiology in Sub-Saharan Africa: A Systematic Review." *The Lancet Infectious Diseases* 11 (3): 223–35.

Global Polio Eradication Initiative. 2013. "Data and Monitoring." http://www.polioeradication.org.

Goldstein, S. T., F. Zhou, S. C. Hadler, B. P. Bell, E. E. Mast, and H. S. Margolis. 2005. "A Mathematical Model to Estimate Global Hepatitis B Disease Burden and Vaccination Impact." *International Journal of Epidemiology* 34 (6): 1329–39.

Grassly, N. C., J. Wenger, S. Durrani, J. Bahi, J. M. Deshpande, and others. 2007. "Protective Efficacy of a Monovalent Oral Type 1 Poliovirus Vaccine." *The Lancet* 369 (9570): 1356–62.

Hadler, S., S. Cochi, J. Bilous, and F. Cutts. 2004. "Vaccination Programs in Developing Countries." In *Vaccines,* 4th ed., edited by S. A. Plotkin and W. A. Orenstein, 1407–42. Philadelphia, PA: Saunders.

Halstead, S. B., J. Jacobson, and K. Dubischar-Kastner. 2013. "Japanese Encephalitis Vaccines." In *Vaccines,* 6th ed., edited by S. A. Plotkin, W. A. Orenstein, and P. A. Offit, 312–51. Philadelphia, PA: Saunders.

Horton, S., and C. Levin. 2016. "Cost-Effectiveness of Interventions for Reproductive, Maternal, Neonatal, and Child Health." In *Disease Control Priorities* (third edition): Volume 2, *Reproductive, Maternal, Newborn, and Child*

Health, edited by R. Black, R. Laxminarayan, M. Temmerman, and N. Walker. Washington, DC: World Bank.

Horton, S., D. Wu, and E. Brouwer. 2015. "Methods and Results for Systematic Search, Cost, and Cost-Effectiveness." Working Paper No. 11, Disease Control Priorities, Seattle, Washington.

Jefferson, T., A. Rivetti, C. Di Pietrantoni, V. Demicheli, and E. Ferroni. 2012. "Vaccine for Preventing Influenza in Healthy Children." *Cochrane Database of Systematic Reviews* 8: CD004879.

Jeuland, M., J. Cook, C. Poulos, J. Clemens, D. Whittington, and DOMI Cholera Economics Study Group. 2009. "Cost-Effectiveness of New-Generation Oral Cholera Vaccines: A Multi-Site Analysis." *Value in Health* 12 (6): 899–908.

Keusch, G. T., C. Fischer Walker, J. K. Das, S. Horton, and D. Habte. 2016. "Diarrheal Diseases." In *Disease Control Priorities* (third edition): Volume 2, *Reproductive, Maternal, Newborn, and Child Health*, edited by R. Black, R. Laxminarayan, M. Temmerman, and N. Walker. Washington, DC: World Bank.

Khan, M. M. 2008. "Economics of Polio Vaccination in the Post-Eradication Era: Should OPV-Using Countries Adopt IPV?" *Vaccine* 26 (16): 2034–40.

Klugman, K. P., S. A. Madhi, R. E. Huebner, R. Kohberger, N. Mbelle, and others. 2003. "A Trial of a 9-Valent Pneumococcal Conjugate Vaccine in Children with and Those without HIV Infection." *New England Journal of Medicine* 349 (14): 1341–48.

Kotloff, K. L., J. P. Nataro, W. C. Blackwelder, D. Nasrin, T. H. Farag, and others. 2013. "Burden and Aetiology of Diarrhoeal Disease in Infants and Young Children in Developing Countries (The Global Enteric Multicenter Study, GEMS): A Prospective, Case-Control Study." *The Lancet* 382 (9888): 209–22.

LaForce, F. M., and J. M. Okwo-Bele. 2011. "Eliminating Epidemic Group A Meningococcal Meningitis in Africa through a New Vaccine." *Health Affairs* 30 (6): 1049–57.

Lee, L. A., L. Franzel, J. Atwell, S. D. Datta, I. K. Friberg, and others. 2013. "The Estimated Mortality Impact of Vaccinations Forecast to Be Administered during 2011–2020 in 73 Countries Supported by the Gavi Alliance." *Vaccine* 31 (Suppl 2): B61–72.

Levine, O. S., R. Lagos, A. Muñoz, J. Villaroel, A. M. Alvarez, and others. 1999. "Defining the Burden of Pneumonia in Children Preventable by Vaccination against *Haemophilus influenzae* Type B." *Pediatric Infectious Disease Journal* 18 (12): 1060–64.

Liu, L., K. Hill, S. Oza, D. Hogan, Y. Chu, and others. 2016. "Levels and Causes of Mortality under Age Five Years." In *Disease Control Priorities* (third edition): Volume 2, *Reproductive, Maternal, Newborn, and Child Health*, edited by R. Black, R. Laxminarayan, M. Temmerman, and N. Walker. Washington, DC: World Bank.

Liu, L., H. L. Johnson, S. Cousens, J. Perin, S. Scott, and others. 2012. "Global, Regional, and National Causes of Child Mortality: An Updated Systematic Analysis for 2010 with Time Trends since 2000." *The Lancet* 379 (9832): 2151–61.

Longini, I. M., A. Nizam, M. Ali, M. Yunus, N. Shenvi, and J. D. Clemens. 2007. "Controlling Endemic Cholera with Oral Vaccines." *PLoS Medicine* 4 (11): E336.

Lucero, M. G., V. E. Dulalia, L. T. Nillos, G. Williams, R. A. Parreño, and others. 2009. "Pneumococcal Conjugate Vaccines for Preventing Vaccine-Type Invasive Pneumococcal Disease and X-Ray Defined Pneumonia in Children Less than Two Years of Age." *Cochrane Database of Systematic Reviews* 4: CD004977.

Lydon, P., R. Levine, M. Makinen, L. Brenzel, V. Mitchell, and others. 2008. "Introducing New Vaccines in the Poorest Countries: What Did We Learn from the GAVI Experience with Financial Sustainability?" *Vaccine* 26 (51): 6706–16.

Madhi, S. A., N. A. Cunliffe, D. Steel, D. Witte, M. Kirsten, and others. 2010. "Effect of Human Rotavirus Vaccine on Severe Diarrhea in African Infants." *New England Journal of Medicine* 362 (4): 289–98.

Mangtani, P., K. Mulholland, S. A. Madhi, K. Edmond, R. O'Loughlin, and R. Hajjeh. 2010. "*Haemophilus influenzae* Type B Disease in HIV-Infected Children: A Review of Disease Epidemiology and Effectiveness of Hib Conjugate Vaccines." *Vaccine* 28 (7): 1677–83.

Martin, S., A. Costa, and W. Perea. 2012. "Stockpiling Oral Cholera Vaccine." *Bulletin of the World Health Organization* 90: 714–14.

Meij, J., A. de Craen, J. Agana, D. Plug, and R. G. Westendorp. 2009. "Low-Cost Interventions Accelerate Epidemiological Transition in Upper East Ghana." *Transactions of the Royal Society of Tropical Medicine and Hygiene* 103 (2): 173–78.

Mintz, E. D., and R. L. Guerrant. 2009. "A Lion in Our Village: The Unconscionable Tragedy of Cholera in Africa." *New England Journal of Medicine* 360 (11): 1060–63.

Mitchell, V., V. J. Dietz, J. M. Okwe-Bele, and F. T. Cutts. 2013. "Poliovirus Vaccine-Inactivated." In *Vaccines*, 6th ed., edited by S. A. Plotkin, W. A. Orenstein, and P. A. Offit, 1371. Philadelphia, PA: Saunders.

Monath, T. P., M. Gershman, J. E. Staples, and A. D. T. Barrett. 2013. "Yellow Fever Vaccine." In *Vaccines*, 6th ed., edited by S. A. Plotkin, W. A. Orenstein, and P. A. Offit, 870–968. Philadelphia, PA: Saunders.

Mulholland, K., S. Hilton, R. Adegbola, S. Usen, A. Oparaugo, and others. 1997. "Randomised Trial of *Haemophilus influenzae* Type-B Tetanus Protein Conjugate Vaccine [Corrected] for Prevention of Pneumonia and Meningitis in Gambian Infants." *The Lancet* 349 (9060): 1191–97.

Mwenda, J. M., K. M. Ntoto, A. Abebe, C. Enweronu-Laryea, I. Amina, and others. 2010. "Burden and Epidemiology of Rotavirus Diarrhea in Selected African Countries: Preliminary Results from the African Rotavirus Surveillance Network." *Journal of Infectious Diseases* 202: S5–11.

Nair, H., E. A. Simoes, I. Rudan, B. D. Gesner, E. Azziz-Baumgartner, and others. 2013. "Global and Regional Burden of Hospital Admissions for Severe Acute Lower Respiratory Infection in Young Children in 2010: A Systematic Analysis." *The Lancet* 381 (9875): 1380–90.

Novak, R. T., J. L. Kambou, F. V. Diomandé, T. F. Tarbando, R. Ouédraogo-Traore, and others. 2012. "Serogroup A

Meningococcal Conjugate Vaccination in Burkina Faso: Analysis of National Surveillance Data." *The Lancet Infectious Diseases* 12 (10): 757–64.

NPC (National Population Commission) [Nigeria] and ICF Macro. 2009. *Nigeria Demographic and Health Survey 2008*. Abuja, Nigeria: National Population Commission and ICF Macro. http://dhsprogram.com/pubs/pdf/FR222 /FR222.pdf.

O'Brien, K. L., L. J. Wolfson, J. P. Watt, E. Henkle, M. Deloria-Knoll, and others. 2009. "Burden of Disease Caused by *Streptococcus pneumoniae* in Children Younger than 5 Years: Global Estimates." *The Lancet* 374 (9693): 893–902.

Ozawa, S., A. Mirelman, M. L. Stack, D. G. Walker, and O. S. Levine. 2012. "Cost-Effectiveness and Economic Benefits of Vaccines in Low- and Middle-Income Countries: A Systematic Review." *Vaccine* 31 (1): 96–108.

Parashar, U. D., E. G. Hummelman, J. S. Bresee, M. A. Miller, and R. I. Glass. 2003. "Global Illness and Deaths Caused by Rotavirus Disease in Children." *Emerging Infectious Diseases Journal* 9 (5): 565–72.

Patel, M. M., A. D. Clark, C. F. Sanderson, J. Tate, and U. D. Parashar. 2012. "Removing the Age Restrictions for Rotavirus Vaccination: A Benefit-Risk Modeling Analysis." *PLoS Medicine* 9 (10): E1001330.

Patel, M. M., V. R. Lopez-Collada, M. M. Bulhões, L. H. De Oliveira, A. Bautista Márquez, and others. 2011. "Intussusception Risk and Health Benefits of Rotavirus Vaccination in Mexico and Brazil." *New England Journal of Medicine* 364 (24): 2283–92.

PHR (Public Health Reports). 2014. "The HHS National Vaccine Program and Global Immunization NVAC Report and Recommendations Approved by the National Vaccine Advisory Committee on September 12, 2013." http://www .publichealthreports.org/issueopen.cfm?articleID=3223.

Reef, S. E., and S. A. Plotkin. 2013. "Rubella Vaccine." In *Vaccines*, 6th ed., edited by S. A. Plotkin, W. A. Orenstein, and P. A. Offit, 688–717. Philadelphia, PA: Saunders.

Ribeiro, G. S., J. B. Lima, J. N. Reis, E. L. Gouveia, S. M. Cordeiro, and others. 2007. "*Haemophilus influenzae* Meningitis 5 Years after Introduction of the *Haemophilus influenzae* Type B Conjugate Vaccine in Brazil." *Vaccine* 25 (22): 4420–28.

RTS,S Clinical Trials Partnership. 2015. "Efficacy and Safety of RTS, S/AS01 Malaria Vaccine with or without a Booster Dose in Infants and Children in Africa: Final Results of a Phase 3, Individually Randomised, Controlled Trial." *The Lancet* 386 (9988): 31–45.

Sack, D. 2014. "Cholera Burden of Disease Estimates." Johns Hopkins School of Public Health, Baltimore, MD.

Simmerman, J. M., J. Lertiendumrong, S. F. Dowell, T. Uyeki, S. J. Olsen, and others. 2006. "The Cost of Influenza in Thailand." *Vaccine* 24 (20): 4417–26.

Simons, E., M. Ferrari, J. Fricks, K. Wannemuehler, A. Anand, and others. 2012. "Assessment of the 2010 Global Measles Mortality Reduction Goal: Results from a Model of Surveillance Data." *The Lancet* 379 (9832): 2173–78.

Sinha, A., O. Levine, M. D. Knoll, F. Muhib, and T. A. Lieu. 2007. "Cost-Effectiveness of Pneumococcal Conjugate Vaccination in the Prevention of Child Mortality: An International Economic Analysis." *The Lancet* 369 (9559): 389–96.

Stack, M. L., S. Ozawa, D. M. Bishai, A. Mirelman, Y. Tam, and others. 2011. "Estimated Economic Benefits during the 'Decade of Vaccines' Include Treatment Savings, Gains in Labor Productivity." *Health Affairs* 30 (6): 1021–28.

Strebel, P. M., M. J. Papania, A. P. Fiebelkorn, and N. A. Halsey. 2012. "Measles Vaccines." In *Vaccines*, 6th ed., edited by S. A. Plotkin, W. A. Orenstein, and P. A. Offit, 352–87. Philadelphia, PA: Saunders.

Sur, D., S. Kanungo, B. Sah, B. Manna, M. Ali, and others. 2011. "Efficacy of a Low-Cost, Inactivated Whole-Cell Oral Cholera Vaccine: Results from 3 Years of Follow-Up of a Randomized, Controlled Trial." *PLoS Neglected Tropical Diseases* 5 (10): E1289.

Tate, J. E., A. H. Burton, C. Boschi-Pinto, A. Duncan Steel, J. Duque, and U. D. Parashar. 2012. "2008 Estimate of Worldwide Rotavirus-Associated Mortality in Children Younger than 5 Years before the Introduction of Universal Rotavirus Vaccination Programmes: A Systematic Review and Meta-Analysis." *The Lancet Infectious Diseases* 12 (2): 136–41.

Trunz, B. B., P. Fine, and C. Dye. 2006. "Effect of BCG Vaccination on Childhood Tuberculous Meningitis and Miliary Tuberculosis Worldwide: A Meta-Analysis and Assessment of Cost-Effectiveness." *The Lancet* 367 (9517): 1173–80.

UN (United Nations). 2015. "UN Millennium Development Goals: Child Health." UN, New York. http://www.un.org /millenniumgoals/childhealth.shtml.

Van Damme, P., J. Ward, D. Shouval, S. Wiersma, and A. Zanetti. 2013. "Hepatitis B Vaccines." In *Vaccines*, 6th ed., edited by S. A. Plotkin, W. A. Orenstein, and P. A. Offit, 205–34. Philadelphia, PA: Saunders.

van Loon, F. P. L., J. D. Clemens, J. Chakraborty, M. R. Rao, B. A. Kay, and others. 1996. "Field Trial of Inactivated Cholera Vaccines in Bangladesh: Results from 5 Years of Follow-Up." *Vaccine* 14 (2): 162–66.

Vynnycky, E., N. Gay, and F. T. Cutts. 2003. "The Predicted Impact of Private Sector MMR Vaccination on the Burden of Congenital Rubella Syndrome." *Vaccine* 21 (21): 2708–19.

Walsh, J. A., and K. S. Warren. 1979. "Selective Primary Health Care: An Interim Strategy for Disease Control in Developing Countries." *New England Journal of Medicine* 301 (18): 967–74.

Watt, J. P., L. J. Wolfson, K. L. O'Brien, E. Henkle, M. Deloria-Knoll, and others. 2009. "Burden of Disease Caused by *Haemophilus influenzae* Type B in Children Younger than 5 Years: Global Estimates." *The Lancet* 374 (9693): 903–11.

WHO (World Health Organization). 1974. *Handbook of Resolutions*. Geneva: World Health Assembly, Fourteenth Plenary Meeting.

———. 2001. *Macroeconomics and Health: Investing in Health for Economic Development*. Geneva: WHO. http://whqlibdoc .who.int/publications/2001/924154550x.pdf.

———. 2004. "BCG Vaccine. WHO Position Paper." *Weekly Epidemiological Record* 4 (79): 25–40.

———. 2006a. "Japanese Encephalitis Vaccines." *Weekly Epidemiological Record* 81 (34/35): 331–40.

———. 2006b. "WHO Position Paper on *Haemophilus influenzae* Type B Conjugate Vaccines." *Weekly Epidemiological Record* 81 (47): 445–52.

———. 2009. "Meeting of the Immunization Strategic Advisory Group of Experts, April: Conclusions and Recommendations." *Weekly Epidemiological Record* 84 (23): 220–36.

———. 2010a. "Cholera Vaccines: WHO Position Paper." *Weekly Epidemiological Record* 85 (13): 117–28.

———. 2010b. "Hepatitis B Vaccines: WHO Position Paper— Recommendations." *Vaccine* 28 (3): 589–90.

———. 2011a. "Meningococcal Vaccines: WHO Position Paper." *Weekly Epidemiological Record* 86 (47): 521–40.

———. 2011b. "Rubella Vaccines: WHO Position Paper." *Weekly Epidemiological Record* 86 (29): 301–16.

———. 2012a. "Proposed Revisions to the 2005 WHO Position Paper on Influenza Vaccines, 2012." WHO, Geneva.

———. 2012b. "Vaccines against Influenza." *Weekly Epidemiological Record* 87 (47): 461–76.

———. 2013a. "Diphtheria Reported Cases." http://apps.who .int/immunization_monitoring/globalsummary/timeseries /tsincidencediphtheria.html.

———. 2013b. "Immunization Surveillance, Assessment and Monitoring." http://www.who.int/immunization_monitoring /burden/pneumo_hib_estimates/en/index.html.

———. 2013c. "Japanese Encephalitis: Status of Surveillance and Immunization in Asia and the Western Pacific, 2012." *Weekly Epidemiological Record* 88 (34): 357–64.

———. 2013d. "Measles Fact Sheet." http://www.who.int /mediacentre/factsheets/fs286/en/.

———. 2013e. "Meeting of the Strategic Advisory Group of Experts on Immunization, April 2013: Conclusions and Recommendations." *Weekly Epidemiological Record* 88 (20): 201–16.

———. 2013f. "Meningococcal Disease in Countries of the African Meningitis Belt, 2012: Emerging Needs and Future Perspectives." *Weekly Epidemiological Record* 88 (12): 129–36.

———. 2013g. "Newly Accessible Japanese Encephalitis Vaccine Will Make Saving Children Easier in Developing Countries." http://www.who.int/mediacentre/news/releases/2013 /japanese_encephalitis_20131009/en/.

———. 2013h. "Practices to Improve Coverage of the Hepatitis B Birth Dose Vaccine." Department of Immunization, Vaccines and Biologicals, WHO, Geneva. http://www.who .int/immunization/documents/control/who_ivb_12.11/en/.

———. 2014a. "Global Burden of Disease." http://www.who .int/healthinfo/global_burden_disease/gbd/en/index.html.

———. 2014b. *Poliomyelitis: Intensification of the Global Eradication Initiative: Report by the Secretariat.* Geneva: WHO. http://apps.who.int/gb/ebwha/pdf_files/wha67/a67 _38-en.pdf.

———. 2014c. "Polio Vaccines. WHO Position Paper." *Weekly Epidemiological Record* 89: 73–92.

———. 2015a. "Multidrug-Resistant Tuberculosis (MDR-TB)." Progammes and Projects, WHO, Geneva. http://www .who.int/tb/challenges/mdr/en/.

———. 2015b. "Meningococcal, A Conjugate Vaccine: Updated Guidance." *Weekly Epidemiological Record* 90: 57–68. http:// www.who.int/wer/2015/wer9008.pdf.

———. 2015c. *World Malaria Report 2014.* Geneva: WHO.

———. 2015d. Background brief. http://www.who.int/malaria /news/2015/background-brief-malaria-vaccine/en/.

WHO and UNICEF (United Nations Children's Fund). 2014. "Progress Towards Global Immunization Goals 2012: Summary Presentation of Key Indicators." WHO, Geneva.

WHO, UNICEF, and World Bank. 2002. *State of the World's Vaccines and Immunization.* Geneva. http://reliefweb.int /sites/reliefweb.int/files/resources/5520E2761424B54EC 1256C7F00505EF7-who-immunisation-oct02.pdf.

Zaman, K., E. Roy, S. E. Arifeen, M. Rahman, R. Raqib, and others. 2008. "Effectiveness of Maternal Influenza Immunization in Mothers and Infants." *New England Journal of Medicine* 359 (15): 1555–64.

Zanella, R. C., S. Bokermann, A. L. Andrade, B. Flannery, and M. C. Brandileone. 2011. "Changes in Serotype Distribution of *Haemophilus influenzae* Meningitis Isolates Identified through Laboratory-Based Surveillance Following Routine Childhood Vaccination against *H. influenzae* Type B in Brazil." *Vaccine* 29 (48): 8937–42.

Zhou, F., J. Santoli, M. L. Messonnier, H. R. Yusuf, A. Shefer, and others. 2005. "Economic Evaluation of the 7-Vaccine Routine Childhood Immunization Schedule in the United States, 2001." *Archives of Pediatrics and Adolescent Medicine* 159 (12): 1136–44.

Management of Severe and Moderate Acute Malnutrition in Children

Lindsey Lenters, Kerri Wazny, and Zulfiqar A. Bhutta

INTRODUCTION

Each year, approximately 5.9 million children around the world die before their fifth birthday (You and others 2015). The leading killers are prematurity and pneumonia, responsible for 17.8 percent and 15.5 percent of all deaths in this age group, respectively (Liu and others 2014, 2016). Degrees of malnutrition are associated with increased risk of all-cause mortality and increased risk of death due to diarrhea, pneumonia, and measles (Black and others 2013).

Defining Malnutrition

The term *malnutrition* is multifaceted. It encompasses both overnutrition, associated with overweight and obesity, and undernutrition, referring to multiple conditions including acute and chronic malnutrition and micronutrient deficiencies.

Chronic malnutrition results from insufficient intake or absorption of essential nutrients over a protracted period. Stunting (short stature for age), the most commonly used indicator of chronic malnutrition, is associated with developmental impairments and reduced economic potential later in life (Black and others 2008; Grantham-McGregor and others 2007). Micronutrient deficiencies are a form of chronic malnutrition that can have marked impacts

on health, development, and productivity over the lifespan. Because visible signs are not always present, micronutrient deficiencies are often referred to as *hidden hunger* (see Das and others [2015], chapter 12 in this volume). The impacts of chronic malnutrition are particularly pronounced when they occur in the first years of life, a period of rapid growth and development.

Acute malnutrition results from sudden reductions in food intake or diet quality and is often combined with pathological causes. Acute malnutrition has been defined in various ways and has been referred to by various names with partially overlapping definitions, including protein-energy malnutrition, wasting, kwashiorkor, and marasmus. In this chapter, we use *acute malnutrition* and *wasting* interchangeably. Acute malnutrition, or wasting, is defined using anthropometric cutoffs and clinical signs. The currently accepted definitions, set out by the WHO, are as follows:

- *Moderate acute malnutrition (MAM),* defined as weight-for-height[1] z-score (WHZ) between −2 and −3 or mid-upper arm circumference (MUAC) between 115 millimeters and <125 millimeters (WHO 2012)
- *Severe acute malnutrition (SAM),* defined as WHZ < −3 or MUAC < 115 millimeters, or the presence of bilateral pitting edema, or both (WHO 2013)

Corresponding author: Zulfiqar A. Bhutta, Centre for Global Child Health, The Hospital for Sick Children, Toronto, Canada, zulfiqar.bhutta@sickkids.ca.

- **Global acute malnutrition (GAM)** refers to MAM and SAM together; it is used as a measurement of nutritional status at a population level and as an indicator of the severity of an emergency situation (GNC 2014).

Marasmus and kwashiorkor are common terms historically used to differentiate between types of SAM. Marasmus refers to children who are very thin for their height (that is, they meet the WHZ or MUAC cutoff) but do not have bilateral pitting edema; kwashiorkor refers to edematous malnutrition. The most recent WHO terminology for SAM has replaced these terms.

Risk Factors and Causes of Undernutrition

Undernutrition results from the complex interplay of a range of distal and proximal factors, as illustrated by the United Nations Children's Fund's (UNICEF) conceptual framework for undernutrition (figure 11.1) (UNICEF 2013). The framework defines basic, underlying, and immediate causes of undernutrition and demonstrates how these causes are interconnected. This general framework also aids in conceptualizing the reasons why children might develop acute malnutrition.

Based on scientific literature investigating the relationships among specific individual, household, and environmental factors and the development of acute malnutrition in children, the following are significant risk factors for MAM and SAM:

- Inadequate dietary intake
- Inappropriate feeding
- Fetal growth restriction
- Inadequate sanitation
- Lack of parental education
- Family size
- Incomplete vaccination
- Poverty
- Economic, political, and environmental instability and emergency situations.

Figure 11.1 Conceptual Framework of Determinants of Undernutrition

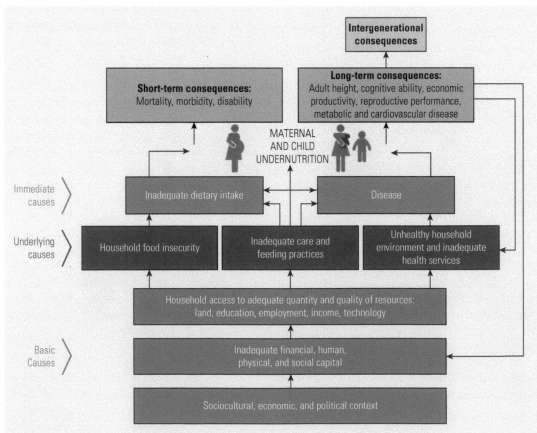

Source: UNICEF 2013.

A study in India demonstrates the impact of infant and young child feeding as well as water, sanitation, and hygiene (WASH) on wasting (Menon and others 2013). The authors found that improved dietary diversity and improved WASH were associated with better nutritional outcomes in children in India; they concluded that integrated interventions targeted to both these risk factors would have a greater impact than single interventions (Menon and others 2013).

Poverty is another risk factor for wasting (Islam and others 2013; Meshram and others 2012), as are unsafe drinking water sources and lack of latrines (Islam and others 2013). Economically disadvantaged families are less likely to have access to improved sources of drinking water, such as water from pipes or tubewells, and are less likely to have access to latrines. One study finds these to be risk factors independent of the wealth index (Islam and others 2013). Another study, which does not assess WASH indicators, finds that the family wealth index to be significantly associated with wasting (Meshram and others 2012). Both studies also find larger family sizes to be associated with an increased risk of wasting (Islam and others 2013; Meshram and others 2012), as does a study in Pakistan (Laghari and others 2013).

Several studies in Bangladesh, India, and Pakistan demonstrate a correlation between low parental education and increased risk of wasting in children (Islam and others 2013; Laghari and others 2013; Long and others 2013; Menon and others 2013; Meshram and others 2012).

A study in Burkina Faso finds incomplete vaccinations and maternal literacy status to be risk factors for wasting relapse (Somasse and others 2013).

Finally, investigators studying the correlation between fetal growth restriction and child wasting find that infants born small for gestational age or those with low birth weight were at a significantly increased risk of being wasted at 24 months (Cao, Wang, and Zeng 2013). Additionally, low birth weight was found to be a risk factor for SAM in children under age five years in Pakistan (Laghari and others 2013).

Incidence of SAM is exacerbated during emergencies, such as drought, famine, or conflict (Hall, Blankson, and Shoham 2011). Indicators such as household food consumption, harvest yield, and staple food prices are early warning signs of imminent food insecurity, followed by increases in the incidence of SAM or GAM (Hall, Blankson, and Shoham 2011).

Consequences of Acute Malnutrition

SAM and MAM are significant public health concerns and disproportionately affect populations in low- and middle-income countries (LMICs). MAM affects 32.8 million children worldwide, 31.8 million of whom reside in LMICs (Black and others 2013). SAM affects 18.7 million children worldwide; 18.5 million of those children reside in LMICs (Black and others 2013).

Map 11.1 shows the prevalence of wasting in children under age five years worldwide. The rates

Map 11.1 Percentage of Children under Age Five Years Who Are Moderately or Severely Wasted, 2007–11

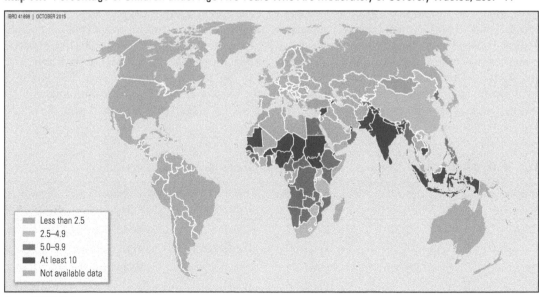

Source: UNICEF 2013.
Note: Data for India are not for the same period as the other countries.

of SAM and MAM are highest in the South-East Asia region and parts of the Africa region; indeed, 70 percent of all wasted children reside in Asia (Black and others 2013).

National wasting statistics can be accessed online through the Joint Malnutrition data set published by UNICEF, the WHO, and the World Bank (UNICEF 2014b; UNICEF, WHO, and World Bank 2012). Rates of SAM and MAM vary widely at subnational levels, particularly where large disparities in income and food security exist; the availability of subnational statistics on wasting also varies widely.

The degree of wasting is positively correlated with an increase in the risk of death (Black and others 2013). Table 11.1 shows all-cause and cause-specific hazard ratios for mortality by degree of wasting. Of the deaths under age five years, 11.5 percent, or approximately 800,000, can be attributed to acute malnutrition (Black and others 2013); SAM is responsible for 540,000 of these deaths (Black and others 2013). Children with acute malnutrition have severely disturbed physiology and metabolism and need to be treated with caution. Simple refeeding can lead to high rates of mortality, and cases can be especially difficult to manage if additional medical complications are present (discussed further under "Treatment of Severe Acute Malnutrition"). Specific guidelines, supported by available evidence and expertise, have been developed for managing these cases and are discussed later in this chapter.

In addition to increasing the risk of death due to infectious illness, wasting increases a child's susceptibility to infections and the severity of illnesses (Laghari and others 2013; Long and others 2013; Meshram and others 2012; UNICEF 2013). Malnutrition has serious physiological consequences, including reductive adaptation, marked immunosuppression, and concurrent infection (Collins, Dent, and others 2006). The relationship between malnutrition and infection is often described as a vicious cycle that begins with infections,

especially diarrhea, and progresses to undernourishment. The undernourishment, in turn, increases the risk of prolonged illness and the susceptibility to additional infection. Human immunodeficiency virus (HIV) infection exacerbates the risk of wasting as well as mortality due to wasting (Sadler and others 2006).

PREVENTION OF ACUTE MALNUTRITION

Providing Adequate Nutrition and Disease Prevention Strategies

Key interventions to prevent the development of acute malnutrition include appropriate breastfeeding[2] and complementary feeding practices[3] (Bhutta, Das, Rizvi, and others 2013). Disease prevention strategies are important in breaking the infection-malnutrition cycle, particularly related to diarrhea and repeated respiratory infections (Bhutta, Das, Walker and others 2013). The evidence on effective approaches to preventing malnutrition focuses on stunting and underweight as outcomes and may not be completely transferrable to prevention of wasting. However, an integrated approach to optimizing healthy growth in infants and children can have an important impact on reducing rates of wasting.

Therapeutic Foods for Preventing and Treating Acute Malnutrition

Treatment approaches are discussed in detail in subsequent sections; here we introduce some of the commonly used specially formulated therapeutic foods.

F75 and F100 are specially formulated milks used in inpatient settings to treat SAM. F75 is given in the stabilization phase of inpatient treatment; children are provided with approximately 80–100 kilocalories per kilogram per day (kcal/kg/d) spread over 8–12 meals per day for three to seven days. F75 is not designed for weight gain (personal communication, Nutriset; UNICEF 2014a). F100 is given during the rehabilitation

Table 11.1 Hazard Ratios of All-Cause and Cause-Specific Deaths, by Degree of Wasting

Weight-for-height z-score	All deaths HR (95% CI)	Pneumonia deaths HR (95% CI)	Diarrhea deaths HR (95% CI)	Measles deaths HR (95% CI)	Other infectious deaths HR (95% CI)
<−3	11.6 (9.8, 13.8)	9.7 (6.1, 15.4)	12.3 (9.2, 16.6)	9.6 (5.1, 18.0)	11.2 (5.9, 21.3)
−3 to −2	3.4 (2.9, 4.0)	4.7 (3.1, 7.1)	3.4 (2.5, 4.6)	2.6 (1.3, 5.1)	2.7 (1.4, 5.5)
−2 to <−1	1.6 (1.4, 1.9)	1.9 (1.3, 2.8)	1.6 (1.2, 2.1)	1.0 (0.6, 1.9)	1.7 (1.0, 2.8)
≥−1	1.0	1.0	1.0	1.0	1.0

Sources: Black and others 2013; Olofin and others 2013.

Note: CI = confidence interval; HR = hazard ratio.

phase of inpatient treatment of SAM, providing children with approximately 100–200 kcal/kg/d for three to four weeks (personal communication, Nutriset; UNICEF 2014a). Because F75 and F100 require preparation and have high moisture content, they cannot be stored for long at room temperature for food safety reasons, and are not given to caretakers to prepare at home (UNICEF 2014a).

Ready-to-use-foods (RUFs) are specially formulated bars, pastes, or biscuits that provide varying ranges of high-quality protein, energy, and micronutrients. These products are more nutrient dense than available home foods and do not require preparation; they typically have very low moisture content and are resistant to microbes. With use of each of these products, continued breastfeeding is recommended.

- Ready-to-use therapeutic foods (RUTFs), such as Plumpy'Nut are designed for the treatment of uncomplicated SAM.
- Ready-to-use supplementary foods (RUSFs), such as Plumpy'Sup, are designed as a supplement to treat MAM.
- Medium-quantity lipid-based nutrient supplements (LNSs), such as Plumpy'Doz, are designed as a supplement to prevent MAM.[4]

Fortified blended flours (FBFs) are an additional class of specially formulated foods. The most commonly used product is Supercereal Plus, formerly called Corn Soy Blend Plus (CSB++). FBFs require some preparation before consumption and are typically distributed in larger quantities as family rations for treating or preventing MAM.

The nutrient composition of some common formulated foods for treatment and prevention of acute malnutrition are shown in table 11.2. Annan, Webb, and Brown (2014) provide a more comprehensive product list of specially formulated foods for MAM management.

Locally Produced Therapeutic Foods

The bulk of RUFs are commercially prepared by a select number of companies and are then distributed to program sites. Decentralizing production could be beneficial for several reasons. Therapeutic foods are often a significant program cost and could be less expensive to produce in-country. Decentralized production could create valuable local economic opportunities.

RUFs can be safely and easily produced in most settings; however, feasibility of production is limited because of the unavailability of necessary ingredients in some settings (Manary 2005). Lenters and others (2013)

Table 11.2 Nutritional Composition of Commonly Used, Specially Formulated Foods for the Prevention and Treatment of Acute Malnutrition

	F75 (100 g milk powder)	F100 (100 g milk powder)	Plumpy'Sup (100 g)	Plumpy'Doz (100 g)	Plumpy'Nut (100 g)	Supercereal Plus (100 g dry matter)
Used for	SAM	SAM	MAM	MAM	MAM or SAM	Prevention of MAM
Recommended serving size (kcal/kg/d)	80–100	200	75	46.3 g/day	SAM: 200 MAM: 75	200 g/day
Macronutrients						
Energy (kcal)	446	520	520–550	534–587	520–550	410
Protein (g)	5.9	>13	12.6–15.4	13.4–17.7	13–16	>16.4
Lipid (g)	15.6	>26	31.5–38.6	26.7–39.1	26–36	>4.1
Minerals						
Potassium (mg)	775	1,100	980–1,210	660–870	1,100–1,400	140
Calcium (mg)	560	300	300–350	800–980	300–500	452
Phosphorus (mg)	330	300	300–350	530–660	300–600	232
Magnesium (mg)	50	80	80–100	115–140	80–100	—
Zinc (mg)	12.2	11	12–15	8.7	11–14	5

Sources: Nutriset catalogs; Supercereal Plus from USAID specifications.
Note: — = not available; d = day; g = gram; kcal = kilocalorie; kg = kilogram; MAM = moderate acute malnutrition; mg = milligram; SAM = severe acute malnutrition.

find no difference in the effectiveness for promoting weight gain from a pooled analysis of data from two studies (Diop and others 2004; Sandige and others 2004) comparing locally produced and imported RUTF that met the same product specifications.

There is interest among academic, donor, and non-profit communities in developing new formulations of RUFs that make use of locally available ingredients while targeting taste preferences of different populations. For example, RUFs could substitute other legumes for the standard peanut base, or reduce or substitute the milk powder component in areas in which dairy is not commonly consumed (Matilsky and others 2009; Oakley and others 2010; Sandige and others 2004). Research is ongoing with respect to the treatment effectiveness and cost-effectiveness of alternate formulations.

MANAGEMENT OF MODERATE ACUTE MALNUTRITION

Although the typology of interventions for MAM and their indicated uses in different contexts have been topics of considerable discussion, substantial ambiguity remains in practice in the classification of interventions, and evidence gaps persist regarding the effectiveness of interventions. One example of guidelines recently developed is the Global Nutrition Cluster decision-making tool that guides the selection of appropriate programming approaches in emergency situations (GNC 2014).

The management of MAM can be broadly categorized into *prevention* and *treatment* strategies. In general, because wasting results in a loss of body mass relative to height, the standard practice has been to provide the child with additional energy and nutrient-dense foods to promote weight gain. The selection of the particular management approach is context specific; different approaches are warranted for populations that are more stable and food secure than for populations experiencing significant food insecurity or humanitarian emergencies.

Strategies for Prevention

Strategies for the prevention of MAM dovetail with public health interventions promoting optimal child growth and development. These strategies include the promotion of appropriate breastfeeding and complementary feeding practices, access to appropriate health care for the prevention and treatment of disease, and improved sanitation and hygiene practices. Additionally, although micronutrient deficiencies are most commonly linked to stunted linear growth, these deficiencies can also contribute to wasting, for example, through the malnutrition-infection cycle. Undernourished children

tend to be more susceptible to infection, which can contribute to weight loss through increased metabolism, as well as reduced nutrient intake and absorption (Guerrant and others 2008; Petri and others 2008). Multiple-micronutrient powders, small-quantity LNSs, and single-nutrient supplements are used to augment the nutritional content of the home diet.

Strategies for Treatment

Research is ongoing with respect to optimal treatment approaches. In 2008, the WHO established a working group on dietary management of MAM; since then, the emphasis on exploring optimal food-based treatments for MAM has increased (GNC 2014). The 2012 WHO technical note on supplementary foods for managing MAM in children ages 6–59 months calls for providing locally available, nutrient-dense foods to improve nutritional status and prevent SAM (WHO 2012). In situations of food shortage, supplementary foods have been supplied with suboptimal effectiveness. WHO (2012) suggests that an energy intake of 25 kcal/kg/d in addition to the standard nutrient requirements of a nonmalnourished child would support a reasonable rate of weight gain without promoting obesity. However, there is no evidence-informed recommendation for the composition of specially formulated foods for treatment (WHO 2012).

The Community-Based Management of Acute Malnutrition (CMAM) Forum published a technical brief in 2014 that echoed the WHO guidelines and discussed recommendations for diets suitable for children with MAM, approaches to counseling caregivers, and a decision-making framework for selecting appropriate supplementary feeding program (SFP) approaches (Annan, Webb, and Brown 2014).

Food-Secure Populations

In food-secure populations, caregivers can be counseled and supported in using high-quality, home-available foods to promote recovery in acutely malnourished children (Bhutta, Das, Rizvi, and others 2013). This intervention can be coupled with general health-promotion approaches to mitigate the underlying factors contributing to acute malnutrition, for example, WASH and health-seeking behaviors.

Two systematic reviews (Lazzerini, Rupert, and Pani 2013; Lenters and others 2013) find no significant differences in mortality between the provision of any type of specially formulated food and standard care, which consists of medical care and counseling without food provision. Children provided with food were significantly more likely to recover, based on two studies in the meta-analysis

(Lazzerini, Rupert, and Pani 2013). This systematic review could not identify any trials investigating the effect of improving the adequacy of local diets.

The literature search conducted by Lenters and others (2013) identifies very few rigorous trials that compare the provision of RUTFs or RUSFs with other types of interventions to modify household- and community-level factors that contribute to the development of wasting. In one study, the mean weight gain was significantly higher in the group provided with RUTFs than in the standard care group in which mothers were taught to prepare a high-calorie cereal milk (Singh and others 2010). However, because this study assessed nutritional status using weight-for-age, children who were not wasted may have been included in the study.

Ashworth and Ferguson (2009) review dietary counseling for treatment of MAM and use programmatic data from United Nations agencies, nongovernmental organizations, and national programs to assess whether the counseling and recommendations given were likely to meet children's dietary needs. The authors conclude that messages tended to be vague and were unlikely to be effective. Their review also aims to assess the effectiveness of dietary counseling in the management of MAM; based on an analysis of 10 studies, they suggest that counseling families on the consumption of family foods can have a positive effect on weight gain. However, this review does not contain a meta-analysis; the studies included are a mix of quasi-experimental and observational data and employ a variety of indices to measure malnutrition.

Food-Insecure Populations

In food-insecure populations, including humanitarian emergency contexts, SFPs are used to reduce mortality and prevent further deterioration of children's nutritional status. These SFPs are classified as targeted SFPs or blanket SFPs, depending on the recipients. A blanket approach provides supplemental food to everyone within a defined population, regardless of whether children are acutely malnourished; a targeted approach provides supplemental rations only for malnourished children meeting program cut-off criteria.

The standard practice for SFPs is to provide a ration of staple food, such as FBF, commonly Supercereal Plus (GNC 2014). However, a growing range of RUFs have been developed specifically for treating MAM. A Cochrane review (Lazzerini, Rupert, and Pani 2013) compares the effectiveness of LNSs with FBFs for the treatment of MAM. This review concludes that both products appear to be effective; there is insufficient evidence to recommend the use of LNS over corn-soy blend (CSB), despite the growing interest from the policy

and programming community in these new specially formulated foods. No reduction in mortality, differences in numbers of children progressing to SAM, or dropping out of the study were found when comparing LNS with CSB for the five studies included in the meta-analysis. Yet, treatment with LNS led to a 10 percent increase in recovery compared with CSB, and slightly improved nutritional status among those recovered. No significant differences were seen when Supercereal Plus was compared with LNS. These findings are echoed in the systematic review conducted by Lenters and others (2013) as part of *The Lancet* series on maternal and child nutrition, as well as in a review conducted by the Food Aid Quality Review group (Webb and others 2011).

In situations that warrant the provision of supplemental foods, there is growing recognition of the need to use integrated approaches to address the immediate need for an improved diet to treat MAM and prevent the progression to SAM, while simultaneously addressing the underlying factors. Livelihood diversification, social protection schemes, and conditional cash transfers are some of the approaches being explored in these contexts (Bhutta, Das, Rizvi, and others 2013).

Seasonal Supplementation

Seasonal blanket feeding programs are an emerging approach aimed at suppressing predictable increases in the rates of SAM and MAM. In chronically food-insecure settings, a spike in the incidence of MAM and SAM is seen in the period before the harvest, known as the "lean season." Seasonal SFPs, which may be targeted by geographic region or age group, tend to include all children who either have, or are at risk for, MAM. The evidence remains limited on the effectiveness or cost-effectiveness of such approaches for prevention; however, several studies investigate the use of RUF supplementation for nonwasted children to reduce seasonal increases in population-wide prevalence rates of wasting (Defourny and others 2009; Grellety and others 2012; Hall and others 2011; Huybregts and others 2012; Isanaka and others 2009; Karakochuk, Stephens, and Zlotkin 2012).

A blanket SFP in Niger provided children ages 6–26 months (MUAC < 110 millimeters millimeters) with roughly 50 grams per day of RUSFs (Defourny and others 2009). Fewer children in the target locality presented in need of therapeutic care than in previous years; however, it was not possible to rule out overall improvements in food security in the absence of a comparison group in the study.

Another study in Niger randomized villages to receive the intervention (one packet of RUTF per day for children) versus no intervention. The intervention led to an estimated 36 percent difference in the incidence of wasting and a 58 percent difference in the incidence of severe wasting (Isanaka and others 2009). Although the authors claim that the difference represented a reduction in wasting, some reviewers argue that the statistically significant difference could be ascribed to increased incidence of wasting in the control villages coupled with no change in the intervention sites (Hall and others 2011).

Where markets are viable, interventions that aim to stimulate the local economy through cash transfers, voucher schemes, or the provision of locally available food rations may be more sustainable and acceptable than the provision of imported RUFs.

TREATMENT OF SEVERE ACUTE MALNUTRITION

Approaches to identifying, referring, and treating SAM cases have been evolving, and a mix of programmatic approaches can be found globally. The WHO endorses community-based management of uncomplicated SAM and recommends that children with poor appetite, severe edema (Grade III), and any of the Integrated Management of Childhood Illness danger signs or medical complications (table 11.3) be treated in inpatient facilities in accordance with their 10-step model (figure 11.2) (WHO 2013).

This section focuses on the WHO-endorsed treatment approaches. Although these approaches are evidence informed, many of the recommendations are rooted in imperfect evidence and supplemented by best practices and expert opinion.

From the 1950s through the 1990s, case fatality rates (CFRs) for the treatment of SAM in health facilities remained static and were typically 20 percent to 30 percent (Ashworth and others 2003; Collins, Dent, and others 2006); specialized treatment centers were able to achieve CFRs of less than 5 percent (Collins, Dent, and others 2006). As a response to the high CFRs and high opportunity costs of inpatient treatment, a community-based approach to treating acute malnutrition has received growing attention from the academic and humanitarian sectors. Community-based treatment of malnutrition was initially referred to as the community therapeutic care model, but it may also be called community management of acute malnutrition (CMAM) and integrated management of acute malnutrition. For clarity, this chapter refers to community-based management as CMAM.

Table 11.3 Common Medical Complications in Severe Acute Malnutrition

Medical complication	Case definition
Anorexia, poor appetite[a]	Child is unable to drink or breastfeed; failed RUTF appetite test.
Intractable vomiting[a]	Child vomits after every oral intake.
High fever	Child has high body temperature, or axillary temperature > 38.5°C, rectal temperature > 39°C.
Hypothermia	Child has low body temperature, or axillary temperature < 35.0°C, rectal temperature < 35.5°C.
Lower respiratory tract infection	Child has a cough with difficult breathing, fast breathing (if child is age 2–12 months: 50 breaths per minute or more; if child is age 12 months to 5 years: 40 breaths per minute or more), or chest indrawing.
Severe anemia	Child has palmar pallor or unusual paleness of the skin (compare the color of the child's palm with your own palm and with the palms of other children).
Skin lesion	Child has broken skin, fissures, flaking of skin.
Unconsciousness[a]	Child does not respond to painful stimuli (for example, injection).
Lethargy, not alert[a]	Child is difficult to wake. Ask the mother if the child is drowsy, shows no interest in what is happening around him or her, does not look at the mother or watch your face when talking, is unusually sleepy.
Hypoglycemia	There are often no clinical signs of hypoglycemia. One sign that does occur in a child with SAM is eyelid retraction: child sleeps with eyes slightly open.
Convulsions[a]	During a convulsion, child's arms and legs stiffen because the muscles are contracting. Ask the mother if the child had convulsions during this current illness.
Severe dehydration	Child with SAM has a recent history of diarrhea, vomiting, high fever or sweating, and recent appearance of clinical signs of dehydration as reported by the caregiver.

Source: Saboya, Khara, and Irena 2011.
Note: °C = degrees centigrade; RUTF = ready-to-use therapeutic food; SAM = severe acute malnutrition.
a. Integrated Management of Childhood Illness danger signs.

Figure 11.2 World Health Organization's 10-Step Plan for the Management of Severe Acute Malnutrition

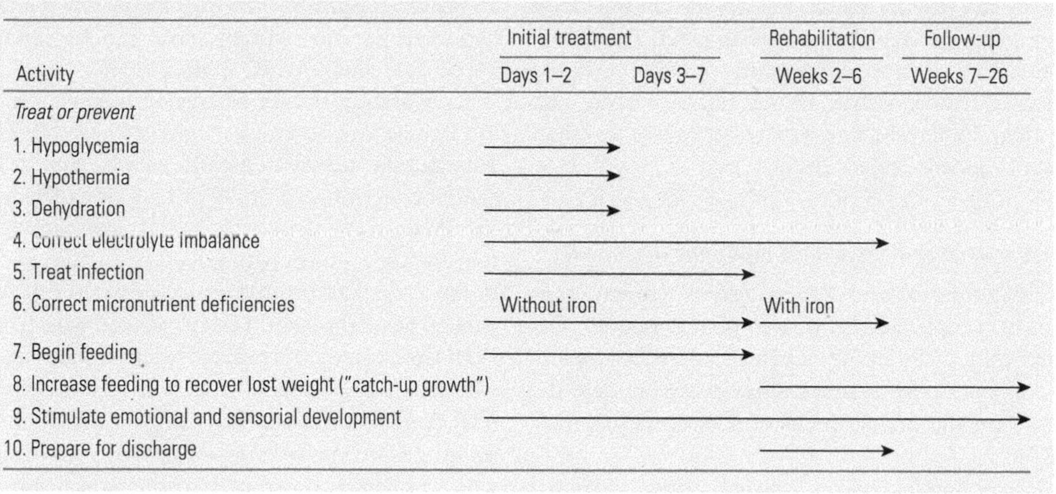

Activity	Initial treatment		Rehabilitation	Follow-up
	Days 1–2	Days 3–7	Weeks 2–6	Weeks 7–26
Treat or prevent				
1. Hypoglycemia	⟶			
2. Hypothermia	⟶			
3. Dehydration	⟶			
4. Correct electrolyte imbalance	⟶			
5. Treat infection	⟶			
6. Correct micronutrient deficiencies	Without iron		With iron ⟶	
7. Begin feeding	⟶			
8. Increase feeding to recover lost weight ("catch-up growth")			⟶	
9. Stimulate emotional and sensorial development	⟶			
10. Prepare for discharge			⟶	

Sources: Picot and others 2012; WHO 2003.

Community-Based Treatment

The first CMAM programs, developed under the community therapeutic care model and implemented in the early 2000s, achieved recovery rates of almost 80 percent and CFRs of less than 5 percent (Collins, Sadler, and others 2006). More than 75 percent of children treated for malnutrition in these programs were treated on an outpatient basis, reducing opportunity costs to caregivers (less time away from income-generating activities and responsibilities as caregiver to additional children).

The community therapeutic care model of treatment rests on the four following principles:

- Maximum coverage and access
- Timeliness
- Appropriate care
- Care for as long as it is needed (Collins, Sadler, and others 2006).

This model strives to reach all severely malnourished children before the development of medical complications and to provide appropriate care until recovery. The model uses community health workers or volunteers (CHWs or CHVs) to actively find cases of wasting within the community. Children are screened to assess their nutritional status, typically using MUAC cutoffs and simple algorithms to assess the presence of medical complications, which would necessitate referral to a facility-based treatment program.

The most commonly seen medical complications in SAM are outlined in table 11.3. Only about 15 percent of children with SAM have medical complications that require inpatient treatment (Collins, Sadler, and others 2006). Substantial programmatic evidence has demonstrated that the community-based model can achieve low mortality rates and decrease opportunity costs to caregivers, resulting in lower default rates (Collins, Sadler, and others 2006; Guerrero and Rogers 2013). *Defaulters* are children who are lost to follow-up (Sphere Project 2011).

In the CMAM model, mothers administer the RUTFs to their children. The rapid changes in the children's condition provide positive feedback to those associated with the recovery process and strengthens community motivation for case-finding, foreseeably increasing coverage (Collins, Sadler, and others 2006).

The 2013 WHO guidelines (WHO 2013) recommend that children should be enrolled and discharged from treatment using the same mode of classification. Children who were admitted based on MUAC should be discharged once their MUAC is ≥ 125 millimeters for at least two weeks or their WHZ is ≥ −2 for at least two weeks. Children who were admitted based on their edema should be discharged based on the measurement routinely used in the program. Once discharged, the children should be followed up periodically to avoid relapse.

The 2013 WHO guidelines (WHO 2013) include several additional updates:

- Children who are not treated with fortified therapeutic foods should receive a high dose of vitamin A on admission; children who receive therapeutic food do not need the high dose of vitamin A.
- RUTFs should be given to children regardless of whether they have diarrhea (WHO 2013).

The CMAM model is endorsed in the Sphere Project guidelines, an evidence-based, sector-wide consensus on minimum standards for humanitarian relief. The guidelines state that treatment programs for SAM should achieve a CFR of less than 10 percent, a recovery rate greater than 75 percent, and a defaulter rate of less than 15 percent (Sphere Project 2011).

The WHO's 10-Step Program for Inpatient Treatment

The WHO published a 10-step guide for inpatient management of complicated SAM to combat the poor CFRs in some health facilities (WHO 2003) and subsequently undertook a series of systematic reviews to update the guidelines on the management of severe malnutrition (WHO 2013).

These systematic reviews collated evidence related to treatment of SAM, including criteria for identifying SAM, discharge, follow-up, treatment of HIV-positive children with SAM, appropriate hydration, and treatment of infants younger than age six months. Overall, the reviews found low or very low quality evidence to support their recommendations as a result of limited availability of randomized controlled trials (RCTs) investigating the treatment options.

The 10-step plan for inpatient management of SAM is shown in figure 11.2. The 10 steps are divided into three phases; children's emotional and sensorial development should be stimulated throughout all phases:

- *Initial treatment*: Hypoglycemia, hypothermia, dehydration, infections, and electrolyte imbalances are corrected, as are micronutrient deficiencies with the exception of iron deficiency.
- *Rehabilitation*: Electrolyte imbalances and micronutrient deficiencies continue to be corrected, and iron is added. Feeding is increased to stimulate catch-up growth, and children are prepared for discharge.
- *Follow-up*: Increased feeding is continued to recover lost weight (Picot and others 2012; WHO 2003).

Initial Treatment Phase

During the initial treatment phase, frequent feeding is important to prevent both hypoglycemia and hypothermia. Feeding during the initial treatment phase should be approached cautiously because of the fragility of the child's physiological state. F75 should be given every 30 minutes for two hours, followed by F75 every two hours, day and night. Breastfed children should be encouraged to continue breastfeeding. Children with hypothermia should be rewarmed by being clothed, covered with a warmed blanket, placed near a heater or lamp, or placed on the mother's chest (skin-to-skin) and covered. Specific protocols for assessing and treating hypothermia and hypoglycemia can be found in the WHO guidelines (WHO 2003, 2013).

Dehydration should be treated following the WHO's 2013 guidelines; several key updates have been included. For example, dehydrated children who are not in shock should be rehydrated orally or by nasogastric tube using ReSoMal or half-strength WHO low-osmolarity oral rehydration solution with added potassium and glucose. If the child has profuse watery diarrhea or suspected cholera he or she should be rehydrated with full-strength WHO low-osmolarity oral rehydration solution. Children who are severely dehydrated or with signs of shock should be rehydrated intravenously, using half-strength Darrow's solution with 5 percent dextrose, Ringer's lactate solution with 5 percent dextrose, or, if neither is available, 0.45 percent saline with 5 percent dextrose (WHO 2013).

Infections should be treated routinely upon admission by provision of a broad-spectrum antibiotic, and measles vaccination should be given for unimmunized children older than age six months.

Micronutrient deficiencies should be treated by giving vitamin A (200,000 international units [IU] for children older than age 12 months, 100,000 IU for children ages 6–12 months, and 50,000 IU for children ages 0–5 months), coupled with daily multivitamin, folic acid, zinc, and copper supplementation for at least two weeks. Iron supplementation should only be given once children have begun gaining weight.

Rehabilitation Phase

During the rehabilitation phase, F75 should be replaced with F100 in the same amounts for 48 hours before increasing successive feeds by 10 milliliters until some remains unconsumed. If available, children could be transitioned from F75 to RUTF according to the updated WHO guidelines (WHO 2013). Children's respiratory and pulse rates should be monitored closely. After transition to F100, children should receive feedings consisting of 100–200 kcal/kg/d and 4–6 g protein/kg/d at least every four hours. Breastfeeding should continue to be encouraged.

Follow-Up Phase

After recovery, parents should be taught to feed children frequently with energy- and nutrient-dense foods and to continue to stimulate their children's sensorial and emotional development. Parents should be requested to bring children back for regular follow-up checks. Vitamin A supplementation and booster immunizations should be provided.

Managing Infections in Children with SAM

In addition to increased susceptibility to infections, children with SAM are more likely to have more severe illnesses and higher mortality rates than nonwasted children (Jones and Berkley 2014; Laghari and others 2013; Long and others 2013; Meshram and others 2012; UNICEF 2013). Common infections include diarrhea, acute respiratory infection, HIV, tuberculosis, meningitis, anemia, bacteremia, and sepsis (Chisti and others 2014; Irena, Mwambazi, and Mulenga 2011; Jones and Berkley 2014; Kumar and others 2013; Nhampossa and others 2013; Page and others 2013; Schlaudecker, Steinhoff, and Moore 2011). The proportion of children with SAM who have comorbidities varies. For example, 31 percent and 33.6 percent, respectively, of children with SAM in two studies in Mozambique and India had acute diarrhea, compared with 67.1 percent of children with SAM in a study in Zambia (Irena, Mwambazi, and Mulenga 2011; Kumar and others 2013; Nhampossa and others 2013).

Determining the etiology of infections can be difficult because of limited resources and because clinical signs of infection may not be apparent (Jones and Berkley 2014; Page and others 2013). Diagnosis of malaria can be challenging because its symptoms can be indistinguishable from other febrile illnesses; rapid diagnostic tests or microscopic blood examination are recommended for malaria diagnosis. Children with SAM who have radiologic-confirmed pneumonia may not exhibit any typical signs or symptoms (Jones and Berkley 2014). The diagnosis of tuberculosis can be especially challenging (Chisti and others 2014; Jones and Berkley 2014). Laboratory-confirmed tuberculosis through *Mycobacterium tuberculosis* culture is the gold standard, but children with SAM often do not produce suitable sputum samples, and culturing the bacteria is a lengthy procedure. Skin tests have high false negative rates, and scoring systems have been developed. Jones and Berkley (2014) recommend the consideration of clinical response to nutritional rehabilitation, such as weight gain and fever, in the diagnosis of tuberculosis.

Treatment for malnourished children with concurrent infections should follow the WHO guidelines. Severely malnourished children diagnosed with tuberculosis should be treated with a single dose of 5–10 milligrams per day of vitamin B6 along with isoniazid. Antiretroviral therapy (ART) should be initiated in the rehabilitation phase of treatment in HIV-positive children with SAM, and they should be given co-trimoxazole daily. HIV-positive mothers should receive ART or infants should receive prophylaxis, and mothers should be encouraged to breastfeed exclusively for six months and continue for up to two years (Jones and Berkley 2014; WHO 2010). Severely malnourished children infected with malaria should be treated with artesunate; those with diarrhea who are dehydrated or in shock should be managed as described in the WHO 10-step plan for inpatient management of SAM.

The provision of broad-spectrum antibiotics to all outpatient children with SAM would mirror WHO recommendations for treatment of nonmalnourished children with pneumonia (Jones and Berkley 2014), although blanket provision of antibiotics is controversial. Because of the differences in the presentation of infection in malnourished versus well-nourished children, Jones and Berkley (2014) recommend that children who do show abnormal radiology be carefully evaluated for tuberculosis.

Considering Antibiotic Treatment

New evidence is emerging on the importance of managing SAM, including uncomplicated SAM, using a package of care that includes antibiotic treatment. The use of broad-spectrum antibiotics has been conditionally recommended for treatment of uncomplicated SAM in community-based treatment programs (WHO 2007). Local governments and policy makers are asked to make this determination in light of local contexts. Although routine antibiotic treatment at the enrollment stage in CMAM programs is part of the protocols of many organizations, this practice remains controversial.

One systematic review of antibiotics as part of SAM management concludes that the evidence for the addition of antibiotics to therapeutic regimens for uncomplicated SAM is weak and urges further efficacy trials (Alcoba and others 2013). Another review concludes that the evidence was insufficient to recommend antibiotic use (Picot and others 2012). An RCT in Malawi looked at children with uncomplicated SAM treated in a community setting, comparing RUTFs to RUTFs plus antibiotics (either amoxicillin or cefdinir). The trial found a significantly higher mortality rate in children receiving placebo than in either antibiotic arm (amoxicillin: relative risk = 1.55, 95 percent confidence interval 1.07–2.24; cefdinir: relative risk = 1.80, 95 percent confidence interval 1.22–2.64) (Trehan and others 2013). Criticisms have been raised, however, because HIV-infection rates are high in this region and could be a major cause of immunodeficiency; 68 percent of the children enrolled were not tested for HIV (Koumans, Routh, and Davis 2013). Additional questions have been raised about the approach to the analysis (Okeke, Cruz, and Keusch 2013).

Because of the small number of studies with limited generalizability, as well as the costs and resistance risks associated with broad use of antibiotics, this topic requires immediate further investigation.

Treatment of Edematous Acute Malnutrition

Edematous acute malnutrition, referred to as kwashiorkor, is a form of acute malnutrition characterized by stunted growth, generalized edema, dermatologic manifestations, and hepatic steatosis (Garrett 2013). Its etiology is not well understood; it has been attributed to a range of factors, including insufficient dietary protein, excessive oxidative stress, a compromised intestinal wall, and intestinal inflammation (Garrett 2013; Smith and others 2013). The prevailing theory implicates the intestinal microbiota. Certain microflora appear to play a role in the development of kwashiorkor, as indicated by a longitudinal comparative study of Malawian twins by Smith and others (2013), as well as a mouse study (Garrett 2013; Smith and others 2013).

Given that children with severe edema[5] have a higher risk of mortality even in the absence of other medical complications, the recommendation is to treat these children in an inpatient setting (WHO 2013). The treatment protocol for children with edematous malnutrition is largely the same but with several important caveats outlined in the WHO guidelines (WHO 2013). For example, initial refeeding should occur at a rate of 100 milliliters per kilogram per day (ml/kg/d) as opposed to the general recommendation of 130 ml/kg/d, with a tailored schedule for progression after initial refeeding (Ashworth and others 2003).

The optimal setting for managing children with SAM who have mild to moderate edema remains unclear; these children may be treated in outpatient settings or referred to inpatient facilities, depending on the protocol of particular programs. No RCTs have compared inpatient treatment to community-based treatment for this group. An evidence review found eight reports describing outcomes for single cohorts of children with edema treated in the community for SAM (WHO 2013). These reports found an average recovery rate of 88 percent and CFR of less than 4 percent. However, the authors graded the quality of this evidence as very low, stating that it is difficult to make any firm recommendations about the effectiveness and safety of outpatient treatment for children with mild to moderate edema (WHO 2013).

At country and sub-country levels, the prevalence and incidence rates of edematous SAM are not well characterized; experts have called for more data on prevalence to establish the burden as an initial step to shed light on its public health importance (personal communication, CMAM Forum). The proportion of edematous SAM ranges from 0 percent in Albania and Indonesia to greater than 70 percent in the former Yugoslav Republic of Macedonia and Nicaragua (personal communication, CMAM Forum).

COSTS AND COST-EFFECTIVENESS OF TREATMENT OF SEVERE ACUTE MALNUTRITION

The published literature on the cost-effectiveness of SAM is limited; the authors of this chapter were unable to find published cost-effectiveness studies for MAM. Accordingly, the following cost-effectiveness section focuses on SAM.

The maternal and child nutrition series in *The Lancet* (Bhutta, Das, Rizvi, and others 2013) estimated the cost of increasing coverage of SAM treatment to 90 percent in 34 high-burden countries. The overall cost of scaling up SAM treatment to 90 percent in these target countries was US$2.6 billion. Of this amount, approximately 35 percent of the costs were for consumables, which is in line with the costs of other estimates for RUTFs in the treatment of SAM (Bhutta, Das, Rizvi, and others 2013).

Inpatient Treatment Programs

Inpatient treatment programs have several disadvantages for treating children who may not require it. Resource constraints can limit the number of children who can be treated. The centralized nature of the facilities means that the difficulties patients face in transport can result in delayed presentation of cases and lower coverage rates. An evaluation of 21 community-based treatment programs in Ethiopia, Malawi, and Sudan found an average coverage rate of 72.5 percent, compared with less than 10 percent coverage in inpatient programs; coverage is defined as the proportion of children needing treatment who receive it for inpatient programs (Collins, Dent, and others 2006). Moreover, because mothers often need to stay with children for longer than three weeks, inpatient treatment can cost families lost labor and economic productivity, as well as pose challenges for families with other children at home. Finally, hospitalization puts children at risk of cross infection (Bachmann 2010; Collins, Dent, and others 2006; Tekeste and others 2012).

Facility-based treatment, however, is required for complicated cases; approximately 15 percent to 20 percent of SAM cases require such treatment (Bachmann 2010; Collins, Dent, and others 2006). We were unable to find any recent studies reporting the costs of inpatient treatment of SAM other than the assumptions of costs made in the 2013 *Lancet* series on maternal and child nutrition. Costs for inpatient treatment of SAM would be highly context-dependent.

Community-Based Programs

Approximately 75 percent to 80 percent of all SAM cases can be effectively treated in the community (Bachmann 2010). A review of cost of treatment found that community-based treatment of SAM was consistently less expensive and had similar or better outcomes, compared to inpatient treatment; however, because many studies were nonrandomized, this finding could have occurred because more severely ill children were admitted to inpatient care (Bachmann 2010).

According to Horton and colleagues (see Ashok and others [2015], chapter 18 in this volume), CMAM is an attractive strategy from a cost-effectiveness perspective. The high risk of death, coupled with reductions in programming costs, lead to a cost-effective strategy. Of the three studies identified and reviewed by Horton, the cost-effectiveness ranged between US$26 and US$39 per disability-adjusted life year (DALY) averted.

Several studies have examined the costs and cost-effectiveness of CMAM programs. Puett and others (2012) compare the cost-effectiveness of a CMAM program delivered by CHWs in Bangladesh with standard inpatient treatment. The authors find that the CMAM program cost US$26 per DALY averted and US$869 per life saved. The costs of SAM treatment in the control group were US$1,344 per DALY averted and US$45,688 per life saved, respectively.

A study in Ethiopia that retrospectively examined the costs of CMAM versus treatment in a therapeutic feeding center (TFC) finds that costs were substantially lower in the CMAM program, with a cost per recovered child for the CMAM and TFC of US$145.50 and US$320.00, respectively (Tekeste and others 2012). Studies in Malawi (Wilford, Golden, and Walker 2012) and Zambia (Bachmann 2009) examining the costs of CMAM compared with hypothetical simulations of no care both find CMAM to be cost-effective and on par with other child health interventions, including universal salt iodization, iron fortification, immunization, and micronutrient fortification. The study in Zambia also finds CMAM to be cost-effective according to the WHO standards, given that the cost per DALY averted was less than the national per capita gross domestic product (GDP). The study in Malawi finds CMAM to cost US$42 per DALY averted; the study in Zambia finds CMAM to cost US$53 per DALY averted. The authors estimated the cost per child to be US$203 and per life saved to be US$1,760 (Wilford, Golden, and Walker 2012).

Overall, CMAM programs are both less expensive and as effective as inpatient care or TFCs, and accordingly are highly cost-effective for treating children with uncomplicated SAM. Community-based programs have higher coverage rates and the potential to catch cases earlier because CHWs and CHVs actively find cases; these programs present lower opportunity costs for families and caregivers of children with SAM. In many CMAM programs, RUTFs are a major contributor to the cost of treatment, constituting 24 percent to 43 percent of the total cost of treatment per child (Puett and others 2012; Tekeste and others 2012). Exploring the use of local rather than imported constituents could lower their relatively high cost.

LOOKING FORWARD

Addressing Evidence Gaps for Effective Management

Approaches to managing SAM have shifted dramatically since the early 2000s, leading to improvements in coverage rates and treatment outcomes (Collins, Dent, and others 2006; Hall, Blankson, and Shoham 2011; Lenters and others 2013). Greater attention is turning to the need for effective strategies to manage MAM. A remarkable range of specially formulated foods for the management of acute malnutrition has been developed and the need for integrated packages of care that include SAM and MAM management has been increasingly appreciated.

Despite these advances, questions remain with respect to etiology, effective treatment approaches, long-term outcomes, and the most effective modes for implementing and sustaining high-quality programs. Furthermore, interpretations of the existing body of literature are limited by study design issues, as well as by a lack of standardization in measurement and reporting. Box 11.1 highlights key research priorities for the effective management of SAM and MAM.

Enhancing Study Design and Standardizing Reporting

It is also imperative to discuss study design issues in the existing body of literature, as well as issues related to reporting of results. A more coordinated, standardized approach to study design and reporting will enhance the interpretability of individual studies and increase the feasibility of conducting pooled analyses, resulting in a stronger evidence base.

The majority of SAM and MAM trials follow children for a short period and only report on changes during the intervention, providing little insight into what happens after treatment. Studies with a short

Box 11.1

Key Priorities for Enhancing Effectiveness of Severe Acute Malnutrition (SAM) and Moderate Acute Malnutrition (MAM) Management

Research Priorities for Effective Management of SAM

- Develop mid-upper arm circumference cut-offs specific to age: 6–11 months, 12–23 months, and 24–59 months (WHO 2013).
- Understand specialized needs of subgroups (Picot and others 2012; WHO 2013):
  - Identification and management of infants younger than age six months with SAM
  - Treatment and long-term support for children with SAM and human immunodeficiency virus, tuberculosis, or other comorbidities.
- Characterize relapse rates and morbidity later in life through follow-up studies (Hall, Blankson, and Shoham 2011; Lenters and others 2013).
- Understand the etiology of nutritional edema and effective strategies for the management of SAM plus edema (WHO 2013).
- Investigate the role of the microbiome and environmental enteropathy in the development of, and recovery from, acute malnutrition (Petri, Naylor, and Haque 2014).
- Clarify the appropriateness of antibiotics for treatment of uncomplicated SAM (Picot and others 2012; WHO 2013).
- Investigate the efficacy of daily low-dose versus single high-dose vitamin A supplementation in children with SAM who have edema or diarrhea (WHO 2013).
- Establish efficacy and effectiveness of local formulations of therapeutic foods that meet WHO specifications (WHO 2013).
- Determine effective fluid management strategies for children with SAM and dehydration or diarrhea (WHO 2013), as well as effective approaches for managing shock in children with SAM (Picot and others 2012).

Research Priorities for Effective Management of MAM

- Expand understanding of specialized nutrient needs for children with MAM (GNC 2014).
- Investigate effective strategies for improving the home diet using locally available ingredients, where feasible (Lazzerini, Rubert, and Pani 2013), and effective nutrition counseling for the prevention and management of MAM (GNC 2014).
- Investigate effective approaches for management of MAM with diarrhea (Annan, Webb, and Brown 2014).
- Understand specialized needs of subgroups, including identification and management of MAM in infants younger than age six months (Annan, Webb, and Brown 2014).
- Clarify the appropriateness of different specially formulated foods and management strategies for different contexts (GNC 2014).

General Priorities for SAM and MAM Research and Programming

- Define *healthy recovery* and investigate body composition and long-term risk of morbidity in children treated with lipid-based specially formulated foods (Annan, Webb, and Brown 2014).
- Improve national and subnational capacity for accurately and consistently measuring coverage rates of SAM and MAM programs (GNC 2014).
- Enhance active case finding in communities and screening at health centers (WHO 2013).
- Explore whether children experience issues when they make the transition to standard family foods from a therapeutic diet (Hall, Blankson, and Shoham 2011).
- Investigate relative effectiveness and costs of different packages of care that include SAM and MAM management (Lenters and others 2013).
- Investigate effectiveness of seasonal blanket supplementation and other strategies (voucher schemes, cash transfers) for the prevention of SAM and MAM.
- Explore patterns of sharing of specially formulated foods (GNC 2014).
- Conduct research in more locations and contexts to be able to assess regional differences in effectiveness and acceptability of treatment and management approaches (Annan, Webb, and Brown 2014).
- Understand how products are used within community interventions, including rates and patterns of sharing (Annan, Webb, and Brown 2014; GNC 2014).

follow-up time are not able to adequately measure time to recovery, and children who have not recovered by the end of the intervention are simply labeled "nonresponders." This practice fails to give an accurate picture of how long it would have taken for the children to recover—a key element in assessing cost-effectiveness or whether another underlying issue, such as HIV infection, is hindering recovery. Furthermore, most SAM and MAM trials rely on passive recruitment: caregivers bring affected children to a health facility, where they may be recruited into a trial. Thus, study results may not be generalizable and can result in selection bias if the characteristics of caregivers who seek help differ systematically from those who do not bring their children for treatment.

Given the wide range of specially formulated foods for managing SAM and MAM, greater care is needed in trial design to ensure that accurate conclusions are drawn. Intervention arms should be comparable in caloric content and nutrient density, with similar packaging, programming, and promotion associated with the interventions (GNC 2014).

In addition to addressing study design challenges, reporting metrics need to be standardized. The pooling of data in meta-analyses is hindered by variability in the definition of acute malnutrition used across studies as well as the lack of consistent outcome definitions (for example, relapse, nonresponse, and default rates are measured differently across studies). If studies choose to include a mix of children with wasting, stunting, and underweight, disaggregated data should be presented according to type of undernutrition.

The need for standardized metrics extends beyond research and into the programming sphere. There is also a need for programs to standardize enrollment and discharge criteria, and to measure and report program outcomes consistently so that program impacts can be tracked over time and compared between sites (GNC 2014; Hall, Blankson, and Shoham 2011; Lenters and others 2013).

Considering Implementation Research and Integrated Programming

Research has trended toward studying the effectiveness of one specially formulated food versus another through RCTs. Although the relative effectiveness of products is an appropriate field of study, it is important to remember that the products are delivered within the context of a program and that the effectiveness of the treatment depends significantly on the quality of care (Puoane and others 2008). Further implementation research is needed to understand how to effectively deliver high-quality programs to consistently achieve optimal outcomes over a sustained time frame.

Experimental designs are not always feasible given constraints within the context as well as the complexity of the intervention. In such cases, high-quality quasi-experimental studies are an important approach for generating evidence. Additionally, RCTs are not always best suited to answering implementation questions. High-quality studies using quality-improvement methods and observational designs, as well as qualitative research and program reports, are all important investigative approaches.

Additionally, with respect to MAM, it is essential not to lose sight of the need for upstream, integrated approaches in the face of growing interest in specially formulated foods for the treatment of MAM. Lenters and colleagues (2013) conducted a rapid Delphi exercise in tandem with a systematic review and meta-analysis of approaches to managing MAM and found a striking discordance. Intervention trials identified through the systematic literature review all focused on comparing specially formulated food, but a thematic analysis of what experts believe to be the optimal management of MAM demonstrated that a more comprehensive approach is needed. The effectiveness of disease prevention and treatment, WASH interventions, community empowerment, livelihood diversification, and other upstream interventions need to be studied to prevent the development of MAM and its progression to SAM.

The current scientific evidence base and programmatic expertise provide a foundation for making substantial strides toward reducing the prevalence of SAM. However, crucial gaps remain in our understanding of the causes of acute malnutrition; the cost-effectiveness of various treatment approaches, particularly for MAM; and the requirements of particular subpopulations, such as young infants and children with HIV or other serious infections. These gaps and challenges can readily be explored through trials and programmatic research using standardized definitions and metrics. While building the best practices and evidence base for SAM and MAM, it is imperative that effective treatment approaches be considered within context: thus, implementation research on how to deliver and sustain high-quality programs must be given high priority. In addition, research, programs, and policies aimed at addressing the social determinants of health and distal factors that ultimately lead to SAM and MAM must be prioritized.

The global burden of acute malnutrition remains unacceptably high; progress toward reducing the prevalence of SAM and MAM has lagged behind reductions in stunting (Black and others 2013). Programs to reduce SAM are a cost-effective investment that should be given high priority by national governments. Finding the balance of preventive and therapeutic strategies for MAM and SAM in varying contexts is a major global priority and a clear focus of attention on the post-2015 agenda.

NOTES

World Bank Income Classifications as of July 2014 are as follows, based on estimates of gross national income (GNI) per capita for 2013:

- Low-income countries (LICs) = US$1,045 or less
- Middle-income countries (MICs) are subdivided:
  a) lower-middle-income = US$1,046 to US$4,125
  b) upper-middle-income (UMICs) = US$4,126 to US$12,745
- High-income countries (HICs) = US$12,746 or more.

This chapter uses the six World Health Organization (WHO) regions: Africa, the Americas, South-East Asia, Europe, Eastern Mediterranean, and Western Pacific.

1. This chapter refers to weight-for-height for simplicity; however note that weight-for-height is used in children 2 to 5 years of age and weight-for-length used in children under age two years.
2. The WHO defines appropriate breastfeeding as early initiation (within the first hour of life) and exclusive breastfeeding on demand for the first six months of life. http://www.who.int/nutrition/topics /exclusive_breastfeeding/en.
3. Appropriate complementary feeding practices, or infant and young child feeding are outlined by the WHO. http:// www.who.int/mediacentre/factsheets/fs342/en.
4. LNS may also be formulated as "small-quantity LNS"— these products deliver micronutrients and essential fatty acids in a lipid matrix. The primary intention is to prevent stunting and micronutrient deficiencies.
5. The severity of edema is graded as + (mild: both feet), ++ (moderate: both feet, plus lower legs, hands, or lower arms), or +++ (severe/generalized: both feet, legs, hands, arms, and face) (WHO 2013).

REFERENCES

Alcoba, G., M. Kerac, S. Breysse, C. Salpeteur, A. Galetto-Lacour, and others. 2013. "Do Children with Uncomplicated Severe Acute Malnutrition Need Antibiotics? A Systematic Review and Meta-Analysis." *PLoS One* 8 (1): E53184.

Annan, R. A., P. Webb, and R. Brown. 2014. "Management of Moderate Acute Malnutrition: Current Knowledge and Practice." CMAM Forum Technical Brief. http://www .cmamforum.org/Pool/Resources/MAM-management -CMAM-Forum-Technical-Brief-Sept-2014.pdf.

Ashok, A., A. Nandi, and R. Laxminarayan. 2016. "The Benefits of a Universal Home-Based Neonatal Care Package in Rural India: An Extended Cost-Effectiveness Analysis." In *Disease Control Priorities* (third edition): Volume 2, *Reproductive, Maternal, Newborn, and Child Health*, edited by R. Black, R. Laxminarayan, M. Temmerman, and N. Walker. Washington, DC: World Bank.

Ashworth, A., and E. Ferguson. 2009. "Dietary Counseling in the Management of Moderate Malnourishment in Children." *Food and Nutrition Bulletin* 30 (Suppl 3): S405–33.

Ashworth, A., S. Khanum, A. Jackson, and C. Schofield. 2003. *Guidelines for the Inpatient Treatment of Severely Malnourished Children.* Geneva: World Health Organization.

Bachmann, M. O. 2009. "Cost Effectiveness of Community-Based Therapeutic Care for Children with Severe Acute Malnutrition in Zambia: Decision Tree Model." *Cost Effectiveness and Resource Allocation* 7: 2.

———. 2010. "Cost-Effectiveness of Community-Based Treatment of Severe Acute Malnutrition in Children." *Expert Review of Pharmacoeconomics and Outcomes Research* 10 (5): 605–12.

Bhutta, Z. A., J. K. Das, A. Rizvi, M. F. Gaffey, N. Walker, and others. 2013. "Evidence-Based Interventions for Improvement of Maternal and Child Nutrition: What Can Be Done and at What Cost?" *The Lancet* 382 (9890): 452–77.

Bhutta, Z. A., J. K. Das, N. Walker, A. Rizvi, H. Campbell, and others. 2013. "Interventions to Address Deaths from Childhood Pneumonia and Diarrhoea Equitably; What Works and at What Cost?" *The Lancet* 381 (9875): 1417–29.

Black, R. E., L. H. Allen, Z. A. Bhutta, L. E. Caulfield, M. de Onis, and others. 2008. "Maternal and Child Undernutrition: Global and Regional Exposures and Health Consequences." *The Lancet* 371 (9608): 243–60.

Black, R. E., C. G. Victora, S. P. Walker, Z. A. Bhutta, P. Christian, and others. 2013. "Maternal and Child Undernutrition and Overweight in Low-Income and Middle-Income Countries." *The Lancet* 382 (9890): 427–51.

Cao, Y., T. Wang, and L. Zeng. 2013. "Risk of Childhood Malnutrition at 24 Months Related to Small for Gestational Age and Low Birth Weight in Rural Western China." In *Annals of Nutrition and Metabolism*, edited by A. Gil and J. A. Martinez. Grenada: 20th International Congress of Nutrition.

Chisti, M. J., M. A. Salam, H. Ashraf, A. S. G. Faruque, P. K. Bardhan, and others. 2014. "History of Contact with Active TB and Positive Tuberculin Skin Test Still Work as the Best Predictors in Diagnosing Pulmonary TB among Severely Malnourished Pneumonia Children." *Journal of Mycobacterial Diseases* 4 (155).

Collins, S., N. Dent, P. Binns, P. Bahwere, K. Sadler, and others. 2006. "Management of Severe Acute Malnutrition in Children." *The Lancet* 368 (9551): 1992–2000.

Collins, S., K. Sadler, N. Dent, T. Khara, S. Guerrero, and others. 2006. "Key Issues in the Success of Community-Based Management of Severe Malnutrition." *Food and Nutrition Bulletin* 27 (3): S49.

Das, J. K., R. A. Salam, A. Imdad, and Z. A. Bhutta. 2016. "Infant and Young Child Growth." In *Disease Control Priorities* (third edition): Volume 2, *Reproductive, Maternal, Newborn, and Child Health*, edited by R. Black, R. Laxminarayan, M. Temmerman, and N. Walker. Washington, DC: World Bank.

Defourny, I., A. Minetti, G. Harczi, S. Doyon, S. Shepherd, and others. 2009. "A Large-Scale Distribution of Milk-Based Fortified Spreads: Evidence for a New Approach in Regions with High Burden of Acute Malnutrition." *PLoS One* 4 (5): E5455.

Diop, E. I., N. I. Dossou, A. Briend, M. A. Yaya, M. M. Ndour, and others. 2004. "Home Rehabilitation for Severely Malnourished Children Using Locally Made Ready-to-Use Therapeutic Food (RUTF) after 1 Week Inpatient Care." *Pediatric Gastroenterology Hepatology and Nutrition* 39: S50–51.

Garrett, W. S. 2013. "Kwashiorkor and the Gut Microbiota." *New England Journal of Medicine* 368 (18): 1746–67.

GNC (Global Nutrition Cluster). 2014. *Moderate Acute Malnutrition (MAM): A Decision Tool for Emergencies.* New York: GNC.

Grantham-McGregor, S., Y. B. Cheung, S. Cueto, P. Glewwe, L. Richter, and others. 2007. "Developmental Potential in the First 5 Years for Children in Developing Countries." *The Lancet* 369 (9555): 60–70.

Grellety, E., S. Shepherd, T. Roederer, M. L. Manzo, S. Doyon, and others. 2012. "Effect of Mass Supplementation with Ready-to-Use Supplementary Food during an Anticipated Nutritional Emergency." *PLoS One* 7 (9).

Guerrant, R. L., R. B. Oria, S. R. Moore, M. O. B. Oria, and A. M. Lima. 2008. "Malnutrition as an Enteric Infectious Disease with Long-Term Effects on Child Development." *Nutrition Review* 66 (9): 487–505.

Guerrero, S., and E. Rogers. 2013. *Access for All Volume 1: Is Community-Based Treatment of Severe Acute Malnutrition (SAM) at Scale Capable of Meeting Global Needs?* London: Coverage Monitoring Network.

Hall, A., B. Blankson, and J. Shoham. 2011. *The Impact and Effectiveness of Emergency Nutrition and Nutrition-Related Interventions: A Review of Published Evidence 2004–2010.* Oxford, UK: Emergency Nutrition Network.

Hall, A., M. Oirere, S. Thurstans, A. Ndumi, and V. Sibson. 2011. "The Practical Challenges of Evaluating a Blanket Emergency Feeding Programme in Northern Kenya." *PLoS One* 6 (10): E26854.

Huybregts, L., F. Houngbé, C. Salpéteur, R. Brown, D. Roberfroid, and others. 2012. "The Effect of Adding Ready-to-Use Supplementary Food to a General Food Distribution on Child Nutritional Status and Morbidity: A Cluster-Randomized Controlled Trial." *PLoS One* 9 (9): E1001313.

Irena, A. H., M. Mwambazi, and V. Mulenga. 2011. "Diarrhea Is a Major Killer of Children with Severe Acute Malnutrition Admitted to Inpatient Set-Up in Lusaka, Zambia." *Nutritional Journal* 10 (110).

Isanaka, S., N. Nombela, A. Djibo, M. Poupard, D. Van Beckhoven, and others. 2009. "Effect of Preventive Supplementation with Ready-to-Use Therapeutic Food on the Nutritional Status, Mortality, and Morbidity of Children Aged 6 to 60 Months in Niger: A Cluster Randomized Trial." *Journal of the American Medical Association* 301 (3): 277–85.

Islam, M. M., M. Alam, M. Tariquzaman, M. A. Kabir, R. Pervin, and others. 2013. "Predictors of the Number of Under-Five Malnourished Children in Bangladesh: Application of the Generalized Poisson Regression Model." *BMC Public Health* 13: 11.

Jones, K. D. J., and J. A. Berkley. 2014. "Severe Acute Malnutrition and Infection." CMAM Forum Technical Brief, CMAM Forum. http://www.cmamforum.org/Pool/Resources /SAM-and-Infections-Technical-Brief-v2-Jan-2014.pdf.

Karakochuk, C., D. Stephens, and S. Zlotkin. 2012. "Treatment of Moderate Acute Malnutrition with Ready-to-Use Supplementary Food Results in Higher Overall Recovery Rates Compared with a Corn-Soya Blend in Children in Southern Ethiopia: An Operations Research Trial." *American Journal of Clinical Nutrition* 96 (4): 911–16.

Koumans, E. H., J. A. Routh, and M. K. Davis. 2013. "Antibiotics for Uncomplicated Severe Malnutrition." Comment in *The New England Journal of Medicine* 368 (25): 2435–37.

Kumar, R., J. Singh, K. Joshi, H. P. Singh, and S. Bijesh. 2013. "Co-Morbidities in Hospitalized Children with Severe Acute Malnutrition." *Indian Pediatrics* 51: 125–27.

Laghari, G. S., M. Akbar, A. H. Radhan, and Z. Hussain. 2013. "The Analysis of Risk Factors in Severe Protein Energy Malnutrition in Order to Know Their Significance for Outcome in Children from 2 Months to 5 Years of Age." *Journal of Liaquat University of Medical and Health Sciences* 12 (2): 103–38.

Lazzerini, M., L. Rubert, and P. Pani. 2013. "Specially Formulated Foods for Treating Children with Moderate Acute Malnutrition in Low- and Middle-Income Countries." *Cochrane Database of Systematic Reviews* 6: CD009584.

Lenters, L. M., K. Wazny, P. Webb, T. Ahmed, and Z. A. Bhutta. 2013. "Treatment of Severe and Moderate Acute Malnutrition in Low- and Middle-Income Settings: A Systematic Review, Meta-Analysis and Delphi Process." *BMC Public Health* 13 (Suppl 3): S23.

Liu, L., K. Hill, S. Oza, D. Hogan, Y. Chu, and others. 2016. "Levels and Causes of Mortality under Age Five Years." In *Disease Control Priorities* (third edition): Volume 2, *Reproductive, Maternal, Newborn, and Child Health*, edited by R. Black, R. Laxminarayan, M. Temmerman, and N. Walker. Washington, DC: World Bank.

Liu, L., S. Oza, D. Hogan, J. Perin, I. Rudan, and others. 2014. "Global, Regional, and National Causes of Child Mortality in 2000–13, with Projections to Inform Post-2015 Priorities: An Updated Systematic Analysis." *The Lancet* 385 (9966): 430–40. doi: 10.1016/S0140-6736(14)61698-6.

Long, K., Z. Horder, A. Faruque, T. Ahmed, and S. Ahmed. 2013. "Associations between Nutritional Status, Household Factors and Specific Diarrheal Pathogens among Children in Mirzapur, Bangladesh." In *Annals of Nutrition and Metabolism*, edited by A. Gil and J. A. Martinez, 679–80. Granada, Spain: 20th International Conference of Nutrition.

Manary, M. 2005. "Local Production and Provision of Ready-to-Use Therapeutic Food for the Treatment of Severe Childhood Malnutrition." Technical Background Paper, World Health Organization, Geneva. http://www.Who.Int/Nutrition/Topics/Backgroundpapers_Local_Production.pdf.

Matilsky, D. K., K. Maleta, T. Castleman, and M. J. Manary. 2009. "Supplementary Feeding with Fortified Spreads Results in Higher Recovery Rates than with a Corn/Soy Blend in Moderately Wasted Children." *Journal of Nutrition* 139 (4): 773–78.

Menon, P., S. Cyriac, S. J. Coastes, and V. M. Aguavo. 2013. "Diet Quality, Water and Toilets: What Roles for Child Undernutrition in India?" In *Annals of Nutrition and Metabolism*, edited by A. Gil and J. A. Martinez. Granada, Spain: 20th International Congress of Nutrition.

Meshram, I. I., N. Arlappa, N. Balakrishna, K. M. Rao, A. Laxmaiah, and others. 2012. "Trends in the Prevalence of Undernutrition, Nutrient & Food Intake and Predictors of Undernutrition among Under Five Year Tribal Children in India." *Asia Pacific Journal of Clinical Nutrition* 21 (4): 568–76.

Nhampossa, T., B. Sigauque, S. Machevo, E. Macete, P. Alonso, and others. 2013. "Severe Malnutrition among Children Under the Age of 5 Years Admitted to a Rural District Hospital in Southern Mozambique." *Public Health Nutrition* 16 (9): 1565–74.

Oakley, E., J. Reinking, H. Sandige, I. Trehan, G. Kennedy, and others. 2010. "A Ready-to-Use Therapeutic Food Containing 10% Milk Is Less Effective Than One with 25% Milk in the Treatment of Severely Malnourished Children." *Journal of Nutrition* 140 (12): 2248–52.

Okeke, I. N., J. R. Cruz, and G. T. Keusch. 2013. "Antibiotics for Uncomplicated Severe Malnutrition." Comment. *New England Journal of Medicine* 368 (25): 2435–37.

Olofin, I., C. M. McDonald, M. Ezzati, S. Flaxman, R. E. Black, and others for the Nutrition Impact Model. 2013. "Associations of Suboptimal Growth with All-Cause and Cause-Specific Mortality in Children under Five Years: A Pooled Analysis of Ten Prospective Studies." *PLoS One* 8 (5): E64636.

Page, A. L., N. De Rekeneire, S. Sayadi, S. Aberrane, A. C. Janssens, and others. 2013. "Infections in Children Admitted with Complicated Severe Acute Malnutrition in Niger." *PLoS One* 8 (7): E68699.

Petri, Jr., W. A., M. Miller, H. J. Binder, M. M. Levine, R. Dillingham, and others. 2008. "Enteric Infections, Diarrhea, and Their Impact on Function and Development." *Journal of Clinical Investigation* 118 (4): 1277–90.

Petri, Jr., W. A., C. Naylor, and R. Haque. 2014. "Environmental Enteropathy and Malnutrition: Do We Know Enough to Intervene?" *Biomed Central Medicine* 12 (187): 1–5.

Picot, J., D. Hartwell, P. Harris, D. Mendes, A. J. Clegg, and others. 2012. "The Effectiveness of Interventions to Treat Severe Acute Malnutrition in Young Children: A Systematic Review." *Health Technology Assessment* 16 (19): 1–315.

Puett, C., K. Sadler, H. Alderman, J. Coates, J. L. Fiedler, and others. 2012. "Cost-Effectiveness of the Community-Based Management of Severe Acute Malnutrition by Community Health Workers in Southern Bangladesh." *Health Policy and Planning* 28 (4): 386–99.

Puoane, T., K. Cuming, D. Sanders, and A. Ashworth. 2008. "Why Do Some Hospitals Achieve Better Care of Severely Malnourished Children than Others? Five-Year Follow-up of Rural Hospitals in Eastern Cape, South Africa." *Health Policy and Planning* 23 (6): 428–37.

Saboya, M., T. Khara, and A. Irena. 2011. "Harmonized Training Package Version 2 Module 13: Management of Severe Acute Malnutrition." ENN, Oxford. http://www.ennonline.net/ourwork/capacitydevelopment/htpversion2.

Sadler, K., P. Bahwere, S. Guerrero, and S. Collins. 2006. "Community-Based Therapeutic Care in HIV-Affected Populations." *Transactions of The Royal Society of Tropical Medicine and Hygiene* 100 (1): 6–9.

Sandige, H., M. J. Ndekha, A. Briend, P. Ashorn, and M. J. Manary. 2004. "Home-Based Treatment of Malnourished Malawian Children with Locally Produced or Imported Ready-to-Use Food." *Journal of Pediatric Gastroenterology and Nutrition* 39 (2): 141–16.

Schlaudecker, E. P., M. C. Steinhoff, and S. R. Moore. 2011. "Interactions of Diarrhea, Pneumonia, and Malnutrition in Childhood: Recent Evidence from Developing Countries." *Current Opinion in Infectious Diseases* 24: 496–502.

Singh, A. S., G. Kang, A. Ramachandran, R. Sarkar, P. Peter, and others. 2010. "Locally Made Ready to Use Therapeutic Food for Treatment of Malnutrition: A Randomized Controlled Trial." *Indian Pediatrics* 47 (8): 679–86.

Smith, M. I., T. Yatsunenko, M. J. Manary, I. Trehan, R. Mkakosya, and others. 2013. "Gut Microbiomes of Malawian Twin Pairs Discordant for Kwashiorkor." *Science* 339 (6119): 548–54.

Somasse, Y. E., M. Dramaix, P. Bahwere, and P. Donnen. 2013. "Relapses from Acute Malnutrition in a Community-Based Management Program in Burkina-Faso." In *Annals of Nutrition and Metabolism*, edited by A. Gil and J. A. Martinez. Granada, Spain: 20th International Congress of Nutrition.

Sphere Project. 2011. *The Sphere Handbook: Humanitarian Charter and Minimum Standards in Humanitarian Response*. Rugby, UK: Practical Action Publishing. http://www.ifrc.org/PageFiles/95530/The-Sphere-Project-Handbook-20111.pdf.

Tekeste, A., M. Wondafrash, G. Azene, and K. Deribe. 2012. "Cost Effectiveness of Community-Based and In-Patient Therapeutic Feeding Programs to Treat Severe Acute Malnutrition in Ethiopia." *Cost Effectiveness and Resource Allocation* 10 (4): 1–10.

Trehan, I., H. S. Goldbach, L. N. Lagrone, G. J. Meuli, R. J. Wang, and others. 2013. "Antibiotics as Part of the Management of Severe Acute Malnutrition." *New England Journal of Medicine* 368 (5): 425–35.

UNICEF (United Nations Children's Fund). 2013. *Improving Child Nutrition: The Achievable Imperative for Global Progress.* New York: UNICEF.

———. 2014a. "Supply Catalogue." UNICEF, New York. http:// Supply.Unicef.Org.

———. 2014b. "UNICEF Data: Monitoring the Situation of Children and Women." UNICEF, New York. http://Data .Unicef.Org/Nutrition/Malnutrition.

UNICEF, WHO, and World Bank. 2012. *Levels and Trends in Child Malnutrition: UNICEF-WHO-World Bank Joint Child Malnutrition Estimates.* Washington, DC.

Webb, P., B. L. Rogers, I. Rosenberg, N. Schlossman, C. Wanke, and others. 2011. *Improving the Nutritional Quality of U.S. Food Aid: Recommendations for Changes to Products and Programs.* Boston, MA: Tufts University.

WHO (World Health Organization). 2003. *Guidelines for the Inpatient Treatment of Severely Malnourished Children.* Geneva: WHO.

———. 2007. "Community-Based Management of Severe Acute Malnutrition: A Joint Statement by the World Health Organization, the World Food Programme, the United Nations System Standing Committee on Nutrition, and the United Nations Children's Fund." World Health Organization, Geneva; World Food Programme, Rome; United Nations System Standing Committee on Nutrition, Geneva; United Nations Children's Fund, New York. http:// www.who.int/nutrition/topics/Statement_community _based_man_sev_acute_mal_eng.pdf.

———. 2010. *Guidelines on HIV and Infant Feeding: Principles and Recommendations for Infant Feeding in the Context of HIV and a Summary of Evidence.* Geneva: WHO.

———. 2012. "Supplementary Foods for the Management of Moderate Acute Malnutrition in Infants and Children 6–59 Months of Age." Technical Note, WHO, Geneva.

———. 2013. *Guideline: Updates on the Management of Severe Acute Malnutrition in Infants and Children.* Geneva: WHO.

Wilford, R., K. Golden, and D. G. Walker. 2012. "Cost-Effectiveness of Community-Based Management of Acute Malnutrition in Malawi." *Health Policy Planning* 27 (2): 127–37.

You, D., S. Ejdemyr, P. Idele, D. Hogan, C. Mathers, and others. 2015. "Global, Regional, and National levels and Trends in Under-5 Mortality between 1990 and 2015, with Scenario-Based Projections to 2030: A Systematic Analysis by the UN Inter-Agency Group for Child Mortality Estimation." *The Lancet* 385: 2275–86.

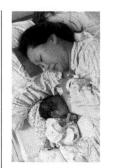

Chapter 12

Infant and Young Child Growth

Jai K. Das, Rehana A. Salam, Aamer Imdad, and
Zulfiqar A. Bhutta

INTRODUCTION

Each year, undernutrition—including fetal growth restriction, stunting, wasting, and micronutrient deficiencies—and suboptimum breastfeeding (BF) underlie nearly 3.1 million deaths of children younger than age five years worldwide, accounting for 45 percent of all deaths in this age group (Liu and others 2012). Fetal growth restriction and suboptimum BF together are responsible for more than 1.3 million deaths, or 19.4 percent of all deaths among children younger than age five years.

Although the prevalence of stunted children has decreased from 40 percent in 1990 to 26 percent in 2011, an estimated 165 million children younger than age five years globally are stunted, based on the World Health Organization's (WHO's) Child Growth Standards (map 12.1). South Asia and Sub-Saharan Africa have the highest estimated prevalence; 68.0 million and 55.8 million stunted children live in South Asia and Sub-Saharan Africa, respectively (UNICEF, WHO, and World Bank 2012). Stunting prevalence among children younger than age five years is substantially higher in the poorest population quintiles and in rural areas, compared with the richest quintiles and urban areas, respectively (Black and others 2013). The complex interplay of social, economic, and political determinants of undernutrition results in substantial inequalities among population subgroups (Black and others 2013).

Optimum nutrition during the crucial periods of pregnancy and the first two years of life, known as the 1,000 days window of opportunity, is essential to health and growth, and its benefits can extend throughout life. A major component of infant and young child feeding (IYCF) in the early years of life is the provision of breast milk and appropriate, nutrient-dense complementary foods (PAHO and WHO 2003). In 2003, the WHO and the United Nations Children's Fund (UNICEF) published a jointly developed global strategy for IYCF to refocus attention on the impact that feeding practices have on infant nutrition and health (WHO and UNICEF 2003). In 2008, the WHO published a set of population-level IYCF indicators developed in response to the need for simple, practical indicators of appropriate feeding practices in children ages 6–23 months (WHO 2002; WHO and UNICEF 2008). A core set of eight indicators (three for BF and five for complementary feeding [CF]) includes measures of dietary diversity, feeding frequency, and consumption of iron-rich or iron-fortified foods, as well as indicators of appropriate BF practices (table 12.1) (Jones and others 2014).

This chapter discusses key concepts in nutrition and growth during this early phase of life, intrauterine growth and maternal interventions (balanced energy and micronutrient supplementation), nutrition interventions to improve infant and child feeding

Corresponding author: Zulfiqar A. Bhutta, Robert Harding Chair in Global Child Health and Policy, the Centre for Global Child Health, The Hospital for Sick Children, Toronto, Canada, and Founding Director, Center of Excellence in Women and Child Health, Aga Khan University, Karachi 74800, Pakistan; zulfiqar.bhutta@sickkids.ca.

(BF, CF, and micronutrient supplementation), other nutrition-related interventions, and challenges in infant and child feeding.

CONSEQUENCES OF UNDERNUTRITION

Good nutrition early in life is essential for children to be able to attain their full developmental potential. Malnutrition leads to early physical growth failure; delayed motor, cognitive, and behavioral development; diminished immunity; and increased morbidity and mortality (Black and others 2013). Deficiencies of essential vitamins and minerals are widespread and have substantial adverse effects on child survival and development. Deficiencies of vitamin A and zinc adversely affect child health and survival; deficiencies of iodine and iron can, together with causing stunting, limit the ability of children to realize their developmental potential.

Mortality and Morbidity

Black and others (2013) demonstrate that all degrees of stunting, wasting, and underweight are associated with increased hazards of death from diarrhea, pneumonia, measles, and other infectious diseases, with the exception of malaria; this analysis confirms the complex interplay between undernutrition and infection. In addition to anthropometric measures, the association between micronutrient deficiencies, such as vitamin A deficiency, and the increased risk of childhood infections and mortality is well established (Black and others 2013). Vitamin A deficiency increases the risk of severe diarrhea and diarrhea mortality, but it is not an important risk factor for the incidence of diarrhea or pneumonia or for pneumonia-related mortality. Other micronutrient deficiencies, such as zinc and iron deficiencies, are widespread in low- and middle-income countries (LMICs). Zinc is associated with increased risk of morbidity and mortality (Black 2003).

Growth and Development

Undernutrition has important consequences for physical and cognitive growth and development. Malnutrition leads to early physical growth failure; delayed motor, cognitive, and behavioral development; diminished immunity; and increased morbidity and mortality. Those who survive the initial and direct consequences of malnutrition in early childhood grow to adulthood, but with disadvantages compared with those who have had adequate nutrition and enjoyed a healthy environment in the initial crucial years of life. Undernutrition is strongly associated with shorter adult height, less schooling, and reduced economic productivity; in women, it is associated with offspring with lower birth weights. Fetal growth restriction, lower birth weight, and undernutrition in childhood have also been associated with long-term consequences, including increased risk of developing metabolic syndrome and cardiovascular disease, systolic hypertension, obesity, insulin resistance, and diabetes type II in adulthood (Greer, Sicherer, and Burks 2008; Salam, Das, and Bhutta 2014). The later consequences of childhood malnutrition also include diminished intellectual performance, low work capacity, and increased risk of delivery complications (Waddington and others 2009).

MATERNAL NUTRITION AND FETAL GROWTH

The determination of child nutrition status starts before birth; maternal nutritional status and fetal growth restriction have been found to be closely associated with child health. Maternal stunting and underweight lead to small for gestational age (SGA) and prematurity. Fetal growth restriction, in turn, is an important contributor to stunting and wasting in children; approximately 20 percent of childhood stunting could have its origins in the fetal period (Black and others 2013). Undernutrition can only be tackled through a multipronged approach with involvement of relevant sectors other than health. This approach was highlighted in the undernutrition series in *The Lancet* (Black and others 2013). The series underscores that nutrition-specific interventions can only reduce the current burden of undernutrition by a fraction; a more holistic approach is required that involves relevant sectors, including agriculture and food security, social safety nets, early child development, maternal mental health, women's empowerment, child protection, classroom education, water and sanitation, and health and family planning services. The conceptual framework in figure 12.1 highlights the risk factors and the nutrition-specific interventions for childhood stunting and wasting.

Definitions

Intrauterine growth restriction (IUGR) describes the pathological inhibition of fetal growth. Although there is no standard definition of IUGR, two terms have been used to describe it: *SGA* and *low birth weight* (LBW):

- *SGA*, the most commonly used term for IUGR, is defined as babies born with weight of less than the 10th percentile of recommended gender-specific weight for gestational age for that population (WHO 1995; Yakoob and Bhutta 2011).
- *LBW* is defined as birth weight less than 2,500 grams, irrespective of gestational age.

Figure 12.1 Malnutrition Risk Factors and Nutrition-Specific Interventions

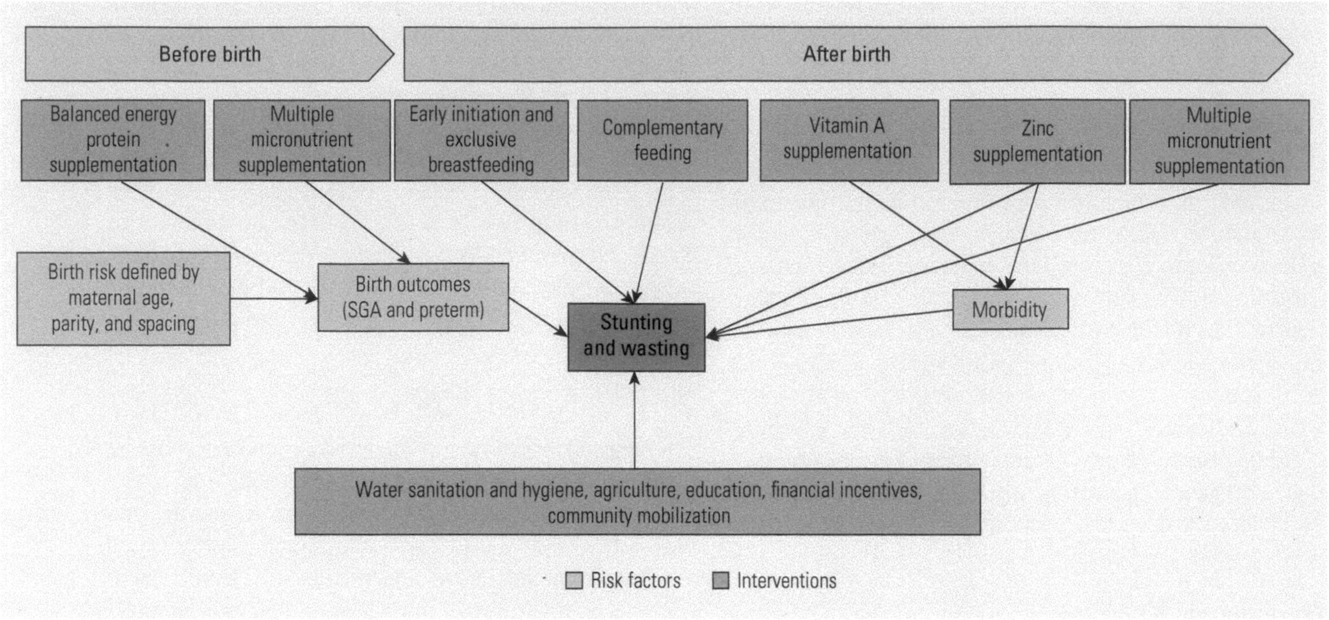

Note: SGA = small for gestational age.

Because birth size depends on both gestational age and growth velocity, the term *SGA* is preferred to LBW. A baby born with LBW but appropriate for gestational age is expected to have better outcomes compared with a baby born SGA. However, LBW has been the most commonly used indicator to describe fetal growth because it can be difficult to determine true gestational age in LMICs (WHO 1995). In this chapter, SGA is used as a proxy indicator for IUGR.

Causes of Intrauterine Growth Restriction

IUGR can have multiple causes. Some of the known risk factors include maternal malnutrition, congenital malformations, congenital infections, maternal smoking, and maternal medical comorbidities such as primary hypertension and diabetes mellitus (Romo, Carceller, and Tobajas 2009). In LMICs, maternal malnutrition is an important risk factor for SGA babies; however, in high-income countries (HICs), cigarette smoking is the most important single factor implicated in IUGR, followed by poor gestational nutrition (Bhutta and others 2013; Salam, Das, and Bhutta 2014). The major nongenetic factor determining the size of the fetus at term is maternal constraint, which is a set of maternal and uteroplacental factors that act to limit the growth of the fetus by limiting nutrient availability or the metabolic-hormonal drive to grow; these factors

are more pronounced in pregnancies involving young mothers, small maternal size, nulliparous, and multiple pregnancies (Gluckman and Hanson 2004). Maternal nutrition influences the availability of nutrients for transfer to the fetus; during starvation, it is likely that low food intake results in a reduced nutrient stream from mother to fetus, giving rise to fetal growth restriction. Maternal undernutrition (body mass index of less than 18.5 kilograms/square meter) has decreased overall since 1980 but remains greater than 10 percent in South Asia and Sub-Saharan Africa (Black and others 2013).

Consequences of Intrauterine Growth Restriction

IUGR is associated with a higher risk of preterm delivery and higher rates of fetal and neonatal morbidity and mortality (Arcangeli and others 2012; Baschat 2011). This higher rate of neonatal mortality in IUGR infants is due to conditions that include birth asphyxia and infections (such as sepsis, pneumonia, and diarrhea), which lead to mortality and together account for about 60 percent of all neonatal deaths (Salam, Das, and Bhutta 2014).

The short-term consequences of IUGR involve metabolic and hematological disturbances, as well as disrupted thermoregulation, which lead to morbidities such as respiratory distress syndrome, necrotizing enterocolitis, and retinopathy of prematurity (Salam,

Das, and Bhutta 2014). The adverse consequences of IUGR are not limited to infancy and childhood; they extend throughout the lifespan. IUGR leads to stunting and wasting, and an estimated 20 percent of stunted children in LMICs were born SGA (Black and others 2013). Evidence indicates that adverse changes in the fetal nutritional environment are associated with increased risk of developing metabolic syndrome and cardiovascular disease, systolic hypertension, obesity, insulin resistance, diabetes type II, and neuropsychological and cognitive deficiencies, as well as with impairments in renal and lung development in adulthood (Bjarnegard and others 2013; Salam, Das, and Bhutta 2014). It has also been shown that early developmental conditions affect all children and their predispositions to long-term consequences, including noncommunicable diseases (Hanson and Gluckman 2011).

Prevention of Intrauterine Growth Restriction

No effective therapies exist to reverse IUGR. Accordingly, initiatives focus on prevention through optimizing the nutritional status of women at the time of conception to establish the foundation for healthy fetal growth and development. Pregnancy is a state of higher metabolic requirements, and both macronutrients and micronutrients play important roles. Multiple nutrition interventions to address maternal nutritional requirements have been studied. These include nutritional counseling; isocaloric (maternal nutrition supplement given during pregnancy in which protein provides 25 percent of total energy content), high (protein provides more than 25 percent of total energy content), and balanced protein energy (BEP) (protein provides less than 25 percent of total energy content) supplementation; micronutrient supplementation; and low-energy supplementation for obese women.

Of these interventions, only BEP supplementation has been shown to affect the incidence of SGA (Bhutta and others 2013). A meta-analysis of 16 studies shows that BEP supplementation increased birth weight (mean difference [MD]: 73 grams; 95 percent confidence interval [CI]: 30–117) and decreased the incidence of SGA (relative risk [RR]: 0.66; 95 percent CI: 0.49–0.89); these effects were more pronounced in malnourished women compared with adequately nourished women. BEP supplementation also decreased the risk of stillbirth; however, the number of patients included in the meta-analysis was small (Imdad and Bhutta 2012).

Micronutrient supplementation during pregnancy has been studied with regard to individual and multiple micronutrients and their beneficial effects for mothers and the developing fetuses. Calcium supplementation has been shown to reduce the incidence of preeclampsia in populations with low calcium intake. Folic acid supplementation during and before pregnancy reduces the incidence of neural tube defects (Bhutta and others 2013). Among micronutrient interventions, iron or iron and folate supplementation has been shown to reduce the incidence of LBW and improve birth weight but has no impact on SGA or IUGR (Peña-Rosas and others 2012; Peña-Rosas and Viteri 2009). Multiple micronutrient supplementation, when compared with iron and folate supplementation, has reduced the incidence of SGA babies by 13 percent (Haider and Bhutta 2012). The effects of supplementation in reducing the incidence of IUGR are clear; moreover, these benefits may extend into early childhood and affect growth and development. The effects of supplementation are not only apparent in reduced IUGR but also in its possible translation into early childhood development (Vaidya and others 2008).

BREASTFEEDING

Timing

The exact scientific basis for the absolute early time window of feeding within the first hour after birth is weak (Edmond and others 2006; Mullany and others 2008). A systematic review suggests that BF initiation within 24 hours of birth is associated with a 44 percent to 45 percent reduction in all-cause and infection-related neonatal mortality and is thought to primarily operate through the effects of exclusive breastfeeding (EBF) (Debes and others 2013).

Interventions to promote BF are a key component of expanding its use. A review of the effects of promotion interventions on occurrence of BF concludes that counseling or educational interventions increased EBF by 43 percent at day one, by 30 percent until age one month, and by 90 percent from age one month to age five months. Significant reductions in the occurrence of mothers not BF were also noted; 32 percent reduction at day one, 30 percent until one month, and 18 percent for one month to five months (Haroon and others 2013). Combined individual and group counseling seemed to be better than individual or group counseling alone.

Prevalence of Breastfeeding

BF provides numerous immunologic, psychological, social, economic, and environmental benefits. It results in improved infant and maternal health outcomes in both LMICs and HICs (Eidelman and others 2012). The WHO recommends EBF for infants until age six months to achieve optimum growth (Kramer and Kikuma 2001). In LMICs, one out of every three children is exclusively breastfed for the first six months of life, although considerable variations exist across regions (UNICEF 2006). Recent data show that the prevalence of EBF in LMICs has increased from 33 percent in 1995 to 39 percent in 2010 (Cai, Wardlaw, and Brown 2012). The prevalence of EBF increased in almost all regions in LMICs, with a major improvement seen in central and west Africa, where the prevalence more than doubled from 12 percent to 28 percent. More modest improvements were observed in South Asia, where the prevalence increased from 40 percent in 1995 to 45 percent in 2010. The median coverage of EBF has increased from 26 percent in 2000–05 to 40 percent in 2006–11 in the 48 Countdown countries (countries with the highest burden of maternal and child deaths) (WHO and UNICEF 2012).

EBF reduces the risk of hospitalization for lower respiratory tract infections in the first year by 72 percent (Ip and others 2007; Ip and others 2009). Any BF compared with exclusive commercial infant formula feeding can reduce the incidence of otitis media by 23 percent, and EBF for more than three months reduces the risk of otitis media by 50 percent (Ip and others 2007). Any BF is associated with a 64 percent reduction in the incidence of nonspecific gastrointestinal tract infections; this effect lasts for two months after cessation of BF (Ip and others 2007; Duijts and others 2010; Ip and others 2009; Quigley, Kelly, and Sacker 2007). BF is also beneficial for preterm infants; it is associated with a 58 percent reduction in the incidence of necrotizing enterocolitis (Ip and others 2007). EBF offers a protective effect for three to four months against the incidence of clinical asthma, atopic dermatitis, and eczema by 27 percent in a low-risk population and up to 42 percent in infants with positive family history (Ip and others 2007; Greer, Sicherer, and Burks 2008). BF can improve nutrition status directly or by reducing infections and morbidity. Promoting EBF is reported to be important in preventing both stunting and overweight among children (Keino and others 2014). A systematic review shows that breastfeeding up to two years of age or beyond had no significant impact on child growth; however, further research is needed (Delgado and Matijasevich 2013).

Supportive Strategies

Although these results show the potential for scaling up BF, none of these trials addresses the issues of barriers in work environments and supportive strategies to overcome them, such as provisions for maternity leave. A Cochrane review of interventions in the workplace to support BF for women found no trials (Abdulwadud and Snow 2012), so much more needs to be done to assess innovations and strategies to promote BF in working women, especially in low-income communities.

COMPLEMENTARY FEEDING

CF for infants refers to the timely introduction of safe and nutritional foods in addition to BF, specifically, clean and nutrient-dense additional foods introduced at age six months and typically provided until age 24 months (Imdad, Yakoob, and Bhutta 2011; WHO 2002). It has been suggested that in addition to disease-prevention strategies, CF interventions targeting this critical window are most efficient in reducing malnutrition and promoting adequate growth and development (WHO 2002).

According to the WHO, CF should be timely, adequate, appropriate, and given in sufficient quantity (WHO 2002). Several strategies have been used to improve CF practices (Dewey and Adu-Afarwuah 2008). These include providing nutritional counseling for mothers to promote healthy feeding practices; providing complementary foods offering extra energy, with or without micronutrient fortification; and increasing the nutrient density of complementary foods through simple technology (Dewey and Adu-Afarwuah 2008).

Inadequacy and insufficiency of complementary foods, poor feeding practices, and high rates of infections have unfavorable impacts on health and growth among children. Sufficient quantities of adequate, safe, and appropriate CF after age six months are essential to meet nutritional requirements when breast milk alone is no longer sufficient. However, estimates indicate that in LMICs, only 39 percent of children younger than age six months were exclusively breastfed in 2010 (Cai, Wardlaw, and Brown 2012); only 58 percent of babies ages six months to nine months were breastfed and given complementary foods; and only 50 percent of babies ages 10 months to 23 months were provided with complementary food and continued BF (UNICEF 2013).

Several strategies have been used to improve CF practices. However, the diversity in types of food, duration, and interventions used makes it difficult to conclude that one particular type of CF intervention is the most effective (Dewey and Adu-Afarwuah 2008). A review (Lassi and others 2013) of two CF strategies—nutritional education and CF with or without nutritional education—shows a significant impact of CF education on height-for-age z-score (HAZ) (MD: 0.23; 95 percent CI: 0.09–0.36), weight-for-age z-score (WAZ)

(MD: 0.16; 95 percent CI: 0.05–0.27), and rates of stunting (RR: 0.71; 95 percent CI: 0.56–0.91). Impacts were even more dramatic when education on CF was provided in combination with actual complementary food in food-insecure populations (HAZ scores: RR: 0.39; 95 percent CI: 0.05–0.73).

Education for improved feeding practices is essential to improve maternal knowledge and to prepare culturally acceptable enriched complementary foods that can lead to increased dietary intake and growth of infants. Maternal counseling in health system and community settings is critical to safeguarding optimal CF practices. Educational messages should be clear and should include the promotion of nutrient-rich animal products. However, in food-insecure populations, these messages need to be combined with food provision or use of protein-rich plant food sources (Lassi and others 2013). Financial constraints may limit the possibility of including adequate amounts of animal products in children's diets, particularly among food-insecure populations (Lassi and others 2013). Measures should be taken at the community level to support activities involving community health workers, lay counselors, and mothers to build community or mother support groups. Communication and advocacy activities on CF could lay the foundation for improved growth and health.

MICRONUTRIENT SUPPLEMENTATION

Micronutrient Deficiencies

According to WHO global estimates, 190 million preschool children and 19.1 million pregnant women have vitamin A deficiencies, defined as serum retinol of less than 0.70 micromoles per liter (Bjarnegard and others 2013). Globally, an estimated 5.17 million preschool-age children (0.9 percent) have night blindness, and 90 million (33.3 percent) have subclinical vitamin A deficiencies (WHO 2009). Approximately 100 million women of reproductive age have iodine deficiencies, and an estimated 82 percent of pregnant women worldwide have inadequate zinc intakes to meet the normal needs of pregnancy (WHO and UNICEF 2003). Iron deficiencies are widespread; about 1.62 billion people have anemia (de Benoist and others 2008); 18.1 percent and 1.5 percent of children have anemia and severe anemia, respectively (Salam, Das, and others 2013). South Asia and Sub-Saharan Africa have the highest prevalence of all iron deficiency anemia, and Sub-Saharan Africa has the highest prevalence of severe iron deficiency anemia (Black and others 2013). Suboptimal vitamin B6 and B12 statuses have also been observed in many LMICs (McLean, de Benoist, and Allen 2008).

Zinc

Zinc deficiency has been associated with growth failure and increased risk of morbidity and mortality due to diarrheal and respiratory illness (Black and others 2013). Multiple randomized trials have studied the role of preventive zinc supplementation to promote linear growth; the findings vary across the study populations (Brown and others 2009; Ramakrishnan, Nguyen, and Martorell 2009). Meta-analyses have shown an overall beneficial effect of zinc supplementation to promote linear growth (Brown and others 2009; Imdad and Bhutta 2011). This effect is more pronounced when zinc is supplemented alone compared with when it is administered in combination with iron (Imdad and Bhutta 2011). The effect is also more pronounced for children with baseline stunting (Umeta and others 2000). No standard dose and duration of zinc supplementation has been recommended to promote linear growth; however, combined data from multiple trials in one of the meta-analyses show that a dose of 10 milligrams per day for 24 weeks led to net gains of 0.37 centimeters (standard deviation ± 0.25) in the intervention group compared with the control (Imdad and Bhutta 2011). Therapeutic zinc given to children with diarrhea has also been shown to reduce the duration and severity of illness (Walker and Black 2010).

Vitamin A

Vitamin A deficiency, a risk factor for increased incidence of infections, is the most common nutritional cause of blindness in the world. It is well established that vitamin A supplementation during childhood decreases all-cause mortality and mortality due to diarrhea and measles (Imdad and others 2010). Studies have also evaluated its role in promotion of linear growth; results have shown that vitamin A supplementation does not have any significant role in this respect. A meta-analysis by Ramakrishnan, Nguyen, and Martorell (2009) analyzes data from 17 studies and finds no statistically significant effect of vitamin A on growth. A large randomized trial conducted in India also does not show any positive effect of vitamin A supplementation on height gain (Awasthi and others 2013).

Iron

The proportion of all childhood anemia corrected by iron supplementation ranges from 63 percent in Europe to 34 percent in Sub-Saharan Africa. A review of 33 studies shows that intermittent iron supplementation in children younger than age two years reduced the risk of anemia by 49 percent and iron deficiency by

76 percent (De-Regil and others 2011). The findings also suggest that intermittent iron supplementation could be a viable public health intervention in settings in which daily supplementation has not been implemented or is not feasible.

A review of the effect of iron supplementation in children on mental and motor development shows only small gains in the mental development and intelligence scores in supplemented school-age children who were initially anemic or iron deficient (Sachdev, Gera, and Nestel 2005). There is no convincing evidence that iron treatment has an effect on the mental development of children younger than age 27 months. Because it has been demonstrated that there is an increased risk of admission to hospital and serious illnesses with iron supplementation in malaria-endemic areas (Sazawal and others 2006), the WHO recommends administration of routine prophylactic iron supplements in malaria-endemic areas on the stipulation that malaria prevention and treatment are made available (WHO 2011, 2014).

Multiple Micronutrient Supplementation

In many LMICs, micronutrient deficiencies coexist, suggesting the need for simple approaches that evaluate and address multiple micronutrient supplementation. These approaches include education, dietary modification, food provision, agricultural interventions, supplementation, and fortification, either alone or in combination. Food fortification can be a potentially cost-effective public health intervention and target a larger population through a single strategy. A meta-analysis of multiple micronutrient fortification in children shows an increase in hemoglobin levels by 0.87 grams per deciliter (95 percent CI: 0.57–1.16) and 57 percent reduced risk of anemia (RR: 0.43; 95 percent CI: 0.26–0.71). Multiple micronutrient food fortification also increased vitamin A serum levels (retinol increase of 3.7 milligrams per deciliter; 95 percent CI: 1.3–6.1) (Eichler and others 2012).

In the past decade, point-of-use or home fortification of child diets has emerged to address widespread micronutrient deficiencies. Multiple micronutrient powders (MNPs) or sprinkles are powdered encapsulated vitamins and minerals that can be added to prepared foods with little change to the food's taste or texture. MNPs are designed to provide the recommended daily nutrient intake of two or more vitamins and minerals to their target populations. A review has established that MNPs appear to be effective for reducing anemia and iron deficiency in children younger than age two years (De-Regil and others 2013). Another review of MNPs suggests benefit in improving anemia and hemoglobin among children; however, it shows no impact on growth

and evidence of increased diarrhea, suggesting further consideration is needed before large-scale implementation (Salam and others 2013).

NUTRITION-SENSITIVE INTERVENTIONS

Complementing the nutrition-specific interventions are nutrition-sensitive interventions to aid the implementation of these primary interventions. Although the direct impact of nutrition-sensitive interventions is limited, they have huge potential. These programs include the following:

- Water, sanitation, and hygiene (WASH) strategies
- Financial incentives at multiple levels
- Community-based nutrition education and mobilization programs.

These strategies can be delivered through health systems, agriculture-based programs, market-based approaches, or other community-based platforms.

WASH Strategies

Consensus has emerged on the importance of improved water supply and excreta disposal for prevention of diseases, especially diarrheal diseases. Provision of safe and clean water, as well as enhanced facilities for excreta disposal and promotion of hygiene, not only aim to improve the quality of life, but also help reduce the incidence of infectious diseases, particularly in children. In 2011, 89 percent of the world's population used improved drinking-water sources, and 55 percent had a piped supply on the premises. In the same year, 1 billion people still defecated in the open (WHO 2013). Although geographic disparities exist, rural and urban disparities within countries are also striking: 83 percent of the rural population has no access to safe water and 71 percent lives without sanitation (WHO 2013). Despite the declining open defecation rates globally, some countries, such as Cambodia and Benin, still have open defecation rates as high as 58 percent and 54 percent, respectively (WHO 2013). Ensuring safe WASH practices is urgently needed at household and community levels.

A review (Dangour and others 2013) of the effect of WASH interventions on the nutritional status of children younger than age 18 years finds no impact on WAZ scores (MD 0.05; 95 percent CI: −0.01–0.12) and weight-for-height z-score scores (MD: 0.02; 95 percent CI: −0.07–0.11), but a small impact on HAZ scores (MD 0.08; 95 percent CI 0.00–0.16). Another review (Cairncross and others 2010) highlights promising impacts of handwashing on reducing diarrhea morbidity by 47 percent (RR: 0.53; 95 percent CI: 0.37–0.67). Water quality improvement also showed significant impacts on reducing the incidence of diarrhea by 42 percent (RR 0.58; 95 percent CI: 0.46–0.72). Another review (Waddington and others 2009) of the effectiveness of these interventions concludes that interventions for water quality (protection or treatment of water at source or point of use) were more effective than interventions to improve water supply (improved source of water, improved distribution, or both). Interventions for water quality were associated with a 42 percent relative reduction in diarrhea morbidity in children younger than age five years, whereas those for water supply had no significant effects.

Overall, sanitation interventions led to a 37 percent reduction in childhood diarrhea morbidity, and hygiene interventions led to a 31 percent reduction. Subgroup analysis suggests that provision of soap with education was more effective than education only. The results suggest that interventions to improve the microbial quality of water, adequate excreta disposal, and behavior change interventions for promotion of hand washing and hygiene play their parts very efficiently in reducing the occurrence of infectious diseases and improving nutrition. Disease prevention and management interventions also have a role in improving nutrition, especially interventions targeting diarrhea and pneumonia (Bhutta and others 2013; Hutton and Chase, forthcoming).

Financial Incentives

Financial incentives are increasingly used as policy strategies to counter poverty, reduce financial barriers, and improve population health. A review of the effect of financial incentives on the coverage of health and nutrition interventions and behaviors targeting children younger than age five years (Bassani and others 2013) concludes that financial incentives have the potential to promote increased coverage of several important child health interventions. More pronounced effects seemed to be achieved by programs that directly removed user fees for access to health services. Some indication of effect was noted for programs that conditioned financial incentives on participation in health education and attendance at health care visits.

Community-Based Programs

A full spectrum of promotive, preventive, and curative interventions to improve child nutrition can be delivered via community platforms. A review (GHWA 2010) of community-based packages of care suggests

that these interventions can double the rate of initiation of BF within one hour of birth (RR: 2.25; 95 percent CI: 1.70–2.97). Lewin and others (2010) review 82 studies with lay health workers and show moderate-quality evidence of the effect on the initiation of BF (RR: 1.36; 95 percent CI: 1.14–1.61), any BF (RR: 1.24; 95 percent CI: 1.10–1.39), and EBF (RR: 2.78; 95 percent CI: 1.74–4.44), compared with usual care.

Although much of the evidence from large-scale programs using community health workers is of poor quality, process indicators and assessments do suggest that community health workers are able to implement many of these projects at scale, and they have substantial potential to improve the uptake of child health and nutrition outcomes in difficult-to-reach populations (GHWA 2010). It is important to underscore the crucial importance of community engagement and buy-in to ensure effective community outreach programs, behavior change, and access (chapter 14 in this volume, [Lassi, Kumar, and Bhutta 2016]).

CHALLENGES AND THE WAY FORWARD

Existing Evidence

The nutrition series in *The Lancet* highlights the existing promising nutrition-specific interventions to reduce fetal growth restriction and SGA births and improve nutrition among children younger than age five years in LMICs (table 12.2) (Bhutta and others 2013). These interventions include the following:

- Periconceptional folic acid supplementation or fortification
- Maternal BEP
- Iron-folate supplementation
- Multiple micronutrient supplementation
- Calcium supplementation for preeclampsia
- BF promotion
- Appropriate CF
- Preventive zinc and vitamin A supplementation
- Management of malnutrition in children.

Scaling up these identified interventions to 90 percent coverage could reduce deaths among children younger than age five years by nearly 15 percent and could reduce stunting by 20 percent and severe wasting by 61 percent (figure 12.2) (Bhutta and others 2013).

Geographic Disparities

Despite the existence of proven interventions and relative improvements in nutrition indicators overall,

Table 12.2 Interventions to Improve Nutrition in Mothers and Children Younger than Age Five Years

Intervention	Estimates
Maternal interventions	
Iron or iron-folate supplementation	• LBW (RR: 0.80; 95 percent CI: 0.68–0.97)
	• Birth weight (MD: 30.81 g; 95 percent CI: 5.94–55.68)
	• Serum hemoglobin concentration at term (MD: 8.88 g/l; 95 percent CI: 6.96–10.80)
	• Anemia at term (RR: 0.31; 95 percent CI: 0.19–0.46)
	• Iron deficiency (RR: 0.43; 95 percent CI: 0.27–0.66)
	• Iron deficiency anemia (RR: 0.34; 95 percent CI: 0.16–0.69)
	• Side effects (RR: 2.36; 95 percent CI: 0.96–5.82)
	• Nonsignificant impacts on premature delivery, neonatal death, congenital anomalies
Maternal multiple micronutrient supplementation	• LBW (RR: 0.89; 95 percent CI: 0.83–0.94)
	• SGA (RR: 0.87; 95 percent CI: 0.81–0.95)
	• Nonsignificant impacts on preterm birth, miscarriage, maternal mortality, perinatal mortality, stillbirths, and neonatal mortality
Maternal balanced energy protein supplementation	• Risk of SGA reduced by 34 percent (RR: 0.66; 95 percent CI: 0.49–0.89)
	• Stillbirths reduced by 38 percent (RR: 0.62; 95 percent CI: 0.40–0.98)
	• Birth weight increased (MD: 73 g; 95 percent CI: 30–117)
Child interventions	
Breastfeeding	• Exclusive breastfeeding rates increased by 43 percent at four to six weeks, with 89 percent and 20 percent significant increases in LMICs and HICs, respectively. Exclusive breastfeeding improved at age six months by 137 percent, with a sixfold increase in LMICs.
Complementary and supplementary feeding	• Statistically significant difference of effect for length during the intervention in children
Iron supplementation	• Anemia (RR: 0.51; 95 percent CI: 0.37–0.72)
	• Iron deficiency (RR: 0.24; 95 percent CI: 0.06–0.91), hemoglobin (MD: 5.20 g/l; 95 percent CI: 2.51–7.88), ferritin (MD: 14.17 mcg/l; 95 percent CI: 3.53–24.81)
Vitamin A supplementation	• All-cause mortality reduced by 24 percent (RR: 0.76; 95 percent CI: 0.69–0.83)
	• Diarrhea-related mortality reduced by 28 percent (RR: 0.72; 95 percent CI: 0.57–0.91)
	• Incidence of diarrhea reduced by 15 percent (RR: 0.85; 95 percent CI: 0.82–0.87)
	• Incidence of measles reduced by 50 percent (RR = 0.50; 95 percent CI 0.37–0.67)
	• Nonsignificant impacts on measles and ARI-related mortality
Zinc supplementation	• Height improved by 0.37 centimeters (SD 0.25) in children supplemented for 24 weeks
	• Diarrhea reduced by 13 percent
	• Pneumonia reduced by 19 percent
	• Nonsignificant impacts on mortality
Disease prevention and management	
WASH interventions	• Diarrhea reduced by 48 percent (RR: 0.52; 95 percent CI: 0.34–0.65) with handwashing with soap, 17 percent with improved water quality, and 36 percent with excreta disposal
Deworming	• Prophylactic single and multiple dose deworming had a nonsignificant effect on hemoglobin and weight gain.
	• Treating children with proven infection showed that single dose of deworming drugs increases weight (0.58 kg; 95 percent CI: 0.40–0.76) and hemoglobin (0.37 g/dL; 95 percent CI: 0.1–0.64).

table continues next page

Table 12.2 Interventions to Improve Nutrition in Mothers and Children Younger than Age Five Years (continued)

Intervention	Estimates
Malaria prevention and treatment	• Antimalarials to prevent malaria in pregnant women reduced antenatal parasitemia (RR: 0.53; 95 percent CI: 0.33–0.86)
	• Birth weight increased (MD: 126.7 g; 95 percent CI: 88.64–164.75)
	• LBW and severe antenatal anemia reduced by 43 percent and 38 percent, respectively
	• ITNs in pregnancy reduced LBW by 23 percent (RR: 0.77; 95 percent CI: 0.61–0.98) and reduced fetal loss (first to fourth pregnancies) by 33 percent (RR: 0.67; 95 percent CI: 0.47–0.97)
	• Nonsignificant impacts on anemia and clinical malaria

Source: Bhutta and others 2013.
Note: ARI = acute respiratory infection; CI = confidence interval; g = grams; g/dL = grams per deciliter; g/l = grams per liter; HIC = high-income country; ITNs = insecticide treated bednets; kg = kilogram; LBW = low birth weight; LMICs = low- and middle-income countries; mcg/l = micrograms per liter; MD = mean difference; RR = relative risk; SD = standard deviation; SGA = small for gestational age; WASH = water, sanitation, and hygiene.

nutrition data indicate considerable disparities among geographic regions, with South Asia bearing the highest burden (Stevens and others 2012). Almost 75 percent of all the world's LBW infants are born in South Asia. In the 75 Countdown countries, more than one child in three is stunted, and the median prevalence of wasting is 7.1 percent. Within countries, wide disparities exist between the richest and poorest wealth quintiles; in 20 percent of the Countdown countries, more than 50 percent of the children in the poorest 20 percent of all families is stunted. With these existing disparities, another challenge is the human immunodeficiency virus epidemic in the Countdown countries, especially those in Sub-Saharan Africa, which threatens to reverse all the nutrition gains achieved through large-scale programs.

Way Forward

Optimal IYCF means that mothers receive optimal antenatal care, are empowered to initiate BF within one hour of birth, BF exclusively for the first six months, and continue BF for two years or more, complemented by nutritionally adequate, nutrient-dense, safe and age-appropriate feeding of solid, semisolid, and soft foods starting in the sixth month (UNICEF 2014). Despite the existing guidelines, early cessation of BF and untimely introduction and poor-quality CF prevail. Strategies to protect, promote, and support EBF are needed at the national, health systems and community levels.

• **At the national level**, creating appropriate structures that ensure the adoption and implementation of the proper policies and legislation is vital (UNICEF 2014). This approach includes the development and implementation of national IYCF policies and strategy frameworks, as well as the development

Figure 12.2 Deaths Younger than Age Five Years Averted by the Scale-Up of Selected Nutrition Interventions per Year by 2025

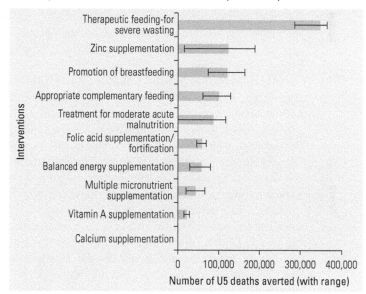

Source: Bhutta and others 2013.
Note: U5 = under age five years.

and enforcement of legislation that relates to the International Code of Marketing of Breast-milk Substitutes and maternity protection.

• **At the health systems level**, strategies include implementation of the Baby-Friendly Hospital Initiative, the education of health staff about adherence to the International Code of Marketing of Breast-milk Substitutes, as well as capacity building for health workers in areas such as BF counseling (UNICEF 2014).

• **At the community level**, maternal support activities involving community health workers, lay counselors, and mother-to-mother support groups are crucial. Promoting the importance of BF possibilities at the workplace is vital. Implementation of an evidence-based communication strategy using multiple channels, connecting and coordinating the efforts at the three levels, is also vital for the successful protection, promotion, and support of BF.

Appropriate CF is a proven intervention that can significantly reduce stunting during the first two years of life. An important issue is that the quality of the food received is often inadequate, failing to provide sufficient protein, fat, or micronutrients for optimal growth and development. Meeting the minimum required dietary quality is a challenge in many countries and has not been emphasized enough. Children may not receive complementary foods at the right age, may not be fed frequently enough during the day, or may receive poor-quality food. A comprehensive approach includes both counseling for caregivers on the best use of available foods (both local and commercially available) and feeding and care practices, and the provision of micronutrient and food supplements, when needed.

The ability to measure and monitor BF and CF practices might help raise awareness of their importance and facilitate progress in achieving improvements in BF practices worldwide (UNICEF 2006). Understanding the extent to which indicators of dietary quality predict anthropometric outcomes is important for interpreting the meaning of the measurements arising from these indicators (Jones and others 2014). Relatively simple indicators for assessing BF practices have been in wide use since the early 1990s (WHO 1991). However, defining simple CF indicators has proved to be challenging because of its multiple dimensions, the variation in these practices across contexts, and the changes in recommended practices that occur from ages 6 months to 23 months (Arimond, Daelmans, and Dewey 2008; WHO 2008). The WHO IYCF indicators are designed not only for describing trends in IYCF practices over time but also for identifying populations at risk and for evaluating the impacts of interventions. A literature review examining the eight core WHO IYCF indicators (table 12.1) and their relationships with child anthropometry using country-level data suggests that these indicators are especially well suited for monitoring trends in diet quality in large-scale data sets where detailed dietary data cannot be collected; however, they may not be highly sensitive or specific measures of dietary quality in the analysis of the causal pathways to child growth (Jones and others 2014).

The importance of maternal nutrition and its impact on child nutrition and health cannot be sufficiently underscored. To tackle the existing burden of child nutrition, strong emphasis should be focused on improving maternal nutrition even before pregnancy so that women enter pregnancy in the optimal state of health and nutrition. The current global emphasis on adolescence can address a multitude of problems and be the impetus for better women and child health and nutrition.

CONCLUSIONS

Infant and young child nutrition is dependent on the direct determinants of nutrition and growth, including diet, behavior, and health. It is also greatly affected by indirect determinants such as food security, education, environment, economic and social conditions, resources, and governance. Hence, the agenda for combating malnutrition requires a multifaceted approach involving both the interventions directed at the more immediate causes of suboptimum growth and development (nutrition specific) and the large-scale nutrition-sensitive programs that broadly address the underlying determinants of malnutrition.

NOTE

World Bank Income Classifications as of July 2014 are as follows, based on estimates of gross national income (GNI) per capita for 2013:
- Low-income countries (LICs) = US$1,045 or less
- Middle-income countries (MICs) are subdivided:
  a) lower-middle-income = US$1,046 to US$4,125
  b) upper-middle-income (UMICs) = US$4,126 to US$12,745
- High-income countries (HICs) = US$12,746 or more.

REFERENCES

Abdulwadud, O. A., and M. E. Snow. 2012. "Interventions in the Workplace to Support Breastfeeding for Women in Employment." *Cochrane Database of Systematic Reviews* 18 (3): 10:CD006177.

Arcangeli, T., B. Thilaganathan, R. Hooper, K. S. Khan, and A. Bhide. 2012. "Neurodevelopmental Delay in Small Babies at Term: A Systematic Review." *Ultrasound in Obstetrics and Gynecology* 40 (3): 267–75.

Arimond, M., B. Daelmans, and K. Dewey. 2008. "Indicators for Feeding Practices in Children." *The Lancet* 371 (9612): 541–42.

Awasthi, S., R. Peto, S. Read, S. Clark, V. Pande, and others. 2013. "Vitamin A Supplementation Every 6 Months with Retinol in 1 Million Pre-School Children in North India: DEVTA, A Cluster-Randomised Trial." *The Lancet* 381 (9876): 1469–77.

Baschat, A. A. 2011. "Neurodevelopment Following Fetal Growth Restriction and Its Relationship with Antepartum Parameters of Placental Dysfunction." *Ultrasound in Obstetrics and Gynecology* 37 (5): 501–14.

Bassani, D. G., P. Arora, K. Wazny, M. F. Gaffey, L. Lenters, and others. 2013. "Financial Incentives and Coverage of Child Health Interventions: A Systematic Review and Meta-Analysis." *BMC Public Health* 13 (Suppl 3): S30.

Bhutta, Z. A., J. K. Das, A. Rizvi, M. F. Gaffey, N. Walker, and others. 2013. "Evidence-Based Interventions for Improvement of Maternal and Child Nutrition: What Can Be Done and at What Cost?" *The Lancet* 382 (9890): 452–77.

Bjarnegard, N., E. Morsing, M. Cinthio, T. Lanne, and J. Brodszki. 2013. "Cardiovascular Function in Adulthood Following Intrauterine Growth Restriction with Abnormal Fetal Blood Flow." *Ultrasound in Obstetrics and Gynecology* 41 (2): 177–84.

Black, R. 2003. "Micronutrient Deficiency: An Underlying Cause of Morbidity and Mortality." *Bulletin of the World Health Organization* 81 (2): 79.

———, C. G. Victora, S. P. Walker, Z. A. Bhutta, P. Christian, and others. 2013. "Maternal and Child Undernutrition and Overweight in Low-Income and Middle-Income Countries." *The Lancet* 382 (9890): 427–51.

Brown, K. H., J. M. Peerson, S. K. Baker, and S. Y. Hess. 2009. "Preventive Zinc Supplementation among Infants, Preschoolers, and Older Prepubertal Children." *Food and Nutrition Bulletin* 30 (1 Suppl): S12–40.

Cai, X., T. Wardlaw, and D. W. Brown. 2012. "Global Trends in Exclusive Breastfeeding." *International Breastfeeding Journal* 7 (1): 12.

Cairncross, S., C. Hunt, S. Boisson, K. Bostoen, V. Curtis, and others. 2010. "Water, Sanitation and Hygiene for the Prevention of Diarrhoea." *International Journal of Epidemiology* 39 (Suppl 1): i193–205.

Dangour, A. D., L. Watson, O. Cumming, S. Boisson, Y. Che, and others. 2013. "Interventions to Improve Water Quality and Supply, Sanitation and Hygiene Practices, and Their Effects on the Nutritional Status of Children." *Cochrane Database of Systematic Reviews* 8: CD009382.

de Benoist, B., E. McLean, I. Egll, and M. Cogswell. 2008. *Worldwide Prevalence of Anaemia 1993–2005: WHO Global Database on Anaemia*. Geneva: World Health Organization.

Debes, A. K., A. Kohli, N. Walker, K. Edmond, and L. C. Mullany. 2013. "Time to Initiation of Breastfeeding and Neonatal Mortality and Morbidity: A Systematic Review." *BMC Public Health* 13 (3): 1–14.

Delgado, C., and A. Matijasevich. 2013. "Breastfeeding up to Two Years of Age or beyond and Its Influence on Child Growth and Development: A Systematic Review." *Cadernos de saude publica* 29 (2): 243–65.

De-Regil, L. M., M. E. Jefferds, A. C. Sylvetsky, and T. Dowswell. 2011. "Intermittent Iron Supplementation for Improving Nutrition and Development in Children under 12 Years of Age." *Cochrane Database of Systematic Reviews* 12: CD009085.

De-Regil, L. M., P. S. Suchdev, G. E. Vist, S. Walleser, and J. P. Peña-Rosas. 2013. "Home Fortification of Foods with Multiple Micronutrient Powders for Health and Nutrition in Children under Two Years of Age (Review)." *Evidence-Based Child Health: A Cochrane Review Journal* 8 (1): 112–201.

Dewey, K. G., and S. Adu-Afarwuah. 2008. "Systematic Review of the Efficacy and Effectiveness of Complementary Feeding Interventions in Developing Countries." *Maternal and Child Nutrition* 4 (Suppl 1): 24–85.

Duijts, L., V. W. Jaddoe, A. Hofman, and H. A. Moll. 2010. "Prolonged and Exclusive Breastfeeding Reduces the Risk of Infectious Diseases in Infancy." *Pediatrics* 126 (1): e18–25.

Edmond, K. M., C. Charles Zandoh, M. A. Quigley, S. Amenga-Etego, S. Owusu-Agyei, and B. R. Kirkwood. 2006. "Delayed Breastfeeding Initiation Increases Risk of Neonatal Mortality." *Pediatrics* 117 (3): e380–86.

Eichler, K., S. Wieser, I. Rüthemann, and U. Brügger. 2012. "Effects of Micronutrient Fortified Milk and Cereal Food for Infants and Children: A Systematic Review." *BMC Public Health* 12 (1): 506.

Eidelman, A. I., R. J. Schanler, M. Johnston, S. Landers, L. Noble, and others. 2012. "Breastfeeding and the Use of Human Milk." *Pediatrics* 129 (3): e827–41.

GHWA (Global Health Workforce Alliance). 2010. *Global Experience of Community Health Workers for Delivery of Health Related Millennium Development Goals: A Systematic Review, Country Case Studies, and Recommendations for Integration into National Health Systems*. Geneva: Global Health Workforce Alliance.

Gluckman, P. D., and M. A. Hanson. 2004. "Maternal Constraint of Fetal Growth and Its Consequences." *Seminars in Fetal and Neonatal Medicine* 9 (5): 419–25.

Greer, F. R., S. H. Sicherer, and A. W. Burks. 2008. "Effects of Early Nutritional Interventions on the Development of Atopic Disease in Infants and Children: The Role of Maternal Dietary Restriction, Breastfeeding, Timing of Introduction of Complementary Foods, and Hydrolyzed Formulas." *Pediatrics* 121 (1): 183–91.

Hanson, M., and P. Gluckman. 2011. "Developmental Origins of Noncommunicable Disease: Population and Public Health Implications." *American Journal of Clinical Nutrition* 94 (Suppl 6): 1754S–8S.

Haider, B. A., and Z. A. Bhutta. 2012. "Multiple-Micronutrient Supplementation for Women during Pregnancy." *Cochrane Database of Systematic Reviews* 11: CD004905.

Haroon, S., J. K. Das, R. A. Salam, A. Imdad, and Z. A. Bhutta. 2013. "Breastfeeding Promotion Interventions and Breastfeeding Practices: A Systematic Review." *BMC Public Health* 13 (3): 1–18.

Hutton, G., and C. Chaise. Forthcoming. "Water Supply, Sanitation, and Hygiene." In *Disease Control Priorities* (third edition): Volume 7, *Injury Prevention and Environmental Health*, edited by C. Mock, R. Nugent, and O. Kobusingye. Washington, DC: World Bank.

Imdad, A., and Z. A. Bhutta. 2011. "Effect of Preventive Zinc Supplementation on Linear Growth in Children under 5 Years of Age in Developing Countries: A Meta-Analysis of Studies for Input to the Lives Saved Tool." *BMC Public Health* 11 (Suppl 3): S22.

———. 2012. "Maternal Nutrition and Birth Outcomes: Effect of Balanced Protein-Energy Supplementation." *Paediatric and Perinatal Epidemiology* 26 (Suppl 1): 178–90.

Imdad, A., K. Herzer, E. Mayo-Wilson, M. Y. Yakoob, and Z. A. Bhutta. 2010. "Vitamin A Supplementation for Preventing Morbidity and Mortality in Children from 6 Months to 5 Years of Age." *Cochrane Database of Systematic Reviews* 12: CD008524.

Imdad, A., M. Y. Yakoob, and Z. A. Bhutta. 2011. "Impact of Maternal Education about Complementary Feeding and Provision of Complementary Foods on Child Growth in Developing Countries." *BMC Public Health* 11 (Suppl 3): S25.

Ip, S., M. Chung, G. Raman, P. Chew, N. Magula, and others. 2007. "Breastfeeding and Maternal and Infant Health Outcomes in Developed Countries." Evidence Report/Technology Assessment No. 153, AHRQ Publication No. 7-E007, Agency for Healthcare Research and Quality, Rockville, Maryland.

Ip, S., M. Chung, G. Raman, T. A. Trikalinos, and J. Lau. 2009. "A Summary of the Agency for Healthcare Research and Quality's Evidence Report on Breastfeeding in Developed Countries." *Breastfeeding Medicine* 4 (S1): S17–30.

Jones, A. D., S. B. Ickes, L. E. Smith, M. N. Mbuya, B. Chasekwa, and others. 2014. "Infant and Young Child Feeding Indicators and Their Associations with Child Anthropometry: A Synthesis of Recent Findings." *Maternal and Child Nutrition* 10 (1): 1–17.

Keino, S., G. Plasqui, G. Ettyang, and B. van den Borne. 2014. "Determinants of Stunting and Overweight among Young Children and Adolescents in Sub-Saharan Africa." *Food and Nutrition Bulletin* 35 (2): 167–78.

Kramer, M. S., and R. Kikuma. 2001. "The Optimal Duration of Exclusive Breastfeeding: Report of an Expert Consultation." WHO, Geneva.

Lassi, Z. S., J. K. Das, G. Zahid, A. Imdad, and Z. A. Bhutta. 2013. "Impact of Education and Provision of Complementary Feeding on Growth and Morbidity in Children Less Than 2 Years of Age in Developing Countries: A Systematic Review." *BMC Public Health* 13 (Suppl 3): S13.

Lassi, Z. S., R. Kumar, and Z. A. Bhutta. 2016. "Community-Based Care to Improve Maternal, Newborn, and Child Health." In *Disease Control Priorities* (third edition): Volume 2, *Reproductive, Maternal, Newborn, and Child Health*, edited by R. Black, R. Laxminarayan, M. Temmerman, and N. Walker. Washington, DC: World Bank.

Lewin, S., S. Munabi-Babigumira, C. Glenton, K. Daniels, X. Bosch-Capblanch, and others. 2010. "Lay Health Workers in Primary and Community Health Care for Maternal and Child Health and the Management of Infectious Diseases." *Cochrane Database of Systematic Reviews* 3: CD004015.

Liu, L., H. L. Johnson, S. Cousens, J. Perin, S. Scott, and others. 2012. "Global, Regional, and National Causes of Child Mortality: An Updated Systematic Analysis for 2010 with Time Trends Since 2000." *The Lancet* 379 (9832): 2151–61.

McLean, E., B. de Benoist, and L. H. Allen. 2008. "Review of the Magnitude of Folate and Vitamin B12 Deficiencies Worldwide." *Food and Nutrition Bulletin* 29 (Suppl 1): 38–51.

Mullany, L. C., J. Katz, Y. M. Li, S. K. Khatry, S. C. Leclerq, and others. 2008. "Breast-Feeding Patterns, Time to Initiation, and Mortality Risk among Newborns in Southern Nepal." *Journal of Nutrition* 138 (3): 599–603.

PAHO (Pan American Health Organization) and WHO (World Health Organization). 2003. "Guiding Principles for Complementary Feeding of the Breastfed Child." PAHO and WHO, Washington, DC.

Peña-Rosas, J. P., L. M. De-Regil, T. Dowswell, and F. E. Viteri. 2012. "Daily Oral Iron Supplementation during Pregnancy." *Cochrane Database of Systematic Reviews* 12: CD004736. doi:10.1002/14651858.CD004736.Pub4.

Peña-Rosas, J. P., and F. E. Viteri. 2009. "Effects and Safety of Preventive Oral Iron or Iron+Folic Acid Supplementation for Women during Pregnancy." *Cochrane Database of Systematic Reviews* 2: CD004736. doi:10.1002/14651858.CD004736.Pub3.

Quigley, M. A., Y. J. Kelly, and A. Sacker. 2007. "Breastfeeding and Hospitalization for Diarrheal and Respiratory Infection in the United Kingdom Millennium Cohort Study." *Pediatrics* 119 (4): E837–42.

Ramakrishnan, U., P. Nguyen, and R. Martorell. 2009. "Effects of Micronutrients on Growth of Children under 5 Y of Age: Meta-Analyses of Single and Multiple Nutrient Interventions." *American Journal of Clinical Nutrition* 89 (1): 191–203.

Romo, A., R. Carceller, and J. Tobajas. 2009. "Intrauterine Growth Retardation (IUGR): Epidemiology and Etiology." *Pediatric Endocrinology Reviews* 6 (Suppl 3): 332–36.

Sachdev, H., T. Gera, and P. Nestel. 2005. "Effect of Iron Supplementation on Mental and Motor Development in Children: Systematic Review of Randomised Controlled Trials." *Public Health Nutrition* 8 (2): 117–32.

Salam, R. A., J. K. Das, and Z. A. Bhutta. 2014. "Impact of Intrauterine Growth Restriction on Long-Term Health." *Current Opinion in Clinical Nutrition and Metabolic Care* 17 (3): 249–54.

Salam, R. A., J. K. Das, A. Ali, Z. Lassi, and Z. A. Bhutta. 2013. "Maternal Undernutrition and Intrauterine Growth Restriction." *Expert Review of Obstetrics and Gynecology* 8 (6): 559–67.

Salam, R. A., C. MacPhail, J. K. Das, and Z. A. Bhutta. 2013. "Effectiveness of Micronutrient Powders (MNP) in Women and Children." *BMC Public Health* 13 (Suppl 3): S22.

Sazawal, S., R. E. Black, M. Ramsan, H. M. Chwaya, R. J. Stoltzfus, and others. 2006. "Effects of Routine Prophylactic Supplementation with Iron and Folic Acid on Admission to Hospital and Mortality in Preschool Children in a High Malaria Transmission Setting: Community-Based, Randomised, Placebo-Controlled Trial." *The Lancet* 367 (9505): 133–43.

Stevens, G. A., M. M. Finucane, C. J. Paciorek, S. R. Flaxman, R. A. White, and others. 2012. "Trends in Mild, Moderate, and Severe Stunting and Underweight, and Progress towards MDG 1 in 141 Developing Countries: A Systematic Analysis of Population Representative Data." *The Lancet* 380: 824–34.

Umeta, M., C. E. West, J. Haidar, P. Deurenberg, and J. G. Hautvast. 2000. "Zinc Supplementation and Stunted Infants in Ethiopia: A Randomised Controlled Trial." *The Lancet* 355 (9220): 2021–26.

UNICEF (United Nations Children's Fund). 2006. "Progress for Children: A Report Card on Nutrition: Number 4." United Nations, New York. http://www2.unicef.org:60090/publications/index_33685.html.

UNICEF. 2013. *Improving Child Nutrition: The Achievable Imperative for Global Progress.* New York: United Nations. http://www.data.unicef.org/corecode/uploads/document6/uploaded_pdfs/corecode/NutritionReport_April2013_Final_29.pdf.

———. 2014. "Infant and Young Child Feeding." New York. http://www.unicef.org/nutrition/index_breastfeeding.html.

UNICEF, WHO, and World Bank. 2012. "Levels and Trends in Child Malnutrition. Joint Child Malnutrition Estimates." New York, NY: UNICEF; Geneva: WHO; Washington, DC: World Bank.

Vaidya, A., N. Saville, B. P. Shrestha, A. M. Costello, D. S. Manandhar, and others. 2008. "Effects of Antenatal Multiple Micronutrient Supplementation on Children's Weight and Size at 2 Years of Age in Nepal: Follow-Up of a Double-Blind Randomised Controlled Trial." *The Lancet* 371 (9611): 492–99.

Waddington, H., B. Snilstveit, H. White, and L. Fewtrell. 2009. *Water, Sanitation and Hygiene Interventions to Combat Childhood Diarrhoea in Developing Countries.* Delhi: International Initiative for Impact Evaluation.

Walker, C. L. F., and R. E. Black. 2010. "Zinc for the Treatment of Diarrhoea: Effect on Diarrhoea Morbidity, Mortality and Incidence of Future Episodes." *International Journal of Epidemiology* 39 (Suppl 1): i63–69.

WHO (World Health Organization). 1991. "Indicators for Assessing Breastfeeding Practices." Division of Child Health and Development, WHO, Geneva.

———. 1995. *Expert Committee Report: Physical Status: The Use and Interpretation of Anthropometry.* Technical Report Series 854. Geneva: WHO.

———. 2002. "Report of Informal Meeting to Review and Develop Indicators for Complementary Feeding." Department of Child and Adolescent Health and Development and Department of Nutrition for Health and Development, WHO, Geneva; Food and Nutrition Program and Regional Office for the Americas, WHO, Washington, DC.

———. 2003. *Global Strategy for Infant and Young Child Feeding.* Geneva: WHO. http://www.who.int/nutrition/topics/global_strategy/en/.

———. 2008. "Indicators for Assessing Infant and Young Child Feeding Practices: Conclusions of a Consensus Meeting." Washington, DC, November 6–8, 2007, WHO, Geneva.

———. 2009. "Global Prevalence of Vitamin A Deficiency in Populations at Risk 1995–2005." WHO Global Database on Vitamin A Deficiency. WHO, Geneva.

———. 2011. *Guideline: Intermittent Iron Supplementation in Preschool and School-Age Children.* Geneva: WHO. http://apps.who.int/iris/bitstream/10665/44648/1/9789241502009_eng.pdf.

———. 2013. "2.4 Billion People Will Lack Improved Sanitation in 2015: World Will Miss MDG Target." Note for Media, WHO, Geneva. http://www.who.int/mediacentre/news/notes/2013/sanitation_mdg_20130513/en/.

———. 2014. "Intermittent Iron Supplementation in Children in Malaria-Endemic Regions." WHO, Geneva. http://www.who.int/elena/titles/iron_infants_malaria/en/.

WHO and UNICEF. 2003. *Global Strategy for Infant and Young Child Feeding.* Geneva: WHO.

———. 2008. "Indicators for Assessing Infant and Young Child Feeding Practices: Part 1 Definitions." WHO, Geneva.

———. 2012. *Building a Future for Women and Children: The 2012 Report.* Geneva: WHO and UNICEF.

Yakoob, M. Y., and Z. A. Bhutta. 2011. "Effect of Routine Iron Supplementation with or without Folic Acid on Anemia during Pregnancy." *BMC Public Health* 11 (Suppl 3): S21.

Chapter **13**

Very Early Childhood Development

Frances E. Aboud and Aisha K. Yousafzai

INTRODUCTION

Developmental potential is the ability to think, learn, remember, relate, and articulate ideas appropriate to age and level of maturity, and an estimated 39 percent of the world's children under age five years do not attain this potential (Grantham-McGregor and others 2007).

The main reason for giving prominent attention to mental development from conception through the first 24 months of life is that early unfavorable conditions can impair the normal development of the brain. The impairment is often incremental and unnoticed until schooling begins. The most striking example of impairment is the gradual deletion of unused brain synapses. The lack of use may be due to the absence of stimulation in the family environment or lack of available energy for brain activity. Regenerating those lost synapses may occur at an older age but with additional costs. For example, children who do not acquire a good vocabulary in the early years will have difficulty learning how to read; children who do not acquire simple problem-solving strategies in the first 24 months will have difficulty understanding math concepts; children who do not develop secure emotional attachments to adults will have difficulty coping with stresses and challenges throughout life. The plasticity of the brain diminishes with age, but greater plasticity in the very early years suggests that brain development has a greater chance of being modified by protective interventions than by interventions later in life (Werker and Hensch 2015).

A second reason for attending to early mental development is that individuals, communities, and societies are healthier and more productive if they have mature mental skills. More educated adults are healthier and wealthier than less educated adults. Educated mothers have healthier children and are more likely to recognize symptoms of illness, follow medical advice, feed their children nutritious foods, and keep their homes clean (Boyle and others 2006; Cleland and van Ginneken 1988). Educated husbands are less likely to condone or use violence to resolve domestic conflicts (Abraham and others 2006). Follow-up data of adults who participated in early psychosocial stimulation programs demonstrate some of these long-term benefits (Gertler and others 2014).

This chapter discusses mental development from birth to age 24 months in low- and middle-income countries (LMICs). We include recent literature published since the 2011 child development series in *The Lancet*. Although we focus on cognitive and language domains, we touch on socioemotional, fine motor, and gross motor development. First, a description of how these domains are measured provides an operational definition of the term *mental development*. Second, conditions that derail early child development are examined. These conditions arise during the prenatal period and continue throughout the next 24 months; they include psychosocial stimulation, prenatal and postnatal nutrition, the physical environment, and

Corresponding author: Frances E. Aboud, McGill University, Department of Psychology, Montreal, frances.aboud@mcgill.ca.

maternal mental health. Finally, the results of several systematic reviews and meta-analyses are presented to show the effects of stimulation and nutrition, along with disease-related interventions to promote mental development. Maternal interventions related to nutrition and mental health are also reviewed. A framework of critical components to include in programs is outlined.

PREVALENCE AND MEASUREMENT: WHAT DOES MENTAL DEVELOPMENT ENTAIL AT THIS AGE?

In the absence of well-validated international indicators, the Ten Questions Survey was used in 18 countries as part of the Multiple Indicator Cluster Survey 2005–06. Included were countries in the Caribbean, west Asia, southeast Asia, and Sub-Saharan Africa. The survey screens for disabilities by asking mothers of children ages 2–9 years two cognitive questions (for example, does your child learn to do things like other children his or her age?) and four language questions (for example, can your child name at least one object?). Results indicate that 7 percent of children had a cognitive disability, and 21 percent had a language disability. Overall, 27 percent of children screened positive for one of the sensory-motor-mental-social disabilities (Gottlieb and others 2009). However, because the answers depend on the ability of the mothers to notice disabilities, screening is likely to reveal only the tip of the iceberg (Yousafzai, Lynch, and Gladstone 2014). Also, because the items address disabilities rather than expected development, measurement experts are working to create a list of 30 or so mental milestones specific to the under-24-month age group to be asked of mothers (see, for example, Prado and others 2014).

The mental competencies of children during the first 24 months can now be directly assessed with behavioral tests and brain recordings. Both tools show that by the end of the first month, newborns respond to language more than to other sounds; they like looking at bright contrasts, movement, and color. The Brazelton Neonatal Behavioral Assessment Scale (Brazelton and Nugent 1995) assesses these competencies through observations of newborns interacting with others. Healthier newborns show better regulation of physiological states by self-soothing; better habituation to repeated sensory inputs, such as ringing bells; and greater response to social speech. The measured competencies are expected to facilitate engagement with physical and social environments in ways that will promote mental development. Impairments during the neonatal period

due to fetal lead contamination and deficits in iodine can be detected with this early assessment (Kooistra and others 2006; Patel and others 2006).

The most common measures of mental development after the newborn period are standardized behavioral tests, such as the Bayley Scales of Infant and Toddler Development, Third Edition (Bayley 2006) and the Griffiths Mental Development Scales (Griffiths and Huntley 1996). Both measure cognitive, receptive language, expressive language, fine motor, and gross motor development from birth to age 3.5 years using a number of items of increasing difficulty. The cognitive items mainly concern the ability to solve small problems. Receptive language items test the ability to understand the meaning of words, sentences, and abstract categories. Expressive language items assess the ability to use sounds, gestures, and the spoken word to communicate. Fine motor items include eye-hand coordination tasks. Gross motor development, such as sitting and walking, is not strongly related to mental development (Hamadani and others 2013) and so is not addressed here.

Social and emotional skills are an important domain of mental development, but measures for this age are not commonly applied in research, and determinants are not widely known. The Griffiths Scales include items that address personal-social skills, such as recognition of one's mother, enjoying playmates, and feeding and dressing oneself. The Bayley Scales also include a social-emotional subscale, with questions for parents that reveal the purposeful and social expression of emotions and interactive behaviors. However, secure attachment is the most important capability acquired in the first two years (Sroufe 2005). It is measured by the Strange Situation, in which observers note how much emotional security children derive from parents when under some stress due to the presence of strange people and objects. Malnourished children and those who receive less responsive warmth appear to be less emotionally secure than well-nourished and supported children (Cooper and others 2009; Isabella 1993; Valenzuela 1990).

CONDITIONS THAT AFFECT CHILD DEVELOPMENT

Many of the conditions that affect the health and growth of children in the first 1,000 days could affect mental development. These factors include the preconception and pregnancy nutritional status of the mother, birth weight and linear growth of the infant, and conditions of labor and delivery; maternal mental health; and environmental conditions. However, we start with the condition most specific to mental development, namely, psychosocial stimulation. Many of these conditions co-occur, as will the impairments they cause.

Psychosocial Stimulation

Psychosocial stimulation refers to an external object or event that elicits a physiological and psychological response in the child. A specific measure of psychosocial stimulation is the Home Observation for Measurement of the Environment (HOME) Inventory (Bradley and Corwyn 2005). The infant and toddler version for children younger than age 24 months includes 45 items that are assessed through observation and interview. The essence of stimulation is observed in mother-child interaction that is verbal and responsive to the child's state, and in play materials that can be manipulated in different ways by the child. The caregiver is also questioned about activities that expose the child to places, people, and conversation. The focus is on opportunities to play and converse in ways that stretch thinking and understanding of speech. Scores on the HOME Inventory from around the world have ranged from a low of 20 (Boivin and others 2013) to a high of 31 (Lozoff and others 2010); in other words, the scores satisfied less than half to two-thirds of the items (figure 13.1). All studies showed very strong correlations between HOME scores and children's mental development, with low HOME scores associated with poor mental development.

A brief version of the inventory called the Family Care Indicators is available for use in national surveys. Consisting of 10 interview questions for the caregiver, it has been validated in South Asia and Sub-Saharan Africa (Hamadani, Tofail, and others 2010; Kariger and others 2012) and used to evaluate responsive and stimulating caregiving in 28 LMICs (Bornstein and Putnick 2012). Mothers (caregivers) were asked what they had done with their children under age five years in the past three days. Items largely focus on the variety of play materials available for the child (for example, things for making music, things for pretending, things for drawing) and play activities (for example, reading or looking at pictures, telling stories, singing songs). Only 25 percent of mothers said they had read to their children in the past three days, 25 percent had sung songs, and 35 percent had told stories. Scores did not vary by child's gender but were lower in families with more children. Thus, the presence of more children does not necessarily mean more of the right kind of stimulation. It is often mistakenly believed that older siblings provide sufficient stimulation and supervision. However, older

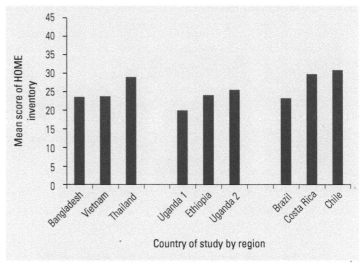

Figure 13.1 Mean HOME Inventory Score and Study

Y-axis: Mean score of HOME inventory

X-axis: Country of study by region (Bangladesh, Vietnam, Thailand, Uganda 1, Ethiopia, Uganda 2, Brazil, Costa Rica, Chile)

Sources: Bangladesh: 23.5 (Aboud and Akhter 2011); Vietnam: 23.6 (Williams and others 2003); Thailand: 28.9 (Williams and others 2003); Uganda 1: 19.8 (Boivin and others 2013); Ethiopia: 24.0 (Bougma 2014); Uganda 2: 25.4 (Singla, Kumbakumba, and Aboud 2015); Brazil: 23.1 (Eickmann and others 2003); Costa Rica: 29.8 (Lozoff and others 1987); Chile: 30.8 (Lozoff and others 2010).
Note: HOME = Home Observation for Measurement of the Environment.

siblings are not able to deliver the sophisticated language of adults or accurately perceive when young children are in danger (Morrongiello, Schell, and Schmidt 2010). Across all 28 LMICs surveyed, the average number of caregiving practices out of six performed in the past three days with a child under age five years was 3.03. Many parents from countries in South Asia and Sub-Saharan Africa practiced only one or two. Although no threshold score is available to identify inadequate levels of stimulation, low levels such as these are unlikely to support expected levels of mental development (Bradley and Corwyn 2005).

Both the HOME Inventory and its briefer version are highly correlated with children's mental development, ranging from $r = 0.20$ to $r = 0.46$ (Aboud and others 2013; Boivin and others 2013; Hamadani, Tofail, and others 2010; Tofail and others 2012). These correlations and the theoretical framework presented here (figure 13.2) support the design of stimulation interventions to enhance mental development. One hypothesized pathway proposes that an adult's child-directed conversation stimulates speech perception sites in the brain, thereby maintaining neural connections throughout language sites in the brain. Also, if the conversation is directly related to children's current state, it is expected to expand the children's receptive language and grammar. This interaction helps children translate their own thoughts and actions into speech and later into writing and reading. Play materials that children enjoy manipulating and combining in multiple ways help them learn about mass

Figure 13.2 Framework Illustrating Pathways from Psychosocial Stimulation to Mental Development

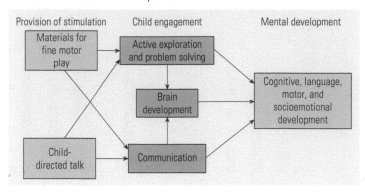

Source: Larson and Yousafzai 2014.

Figure 13.3 Framework Illustrating Pathways from Nutritional Status to Mental Development

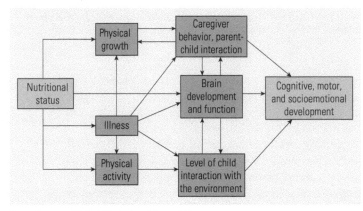

Source: Brown and Pollitt 1996; Prado and Dewey 2014.

and weight, as well as problem solving. The material must be challenging so that children have opportunities to construct the material in new ways.

Child Nutrition

One of the strongest risk factors for poor mental development is short length- or height-for-age (for cross-sectional studies, see Olney and others 2009; Servili and others 2010; for longitudinal studies, see Grantham-McGregor and others 2007). Stunting is a commonly used indicator of chronic undernutrition, defined as more than two standard deviations below the age- and gender-specific norm, that increases rapidly after age six months; by 24 months, 50 percent of children in LMICs are stunted (Victora, de Onis, and Hallal 2010). Children rarely catch up after this age.

It is not clear why length and height are so strongly related to cognitive and language development, except

that linear growth may be a proxy for other critical nutrition processes related to brain and behavioral development. A model of how nutrition contributes to mental development is presented in figure 13.3 (Brown and Pollitt 1996; Prado and Dewey 2014). One pathway is direct in the sense that nutrients support the structure and activity of brain sites responsible for mental development. Other pathways are indirect in that nutrition enhances health and engagement with the environment, which promote mental development. Evidence from nutrition interventions showing effects on growth and health are described here. The next section presents intervention effects on mental development.

Macronutrients

Sufficient macronutrients, such as carbohydrates, proteins, and fats, are important to linear growth and mental development. In the first six months, exclusive breastfeeding provides sufficient nutrients to support healthy rates of growth and immunity (Kramer and others 2001) (see chapter 5 in this volume, Stevens, Finucane, and Paciorek 2016). After age six months, the quality of diet is captured by the term *dietary diversity* and measured as the number of seven different food categories in a daily diet (Daelmans, Dewey, and Arimond 2009). Dietary diversity was positively related to linear growth in five of the nine countries for which these data were analyzed (Jones and others 2014). Improving dietary diversity, especially with animal-source foods, is a critical message in nutrition education interventions (Neumann and others 2007). In eight studies, nutrition education alone for mothers of children ages 6–24 months, usually about foods to feed and number of meals, led to gains in length, with an effect size of $d = 0.21$, where effect size d refers to the number of standard deviations by which intervention children's length exceeded that of control children (Dewey and Adu-Afarwuah 2008; Imdad, Yakoob, and Bhutta 2011). Agricultural improvements at the household level are also being implemented and evaluated (Iannotti and others 2014).

Micronutrients

Micronutrients such as iron and iodine are considered to be important for mental development in the first 24 months (see chapter 11 in this volume, Lenters, Wazny, and Bhutta 2016; and chapter 12, Das and others 2016). Numerous studies have demonstrated high levels of anemia in young children, especially in South Asia and Sub-Saharan Africa, where 20 percent of children younger than age five years are anemic (Black and others 2013). Both an iron-deficient diet and hookworm in contaminated soil are responsible for low levels of hemoglobin. Anemic children are consistently found to have lower levels of mental development than non-anemic children in case-control studies, and differences persist over the long term (Lozoff and others 2006). Anemic children also show a number of socially isolating behaviors, such as wariness and lethargy. However, the nutritional and mental consequences of providing young children with iron are mixed and generally weak (Pasricha and others 2013). In many cases, iron therapy has not sufficiently raised their hemoglobin levels; even when it has, children's mental development scores frequently have not improved. Alternative explanations are being sought for the longitudinal findings, such as low levels of stimulation in the home environment, where the mother may be anemic. Brain functioning, such as speed of processing auditory and visual information, may be a more sensitive measure of the mental effects, especially if iron is an important element in the myelin sheath around neuronal axons (Lozoff and others 2006).

Iodine deficiency is consistently associated with poor school achievement, but much less is known about its effect on the mental development of children younger than age 24 months (Zimmermann 2012; Zimmermann, Jooste, and Pandav 2008). Many countries lack naturally occurring iodine in the soil and water and therefore must fortify a product such as salt. Most of the data on prevalence has been collected from children ages 6–12 years whose urinary iodine levels tend to match that of their parents. Based on these data, an estimated 40 percent of the Sub-Saharan African population and 31.6 percent of the population of East Asia and Pacific and South Asia are iodine deficient (Black and others 2013). Four prospective studies find that mental development scores of children with inadequate iodine levels at birth were half a standard deviation less than those with healthy levels (Bougma and others 2013); this finding translates into a development quotient difference of 8 points on a standard mental test—a meaningful difference.

Multiple Vitamin and Mineral Supplements

Multiple micronutrients constitute the common nutritional supplement provided to young children. Children are often deficient in many minerals, such as iron and zinc, as well as vitamins. All are critical for health and growth, and their effects on mental development are becoming clear. The rationale for studying multiple micronutrients is that they work together to improve health, they appear to be necessary for linear growth, and they are found in many sites in the brain. Most of what is known about the effects of combining multiple micronutrients comes from evaluations of trials in which various combinations are provided in a powder sprinkled on the food daily at mealtime. Alternatively,

researchers weigh meal foods and calculate quantities of different nutrients in each food item.

Linear growth is still the strongest correlate of mental development, so it is important to evaluate the effects of macro- and micronutrient interventions on children's height. The section on Interventions for Mental Development reports effects on cognitive and language outcomes. Systematic reviews have consistently shown that the effect sizes of nutrition interventions on linear growth gains were lowest for micronutrient fortification (about 0.12), and better for energy alone (about 0.25) and the provision of food with extra proteins and nutrients (about 0.28) (Bhutta and others 2013; Dewey and Adu-Afarwuah 2008). The effect sizes for nutrition education were 0.20, especially those programs emphasizing dietary diversity and animal-source foods. Although nutrition education is insufficient on its own, especially in food-insecure sites, it is necessary if benefits from short-term supplementation and fortification are to be sustained, and in some cases leads to better mental development (Vazir and others 2013).

Environmental Conditions

Environmental conditions encompass a broad array of vectors, including contaminated razors used to cut the umbilical cord and leading to tetanus, viruses and bacteria that follow a fecal-oral transmission route starting from poor home sanitation and leading to diarrhea, parasites carried by the female *Anopheles* mosquito leading to malaria, and *Chlamydia trachomitis* brought by moisture-seeking flies to children's eyes that can lead to blindness. Despite a resurgence in some places, deaths due to neonatal tetanus, and sensory-motor disabilities due to polio and measles, are being reduced with the help of vaccines. However, trachoma, diarrhea, and cerebral malaria continue to have major impacts on early mental development.

Trachoma

Trachoma, active in 40.6 million people worldwide, is responsible for blindness in 8.2 million people (Mariotti, Pascolini, and Rose-Nussbaumer 2009). It is endemic in 57 countries, but 80 percent of the cases are in 15 countries, most in Sub-Saharan Africa. One study of southern Sudan found that 64 percent of children ages 1–9 years had active trachoma; 46.2 percent of infants had signs of active trachoma (Ngondi and others 2005). The condition begins in early childhood when the *Chlamydia trachomitis*, passed by hand or flies, leads to inflammation of the conjunctiva of the upper eyelid. The infection may disappear, but repeated reinfection leads to blindness. Although surgery is needed for cases of blindness among adults, the more common approach has been mass azithromycin antibiotic treatment as a primary and secondary prevention (Ogden and Emerson 2012).

Diarrhea

Diarrhea becomes most prevalent between 6 and 24 months of age; children have on average four to five episodes a year (Kosek, Bern, and Guerrant 2003). The most common cause of severe diarrhea is rotavirus, for which vaccines are being given to infants in many countries in East Asia and Pacific and South Asia and Sub-Saharan Africa (Armah and others 2010). Other common causes are bacteria, such as salmonella, shigella, and pathogenic *E. coli*. The main route of transmission is fecal-oral, so the risk is high if families do not use a latrine or improved sources of water. Children become exposed to contaminated soil and water, typically after age six months when they start to crawl and share family meals. Hookworm, one of the geohelminths found in contaminated soil, is responsible for half of the anemia in children, and diarrhea is a common cause of malnutrition and stunting (Checkley and others 2008). Although there is little evidence that worms and diarrhea directly impede mental development, they may diminish important determinants, such as growth and activity (Fischer Walker and others 2012; Taylor-Robinson, Jones, and Garner 2007) (see chapter 9 in this volume, Keusch and others 2016).

Enteropathy

Recent attention has focused on tropical or environmental enteropathy, which results from constantly ingested fecal bacteria, as a subclinical condition. In several studies, fecal bacteria contamination was very high in children's food and in soil and chicken feces found around the home where children play (Ngure and others 2014); these levels are correlated with microbiological data from the children and high levels of inflammation. Constantly high levels of pathogenic bacteria lead to chronic changes in the villi of the small intestines (Humphrey 2009; McKay and others 2010; Weisz and others 2012). The effect of enteropathy is to increase absorption of bacterial products, such as endotoxins, into the system and allow for leakage of nutrients, such as proteins. Consequently, young children experience recurrent infections, with associated loss of appetite and diversion of nutrients to fight infections and inflammation, resulting in inactivity and growth faltering. Jiang and others (2014) find a direct association between mental development scores and the number of days during which an infant experienced fever and elevated levels of pro-inflammatory cytokines. Although preliminary, the work suggests a connection between inflammation and mental development. If enteropathy is as prevalent and severe as feared, how to eliminate sources of contamination in the environment without restricting children's access to psychosocial stimulation around the home must be seriously reconsidered.

Cerebral Malaria

Cerebral malaria has clear but variable consequences for early childhood mental development. There are 104 malaria-endemic countries in the world; most are in Sub-Saharan Africa. The parasite *Plasmodium falciparum*, in particular, is most strongly associated with cerebral malaria leading to high fever, coma, and organ failure. Contracted by pregnant women or young children, malaria is a serious cause of death and disability among children. In one Ugandan study, approximately 10 percent of survivors had severe neurological deficits; the majority had moderate problems that were detected only with psychological testing when the children were older (Bangirana and others 2006). Disabilities are evident in auditory or visual processing, as well as in memory and attention; language problems were not as severely affected. Because impairments vary, many researchers report the number of subtests on which cerebral malaria survivors show deficits compared with controls. For example, a prospective study with children ages 5–9 years in Kampala, Uganda, finds that on several tests of attention, working memory, and learning, 36.4 percent showed deficits on at least one measure at hospital discharge; 21.4 percent maintained deficits at six-month and two-year follow-ups, compared with 5.7 percent of healthy controls (Boivin and others 2007; John and others 2008). Deficits in attention and memory were most common and were related to the number of seizures and duration of coma.

Most of this research has been conducted in urban hospitals, although the larger burden of malaria is likely found in rural sites. Consequently, the evidence is strong that a large proportion of children with cerebral malaria and its associated brain complications will show long-term cognitive and perceptual problems.

Maternal Nutrition

The optimum body mass index (BMI) for women at the start of pregnancy is 18.5 to 24 kilograms per meter squared. In LMICs, more than 10 percent of women are less than 18.5, with the highest levels of low BMI found in South Asia and Sub-Saharan Africa (Black and others 2013). BMI is an important benchmark because it highlights the undernutrition of many women before they become pregnant. The failure to meet the benchmark indicates increased risk of difficult deliveries for mothers and children; short maternal stature, defined as less than

145 centimeters, is also problematic. Although the rate of low BMI is declining, the prevalence of unattended home deliveries remains high. Consequently, birth injuries, such as asphyxia, are untreated and leave lasting effects on mental development.

Mothers with low BMI, short stature, or both put their children at risk of being small-for-gestational-age (SGA). SGA, defined as having birth weight less than the 10th percentile for gestational age, includes newborns who are at term (37–40 weeks) but small—less than 2,500 grams at 37 weeks and less than 2,900 grams at 40 weeks, as well as those who are preterm and small. In 2010, an estimated 32.4 million newborns in LMICs, or 27 percent of the 120 million births, were SGA; of these, 30 million were born at term with intrauterine growth restriction (Lee and others 2013). South Asia makes the highest contribution to this figure; 42 percent of its births are SGA. Prematurity tends to be consistent at 18 percent for Sub-Saharan Africa and 12 percent for South Asia (Lawn and others 2014), although very few born younger than 32 weeks survive in LMICs. The group most at risk for neurological and developmental disabilities is the combined group of premature infants and term SGA infants, who together make up 43.3 million or 36 percent of live births (Lee and others 2013). Some experts identify only SGA infants (preterm and term) as high risk.

Increased Risk of Neurodevelopmental Disabilities

Although the first hurdle for SGA and premature newborns is surviving respiratory distress, hypothermia, and infections during the first month, the second hurdle is early neurodevelopmental disabilities (Blencowe and others 2013). These issues include cognitive impairment, hearing and vision problems, and motor and behavioral problems. A systematic review of surviving preterm children, mainly from high-income countries (HICs), indicates that approximately 7 percent showed mild or moderate-to-severe impairment in one of these areas. Those with very short gestational age fared worse: 24.5 percent of those with less than 32 weeks' gestation had moderate-to-severe impairment, whereas 1.8 percent of those between 32 and 37 weeks had impairments (Blencowe and others 2013; Platt 2014). One hospital-based assessment of surviving preterm Bangladeshi infants with gestational age of less than 33 weeks finds that 73 percent had mild or serious impairments when tested at younger than age two years; 66 percent were reported as having impairments between ages two and four years (Khan and others 2009); most of the impairments were cognitive. Although most data come from studies in HICs, conclusions and applications to East Asia and Pacific and South Asia and Sub-Saharan Africa

are clear, especially for the 12.6 million children born at ages 32–37 weeks who need facility and family care but not necessarily a high-technology intensive care unit. More research is needed to identify the range of disabilities they may experience related to sensory development, learning, mental health, and executive function. Programs to prevent and treat these disabilities have received little attention in LMICs.

Increased Risk of Delayed Mental Development

The third hurdle for SGA and premature newborns is linear growth restriction, an important determinant of mental development. SGA newborns have experienced fetal growth restriction and are unlikely to catch up because of problems starting breastfeeding and the usual decline in growth rates found in the first 24 months (Christian and others 2013). In 19 longitudinal cohort studies from LMICs that followed children from birth to between ages 12 and 60 months, low birth weight (LBW) children were almost three times more likely to be stunted (< −2.00 height-for-age z-score) than normal birth weight children, but this likelihood varied according to gestational age. The risks were highest for preterm SGA newborns (odds ratio: 4.51), next for term-SGA (odds ratio: 2.43), and lowest for preterm average-for-gestational-age (odds ratio: 1.93). Accordingly, although prematurity was the stronger determinant of neonatal mortality, weight-for-gestational-age had more lasting effects on linear growth. The mental development of SGA newborns may be compromised in the short term, but their longer-term prospects in LMICs are unclear. For example, Tofail and others (2012) find that at age 10 months, LBW Bangladeshi infants, most of whom were term, had lower mental and motor Bayley scores than normal birth weight children, after controlling for a range of covariates, such as weight, length, and gestational age. Similarly, Walker and others (2004) find lower Griffiths scores at ages 15 and 24 months on cognitive and motor subscales for term-LBW Jamaican children compared with normal-weight peers. Thus, preterm- and term-SGA babies are likely to have lower mental development if they continue to have poor health and growth, and inadequate nutrition during fetal growth may be partly responsible.

Maternal Mental Health

Maternal depression is increasingly recognized as an important risk factor for poor child development (Tomlinson and others 2014; Walker and others 2011) (see chapter 3 in this volume, Filippi and others 2016). A systematic review reports that the prevalence of maternal depression among pregnant women in low-income and lower-middle-income countries was 15.9 percent, and in the postpartum period was 19.8 percent; these rates are higher than those for women in HICs, which are, on average, 10 percent and 13 percent, respectively (Fisher and others 2012). Prevalence is higher in many South Asian countries, for example, in Pakistan, where one study reports a 25 percent prevalence of maternal depression in the antenatal period and 28 percent in the postnatal period (Rahman, Iqbal, and Harrington 2003). Recognizing that depression may not be confined to the prenatal and postnatal periods, many researchers monitoring maternal depression for 24 months after birth and beyond find it to be high in South Asia and Sub-Saharan Africa, from 20 percent to 30 percent, using the WHO's 20-item Self-Reporting Questionnaire (Harpham and others 2005; Servili and others 2010; Weobong and others 2009).

Important determinants of maternal mental health include intimate partner violence (Ludermir and others 2008); social support (Rahman and Creed 2007); the quality of her relationships with her husband (Oweye, Aina, and Morakinyo 2006) and other close relatives, such as in-laws (Chandran and others 2002); and her coping strategies (Faisal-Cury and others 2003). Nutritional status may be implicated. Evidence suggests that iron-deficiency anemia contributes to a depressed mood at levels lower than required for a diagnosis of depression, as might iodine deficiency (Beard and others 2005). Illness, fatigue, and lethargy are likely to reduce a mother's ability to cope as well as to care for her young child. Infants with special needs requiring higher levels of care have been linked to higher levels of maternal distress (Yousafzai, Lynch, and Gladstone 2014).

Studies from South Asia have shown that young children of depressed mothers are at risk of poor health, growth, and development outcomes. Rural Pakistani children of depressed mothers were twice as likely to have five or more episodes of diarrhea per year than children of nondepressed mothers (Rahman, Bunn, and others 2007). Studies from India and Pakistan have shown that infants born to depressed mothers are 2.3 to 7.4 times more likely to be underweight (Patel and others 2004); in India, they were more likely to be stunted, but not in Vietnam, Ethiopia, or Peru (Harpham and others 2005). Evidence for the effect of maternal depression on mental development is mixed in LMICs. Some hospital samples show a link (for example, Hamadani and others 2012), but in rural Ethiopia, maternal depression was not associated with poor mental development in children (Servili and others 2010). In Bangladesh, maternal depression was found to be linked to poor mental development outcomes only if depressed mothers perceived their children as irritable (Black and others 2007). Maternal depression has a potentially detrimental impact on children and needs to be examined more carefully.

INTERVENTIONS TO ENHANCE MENTAL DEVELOPMENT

This section describes key protective interventions that promote healthy early child development. We consider each intervention's outcome (figure 13.4), organizing the interventions into development-specific interventions that focus on the child, including psychosocial stimulation, child nutrition, and reduction of infections, followed by development-sensitive interventions that focus on the mother, including maternal nutrition and maternal mental health, that might indirectly affect the child.

Development-Specific Interventions

Psychosocial Stimulation

One of the strongest protective factors for mental development is the amount and quality of psychosocial stimulation provided in the home. A systematic review and meta-analysis of stimulation intervention outcomes from 21 studies finds positive effects: the mean effect size for cognitive outcomes was $d = 0.420$ and for language outcomes was $d = 0.468$ (Aboud and Yousafzai 2015). These effects are considerably higher than for other interventions, such as nutrition and hygiene. However, stimulation programs require considerably more manpower, training, and supervision. Four models of delivery have been implemented and evaluated (box 13.1), but all require special training of professionals or paraprofessionals and a method of instruction that encourages parents to actively learn new practices and be able to generalize what they learn as their children grow.

Changing behavior is difficult, but one review identifies several techniques that are more successful than others (Aboud and Yousafzai 2015). The traditional technique of simply educating or informing parents about what to do and why has not worked (Aboud 2007). Behavior change requires more than communication; it requires active learning techniques, such as demonstrations, practicing with children and receiving coaching and feedback, identifying and solving problems with enacting the practice, providing visual reminders, and engaging social support from peers and family members. Actual changes to parents' behavior can be evaluated using the HOME Inventory; effect sizes for better HOME scores in intervention groups tend to be higher whenever mental scores are high, thus confirming a strong relationship between changes to stimulation

Figure 13.4 Conditions That Put Children at Risk of Poor Mental Development, and Solutions Entailing Health Provider Support and Parental Behavior Changes

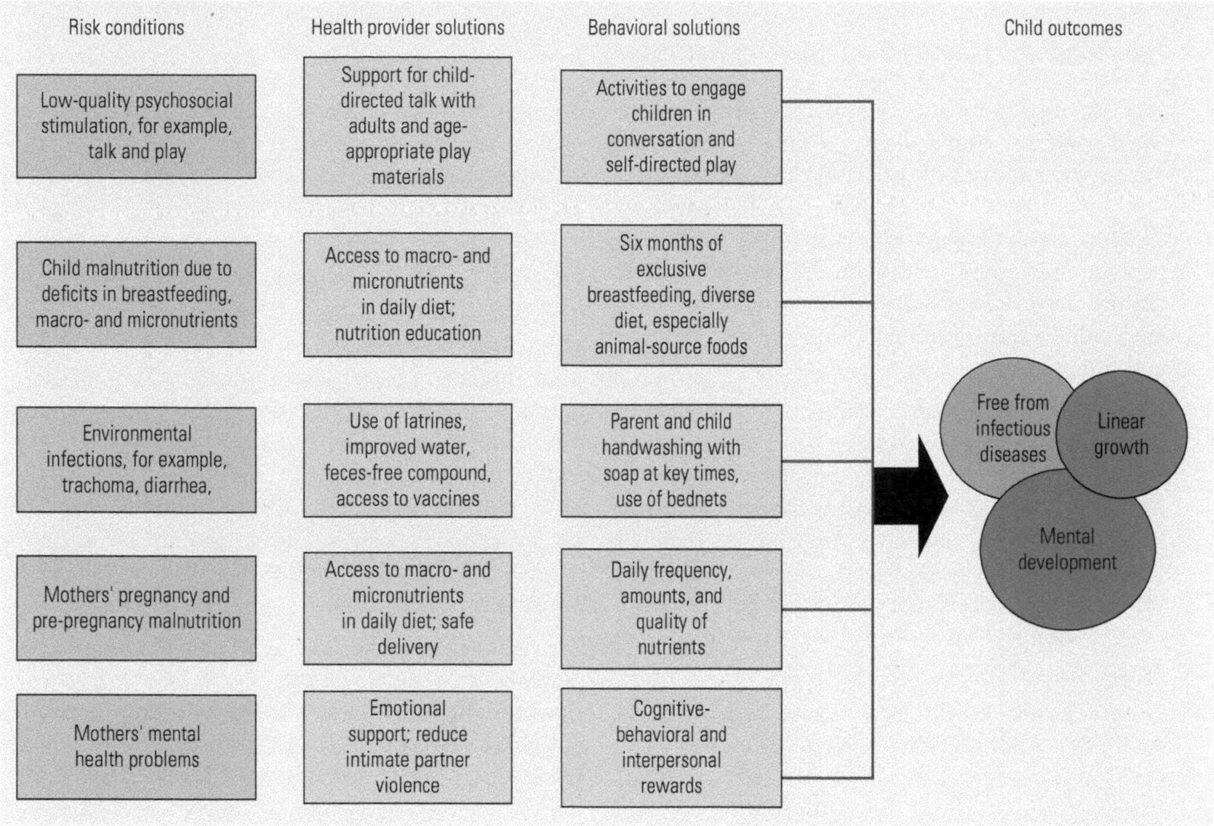

Source: Compilation based on sources cited in this chapter.

and mental development (figure 13.5). Typically changes are small, although significantly greater than changes in the control group. There are too few longitudinal studies yet to confirm that parents are able to sustain the new practices and adapt them as children age.

Overall, stimulation interventions, regardless of their delivery strategy, successfully improved mental development. This success may be partly attributed to the effect of the interventions on raising parental stimulation practices, which, in addition to linear growth, is one of the strongest correlates of mental development.

Child Nutrition

Exclusive breastfeeding from birth to six months is known to support healthy rates of growth and immunity. Correlational evidence argues that breastfed babies also have better mental development (Anderson, Johnson, and Remley 1999). This claim was affirmed by a trial in Belarus, in which half of the hospitals were randomly assigned to start the World Health Organization–supported Baby-Friendly Hospital Initiative activities sooner than others. Mothers who delivered in these hospitals breastfed longer, and their children had higher verbal intelligence at age six years (Kramer and others 2008).

One important nutrient in breast milk, fatty acids, has been studied in relation to mental development but mainly in HICs. Long-chain polyunsaturated fatty acids (PUFA), particularly n-3, that are present in the brain and breast milk are considered to be a promising candidate to support mental development. Multiple trials, conducted mainly in HICs where it is possible to provide infants with formula milk with varying amounts of fatty acids, found no effects on Bayley mental or motor scores (Beyerlein and others 2010; Qawasmi and others 2012; Smithers and others 2008). Similar tests of fatty acids found in fish and fish oil have shown no advantage to Bangladeshi children whose mothers received fish oil during pregnancy (Tofail and others 2006). However, research on fatty acids continues to follow children as

---

Box 13.1

Four Models of Stimulation Program Delivery

Four delivery formats for stimulation programs are most common: home visits, group sessions, clinic appointments, and one of these three piggybacked onto conditional cash transfer (CCT) programs. A fifth, combining group with home visits, has become increasingly common. All delivery models require a curriculum manual for providers. Those employing paraprofessionals require more training and supervision.

Home visits entail weekly or fortnightly visits by a paraprofessional to the children's homes. The home visitors engage in specific age-appropriate play activities with the children, demonstrate these activities to watching mothers, and leave play materials that will be replaced at the next session. Interventions based on home visits usually entailed more than 24 visits over 12 months (Lozoff and others 2010; Tofail and others 2013; Vazir and others 2013).

Group sessions consist of meetings with 8 to 20 mothers, and sometimes fathers, with their children at convenient locations in communities. Paraprofessionals from the community or local community health workers conduct the sessions. Group leaders demonstrate specific activities and coach mothers as they practice with their children. Groups could engage in discussions and general problem solving. Interventions using groups usually had fewer sessions than those using home visits (Aboud and Akhter 2011). Many interventions combined home visits with group sessions (Aboud and others 2013; Eickmann and others 2003; Yousafzai and others 2014). Informational and social needs

common to all parents are addressed during group sessions, and family-specific problems are addressed during home visits. These combined interventions usually had more than 15 contacts over 12 or 24 months.

The third model uses well- or sick-baby clinic visits to inquire about what mothers know about stimulating their children with toys and talk and counseling them on improved practices. This advice is usually provided by professionals, sometimes with two to four contacts (Jin and others 2007; Potterton and others 2010) and with at most 12 monthly contacts (Nair and others 2009). Group and clinic models explicitly aim to change parents' behavior, particularly the opportunities that parents provide for play and conversation.

The final model is the scale up of stimulation interventions using the infrastructure of a CCT program. One example is the home-visiting program attached to Colombia's Familias en Acción program. Mother Leaders from the community were trained to make weekly visits to the homes of children ages 12–24 months to provide guidance on play (Attanasio and others 2014). Another Colombian example is the home-based group care offered to CCT beneficiaries, whereby mothers were trained to provide stimulation weekdays to 15 children (most under age three years) in their homes (Bernal and Fernández 2013). Both large-scale effectiveness evaluations showed positive effects on the order of 0.2 to 0.3 standard deviation difference on children's cognitive and language abilities.

---

they age (Colombo and others 2013). Supplementation with a milk lipid, ganglioside, was found to have positive effects on early mental development in Indonesia (Gurnida and others 2012). Furthermore, research has found mental development benefits of fatty acids in colostrum; 14-month-old children whose mothers had high levels of n-3 PUFA in colostrum and who were breastfed with greater intensity or duration had higher mental development scores (Guxens and others 2011). Thus, the clear cognitive benefits to breastfeeding appear to stem from high levels of n-3 PUFA and cumulative amounts of ingested breast milk.

Research is being conducted on multiple micronutrients with and without lipids. Some studies use vitamin A as the baseline and compare it with five other micronutrients (Black and others 2004); others provide a porridge with carbohydrates and add micronutrients (Manno and others 2012; Rosado and others 2011). Pollitt and others (2000) gave all children eight micronutrients (vitamins and minerals) with high-energy milk added to the diet of intervention children only. The fortification in many cases was available for a period of six to eight months; the effects on mental development scores were small. A review of 21 interventions examining the effects of multiple micronutrients on mental development yielded a very small overall effect size of $d = 0.082$ (Larson and Yousafzai in press). In many cases, children showed benefits, such as reduced anemia, but no benefits in linear growth. Motor development improved in some cases. Currently multiple micronutrients are being combined with a lipid base that provides macronutrients to examine their combined effects on linear growth. This combination has the potential to enhance mental development in food-insecure sites.

Integrated Packages of Psychosocial Stimulation and Child Nutrition

Researchers and program implementers are paying closer attention to optimizing integrated packages of stimulation and nutrition care given the independent and potentially additive benefits to promoting mental development. Although most small- and large-scale interventions have found little added benefit to mental development from integrating nutrition with stimulation (Attanasio and others 2014; Grantham-McGregor and others 2014; Yousafzai and others 2014), other benefits of integration, such as cost and task-sharing, are being examined. This combination is illustrated in a completed stimulation and nutrition trial in Pakistan (box 13.2).

Reducing Infection Transmitted by Ground Contamination, Mosquitoes, and Flies

The most commonly implemented solutions to environmental causes of infection are constructing and using latrines, improving access to clean drinking water, promoting facewashing and handwashing with soap, cleaning up animal feces around the home, immunizing all infants with the rotavirus vaccine, and deworming children starting at age 12 months (Dangour and others 2013; Ejemot and others 2008; Fewtrell and others 2005). Places where piped water and sewerage systems are installed have experienced an immediate reduction in diarrheal diseases (Fewtrell and others 2005). However, widespread provision of water and sanitation infrastructure is unrealistic in the near future, especially in rural areas of LMICs. Although 68 percent of urban dwellers in LMICs have latrines, only 40 percent of rural people have them (UNICEF 2013). Improved sources of water are commonly provided at the community level or preferably at point of use, so that the urban-rural gap for improved water is narrower than that for sanitation (94 percent of urban dwellers have access to improved sources of water compared with 76 percent of rural dwellers). Concern about the effects of very high levels of arsenic in drinking water is supported by evidence of fetal loss and infant mortality

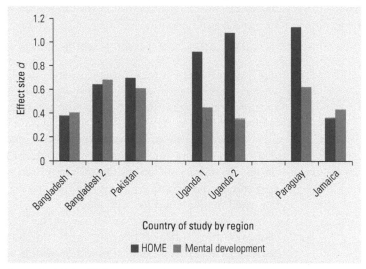

Figure 13.5 HOME Effect Size, Mental Development Effect Size, and Study

Sources: Bangladesh 1: HOME 0.38, Language Development 0.40 (Aboud and Akhter 2011); Bangladesh 2: HOME 0.64, Cognitive Development 0.67 (Aboud and others 2013); Pakistan: HOME 0.69, Cognitive Development 0.60 (Yousafzai and others 2014); Uganda 1: HOME 0.91, Language Development 0.44 (Boivin and others 2013); Uganda 2: HOME 1.07, Cognitive Development 0.35 (Singla, Kumbakumba, and Aboud 2015;) Paraguay: HOME 1.12, Mental Development 0.62 (Peairson and others 2008); Jamaica: HOME 0.36, Cognitive Development 0.42 (Walker and others 2004).
Note: HOME = Home Observation for Measurement of the Environment.

(Rahman, Vahter, and others 2007), but arsenic in water appears to have little effect on mental development in the first 24 months and up to age five years (Hamadani, Grantham-McGregor, and others 2010; Hamadani and others 2011).

Immunization with rotavirus vaccine as part of the national immunization schedule has begun in more than 35 countries, with support from the Global Alliance for Vaccines and Immunization. The rotavirus vaccine has been effective in reducing severe cases of diarrhea, mortality, and hospital and clinic visits, and it provides protection for several years. Mass treatment of children with deworming medication and azithromycin for trachoma can be attached to outreach services that deliver vitamin A drops. However, these are short-term solutions. The WHO's recommended SAFE (surgery, antibiotics, facial cleanliness, and environmental improvements) strategy for trachoma elimination also includes hygiene (facewashing) and environmental management (along with surgery and antibiotics) as the more sustainable approaches (Mecaskey and others 2003).

Environmental management of stagnant water is only one of the means by which to control malaria. Bednets, intermittent preventive treatment, and vaccines are the most studied preventive interventions (Cissé and others 2006; Gies and others 2009). The provision of free insecticide-treated bednets led to high coverage and protection (Alaii and others 2003); and three

Box 13.2

Pakistan Early Child Development Scale-Up Trial: Case Study of a Successful Program

The Pakistan Early Child Development Scale-Up Trial successfully enhanced the cognitive, language, and motor development of children whose parents received counseling in psychosocial stimulation for their children, with or without enhanced nutrition education and multiple micronutrient fortification (Yousafzai and others 2014). The program showed clear benefits from parenting practices that improved mother-child interactions and the quality of home stimulation. Lady Health Workers (LHWs), who every month deliver basic maternal and child health services to rural and remote households as part of the government health system, added counseling on psychosocial stimulation and nutrition to their activities for families with children under age two years.

Psychosocial Stimulation Intervention

The psychosocial stimulation intervention, using the Care for Child Development messages and materials developed by the United Nations Children's Fund (UNICEF) and the World Health Organization, encouraged mother-child play and communication activities (UNICEF and WHO 2009). The LHWs provided information about recommended practices and benefits, suggested developmentally appropriate activities for caregivers to try with their young children, and coached caregivers by providing prompts and encouragement to respond to children's efforts and communication. The goal of the intervention was to enhance the quality of caregiver-child interactions and promote children's cognitive, language, motor, and social-emotional skills.

The intervention was delivered through a combination of home visits and group sessions. The group sessions offered opportunities for problem solving and social support through encouragement, praise, and peer-to-peer learning.

Nutrition Intervention

The nutrition intervention was designed to enrich the existing basic nutrition education curriculum in the LHW program delivered through home visits. This goal was achieved by the addition of responsive feeding messages and the distribution of a multiple micronutrient powder for young children ages 6–24 months. The LHWs were trained to move away from a traditional didactic approach to a counseling strategy for delivering nutrition education. During the home visits, the LHWs provided information about recommended practices and benefits, engaged in problem solving, and provided encouragement.

Critical to the success of the program was the use of supportive supervision, on-the-job coaching, and mentorship for LHWs. It was important for them to integrate the new practices with existing health messages without burdening mothers. Group delivery strategies combined with home visits permitted the LHWs to reach a greater proportion of the community, and the demand for community-based services increased. The cost of integrating the interventions into the existing LHW services was US$4 per month per child.

Source: Gowani and others 2014; Yousafzai and others 2014.

intermittent doses of an antimalarial medication at the time of routine immunization reduced the incidence of malaria by 20 percent (Macete and others 2006). Neither hemoglobin levels nor future immunity were compromised with these preventive antimalarial measures. Psychosocial stimulation interventions appear to be effective at overcoming some of the deficits caused by cerebral malaria.

Latrine use and handwashing habits are very difficult to change. Interventions to increase latrine use and handwashing have met with success mainly in controlled experimental settings (Briscoe and Aboud 2012); they have been less successful when implemented at the community level (Huda and others 2012; Hutton and Chase, forthcoming; Luby and others 2008).

Development-Sensitive Interventions

Maternal Nutrition

Strategies to address the growing number of premature births (Lawn and others 2014) have not yet been identified. High stress during pregnancy is a correlate among African-American women, many of whom deliver preterm-LBW babies (Lobel and others 2008). SGA is thought to be associated with maternal infection (malaria) and malnutrition (Black and others 2013), and preventable through intermittent preventive antimalarial treatment (Gies and others 2009) and maternal nutrition, respectively.

Raising birth weights by providing supplements to pregnant women has received mixed reviews. Iron and folic acid supplementation are clearly beneficial, the latter in reducing neural tube defects that result in mental development impairments. Reviews of studies providing micronutrient supplements, energy-protein supplements, or both found small reductions in the number of SGA newborns (Haider and Bhutta 2012; Imdad, Yakoob, and Bhutta 2011). However, a large study in Bangladesh examined the effects of a daily energy-protein supplement starting either in the first trimester or later in the second trimester, and the effects of an additional 13 micronutrients, compared with the usual iron and folic acid (Persson and others 2012). Gestational age with a mean of 39 weeks was similar across groups, indicating that prematurity was not affected. Birth length and birth weight were not affected, with 31 percent LBW. Infant mortality was lowest among children whose mothers received multiple micronutrients and started energy-protein supplements early. A follow-up on the children from this study, using two items from the Bayley Scale at age seven months, found minimal differences on one item benefiting only those with low BMI mothers who received early energy-protein supplements (Tofail and others 2008). The nonsignificant findings of this study are supported by a preliminary meta-analysis of 10 randomized controlled trials (RCTs) in which pregnant women were given micronutrient or other fortified foods and their children tested before age 24 months. The overall mental development effect size was $d = 0.042$ (Larson and Yousafzai in press). Many scientists conclude that providing nutrition supplements during pregnancy is too late to significantly benefit birth outcomes and mental development, and that maternal nutritional status at conception is critical. More attention needs to be given to nutrition among children and adolescent girls.

Iodine is so important for reproductive and mental development that governments legislate the fortification of salt for general use. Interventions designed to study the effects of iodine on mental development in iodine-deficient areas typically randomize pregnant women to receive capsules that provide sufficient iodine for one year. Ten existing interventions, two of which were RCTs, found a moderate effect size for mental development of $d = 0.50$ (Bougma and others 2013).

Iodine provided during pregnancy was more beneficial than iodine supplementation given to children after birth. Another strategy is to provide the lactating mother with iodine supplements; this indirect supplementation maintained healthy urine and serum levels in the infant better than direct supplementation of the infant (Bouhouch and others 2014). An important test is whether iodine delivered through salt in the diets of mothers and children improves the mental development of children. Careful scrutiny of RCTs in which school-age children were given an iodine capsule or a placebo reveals that the large majority of verbal and nonverbal tests yielded no positive outcomes (Huda, Grantham-McGregor, and Tomkins 2001; van den Briel and others 2000). However, iodized salt had a consistently small but positive effect on the mental development scores of children under age 24 months in Ethiopia (Bougma and others 2014). In short, iodine will have maximum effect on children's mental development if available to women during pregnancy and lactation.

Maternal Mental Health

Integrated packages supporting mothers and children are receiving increasing attention (Tomlinson and others 2014). The postnatal period up to 24 months after birth might be a suitable time to address maternal depression along with child feeding and stimulation practices. This broader focus might benefit children's development and can be provided in a context that does not stigmatize mothers. The available handful of evaluated interventions suggests that alleviating maternal depression may help mothers better meet their children's needs. In Pakistan, the Thinking Healthy program was developed using principles of cognitive-behavioral therapy, although it also includes elements of interpersonal therapy. Cognitive-behavioral and interpersonal therapies are the two therapies for which there is sound evidence in North America and Europe; it is valuable to know that their principles can be adapted for use in LMICs. In Pakistan, community health workers were trained in a structured form of dialogue that covered empathic listening, family engagement, guided discovery using pictures, behavioral activation, and problem solving.

The integration of the Thinking Healthy program in a community-based maternal and child health service resulted in significant reduction of maternal depression in Pakistan. Additional positive benefits in the intervention group were lower rates of infant and young child diarrheal illness, higher rates of young child immunization, higher reported use of contraceptives among women, and increased parental time spent playing with their young children (Rahman and others 2008). It is reasonable that countries with a high prevalence of maternal depression should implement preventive programs for all women by combining risk-reducing skills for depression with child stimulation and nutrition skills. In Uganda, a combined 12-session group program to address maternal depression, child stimulation, and nutrition was effective in preventing depressive symptoms and enhancing children's cognitive and language development (Singla, Kumbakumba, and Aboud 2015).

COST-BENEFIT OF EARLY CHILDHOOD INTERVENTIONS

Recognition of the beneficial societal returns of investing in early childhood is increasing (Kilburn and Karoly 2008). Many of the interventions discussed in this chapter are cost-effective and cost information is available (further detail can be found in chapter 17 in this volume, Horton and Levin 2016). This section focuses on literature not covered elsewhere specific to psychosocial stimulation and maternal depression. Generally, cost analyses are more readily available on the benefits of preschool programs for children ages three years and older (Engle and others 2011); less information is available on the costs of early stimulation interventions for children younger than age two years. There may be several reasons for the meager available data on costs for early stimualtion interventions; for example, Alderman and others (2014) highlight the many challenges in calculating cost-benefits of health and nutrition services with integrated early stimulation, including synergies between the fixed costs (existing costs linked to service delivery) and the additional costs of implementing the new intervention. A recent attempt at a cost and cost-effectiveness analysis points to the challenges that contribute to this lack of data on LMICs (Batura and others 2015). One challenge is that the follow-up is short, and outcomes do not focus on productivity.

One short-term cost-effectiveness analysis compared the costs and benefits of a nutrition education-plus-supplement package with one that counseled psychosocial stimulation (Gowani and others 2014). The former provided micronutrient fortification whereas the latter provided some play and book materials, costing approximately US$4.50 per child per month (approximately US$55[1] per year) using group and home visits. More psychosocial stimulation intervention studies need to conduct cost analyses, as do programs that combine nutrition and hygiene with stimulation and maternal mental health. One cost-benefit study analyzing labor market returns for

a Jamaica cohort studied by Grantham-McGregor and others (1991) finds that adults age 22 years who received early psychosocial stimulation earned 25 percent more than control counterparts (Gertler and others 2014).

Cash transfer or CCT programs that target the most economically disadvantaged families provide a delivery platform that shows promising returns to investment in short- and medium-term outcomes. The two Colombian studies described in this chapter (box 13.1) showing benefits to children who received home visits or home-based group care under three years of age estimated a cost per child of US$516 per year (Attanasio and others 2014) and US$347 per 16 months (Bernal and Fernandez 2013). Evaluations of large-scale and long-running programs in Ecuador (Fernald and Hidrobo 2011; Paxson and Schady 2010), Mexico (Fernald, Gertler, and Neufeld 2008), and Nicaragua (Macours, Schady, and Vakis 2012) have demonstrated benefits to child outcomes in the preschool years. Cash transfers of US$70 monthly, for example, are linked to conditions such as attending health clinics, providing good nutrition, and school enrollment (Fernald, Gertler, and Neufeld 2008). Evaluations of CCT programs show that benefits are greater for the poorest children. Two pathways have been proposed to explain how CCT programs result in benefits to children's development. First, families might invest more in better nutrition for young children and in learning and play materials. For example, mothers who received a cash transfer (nonconditional) in Ecuador were more likely to purchase a toy for their young children (Fernald and Hidrobo 2011). Second, reduced financial pressure and stress may lead to improved psychosocial well-being in the family, leading to improved early child care. These models are primarily from Latin America and the Caribbean, but hold promise for other regions.

CONCLUSIONS

The risk factors of greatest importance concern low-quality psychosocial stimulation at home; inadequate child nutrition; infections from environmental vectors, such as trachoma and malaria; and maternal nutrition and mental health during the first 1,000 days.

- **Psychosocial stimulation**. Programs to promote mental development through stimulation are very effective, especially if they use techniques of active learning to help parents and community paraprofessionals adopt the recommended practices.
- **Child nutrition**. The effects of macro- and micronutrients on development are increasingly clear as the

pathways through health, behavior, and brain development have been clarified.

- **Infectious illnesses.** Significant advances have been made in vaccines, preventive medications, and treatment; access remains a major obstacle. Further research is required to understand how repeated infections, particularly diarrheal illness, affect child nutrition and development outcomes.
- **Maternal nutrition.** Nutrients available to children from the pregnant and lactating mother are being examined. These include iodine, iron, and PUFA.
- **Maternal mental health.** Given the high levels of depressive symptoms among mothers of young children beyond the postnatal period, mental health can no longer be neglected in health and development services. Effective strategies are likely to benefit all mothers with young children in these settings.

Recommendations for future directions include the following:

- Government, community-based, and private organizations can adopt and adapt successful context-specific programs that address four or five critical practices related to stimulation, nutrition, hygiene, and maternal care. Evaluations of outcomes, acceptability, costs, and task-sharing among personnel can clarify whether there are benefits to integrating services.
- Program planners and implementers can adopt a social-ecological approach that improves access to food, a clean environment, and availability of play materials, as well as promotes parent practices that support child development.
- Programs can incorporate a multimode communication strategy of supportive practices so they are seen as normative and approved by respected authorities. The communication modes could include community groups, home visits, clinic visits, and mass media.
- Policy makers and partners can implement cost-effectiveness analyses in LMICs.
- Researchers and other stakeholders can develop and provide advocacy materials for effective programs and disseminate them to government officials, policy makers, health and education professionals, media, and civil society organizations.

NOTE

World Bank Income Classifications as of July 2014 are as follows, based on estimates of gross national income (GNI) per capita for 2013:

- Low-income countries (LICs) = US$1,045 or less

- Middle-income countries (MICs) are subdivided:
  a) lower-middle-income = US$1,046 to US$4,125
  b) upper-middle-income (UMICs) = US$4,126 to US $12,745
- High-income countries (HICs) = US$12,746 or more.

1. For comparability across chapters, we present economic data in U.S. dollars, adjusted to 2012.

REFERENCES

Aboud, F. E. 2007. "Evaluation of an Early Childhood Parenting Program in Rural Bangladesh." *Journal of Health, Population and Nutrition* 25: 3–13.

Aboud, F. E., and S. Akhter. 2011. "A Cluster Randomized Evaluation of a Responsive Stimulation and Feeding Intervention in Bangladesh." *Pediatrics* 127: e1191–97.

Aboud, F. E., D. R. Singla, M. I. Nahil, and I. Borisova. 2013. "Effectiveness of a Parenting Program in Bangladesh to Address Early Childhood Health, Growth and Development." *Social Science and Medicine* 97: 250–58.

Aboud, F. E., and A. K. Yousafzai. 2015. "Global Health and Development in Early Childhood." *Annual Review of Psychology* 66: 433–57.

Abraham, N., R. Jewkes, R. Laubscher, and M. Hoffman. 2006. "Intimate Partner Violence: Prevalence and Risk Factors for Men in Cape Town, South Africa." *Violence and Victims* 21 (2): 247–64.

Alaii, J. A., H. W. van den Borne, S. P. Kachur, H. Mwenesi, J. M. Vulule, and others. 2003. "Perceptions of Bed Nets and Malaria Prevention before and after a Randomized Controlled Trial of Permethrin-Treated Bed Nets in Western Kenya." *American Journal of Tropical Medicine and Hygiene* 68: 142–48.

Alderman, H., J. R. Behrman, S. Grantham-McGregor, F. Lopez-Boo, and S. Urzuas. 2014. "Economic Perspectives on Integrating Early Child Stimulation with Nutritional Interventions." *Annals of the New York Academy of Sciences* 1308: 129–38.

Anderson, J. W., B. M. Johnson, and D. T. Remley. 1999. "Breast-Feeding and Cognitive Development: A Meta-Analysis." *American Journal of Clinical Nutrition* 70 (4): 525–35.

Armah, G. E., S. O. Sow, R. F. Breiman, M. J. Dallas, M. D. Tapia, and others. 2010. "Efficacy of Pentavalent Rotavirus Vaccine against Severe Rotavirus Gastroenteritis in Infants in Developing Countries in Sub-Saharan Africa: A Randomised, Double-Blind, Placebo-Controlled Trial." *The Lancet* 376: 606–14.

Attanasio, O. P., E. O. A. Fitzsimons, S. M. Grantham-McGregor, C. M. Douglas, and M. Rubo-Codina. 2014. "Using the Infrastructure of a Conditional Cash Transfer Program in Colombia: Cluster Randomized Controlled Trial." *British Medical Journal* 349: g5785.

Bangirana, P., R. Idro, C. C. John, and M. J. Boivin. 2006. "Rehabilitation for Cognitive Impairments after Cerebral Malaria in African Children: Strategies and Limitations." *Tropical Medicine and International Health* 11 (9): 1341–49.

Batura, N., Z. Hill, H. Haghparast-Bidgoli, R. Lingam, T. Colburn, and others. 2015. "Highlighting the Evidence Gap: How Cost Effective Are Interventions to Improve Early Childhood Nutrition and Development?" *Health Policy and Planning* 30 (6): 813–21. doi:10.1093/heapol/czu055.

Bayley, N. 2006. *Bayley Scales of Infant Development Manual.* 3rd ed. Antonio, TX: The Psychological Corporation.

Beard, J. L., M. K. Hendricks, E. M. Perez, L. E. Murray-Kolb, A. Berg, and others. 2005. "Maternal Iron Deficiency Anemia Affects Postpartum Emotions and Cognition." *Journal of Nutrition* 135: 265–72.

Bernal, R., and C. Fernández. 2013. "Subsidized Child Care and Child Development in Colombia: Effects of *Hogares Comunitarios de Bienestar* as a Function of Timing and Length of Exposure." *Social Science and Medicine* 97: 241–49.

Beyerlein, A., M. Hadders-Algra, K. Kennedy, M. Fewtrell, A. Singhal, and others. 2010. "Infant Formula Supplementation with Long-Chain Polyunsaturated Fatty Acids Has No Effect on Bayley Developmental Scores at 18 Months of Age—IPD Meta-Analysis of 4 Large Clinical Trials." *Journal of Pediatric Gastroenterology and Nutrition* 50 (1): 79–84.

Bhutta, Z. A., J. K. Das, A. Rizvi, M. F. Gaffey, N. Walker, and others. 2013. "Evidence-Based Interventions for Improvement of Maternal and Child Nutrition: What Can Be Done and at What Cost?" *The Lancet* 382 (9890): 452–77.

Black, M. M., A. H. Baqui, K. Zaman, S. W. McNary, K. Le, and others. 2007. "Depressive Symptoms among Rural Bangladeshi Mothers: Implications for Infant Development." *Journal of Child Psychology and Psychiatry* 48 (8): 764–72.

Black, M. M., A. H. Baqui, K. Zaman, L. A. Persson, S. El Arifeen, and others. 2004. "Iron and Zinc Supplementation Promote Motor Development and Exploratory Behavior among Bangladeshi Infants." *American Journal of Clinical Nutrition* 80 (4): 903–10.

Black, R. E., C. G. Victora, S. P. Walker, Z. A. Bhutta, P. Christian, and others. 2013. "Maternal and Child Undernutrition and Overweight in Low-Income and Middle-Income Countries." *The Lancet* 382 (9890): 427–51.

Blencowe, H., A. C. C. Lee, S. Cousens, A. Bahalim, R. Narwal, and others. 2013. "Preterm Birth-Associated Neurodevelopmental Impairment Estimates at Regional and Global Levels for 2010." *Pediatric Research* 74 (Suppl. 1): 17–34.

Boivin, M. J., P. Bangirana, J. Byarugaba, R. O. Opoka, R. Idro, and others. 2007. "Cognitive Impairment after Cerebral Malaria in Children: A Prospective Study." *Pediatrics* 119 (2): e360–66.

Boivin, M. J., P. Bangirana, N. Nakasujja, C. F. Page, C. Shohet, and others. 2013. "A Year-Long Caregiver Training Program to Improve Neurocognition in Preschool Ugandan HIV-Exposed Children." *Journal of Developmental and Behavioral Pediatrics* 34 (4): 269–78.

Bornstein, M. H., and D. L. Putnick. 2012. "Cognitive and Socioemotional Caregiving in Developing Countries." *Child Development* 83 (1): 46–61.

Bougma, K., F. E. Aboud, K. B. Harding, and G. S. Marquis. 2013. "Iodine and Mental Development of Children 5 Years Old and Under: A Systematic Review and Meta-Analysis." *Nutrients* 5 (4): 1384–416.

Bougma, K., G. S. Marquis, F. E. Aboud, H. Mohammed, D. Singla, and others. 2014. "Iodine and Other Nutritional Predictors of Infant and Preschoolers' Development: Results from a Cluster Randomized Trial in Ethiopia." Micronutrient Forum Conference, Addis Ababa, June 5.

Bouhouch, R. R., S. Bouhouch, M. Cherkaoui, A. Aboussad, S. Stinca, and others. 2014. "Direct Iodine Supplementation of Infants versus Supplementation of their Breastfeeding Mothers: A Double-Blind, Randomized, Placebo-Controlled Trial." *The Lancet Diabetes and Endocrinology* 2: 197–209.

Boyle, M. H., Y. Racine, K. Georgiades, D. Snelling, S. Hong, and others. 2006. "The Influence of Economic Development Level, Household Wealth and Maternal Education on Child Health in the Developing World." *Social Science and Medicine* 63 (8): 2242–54.

Bradley, R. H., and R. F. Corwyn. 2005. "Caring for Children around the World: A View from HOME." *International Journal of Behavioral Development* 29 (6): 468–78.

Brazelton, T. B., and J. K. Nugent. 1995. *Neonatal Behavioral Assessment Scale.* 3rd ed. London: McKeith Press.

Briscoe, C., and F. E. Aboud. 2012. "Behaviour Change Communication Targeting Four Health Behaviours in Developing Countries: A Review of Change Techniques." *Social Science and Medicine* 75 (4): 612–21.

Brown, J. L., and E. Pollitt. 1996. "Malnutrition, Poverty and Intellectual Development." *Scientific American* 274 (2): 38–43.

Chandran, M., P. Tharyan, J. Muliyil, and S. Abraham. 2002. "Post-Partum Depression in a Cohort of Women from a Rural Area of Tamil Nadu, India: Incidence and Risk Factors." *British Journal of Psychiatry* 181: 499–504.

Checkley, W., G. Buckley, R. H. Gilman, A. M. O. Assis, R. L. Guerrant, and others. 2008. "Multi-Country Analysis of the Effects of Diarrhoea on Childhood Stunting." *International Journal of Epidemiology* 37 (4): 816–30.

Christian, P., S. E. Lee, M. D. Angel, L. S. Adair, S. E. Aifeen, and others. 2013. "Risk of Childhood Undernutrition Related to Small-for-Gestational Age and Preterm Birth in Low- and Middle-Income Countries." *International Journal of Epidemiology* 42 (5): 1340–55.

Cissé, B., C. Sokhna, D. Boulanger, J. Milet, E. H. Bâ, and others. 2006. "Seasonal Intermittent Preventive Treatment with Artesunate and Sulfadoxine-Pyrimethamine for Prevention of Malaria in Senegalese Children: A Randomised, Placebo-Controlled, Double-Blind Trial." *The Lancet* 367 (9511): 659–67.

Cleland, J., and J. K. van Ginneken. 1988. "Maternal Education and Child Survival in Developing Countries: The Search for Pathways of Influence." *Social Science and Medicine* 27 (12): 1357–68.

Colombo, J., S. E. Carlson, C. L. Cheatham, D. L. Shaddy, E. H. Kerling, and others. 2013. "Long-Term Effects of LCPUFA Supplementation on Childhood Cognitive Outcomes." *American Journal of Clinical Nutrition* 98 (2): 403–12.

Cooper, P. J., M. Tomlinson, L. Swartz, M. Landman, C. Molteno, and others. 2009. "Improving Quality of Mother-Infant Relationship and Infant Attachment in Socioeconomically Deprived Community in South Africa: Randomised Controlled Trial." *British Medical Journal* 338: b974.

Daelmans, B., K. Dewey, and M. Arimond. 2009. "New and Updated Indicators for Assessing Infant and Young Child Feeding." *Food and Nutrition Bulletin* 30 (2): S256–62.

Dangour, A. D., L. Watson, O. Cumming, S. Boisson, Y. Che, and others. 2013. "Interventions to Improve Water Quality and Supply, Sanitation and Hygiene Practices, and Their Effects on the Nutritional Status of Children." *Cochrane Database of Systematic Reviews* 8: CD009382. doi:10.1002/14651858.

Das, J. K., R. A. Salam, A. Imdad, and Z. A. Bhutta. 2016. "Infant and Young Child Growth." In *Disease Control Priorities* (third edition): Volume 2, *Reproductive, Maternal, Newborn, and Child Health*, edited by R. Black, R. Laxminarayan, M. Temmerman, and N. Walker. Washington, DC: World Bank.

Dewey, K., and S. Adu-Afarwuah. 2008. "Systematic Review of the Efficacy and Effectiveness of Complementary Feeding Interventions in Developing Countries." *Maternal and Child Nutrition* 4 (Suppl. 1): 24–85.

Eickmann, S. H., A. Lima, M. Guerra, M. Lima, P. Lira, and others. 2003. "Improved Cognitive and Motor Development in a Community-Based Intervention of Psychosocial Stimulation in Northeast Brazil." *Developmental Medicine and Child Neurology* 45 (8): 536–41.

Ejemot, R., J. Ehiri, M. Meremikwu, and J. Critchley. 2008. "Hand Washing for Preventing Diarrhoea." *Cochrane Database Systematic Review* (1): CD004265.

Engle, P. L., C. H. Fernald, J. R. Behrman, C. O'Gara, A. K. Yousafzai, and others. 2011. "Strategies for Reducing Inequalities and Improving Developmental Outcomes for Young Children in Low-Income and Middle-Income Countries." *The Lancet* 378 (9799): 1339–53.

Faisal-Cury, A., J. J. A. Tedesco, S. Kahhale, P. R. Menezes, and M. Zugaib. 2003. "Postpartum Depression: In Relation to Life Events and Patterns of Coping." *Archives of Women Mental Health* 7: 123–31.

Fernald, L. C. H., P. J. Gertler, and L. M. Neufeld. 2008. "Role of Cash in Conditional Cash Transfer Programmes for Child Health, Growth, and Development: An Analysis of Mexico's Oportunidades." *The Lancet* 371 (9615): 828–37.

Fernald, L. C. H., and M. Hidrobo. 2011. "Effect of Ecuador's Cash Transfer Program (*Bono de Desarrollo Humano*) on Child Development in Infants and Toddlers: A Randomized Effectiveness Trial." *Social Science and Medicine* 72 (9): 1437–46.

Fewtrell, L., R. B. Kaufmann, D. Kay, W. Enanoria, L. Haller, and others. 2005. "Water, Sanitation, and Hygiene Interventions to Reduce Diarrhoea in Less Developed Countries: A Systematic Review and Meta-Analysis." *The Lancet Infectious Diseases* 5 (1): 42–52.

Filippi, V., D. Chou, C. Ronsmans, W. Graham, and L. Say. 2016. "Levels and Causes of Maternal Morbidity and Mortality." In *Disease Control Priorities* (third Edition): Volume 2, *Reproductive, Maternal, Newborn, and Child Health*, edited by R. Black, R. Laxminarayan, M. Temmerman, and N. Walker. Washington, DC: World Bank.

Fischer Walker, C. L., L. Lamberti, L. Adair, R. L. Guerrant, A. G. Lescano, and others. 2012. "Does Childhood Diarrhea Influence Cognition beyond the Diarrhea-Stunting Pathway?" *PLoS One* 7 (10): e47908.

Fisher, J., M. Cabral de Mello, V. Patel, A. Rahman, T. Tran, and others. 2012. "Prevalence and Determinants of Common Perinatal Mental Disorders in Women in Low- and Lower-Middle-Income Countries: A Systematic Review." *Bulletin of the World Health Organization* 90 (2): 139–49G.

Gertler, P., J. Heckman, R. Pinto, A. Zanolini, C. Vermeersch, and others. 2014. "Labour Market Returns to an Early Childhood Stimulation Intervention in Jamaica." *Science* 344: 998–1001.

Gies, S., S. O. Coulibaly, C. Ky, F. T. Ouattara, B. J. Brabin, and others. 2009. "Community-Based Promotional Campaign to Improve Uptake of Intermittent Preventive Antimalarial Treatment in Pregnancy in Burkina Faso." *American Journal of Tropical Medicine and Hygiene* 80 (3): 460–69.

Gottlieb, C. A., M. J. Maenner, C. Cappa, and M. S. Durkin. 2009. "Child Disability Screening, Nutrition, and Early Learning in 18 Countries with Low and Middle Incomes: Data from the Third Round of UNICEF's Multiple Indicator Cluster Survey (2005–06)." *The Lancet* 374 (9704): 1831–39.

Gowani, S., A. K. Yousafzai, R. Armstrong, and Z. A. Bhutta. 2014. "Cost Effectiveness of Responsive Stimulation and Nutrition Interventions on Early Child Development Outcomes in Pakistan." *Annals of the New York Academy of Sciences* 1308: 149–61.

Grantham-McGregor, S. M., Y. Cheung, S. Cueto, P. Glewwe, L. Richter, and others. 2007. "Developmental Potential in the First 5 Years for Children in Developing Countries." *The Lancet* 369 (9555): 60–70.

Grantham-McGregor, S. M., L. C. H. Fernald, R. M. C. Kagawa, and S. Walker. 2014. "Effects of Integrated Child Development and Nutrition Interventions on Child Development and Nutritional Status." *Annals of the New York Academy of Sciences* 1308: 1–22.

Grantham-McGregor, S. M., C. A. Powell, S. P. Walker, and J. H. Himes. 1991. "Nutritional Supplementation, Psychosocial Stimulation, and Mental Development of Stunted Children: The Jamaican Study." *The Lancet* 338 (8758): 1–5.

Griffiths, R., and M. Huntley. 1996. *GMDS 0-2. Griffiths Mental Development Scales–Revised: Birth to 2 Years.* Oxford: Hogrefe.

Gurnida, D. A., A. M. Rowan, P. Idradinata, D. Muchtadi, and N. Sekarwa. 2012. "Association of Complex Lipids Containing Gangliosides with Cognitive Development of 6-Month-Old Infants." *Early Human Development* 88 (8): 595–601.

Guxens, M., M. A. Mendez, C. Molto-Puigmarti, J. Julvez, R. Garcia-Esteban, and others. 2011. "Breastfeeding, Long-Chain Polyunsaturated Fatty Acids in Colostrum, and Infant Mental Development." *Pediatrics* 128 (4): e880.

Haider, B. A., and Z. A. Bhutta. 2012. "Multiple-Micronutrient Supplementation for Women during Pregnancy." *Cochrane Database of Systematic Reviews* 11: CD004905. doi:0.1002/14651858.CD004905.pub3.

Hamadani, J. D., S. M. Grantham-McGregor, F. Tofail, B. Nermell, B. Fangstrom, and others. 2010. "Pre- and Postnatal Arsenic Exposure and Child Development at 18 Months of Age: A Cohort Study in Rural Bangladesh." *International Journal of Epidemiology* 39 (5): 1206–16.

Hamadani, J. D., F. Tofail, T. Cole, and S. Grantham-McGregor. 2013. "The Relation between Age of Attainment of Motor Milestones and Future Cognitive and Motor Development in Bangladeshi Children." *Maternal and Child Nutrition* 9 (Suppl. 1): 89–104.

Hamadani, J. D., F. Tofail, A. Hilaly, S. N. Huda, P. Engle, and others. 2010. "Use of Family Care Indicators and Their Relationship with Child Development in Bangladesh." *Journal of Health, Population and Nutrition* 28 (1): 23–33.

Hamadani, J. D., F. Tofail, A. Hilaly, F. Mehrin, S. Shiraji, and others. 2012. "Association of Postpartum Maternal Morbidities with Children's Mental, Psychomotor and Language Development in Rural Bangladesh." *Journal of Health, Population, and Nutrition* 30 (2): 193–204.

Hamadani, J. D., F. Tofail, B. Nermell, R. Gardner, S. Shiraji, and others. 2011. "Critical Windows of Exposure for Arsenic-Associated Impairment of Cognitive Function in Pre-School Girls and Boys: A Population-Based Cohort Study." *International Journal of Epidemiology* 40 (6): 1593–604.

Harpham, T., S. Huttly, M. J. De Silva, and T. Abramsky. 2005. "Maternal Mental Health and Child Nutritional Status in Four Developing Countries." *Journal of Epidemiology and Community Health* 59: 1060–64.

Horton, S., and C. Levin. 2016. "Cost-Effectiveness of Interventions for Reproductive, Maternal, Neonatal, and Child Health." In *Disease Control Priorities* (third edition): Volume 2, *Reproductive, Maternal, Newborn, and Child Health*, edited by R. Black, R. Laxminarayan, M. Temmerman, and N. Walker. Washington, DC: World Bank.

Huda, S. N., S. M. Grantham-McGregor, and A. Tomkins. 2001. "Cognitive and Motor Functions of Iodine-Deficient but Euthyroid Children in Bangladesh Do Not Benefit from Iodized Poppy Seed Oil." *Journal of Nutrition* 131 (1): 72–77.

Huda, T. M. N., L. Unicomb, R. B. Johnston, A. K. Halder, M. A. Y. Sharker, and others. 2012. "Interim Evaluation of a Large Scale Sanitation, Hygiene and Water Improvement Programme on Childhood Diarrhea and Respiratory Disease in Rural Bangladesh." *Social Science and Medicine* 75 (4): 604–11.

Humphrey, J. H. 2009. "Child Undernutrition, Tropical Enteropathy, Toilets, and Handwashing." *The Lancet* 374: 1032–35.

Hutton, G., and C. Chase. Forthcoming. "Water and Sanitation." In *Disease Control Priorities* (third edition): Volume 7, *Injury Prevention and Environmental Health*, edited by C. N. Mock, R. Nugent, and O. Kobusingye. Washington, DC: World Bank.

Iannotti, L. L., C. K. Lutter, D. A. Bunn, and C. P. Stewart. 2014. "Eggs: The Uncracked Potential for Improving Maternal and Young Child Nutrition among the World's Poor." *Nutrition Reviews* 72 (6): 355–68.

Imdad, A., M. Y. Yakoob, and Z. A. Bhutta. 2011. "Impact of Maternal Education about Complementary Feeding and Provision of Complementary Foods on Child Growth in Developing Countries." *BMC Public Health* 11 (Suppl. 3): S25.

Isabella, R. A. 1993. "Origins of Attachment: Maternal Interactive Behavior across the First Year." *Child Development* 64 (2): 605–21.

Jiang, N. M., F. Tofail, S. N. Moonah, R. J. Scharf, M. Taniuchi, and others. 2014. "Febrile Illness and Pro-Inflammatory Cytokines Are Associated with Lower Neurodevelopmental Scores in Bangladeshi Infants Living in Poverty." *BMC Pediatrics* 14: 50.

Jin, X., Y. Su, F. Jiang, J. Ma, C. Morgan, and X. Shen. 2007. "'Care for Development' Intervention in Rural China: A Prospective Follow-Up Study." *Journal of Developmental and Behavioral Pediatrics* 28 (3): 213–18.

John, C. C., P. Bangirana, J. Byarugaba, R. O. Opoka, R. Idro, and others. 2008. "Cerebral Malaria in Children Is Associated with Long-Term Cognitive Impairment." *Pediatrics* 122 (1): e92–99.

Jones, A. D., B. I. Scott, L. E. Smith, M. M. N. Mbuya, B. Chasekwa, and others. 2014. "World Health Organization Infant and Young Child Feeding Indicators and their Associations with Child Anthropometry: A Synthesis of Recent Findings." *Maternal and Child Nutrition* 10 (1): 1–17.

Kariger, P., E. A. Frongillo, P. Engle, P. M. Rebello Britto, S. M. Sywulka, and others. 2012. "Indicators of Family Care for Development for Use in Multicountry Surveys." *Journal of Health, Population and Nutrition* 30 (4): 472–86.

Keusch, G. T., C. Fischer Walker, J. K. Das, S. Horton, and D. Habte. 2016. "Diarrheal Diseases." In *Disease Control Priorities* (third edition): Volume 2, *Reproductive, Maternal, Newborn, and Child Health*, edited by R. Black, R. Laxminarayan, M. Temmerman, and N. Walker. Washington, DC: World Bank.

Khan, N. Z., H. Muslima, M. Parveen, M. Bhattcharya, N. Begun, and others. 2009. "Neurodevelopmental Outcomes of Preterm Infants in Bangladesh." *Pediatrics* 118 (1): 280–89.

Kilburn, R. M., and L. A. Karoly. 2008. *The Economics of Early Childhood Policy: What the Dismal Science Has to Say about Investing in Children*. Santa Monica, CA: RAND Cooperation.

Kooistra, L., S. Crawford, A. L. van Baar, E. O. Brouwers, and V. J. Pop. 2006. "Neonatal Effects of Maternal Hypothyroxinemia during Early Pregnancy." *Pediatrics* 117 (1): 161–67.

Kosek, M., C. Bern, and R. L. Guerrant. 2003. "The Global Burden of Diarrhoeal Disease, as Estimated from Studies Published between 1992 and 2000." *Bulletin of the World Health Organization* 81 (3): 197–204.

Kramer, M. S., F. E. Aboud, E. Mironova, I. Vanilovich, R. W. Platt, and others. 2008. "Breastfeeding and Child Cognitive Development: New Evidence from a Large Randomized Trial." *Archives of General Psychiatry* 65 (5): 578–84.

Kramer, M. S., B. Chalmers, E. D. Hodnett, Z. Sevkovskaya, I. Dzikovich, and others. 2001. "Promotion of Breastfeeding Intervention Trial (PROBIT): A Randomized Trial in the

Republic of Belarus." *Journal of the American Medical Association* 285 (4): 413–20.

Larson, L. M., and A. K. Yousafzai. 2014. "Meta-Analyses of Nutrition and Stimulation Interventions: Effects on Child Development." Micronutrient Forum Conference, Addis Ababa, June 2.

Larson, L. M., and A. K. Yousafzai. Forthcoming. "A Meta-analysis of Nutrition Interventions on Mental Development of Children Under-Two in Low- and Middle-Income Countries." *Maternal & Child Nutrition.*

Lawn, J. E., H. Blencowe, S. Oza, D. You, A. C. C. Lee, and others. 2014. "Every Newborn: Progress, Priorities, and Potential beyond Survival." *The Lancet* 384 (9938): 189–205.

Lee, A. C. C., J. Katz, H. Blencowe, S. Cousens, N. Kozuki, and others. 2013. "National and Regional Estimates of Term and Preterm Babies Born Small for Gestational Age in 138 Low-Income and Middle-Income Countries in 2010." *The Lancet Global Health* 1: e26–36.

Lenters, L., K. Wazny, and Z. A. Bhutta. 2016. "Management of Severe and Moderate Acute Malnutrition in Children." In *Disease Control Priorities* (third edition): Volume 2, *Reproductive, Maternal, Newborn, and Child Health*, edited by R. Black, R. Laxminarayan, M. Temmerman, and N. Walker. Washington, DC: World Bank.

Lobel, M., D. L. Cannella, J. E. Graham, C. DeVincent, J. Schneider, and others. 2008. "Pregnancy-Specific Stress, Prenatal Health Behaviors, and Birth Outcomes." *Health Psychology* 27 (5): 604–15.

Lozoff, B., J. Beard, J. Connor, B. Felt, M. Georgieff, and others. 2006. "Long-Lasting Neural and Behavioral Effects of Iron Deficiency in Infancy." *Nutrition Reviews* 64 (5): S34–43.

Lozoff, B., G. M. Brittenham, A. W. Wolf, D. K. McClish, P. M. Kuhnert, and others. 1987. "Iron Deficiency Anemia and Iron Therapy Effects on Infant Developmental Test Performance." *Pediatrics* 79 (6): 981–95.

Lozoff, B., J. B. Smith, K. M. Clark, C. G. Perales, F. Rivera, and others. 2010. "Home Intervention Improves Cognitive and Social-Emotional Scores in Iron-Deficient Anemic Infants." *Pediatrics* 126 (4): e884–94.

Luby, S. P., C. Mendoza, B. H. Keswick, T. M. Chiller, and R. M. Hoekstra. 2008. "Difficulties in Bringing Point-of-Use Water Treatment to Scale in Rural Guatemala." *American Journal of Tropical Medicine and Hygiene* 78 (3): 382–87.

Ludermir, A. B., L. B. Schraiber, A. F. P. L. D'Oliveira, I. França-Junior, and H. A. Jansen. 2008. "Violence against Women by their Intimate Partner and Common Mental Disorders." *Social Science and Medicine* 66 (4): 1008–18.

Macete, E., P. Aide, J. J. Aponte, S. Sanz, I. Mandomando, and others. 2006. "Intermittent Preventive Treatment for Malaria Control Administered at the Time of Routine Vaccinations in Mozambican Infants: A Randomized, Placebo-Controlled Trial." *Journal of Infectious Diseases* 194 (3): 276–85.

Macours, K., N. Schady, and R. Vakis. 2012. "Cash Transfers, Behavioral Changes, and Cognitive Development in Early Childhood: Evidence from a Randomized Experiment." *American Economic Journal: Applied Economics* 4 (2): 247–73.

Manno, D., P. K. Kowa, H. K. Bwalya, J. Siame, S. Grantham-McGregor, and others. 2012. "Rich Micronutrient Fortification of Locally Produced Infant Food Does Not Improve Mental and Motor Development of Zambian Infants: A Randomized Controlled Trial." *British Journal of Nutrition* 107: 556–66.

Mariotti, S. P., D. Pascolini, and J. Rose-Nussbaumer. 2009. "Trachoma: Global Magnitude of a Preventable Cause of Blindness." *British Journal of Ophthalmology* 93: 563–68.

McKay, S., E. Gaudier, D. I. Campbell, A. M. Prentice, and R. Albers. 2010. "Environmental Enteropathy: New Targets for Nutritional Interventions." *International Health* 2 (3): 172–80.

Mecaskey, J. W., C. A. Knirsch, J. A. Kumaresan, and J. A. Cook. 2003. "The Possibility of Eliminating Blinding Trachoma." *The Lancet Infectious Diseases* 3 (11): 728–34.

Morrongiello, B. A., S. L. Schell, and S. Schmidt. 2010. "'Please Keep an Eye on Your Younger Sister': Sibling Supervision and Young Children's Risk of Unintentional Injury." *Injury Prevention* 16 (6): 398–402.

Nair, M. C. K., E. Philip, G. B. Jeyaseelan, S. Mathews, and K. Padma. 2009. "Effect of Child Development Centre Model Early Stimulation among At-Risk Babies: A Randomized Controlled Trial." *Indian Pediatrics* 46: s20–26.

Neumann, C. G., S. P. Murphy, C. Gewa, M. Grillenberger, and N. O. Bwibo. 2007. "Meat Supplementation Improves Growth, Cognitive, and Behavioural Outcomes in Kenyan Children." *Journal of Nutrition* 137 (4): 1119–23.

Ngondi, J., A. Onsarigo, L. Adamu, I. Matende, S. Baba, and others. 2005. "The Epidemiology of Trachoma in Eastern Equatoria and Upper Nile States, Southern Sudan." *Bulletin of the World Health Organization* 83 (12): 904–12.

Ngure, F. M., B. M. Reid, J. H. Humphrey, M. N. Mbuya, G. Pelto, and others. 2014. "Water, Sanitation, and Hygiene (WASH), Environmental Enteropathy, Nutrition, and Early Child Development: Making the Links." *Annals of the New York Academy of Sciences* 1308: 118–28.

Ogden, S., and P. Emerson. 2012. "How Communities Can Control Trachoma without a Big Budget." *Community Eye Health Journal* 25 (79 & 80): 80–81.

Olney, D., P. Kariger, R. Stoltzfus, S. Khalfan, N. Ali, and others. 2009. "Development of Nutritionally At-Risk Young Children Is Predicted by Malaria, Anemia, and Stunting in Pemba, Zanzibar." *Journal of Nutrition* 139 (4): 763–72.

Oweye, O., F. Aina, and O. Morakinyo. 2006. "Risk Factors of Postpartum Depression and EPDS Scores in a Group of Nigerian Women." *Tropical Doctor* 36 (2): 100–3.

Pasricha, S.-R., E. Hayes, K. Kalumba, and B.-A. Biggs. 2013. "Effect of Daily Iron Supplementation on Health in Children Aged 4–23 Months: A Systematic Review and Meta-Analysis of Randomised Controlled Trials." *The Lancet Global Health* 1 (2): e77–86.

Patel, A. B., M. R. Mamtani, T. P. Thakre, and H. Kulkarni. 2006. "Association of Umbilical Cord Blood Lead with Neonatal Behaviour at Varying Levels of Exposure." *Behavioral and Brain Functions* 2: 22. doi:10.1186/1744-9081-2-22.

Patel, V., A. Rahman, K. S. Jacob, and M. Hughes. 2004. "Effect of Maternal Mental Health on Infant Growth in Low

Income Countries: New Evidence from South Asia." *British Medical Journal* 328 (7443): 820–23.

Paxson, C., and N. Schady. 2010. "Does Money Matter? The Effects of Cash Transfers on Child Health and Development in Rural Ecuador." *Economic Development and Cultural Change* 59 (1): 187–229.

Peairson, S., A. M. B. Austin, C. N. de Aquino, and E. U. de Burró. 2008. "Cognitive Development and Home Environment of Rural Paraguayan Infants and Toddlers Participating in Pastoral del Niño, an Early Child Development Program." *Journal of Research in Childhood Education* 22 (4): 343–62.

Persson, L. A., S. El Arifeen, E.-C. Ekstrom, K. M. Rasmussen, E. A. Frongillo, and others. 2012. "Effects of Prenatal Micronutrient and Daily Food Supplementation on Maternal Hemoglobin, Birth Weight, and Infant Mortality among Children in Bangladesh." *Journal of the American Medical Association* 307 (19): 2050–59.

Platt, M. J. 2014. "Outcomes in Preterm Infants." *Public Health* 128 (5): 399–403. doi:10.1016/j.puhe.2014.03.010.

Pollitt, E., C. Saco-Pollitt, M. A. Husaini, and J. Huang. 2000. "Effects of an Energy and Micronutrient Supplement on Mental Development and Behavior under Natural Conditions in Undernourished Children in Indonesia." *European Journal of Clinical Nutrition* 54: S80–90.

Potterton, J., A. Stewart, P. Cooper, and P. Becker. 2010. "The Effect of a Basic Home Stimulation Programme on the Development of Young Children Infected with HIV." *Developmental Medicine and Child Neurology* 52 (6): 547–51.

Prado, E. L., A. A. Abubakar, S. Abbeddou, E. Y. Jimenez, J. W. Somé, and others. 2014. "Extending the Developmental Milestones Checklist for Use in a Different Context in Sub-Saharan Africa." *Acta Paediatrica* 103 (4): 447–54.

Prado, E. L., and K. G. Dewey. 2014. "Nutrition and Brain Development in Early Life." *Nutrition Reviews* 72 (4): 267–84.

Qawasmi, A., A. Landeros-Weisenberger, J. F. Leckman, and M. H. Bloch. 2012. "Meta-Analysis of Long-Chain Polyunsaturated Fatty Acid Supplementation of Formula and Infant Cognition." *Pediatrics* 129 (6): 1141–49.

Rahman, A., J. Bunn, H. Lovel, and F. Creed. 2007. "Maternal Depression Increases Infant Risk of Diarrhoeal Illness: A Cohort Study." *Archives of Disease in Childhood* 92 (1): 24–28.

Rahman, A., and F. Creed. 2007. "Outcome of Prenatal Depression and Risk Factors Associated with Persistence in the First Postnatal Year: Prospective Study from Rawalpindi, Pakistan." *Journal of Affective Disorders* 100 (1–3): 115–21.

Rahman, A., Z. Iqbal, and R. Harrington. 2003. "Life Events, Social Support and Depression in Childbirth: Perspectives from a Rural Community in the Developing World." *Psychological Medicine* 33 (7): 1161–67.

Rahman, A., A. Malik, S. Sikander, C. Roberts, and F. Creed. 2008. "Cognitive Behaviour Therapy-Based Intervention by Community Health Workers for Mothers with Depression and Their Infants in Rural Pakistan: A

Cluster-Randomised Controlled Trial." *The Lancet* 372 (9642): 902–09.

Rahman, A., M. Vahter, E.-C. Ekstrom, M. Rahman, A. H. Mustafa, and others. 2007. "Association of Arsenic Exposure during Pregnancy with Fetal Loss and Infant Death: A Cohort Study in Bangladesh." *American Journal of Epidemiology* 165 (12): 1389–96.

Rosado, J. L., P. López, O. P. Garcia, J. Alatorre, and C. Alvarado. 2011. "Effectiveness of the Nutritional Supplement Used in the Mexican Opportunidades Programme on Growth, Anaemia, Morbidity and Cognitive Development in Children Aged 12–24 Months." *Public Health Nutrition* 14 (5): 931–37.

Servili, C., G. Medhin, C. Hanlon, M. Tomlinson, B. Worku, and others. 2010. "Maternal Common Mental Disorders and Infant Development in Ethiopia: The P=MaMiE Birth Cohort." *BMC Public Health* 10: 693.

Singla, D. R., E. Kumbakumba, and F. E. Aboud. 2015. "Effects of a Parenting Intervention to Address Both Maternal Psychological Wellbeing and Child Development and Growth in Rural Uganda: A Community-Based, Cluster-Randomised Trial." *The Lancet Global Health* 3 (8): e458–e469.

Smithers, L. G., R. A. Gibson, A. McPhee, and M. Makrides. 2008. "Effect of Long-Chain Polyunsaturated Fatty Acid Supplementation of Preterm Infants on Disease Risk and Neurodevelopment: A Systematic Review of Randomized Controlled Trials." *American Journal of Clinical Nutrition* 87 (4): 912–20.

Sroufe, L. A. 2005. "Attachment and Development: A Prospective, Longitudinal Study from Birth to Adulthood." *Attachment and Human Development* 7 (4): 349–67.

Stevens, G., M. Finucane, and C. Paciorek. 2016. "Levels and Trends in Low Height-for-Age." In *Disease Control Priorities* (third edition): Volume 2, *Reproductive, Maternal, Newborn, and Child Health*, edited by R. Black, R. Laxminarayan, M. Temmerman, and N. Walker. Washington, DC: World Bank.

Taylor-Robinson, D., A. Jones, and P. Garner. 2007. "Deworming Drugs for Treating Soil-Transmitted Intestinal Worms in Children: Effects on Growth and School Performance (Review)." *Cochrane Database of Systematic Reviews* 4: CD000371.

Tofail, F., J. D. Hamadani, A. Z. T. Ahmed, M. Mehrin, M. Hakin, and others. 2012. "The Mental Development and Behavior of Low-Birth-Weight Bangladeshi Infants from an Urban Low-Income Community." *European Journal of Clinical Nutrition* 66 (2): 237–43.

Tofail, F., J. D. Hamadani, F. Mehrin, D. A. Ridout, S. N. Huda, and others. 2013. "Psychosocial Stimulation Benefits Development in Nonanemic Children but Not in Anemic, Iron-Deficient Children." *Journal of Nutrition* 143 (6): 885–93.

Tofail, F., I. Kabir, J. D. Hamadani, F. Chowdhury, S. Yesmin, and others. 2006. "Supplementation of Fish-Oil and Soy-Oil during Pregnancy and Psychomotor Development of Infants." *Journal of Health, Population and Nutrition* 24 (1): 48–56.

Tofail, F., L. A. Persson, S. E. Arifeen, J. D. Hamadani, F. Mehrin, and others. 2008. "Effects of Prenatal Food and

Micronutrient Supplementation on Infant Development: A Randomized Trial from the Maternal and Infant Nutrition Interventions, Matlab (MINIMat) Study." *American Journal of Clinical Nutrition* 87 (3): 704–11.

Tomlinson, M., A. Rahman, D. Sanders, J. Maselko, and M. J. Rotheram-Borus. 2014. "Leveraging Paraprofessionals and Family Strengths to Improve Coverage and Penetration of Nutrition and Early Child Development Services." *Annals of the New York Academy of Sciences* 1308: 162–72.

UNICEF (United Nations Children's Fund). 2013. *The State of the World's Children.* New York: UNICEF.

——— and WHO (World Health Organization). 2009. *Care for Child Development.* New York: UNICEF and WHO.

Valenzuela, M. 1990. "Attachment in Chronically Underweight Young Children." *Child Development* 61 (6): 1984–96.

van den Briel, T., C. E. West, N. Bleichrodt, F. J. R. van de Vijver, E. A. Ategbo, and others. 2000. "Improved Iodine Status Is Associated with Improved Mental Performance of Schoolchildren in Benin." *American Journal of Clinical Nutrition* 72 (5): 1179–85.

Vazir, S., P. Engle, N. Balakrishna, P. L. Griffiths, S. L. Johnson, and others. 2013. "Cluster-Randomized Trial on Complementary and Responsive Feeding Education to Caregivers Found Improved Dietary Intake, Growth and Development among Rural Indian Toddlers." *Maternal and Child Nutrition* 9 (1): 99–117.

Victora, C. G., M. de Onis, and P. C. Hallal. 2010. "Worldwide Timing of Growth Faltering: Revisiting Implications for Interventions Using the World Health Organization Growth Standards." *Pediatrics* 125 (3): e473–80.

Walker, S. P., S. Chang, C. Powell, and S. M. Grantham-McGregor. 2004. "Psychosocial Intervention Improves the Development of Term Low Birth Weight Infants." *Journal of Nutrition* 134 (6): 1417–23.

Walker, S. P., T. D. Wachs, S. Grantham-McGregor, M. M. Black, C. A. Nelson, and others. 2011. "Inequality in Early

Childhood: Risk and Protective Factors for Early Child Development." *The Lancet* 378 (9799): 1325–38.

Weisz, A. J., M. J. Manary, K. Stephenson, S. Agapova, F. G. Manary, and others. 2012. "Abnormal Gut Integrity Is Associated with Reduced Linear Growth in Rural Malawian Children." *Journal of Pediatric Gastroenterology and Nutrition* 55 (6): 747–50.

Weobong, B., B. Akpalu, V. Doku, S. Owusu-Agyei, L. Hurt, and others. 2009. "The Comparative Validity of Screening Scales for Postnatal Common Mental Disorder in Kintampo Ghana." *Journal of Affective Disorders* 113 (1–2): 109–17.

Werker, J. F., and T. K. Hensch. 2015. "Critical Periods in Speech Perception: New Directions." *Annual Review of Psychology* 66: 173–96.

Williams, P., U. Piamjariyakul, A. Williams, P. Hornboonherm, P. Meena, and others. 2003. "Thai Mothers and Children and the HOME Observation for Measurement of the Environment (Home Inventory): Pilot Study." *International Journal of Nursing Studies* 40 (3): 249–58.

Yousafzai, A. K., P. Lynch, and M. Gladstone. 2014. "Moving beyond Prevalence Studies: Screening and Interventions for Children with Disabilities in Low- and Middle-Income Countries." *Archives of Disease in Childhood* 99 (9): 840–48. doi:10.1136/archdischild-2012-302066.

Yousafzai, A. K., M. A. Rasheed, A. Rizvi, R. Armstrong, and Z. A. Bhutta. 2014. "Effect of Integrated Responsive Stimulation and Nutrition Interventions in the Lady Health Worker Programme in Pakistan on Child Development, Growth, and Health Outcomes: A Cluster Randomized Factorial Effectiveness Trial." *The Lancet* 384 (9950): 1282–93. doi:10.1016/S0140-6736(14)60455-4.

Zimmermann, M. B. 2012. "The Effects of Iodine Deficiency in Pregnancy and Infancy." *Paediatric and Perinatal Epidemiology* 26 (Suppl. 1): 108–17.

———, P. L. Jooste, and C. S. Pandav. 2008. "Iodine-Deficiency Disorders." *The Lancet* 372 (9645): 1251–62.

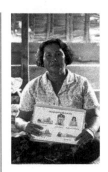

Community-Based Care to Improve Maternal, Newborn, and Child Health

Zohra S. Lassi, Rohail Kumar, and Zulfiqar A. Bhutta

INTRODUCTION

Significant progress has been made in maternal, newborn, and child health (MNCH) in recent decades. Between 1990 and 2015, the global mortality rate for children under age five years dropped by 53 percent, from 90.6 deaths per 1,000 live births in 1990 to 42.5 in 2015 (Liu and others 2016). Maternal mortality is also on the decline globally.[1]

Despite progress, maternal, neonatal, and under-five mortality remain high in many low- and middle-income countries (LMICs). In 2015, approximately 303,000 women died as a result of complications from pregnancy and childbirth (WHO 2015). Globally, an estimated 5.9 million children under age five years die each year, including 2.7 million within the first month of life (Liu and others 2016).

Health indicators differ across countries, regions, and socioeconomic levels (Lozano and others 2011). Approximately 99 percent of all newborn deaths occur in LMICs (Bayer 2001). Maternal mortality is concentrated in Sub-Saharan Africa (Hogan and others 2010), where mortality rates for the poor are double those for the nonpoor, and they are higher among rural populations and women with low levels of education (*PLoS Medicine* Editors 2010). Children living in low-income countries are three times more likely to die before age

five years than children living in high-income countries (HICs) (Black and others 2013).

Pneumonia, diarrhea, malaria, and inadequate nutrition drive early childhood deaths around the world. In 2015, an estimated 526,000 episodes of diarrhea and 922,000 cases of pneumonia in children under age five years led to death (Liu and others 2016). Undernutrition is a primary underlying cause of 3.5 million maternal and child deaths each year (Black and others 2013); stunting, wasting, and micronutrient deficiencies are responsible for approximately 35 percent of the disease burden in children under age five years and 11 percent of the total global disease burden (Lozano and others 2011). Although maternal mortality is caused chiefly by postpartum hemorrhage, preeclampsia and eclampsia, and sepsis, a large proportion of maternal deaths can be attributed to limited access to skilled care during childbirth and the postnatal period (Lozano and others 2011) as well as to limited access to family planning services and safe abortions (UNFPA and Guttmacher Institute 2010).

An appropriate mix of interventions can significantly reduce the burden of maternal and child mortality and morbidity. However, these interventions often do not reach those who need them most (Bayer 2001; Sines, Tinker, and Ruben 2006). An integrated approach that includes community-based care as an essential

Corresponding author: Zulfiqar A. Bhutta, Robert Harding Chair in Global Child Health & Policy, Centre for Global Child Health, Hospital for Sick Children, Toronto, Canada; Zulfiqar.bhutta@sickkids.ca.

component has the potential to substantially improve maternal, newborn, and child health outcomes.

This chapter provides a summary of community-based programs for improving MNCH. The chapter discusses strategies to improve the supply of services, including through community-based interventions and home visitations implemented by community health workers (CHWs), and strategies to increase demand for services, including through community mobilization efforts. The chapter summarizes the evidence about the impact of such interventions, describes contextual factors that affect implementation, and considers issues of cost-effectiveness. It concludes by highlighting research gaps, the challenges of scaling up, and the way forward.

COMMUNITY-BASED CARE

It is widely agreed that communities should take an active part in improving their own health outcomes (WHO 1979, 1986, 2008, 2011) and that CHWs can play a vital role. Since 2000, national governments have realized the substantial potential of CHWs to achieve child survival goals; these governments have or are considering national programs for CHWs. For example, since 2003, Ethiopia has trained thousands of community-based health extension workers to focus on maternal, newborn, and child health (Medhanyie and others 2012).

Although strategies vary considerably, community-based interventions may encompass encouraging healthier practices and care seeking among communities and families; recruiting and training local community members to work alongside trained health care professionals; and community member involvement in service provision, including diagnosis, treatment, and referral. Within these broad categories are a range of approaches, including CHWS, traditional birth attendants (TBAs), health campaigns, school-based health promotion, home-based care, and even community franchise–operated clinics.

Community-based care is an important component of providing a continuum of care for low-resource communities. The health and well-being of women, newborns, and children are inherently linked. When mothers are malnourished, ill, or receive insufficient care, their newborns are at increased risk of disease and premature death. In LMICs, a mother's death during childbirth significantly raises the risk that the child will not survive (Ronsmans and others 2010).

Better health requires that women and children have the ability to access quality services from conception and pregnancy to delivery, the postnatal period, and childhood. Issues such as human immunodeficiency virus/acquired immune deficiency syndrome (HIV/AIDS), sexually transmitted infections, malaria, malnutrition, complications during pregnancy and delivery, and inadequate newborn and child care can be addressed through vertical programs. However, the best results can be obtained if these issues are tackled through interventions that target maternal, newborn, and child health care as a whole. Coordinating care, from preconception to delivery and the health of the child, can lead to profound benefits for the health and well-being of women and children and improve subsequent pregnancy and child health outcomes. A recent review of preconception risks and interventions shows that preconception care in community groups is associated with a lower neonatal mortality rate (risk ratio 0.76; 95 percent confidence interval 0.66–0.88), and a significant increase in antenatal care (ANC) (risk ratio 1.39; 95 percent confidence interval 1.00–1.93), breastfeeding rates (risk ratio 1.20; 95 percent confidence interval 1.07–1.36), and use of clean delivery kits (risk ratio 2.36; 95 percent confidence interval 1.55–3.60) (Dean and others 2011).

There are many approaches to community-based care. This chapter describes interventions aimed at improving the supply of services by delivering them in communities, often through CHWs, and interventions aimed at increasing demand for services and promoting healthy behaviors.

COMMUNITY-BASED CARE TO IMPROVE THE SUPPLY OF SERVICES

Health care provided in communities, as opposed to health facilities, is often provided by CHWs and may include home visitations and other intervention packages. The level of training CHWs receive, whether they are employed by a nongovernmental organization or the government and whether they are paid or volunteer, varies widely between and within countries. In general, they work in conjunction with frontline health workers across the primary health care spectrum to provide health education and promotion, distribute commodities, diagnose and manage illness, and provide referrals.

Substantial evidence suggests that community-based interventions are an important platform for improving health care delivery and outcomes (Bhutta and others 2010; Kerber and others 2007; Lassi, Haider, and Bhutta 2010; Lewin and others 2010; Singh and Sachs 2013).

Home Visits

For both at-risk pregnancies and healthy pregnancies, home visits by CHWs in the pre- and postnatal period to counsel mothers, provide newborn care, and facilitate referral may lead to early detection of complications and appropriate referrals. Studies in Bangladesh, India, and Pakistan suggest that home visits can reduce newborn deaths in high mortality settings by 30 percent to 61 percent (Bang and others 1999; Baqui and others 2008; Bhutta and others 2008).

Community Management of Delivery Complications, Neonatal Care, and Childhood Illnesses

A pilot home-based newborn care intervention in India consisting of sepsis management; support for low-birth-weight (LBW) infants; and primary prevention, health education, and training of TBAs has been shown to decrease newborn and infant mortality rates (Bang and others 1999; Bang, Reddy, and others 2005). Home-based interventions in India to reduce neonatal and infant deaths and stillbirths included surveillance to identify pregnant women, followed by two home visits during pregnancy for birth preparedness and for routine neonatal care. In the event of a high-risk neonate or an LBW infant, extra care was administered. In the trial, 93 percent of neonates in the intervention areas received home-based care (Bang and others 1999). Similarly, results from a study in India show that the asphyxia-specific mortality rate was significantly reduced by 65 percent, comparing periods before and after CHW training with either tube-and-mask or bag-and-mask ventilation, and the case fatality of severe asphyxia was reduced by 48 percent (Bang, Bang, and others 2005). Results from a randomized controlled trial (RCT) in rural India (Bang and others 1999) suggest that implementation

by CHWs of an essential newborn care package, in conjunction with administration of home-based antibiotic therapy for suspected neonatal sepsis, resulted in a 62 percent reduction in the neonatal mortality rate, when 93 percent of newborns in the intervention area were provided with treatment. Another study from an Indian urban slum reports a low case fatality rate of 3.3 percent among babies younger than age two months who were treated for serious infections as outpatients due to family noncompliance with advice for hospitalization (Bhandari and others 1996).

A systematic review of RCTs suggests that home visits for neonatal care by CHWs are associated with a 38 percent reduction in neonatal mortality and a 24 percent reduction in the stillbirth rate (table 14.1) in resource-limited settings with poorly accessible facility-based care, when conducted in conjunction with community mobilization activities (Gogia and Sachdev 2010). The review also shows significant improvements in other care-related outcomes (table 14.1).

Evidence suggests that home visits improve coverage of key newborn care practices such as early initiation of breastfeeding and exclusive breastfeeding; skin-to-skin contact; delayed bathing and attention to hygiene, such as handwashing with soap and water; clean umbilical cord care; immunization; and appropriate management and referral for sepsis and other infections. This evidence complements the experience from HICs, which shows that postnatal home visits are effective in improving parenting skills (Olds and others 2004).

Evidence also suggests that CHWs can effectively perform neonatal resuscitation. Basic neonatal resuscitation,

Table 14.1 Evidence on Community-Based Care through Home Visitations

Study	Interventions assessed	Outcomes	Estimates
Gogia and Sachdev 2010	Randomized controlled trials comparing various intervention packages, one being home visits for neonatal care by community health workers	Neonatal mortality	RR 0.62 (95% CI: 0.44–0.87); five studies
		Stillbirths	RR 0.76 (95% CI: 0.65–0.89); three studies
		Antenatal care visits	RR 1.33 (95% CI: 1.20–1.47); four studies
		Tetanus toxoid immunization	RR 1.11 (95% CI: 1.04–1.18); four studies
		Breastfeeding within one hour of birth	RR 3.35 (95% CI: 1.31–8.59); four studies
		Clean cord care	RR 1.70 (95% CI: 1.39–2.08); four studies
		Delayed bathing after more than 24 hours	RR 4.36 (95% CI: 2.29–9.37); four studies
Bhutta and Lassi 2010	Randomized controlled trials that built community support and advocacy groups for mobilization on issues related to maternal, neonatal, and child health	Neonatal mortality	RR 0.70 (95% CI: 0.61–0.81); six studies, n = 67,808

Note: CI = confidence interval; n = number of observations; RR = risk ratio.

including bag-and-mask ventilation, is adequate for most newborns who require neonatal resuscitation in low-resource settings (Newton and English 2006). The results of a systematic review report that several trials have shown that CHWs can perform neonatal resuscitation with reductions of up to 20 percent in intrapartum-related neonatal deaths (Wall and others 2009).

In integrated community case management (iCCM), CHWs are identified and trained in classification and treatment of key childhood illnesses, including identifying children in need of immediate referral.[2] A systematic review suggests that iCCM of pneumonia could result in a 70 percent reduction in mortality in children younger than age five years (Theodoratou and others 2010). Another systematic review (Das and others 2013) shows that community-based interventions correlate to 13 percent and 9 percent increases in care seeking for pneumonia and diarrhea, respectively (table 14.2). These interventions are also associated with an up to 160 percent increase in the use of oral rehydration solution, an 80 percent increase in the use of zinc for management of diarrhea, and a 32 percent reduction in pneumonia-specific mortality (Das and others 2013). Furthermore, in a meta-analysis of trials of community-based case management of pneumonia (Sazawal and Black 2003), all-cause neonatal mortality was 27 percent lower in the intervention group; pneumonia-specific neonatal mortality in the intervention group was reduced by an even greater amount.

A systematic review carried out to assess the improvement in skills of CHWs shows that workers trained in Integrated Management of Childhood Illness (IMCI), a strategy developed by the World Health Organization (WHO) in the 1990s, were more likely to correctly classify illnesses (risk ratio 1.93; 95 percent confidence interval 1.66–2.24) (Nguyen and others 2013). An RCT in Bangladesh demonstrates that implementation of IMCI improved health worker skills, health system support, and family and community practices, which translated into increased care seeking for illnesses. In IMCI areas, more children younger than age six months were exclusively breastfed (76 percent versus 65 percent; difference of differences 10.1 percent; 95 percent confidence interval 2.65–17.62), and the prevalence of stunting in children ages 24–59 months decreased more rapidly (difference of differences −7.33; 95 percent confidence interval −13.83 to −0.83) than in comparison areas, thereby reducing morbidity (Arifeen and others 2009).

An RCT from Zambia shows that CHWs can be trained to perform rapid diagnostic tests (RDTs) for malaria, treat test-positive children with antimalarials, and treat those with nonsevere pneumonia with amoxicillin. A higher number of children with nonsevere pneumonia received early and appropriate treatment in the intervention arm (treated by CHWs trained to perform RDTs) (risk ratio 5.32; 95 percent confidence interval 2.19–8.94). In the intervention group, only 27.5 percent of children with fever received antimalarial drugs after an RDT was conducted, while 99.1 percent of the children in the fever group received treatment for malaria (Yeboah-Antwi and others 2010).

This successful merger of formal health care systems with community-based efforts has profound effects on the achievement of Millennium Development Goals 4 and 5 to reduce child mortality and improve maternal health. Box 14.1 highlights an example of a CHW-based program.

Table 14.2 Evidence on Community Care through Home Visitations

Study	Interventions assessed	Outcomes	Estimates
Das and others 2013	Effect of community-based interventions, including community case management, on the coverage of various commodities and on mortality due to diarrhea and pneumonia	Health care seeking for pneumonia	RR 1.13 (95% CI: 1.08–1.18); two studies, n = 671
		Health care seeking for diarrhea	RR 1.09 (95% CI: 1.06–1.12); four studies, n = 8,253
		Pneumonia mortality in newborns from birth to age one month	RR 0.58 (95% CI: 0.44–0.77); four studies, n = 1,070
		Pneumonia mortality in children ages 1–4 years	RR 0.58 (95% CI: 0.50–0.67); nine studies, n = 2,507
		Zinc use rates	RR 2.39 (95% CI: 1.45–3.93); four studies, n = 32,676
		Free distribution of oral rehydration solution	RR 3.10 (95% CI: 1.28–7.48); two studies, n = 14,783
Theodoratou and others 2010	Effect of case management of childhood pneumonia on mortality	ALRI-related mortality	RR 0.65 (95% CI: 0.52–0.82); nine studies

Note: ALRI = acute lower respiratory infection; CI = confidence interval; n = number of observations; RR = risk ratio.

Pakistan's Lady Health Workers

Pakistan's lady health worker (LHW) program, a government-supported community health service begun in 1994, has expanded to cover more than 70 percent of the rural population. In the program, LHWs receive a regular salary and are trained to promote health awareness and provide basic care to pregnant mothers, neonates, and children, including ensuring up-to-date immunizations and monitoring nutritional status. LHWs also provide contraceptive and family planning services.

LHWs serve the community, working from home, and attend to approximately 200 households. Approximately 20 percent of the entire population of Pakistan is covered by 69,000 LHWs. Lady health supervisors are responsible for supervising the

LHWs; external evaluations are conducted every three to five years.

Studies show that women are more likely to use modern reversible contraceptive methods if offered by LHWs, and coordination of traditional birth attendants (TBAs) and LHWs led to a reduction in stillbirths and in hemorrhage-related complications. In another study, LHWs were given additional training and were linked with *dais* (TBAs in Pakistan), who were given training for newborn resuscitation and immediate newborn care; this approach also led to reductions in stillbirths, improvements in institutional deliveries, and increased initiation of early and exclusive breastfeeding.

Source: Bhutta and others 2010.

Community-Based Intervention Packages

Data suggest that the introduction of community-based intervention packages has the potential to reduce maternal and neonatal mortality (Ricca and others 2013; Schiffman and others 2010). Community-based care may improve breastfeeding practices and increase referrals to health facilities for pregnancy-related complications and other health care services during pregnancy, such as iron and folic acid supplementation (Lassi and others 2013). Results from a systematic review suggest that implementation of community-based intervention care packages led to a 25 percent reduction in neonatal mortality; referrals to health facilities for pregnancy-related complication increased by 40 percent; rates of early breastfeeding increased by 94 percent; and health care seeking for neonatal illnesses increased by 45 percent, leading to decreases in neonatal and maternal morbidity (tables 14.3 and 14.4) (Lassi, Haider, and Bhutta 2010). Interventions for the topics that follow are covered in more detail in two *DCP3* volumes: *HIV/AIDS, STIs, Tuberculosis, and Malaria* (Volume 6, Bundy and others), and *Child and Adolescent Development* (Volume 8, Holmes and others), both forthcoming in 2016.

Malaria. Community-based interventions may also contribute to prevention of malaria. Bhutta and others (2013) show that intermittent preventive treatment with sulfadoxine-pyrimethamine in pregnancy, delivered

through community-based approaches, is associated with a higher mean birth weight compared with case management (weighted mean difference 108.6 grams; 95 percent confidence interval 55.67–161.54). The review also indicates that ownership of insecticide-treated nets (ITNs) increased by 116 percent and usage increased by 77 percent. The use of ITNs was associated with a 23 percent reduction in the risk of delivering an LBW newborn. A meta-analysis replicates the findings of Bhutta and others (2013) and finds that ITN ownership significantly affects morbidity outcomes, including parasitemia, malaria prevalence, and anemia (Salam, Das, and others 2014).

Helminths. Salam, Maredia, and others (2014) also find that interventions such as preventive chemotherapy, health education to promote general hygiene and sanitation, iron and beta-carotene supplementation, construction of latrines, removal of cattle from residential areas, staff training, and community mobilization can have significant impacts on the prevention and management of worm infestations in children. Evidence suggests that school-based delivery of antihelminths can significantly reduce soil-transmitted helminths prevalence by 55 percent, schistosomiasis prevalence (risk ratio 0.50; 95 percent confidence interval: 0.33–0.75), and anemia prevalence (risk ratio 0.87; 95 percent confidence

Table 14.3 Evidence on Community-Based Intervention Packages

Study	Interventions assessed	Outcomes	Estimates
Lassi, Haider, and Bhutta 2010	Randomized controlled trials undertaken to compare effects of various community-based intervention packages on maternal and newborn care	Neonatal mortality	RR 0.43 (95% CI: 0.27–0.69); 13 studies, n = 136,425
		Stillbirths	RR 0.84 (95% CI: 0.74–0.97); 11studies, n = 113,821
		Perinatal mortality	RR 0.80 (95% CI: 0.71–0.91); 10 studies, n = 110,291
		Maternal morbidity	RR 0.75 (95% CI: 0.61–0.92); 4 studies, n = 138,290
		Institutional deliveries	RR 1.28 (95% CI: 0.98–1.67); 8 studies, n = 80,479
		Rates of early breastfeeding	RR 1.94 (95% CI: 1.56–2.42); 6 studies, n = 20,627
		Referrals to health facility for pregnancy-related complication	RR 1.40 (95% CI: 1.19–1.65); 2 studies, n = 22,800
		Health care seeking for neonatal illnesses	RR 1.45 (95% CI: 1.01–2.08); 5 studies, n = 57,157
Kidney and others 2009	Randomized controlled trials that assess community-level interventions and maternal death as an outcome	Maternal mortality	OR 0.62 (95% CI: 0.39–0.98); 2 studies, n = 26,238
Salam, Das, and others 2014	Effectiveness of community-based delivery of interventions for the prevention and management of malaria, including distribution of ITN, environmental cleaning, and provision of intermittent preventive treatment during pregnancy and childhood	ITN ownership	RR 2.16 (95% CI: 1.86–2.52); 14 studies
		ITN usage	RR 1.77 (95% CI: 1.48–2.11); 14 studies
		Parasitemia	RR 0.56 (95% CI: 0.42–0.74); 10 studies
		Malaria prevalence	RR: 0.46 (95% CI: 0.29–0.73); 9 studies
		Anemia	RR: 0.79 (95% CI: 0.64–0.97); 11 studies
Salam, Maredia, and others 2014	Effectiveness of community-based delivery for the prevention and control of helminthiasis, including soil-transmitted helminthiasis (ascariasis, hookworms and trichuriasis), lymphatic filariasis, onchocerciasis, dracunculiasis, and schistosomiasis	Soil-transmitted helminthic	RR 0.45 (95% CI: 0.38–0.54); 10 studies
		Schistosomiasis	RR 0.40 (95% CI: 0.33–0.50); 13 studies
		Mean hemoglobin levels	SMD 0.24 (95% CI: 0.16–0.32); 11 studies
Salam, Haroon, and others 2014	Effectiveness of community-based interventions for the prevention and management of HIV, including educational activities, counseling, home visits, mentoring, women's groups, peer leadership, street	HIV/AIDS-related knowledge scores	SMD 0.66 (95% CI: 0.25–1.07); 6 studies
		Mean number of times condom used	SMD 0.96 (95% CI: 0.03–1.58); 2 studies
		Protected sex	RR 1.19 (95% CI: 1.13–1.25); 4 studies

table continues next page

Table 14.3 Evidence on Community-Based Intervention Packages (continued)

Study	Interventions assessed	Outcomes	Estimates
	outreach activities, and dramas to increase awareness of HIV/AIDS risk factors and address perceived barriers to counseling and voluntary testing	Treatment adherence	MD 3.88 (95% CI: 2.69–5.07); 1 study
		Stillbirths	RR 0.34 (95% CI: 0.18–0.65); 1 study
Arshad and others 2014	Effectiveness of community-based interventions for the prevention and treatment of tuberculosis, including variants of DOTS; community outreach; training sessions and increased awareness to increase the detection rate and decrease relapse rates	Completion of tuberculosis treatment	RR 1.09 (95% CI: 1.07–1.11); 36 studies
		Tuberculosis detection rates	RR 3.10 (95% CI: 2.92–3.28); 5 studies

Note: CI = confidence interval; DOTS = directly observed treatment short course; HIV/AIDS = human immunodeficiency virus/acquired immune deficiency syndrome; ITN = insecticide-treated net; MD = mean difference; n = number of observations; OR = odds ratio; RR = risk ratio; SMD = standard mean difference.

Table 14.4 Forest Plot on a Community-Based Intervention Package and Its Impact on Health Care Seeking for Neonatal Illnesses

Study or subgroup	Intervention package N	Standard care N	Log [risk ratio] (SE)	Risk ratio IV, random, 95% CI	Weight (%)	Risk ratio IV, random, 95% CI
Azad and others 2010	15,695	15,257	−0.117 (0.12)		22.5	0.89 [0.70, 1.13]
Bari and others 2006	520	548	0.068 (0.03)		24.6	1.07 [1.01, 1.14]
Kumar and others 2008	1,087	1,079	0.657 (0.08)		23.7	1.93 [1.65, 2.26]
Manandhar and others 2004	2,864	3,181	1.044 (0.277)		16.0	2.84 [1.65, 4.89]
Tripathy and others 2010	8,807	8,119	0.425 (0.35)		13.2	1.53 [0.77, 3.04]
Total (95% CI)					100	1.45 [1.01, 2.08]

Heterogeneity: Tau² = 0.14; Chi² = 63.42, df = 4 (P<0.00001); I² = 94%
Test for overall effect: Z = 1.99 (P = 0.047)

0.01   0.1   1   10   100
Favors control   Favors experimental

Source: Lassi, Haider, and Bhutta 2010.
Note: CI = confidence interval; IV = inverse variance; n = number of participants; SE = standard error.

interval 0.81–0.94) in school-going children. It also improves the mean hemoglobin levels significantly (standard mean difference 0.24; 95 percent confidence interval 0.16–0.32) (Salam, Maredia, and others 2014).

HIV/AIDS. Similarly, community-based interventions can significantly improve HIV/AIDS status. Interventions such as educational activities, counseling sessions, home visits, mentoring, women's groups, peer leadership, and street outreach to increase awareness of HIV/AIDS risk factors have shown significant impacts on sexual practices and health outcomes. These interventions improve HIV/AIDS-related knowledge scores (standard mean difference 0.66; 95 percent confidence interval 0.25–1.07) and the frequency of protected sex (risk ratio 1.19; 95 percent confidence interval 1.13–1.25). Home visits can also decrease HIV-related morbidity by significantly increasing treatment adherence scores (mean difference 3.88; 95 percent confidence interval 2.69–5.07). Community delivery of highly active antiretroviral therapy during pregnancy and lactation also led to a 66 percent decrease in stillbirths (risk ratio 0.34; 95 percent confidence interval 0.18–0.65) (Salam, Haroon, and others 2014).

Tuberculosis. Tuberculosis can be managed and prevented through community-based intervention packages, including through variants of the directly observed treatment short course, community outreach, training sessions, and increased awareness to boost the detection rate and decrease relapse rates. Findings from 41 studies on the effectiveness of community-based interventions for tuberculosis show that these interventions were associated with a significant increase in cure and the success and completion of treatment (risk ratio 1.09; 95 percent confidence interval 1.07–1.11). Moreover, detection rates increased with community-based interventions using CHWs as the delivery strategy, with a pooled risk ratio of 3.10 (95 percent confidence interval 2.92–3.28) (Arshad and others 2014).

Nutrition. Evidence suggests that community-based nutrition programs can have a positive impact on health outcomes. India's Tamil Nadu Integrated Nutrition Program delivered nutrition services composed of monthly growth monitoring, short-term supplementary feeding for malnourished children and pregnant and lactating women, deworming and micronutrient supplementation, and education on diarrhea management and feeding. Approximately 25 percent of the project's food requirements were provided by village women's groups in a neighboring state; this arrangement contributed to the incomes of local women and educated them in the production of a low-cost weaning food (Balachander 1993).

A nutrition program in Ethiopia is also illustrative. In the program, monthly community sessions are held to monitor and promote the growth of children ages two years and younger (Getachew 2011; World Bank 2012). The program empowers communities to assess the nutritional status of their children and take action, using their own resources, to prevent malnutrition. Monthly tracking of all children in the community enables the timely identification of severely underweight children and their referral for further examination and treatment. The government of Ethiopia introduced this initiative in 2008 in drought-prone and food-insecure districts. An evaluation jointly undertaken by the World Bank, United Nations Children's Fund, and Tulane University shows that the program contributed to improved feeding and child care and thereby to lower rates of stunting: intervention areas experienced a 3–5 percentage point decrease in stunting compared with the national rate of decline of 1.3 percentage points a year (Getachew 2011; World Bank 2012). The study also finds that the program positively influenced infant and young child feeding, including greater adherence to exclusive breastfeeding for babies younger than age six

months, complementary feeding between ages 6 and 23 months, and dietary diversity for older children, thereby reducing morbidity and mortality related to malnutrition (Getachew 2011; World Bank 2012).

A systemic review of community-based interventions to improve child nutrition status suggests that nutrition education in both food-secure and food-insecure populations is associated with an increase in height-for-age Z scores of 0.22 (95 percent confidence interval 0.01–0.43) and 0.25 (95 percent confidence interval 0.09–0.42), respectively, compared with a control group (annex figure 14A.1). The review also suggests that simple interventions, such as individual counseling and group counseling, increase the odds of exclusive breastfeeding practices (Bhutta and others 2013; Lassi and others 2013). Table 14.5 highlights several community-based nutrition programs.

COMMUNITY-BASED CARE TO INCREASE THE DEMAND FOR SERVICES— EMPOWERING COMMUNITIES

In addition to delivering health services, CHWs and other community facilitators can be involved in education and health promotion activities to empower communities with knowledge and mobilize them to improve their health practices.

One such mechanism for empowering and educating communities is organized women's groups, which gather around particular health issues. For example, women's groups may seek to increase appropriate care seeking (including ANC and institutional delivery) and appropriate home prevention and care practices for mothers and newborns.

A pooled analysis of RCTs from Bangladesh, India, Nepal, and Pakistan—in which community support groups and group advocacy sessions that targeted women were implemented as part of community interventions— suggests that these interventions led to a 30 percent reduction in neonatal mortality (table 14.6). A decrease in neonatal morbidity through benefits of domiciliary practices, such as early initiation of breastfeeding and health-seeking behaviors, was also observed (risk ratio 1.87; 95 percent confidence interval 1.36–2.58) (annex figure 14A.2) (Bhutta and Lassi 2010).

A 2013 systematic review suggests that women's groups practicing participatory learning and action— specifically identifying and prioritizing problems during pregnancy, delivery, and postpartum period—are associated with a nonsignificant 23 percent reduction in maternal mortality and a 20 percent reduction in neonatal mortality (Prost and others 2013) (table 14.6).

Table 14.5 Characteristics of Selected Nutrition Programs

Program	Institution and evaluation year	Sponsors and funds	Staff and service providers	Objectives of the nutrition program	Coverage of the nutrition program	Program evaluation results
Nutrition centers as part of Viva Criança program, Brazil	1992 Evaluation in 1996	World Bank	A trained nutritionist, CHWs, and support staff	Provide nutrition training for center staff and CHWs and identify, treat, and then follow up moderately and severely malnourished children. Also provide up-to-date nutrition information to mothers and others in the community, and mobilize the community to find and implement strategies to prevent child malnutrition.	A total of 35 centers were developed; only 20 were functioning as nutrition centers.	Case fatality in two centers was 40 percent and more. Entry and exit criteria for rehabilitation were ill defined, resulting in some nonmalnourished children being enrolled. Few staff were adequately trained; knowledge was weak, especially about case management; and mothers were not effectively instructed.
Integrated Nutrition Project, Bangladesh	1995 Evaluation in 2000	Ministry of Health and Family Welfare, World Bank, World Food Program	CHWs and trained nutritionists	Improve the capacity of communities, households, and individuals in the project areas to understand their nutritional problems and to take appropriate action; and improve the nutritional status of the population in the project area, with particular emphasis on children and pregnant and lactating women.	Coverage was 55 of the 464 districts in Bangladesh.	The program improved knowledge by about 10–20 percentage points beyond that seen in nonproject areas regarding exclusive breastfeeding. Roughly 60 percent of malnourished women (with BMI < 18.5) received supplementary feeding.
Iringa nutrition project, Tanzania	1984 Evaluation in 1992	Government of Tanzania, UNICEF	CHWs and trained nutritionists	Reduce infant and young child mortality and morbidity through better child growth and development, and improvement of maternal nutrition. This was achieved by training of CHWs, day care programs, educational activities, village campaigns, and cash training programs.	The program began in 168 villages in the Iringa Region of Tanzania, covering an estimated population of 46,000 children under age five years.	The prevalence of total underweight (weight-for-age < 80 percent of WHO standard) decreased from 55.9 percent to 38.0 percent, and the prevalence of severe underweight (weight-for-age < 60 percent) decreased from 6.3 percent to 1.8 percent.

table continues next page

Table 14.5 Characteristics of Selected Nutrition Programs (continued)

Program	Institution and evaluation year	Sponsors and funds	Staff and service providers	Objectives of the nutrition program	Coverage of the nutrition program	Program evaluation results
Integrated Child Development Services (ICDS) scheme, India	1975 Evaluated in 2005	Ministry of Women and Child Development	CHWs	Improve the nutritional and health status of children younger than age six years, and reduce incidence of mortality, morbidity, malnutrition, and school dropouts. Also aims to enhance the capability of the mother to look after the normal health, nutritional, and developmental needs of the child through proper community education. The package of services provided by the ICDS scheme includes supplementary nutrition, immunizations, health checkups, referral services, nutrition and health education, and preschool education. Iron and folic acid tablets and mega doses of vitamin A are distributed.	Started in 33 blocks and now spans the country. It is delivered through a network of more than 1 million CHWs and reaches more than 70 million children and 15 million pregnant and lactating mothers.	Multiple evaluations suggest that although there had been a vast increase in ICDS blocks, there was a lack of infrastructure and basic amenities. Though immunization activities under ICDS have appreciable credibility, nonformal preschool, nutrition, and health education are not fully functioning as planned. A World Bank evaluation in 1999 suggested that the program had no significant impact on nutritional outcomes.

Sources: Balachander 1993; do Monte and others 1998; Gupta, Gupta, and Baridalyne 2013; World Bank 2005; Yambi and Mlolwa 1992.
Note: BMI = body mass index; CHW = community health worker; UNICEF = United Nations Children's Fund; WHO = World Health Organization.

Table 14.6 Evidence on Community-Based Care through Community Mobilization

Study	Interventions assessed	Outcomes	Estimates
Prost and others 2013	Seven randomized controlled trials undertaken on the effects of women's groups practicing participatory learning and action were assessed to identify population-level predictors of effect on maternal mortality, neonatal mortality, and stillbirths.	Maternal mortality	OR 0.77 (95% CI: 0.48–1.23); seven studies, n = 113,911
		Neonatal mortality	OR 0.80 (95% CI: 0.67–0.96); seven studies, n = 113,911
Bhutta and Lassi 2010	Six randomized controlled trials that built community support and advocacy groups for mobilization on issues related to maternal, neonatal, and child health were analyzed.	Neonatal mortality	RR 0.70 (95% CI: 0.61–0.81); six studies, n = 67,808

Note: CI = confidence interval; OR = odds ratio; RR = risk ratio.

A study from Ethiopia showed promising results when a group of women from the community were empowered and mobilized to recognize and treat malaria (Rosato and others 2008). This process led to an overall 40 percent reduction in mortality in children under age five years (Kidane and Morrow 2000). In communities with underresourced health systems, such as in Jharkhand and Orissa, two of the poorest states in eastern India, 55 percent coverage of women's groups formed to facilitate participatory learning, safe delivery practices, and care-seeking behavior was believed to be a factor in reducing maternal depression. Neonatal mortality rates were reduced by 45 percent in the intervention arm (Tripathy and others 2010).

An effective community mobilization program led to a 28 percent reduction in neonatal mortality in a study conducted in Hala, Pakistan, of LHWs who had received training in home-based neonatal care and TBAs who received voluntary training (Bhutta and others 2008).

The Makwanpur trial was conducted in a rural mountainous community in Nepal, where 94 percent of babies are born at home (Pradhan and New 1997) and only 13 percent of births are attended by trained health workers (Central Bureau of Statistics 2001). With the implementation of facilitated monthly group meetings among pregnant women, a decrease in neonatal mortality was seen in the intervention arm, compared with the control arm, with an odds ratio of 0.7 (95 percent confidence interval 0.53–0.94) (Manandhar and others 2004).

QUESTIONS AND CHALLENGES

Expanding the Community Health Worker Mandate

Shortages in human resources and expanding populations have given new relevance to training CHWs in ever-more complex tasks. For countries with limited resources for training or employing paid labor, task shifting may allow CHWs or less trained TBAs to receive training and perform interventions that might have previously been reserved for more highly trained professionals (WHO 2012).

However, no global consensus exists on the appropriate package of services for CHWs. The case of CHWs and misoprostol is illustrative. The WHO recommends the use of oxytocin (10 International Units, intravenous/intramuscular) as the uterotonic drug for the prevention of postpartum hemorrhage, and misoprostol (600 microgram by mouth) administered by CHWs in the absence of a skilled birth attendant (Department of Reproductive Health and Research, WHO 2012).

An RCT from Afghanistan shows that uterotonics such as misoprostol are widely accepted in communities and can potentially decrease significant postpartum hemorrhage-related maternal morbidity and mortality. Results show that of the 1,421 women in the intervention group who took misoprostol, 100 percent correctly took it after birth. In the intervention area where community-based distribution of misoprostol was introduced, near-universal uterotonic coverage (92 percent) was achieved, compared with 25 percent coverage in the control areas (Sanghvi and others 2010).

A systematic review suggests that in the community, misoprostol distribution rates during home visits were higher compared with facility-based ANC distribution. Coverage rates were also higher when CHWs and TBAs distributed misoprostol compared with ANC providers (Smith and others 2013). The review highlights that misoprostol and other uterotonics may very well be widely acceptable within the community and can be delivered by CHWs. Usage is particularly seen more in the South Asia region, with uterotonic usage rates of up to 69 percent (Flandermeyer, Stanton, and Armbruster 2010).

A community-based, cluster-RCT from Ghana evaluates the use of intramuscular oxytocin with a Uniject device delivered by a CHW. In this trial, women receiving oxytocin had a reduced risk of postpartum hemorrhage (risk ratio 0.49; 95 percent confidence interval 0.27–0.88) (Stanton and others 2013), suggesting that, with appropriate training, CHWs can deliver injectable uterotonics.

Neonatal resuscitation, the administration of intravenous antibiotics, and the management of postpartum hemorrhage with uterotonics are some of the interventions that may be appropriate for CHWs. Although promising evidence is emerging for their possible new roles, the data are still insufficient to draw a conclusion as to whether CHWs can be handed these tasks. Investigators should focus on this area of research as a promising approach in low-resource settings. However, increasing the number of tasks required from CHWs has also initiated a debate on the potential for overburdening CHWs and compromising quality.

Improving the Quality of Community-Based Care

Ensuring that care provided in communities meets quality standards is a key concern, and training and supervision are crucial mechanisms for ensuring quality care. However, training and supervisory systems are often deficient in the CHW subsystem in LMICs. Effective supervision requires that supervisors be trained and that they be provided with resources for supervision (Mason and others 2006). Training styles have evolved from being primarily classroom based into more interactive sessions, including small group discussions, clinical vignettes, and field training (Mason and others 2006). These modifications allow CHWs, especially those who are less educated or illiterate, to simulate real-life situations and be better equipped to manage such situations. Training should take into account differences in cultural and religious beliefs and particular practices of communities. A program tailored to communities' specific needs and health concerns is preferable.

Updates to technology or medical methods and practices can be communicated to CHWs through regular refresher training courses or through open lines of communication between CHWs and supervisors. Regular follow-up and evaluation of training courses will reinforce knowledge and skills as well as provide opportunities to acknowledge problems and issues that have arisen.

Poor supervision is often cited as a major constraint to improving the quality of essential health interventions and a factor in the poor performance of frontline health workers (PAIMAN 2006; WHO 2006). Effective supervision, however, can be an opportunity to show CHWs that their work is valued and motivate them (Bhutta and others 2010).

The supervision of CHWs requires that supervisors be aware of the issues and problems that CHWs face and understand gaps in capacity. The majority of CHW programs have been run at a small scale by nongovernmental organizations with the capacity to train and supervise; therefore, it was relatively easy to supervise CHWs in those programs. However, once a program is implemented at scale, government bodies need to ensure that supervision and monitoring are performed effectively and are considered to be a core pillar for successful delivery of the program. National CHW programs, which encompass CHWs in remote, rural areas, may be difficult to monitor and supervise effectively and consistently.

Leveraging Mobile Technology

Limited but increasing evidence indicates that the growing use of mobile health (mHealth) tools may increase the effectiveness of CHWs in resource-constrained settings. Mobile technology can be used for a variety of purposes, from helping CHWs collect comprehensive, timely, and precise health data to providing CHWs with information and reminders about health care practices and protocols via text messaging (Freifeld and others 2010; Guy and others 2012; Jha and others 2009; Mukund and Murray 2010). Mobile technology can also play a role in training, peer-to-peer learning, and monitoring of the performance of CHWs, in the following ways:

- A cluster RCT at rural health facilities in Kenya shows that health workers at dispensaries and rural outpatient services who received text messages on their personal mobile phones about malaria case management for six months as reminders provided better case management for malaria in children (Zurovac and others 2011).
- The Tanzania CommCare project used an automated text-message system to remotely monitor the real-time performance of midwives and provide workers with alerts and reminders to their mobile phones about past-due patient visits (Svoronos and others 2010). Compared with a group of midwives who did not receive alerts and reminders, the midwives who received these messages improved the number of timely visits to expectant mothers.
- In the Aceh-Behar midwives study in Indonesia, the use of mobile phones was positively associated with access to institutional and peer information resources, which, in turn, was positively associated with an increase in knowledge about best practices for providing obstetric care (Lee, Chib, and Kim 2011).
- The k4Health project in Malawi introduced a text-messaging network to improve the exchange and use of reproductive health and HIV/AIDS information among CHWs. After an 18-month pilot, the authors found that CHWs who used the text-message network were more likely to contact supervisors for clinical support from the field (Lemay and others 2012).

The potential for CHWs to use mobile tools to improve health service delivery in resource-limited settings is certainly great; however, a stronger evidence base is necessary to guide global health policy and program implementation.

Improving Referral Systems

CHWs are often the first line of care for many patients, such as in Pakistan, where approximately 17 percent of those who seek health care consult CHWs first. For referral systems to be effective, transportation and communications capabilities must be in place, and CHWs must be integrated into the primary health care system (figure 14.1).

Integrating CHWs into the primary health care system, as well as ensuring sufficient staffing at facilities, is vital for ensuring strong referrals and for alerting facilities of the imminent arrival of patients. The Brazilian Ministry of Health created the Family Health Program in 1993; the program placed health agents (CHWs) in teams of physicians, dentists, nurses, dental assistants, and nursing technicians, thus formally integrating the CHWs into the primary health system (Singh and Sachs 2013).

Enhancing Motivation

In the absence of appropriate compensation, along with weak supervision and monitoring systems, a lack of effort and decline in performance among CHWs has been noted (Bhutta and others 2010). CHWs, especially in low-income countries and lower-middle

income countries, may come from lower socioeconomic groups and would benefit from regular salaries. Although some may serve on a voluntary basis, full-time status would help improve performance and encourage CHWs to exert the effort necessary to deliver quality care.

Some countries are exploring the use of nonfinancial incentives to motivate CHWs. Nonfinancial incentives can also play a key role in the overall satisfaction and motivation of CHWs (Bhutta, Pariyo, and Huicho 2010). One such incentive is the certification of training so that CHWs may gain recognition from peers and work toward building a career. Recognition and the knowledge that career advancement is a possibility motivates CHWs to continually improve the quality of the care they provide. Community support, as well as professional support from superiors, is another motivating factor for overall job security and satisfaction.

Scaling Up

Scaling up health interventions includes expanding interventions, whether on a population or a geographical basis, and sustaining their use. Both require increased resources, funding, and in some cases, technical equipment.

Scale up of community mobilization efforts can be bolstered by partnerships between government and nongovernmental organizations (Coe 2001; CORE Group 2005; Howard-Grabman, Seoane, and Davenport 1994). Strong political will along with mechanisms for monitoring political commitments are essential components of implementing interventions on a large scale. Allowing communities to take an active part in the decision-making and implementation processes permits differences in culture, religion, or beliefs to be addressed and successfully planned for; this approach leads to successful intervention packages and programs that meet the populations' needs and achieve the initial goals for which they are designed. A bottom-up approach from educated communities with adequate support from reliable government and national institutions will be key for sustainable interventions.

Building Links with Community and Local Health Facilities

Primary care services need to be well linked with the community, and effective communication must be present along with feedback mechanisms so that community concerns may be conveyed to higher authorities.

We have developed an evidence-driven framework based on a continuum of care model for reproductive, maternal, neonatal, and child health (figure 14.2), highlighting several approaches that have been recognized

Figure 14.1 Linking the Places Where Care Is Given

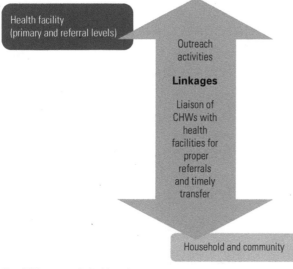

Health facility (primary and referral levels)

Outreach activities

Linkages

Liaison of CHWs with health facilities for proper referrals and timely transfer

Household and community

Note: CHWs = community health workers.

as successfully reaching communities and providing the best possible interventions. The framework (figure 14.3) portrays the essential components of a promising health care system that should be focused on integrating communities with the primary health care system. Unless these two elements can work together effectively, neither can benefit from the available resources and infrastructure. Community mobilization, home visitation, social marketing, community intervention packages, and community-based programs can be the bridge between these two levels. Once the links are firmly established, the health care system can gain substantially from the resources and support provided by national and local governments and nongovernmental organizations.

COSTS AND COST-EFFECTIVENESS OF COMMUNITY-BASED PROGRAMS

Cost-Effectiveness of Community-Based Programs

CHW program costs vary widely from country to country. The introduction of community-based interventions requires personnel, resources, training, management, and infrastructure.

Using the WHO-CHOICE model, Adam and others (2005) estimate the most cost-effective mix of interventions for countries with high adult and child mortality in Sub-Saharan Africa and South-East Asia. Interventions for newborn care at the community level were highly cost-effective, followed by ANC, skilled attendance at birth, maternal and neonatal primary

Figure 14.2 Links between Health Care Professionals and Communities

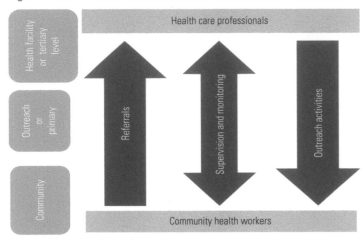

Figure 14.3 Integrated Health Care System and Approaches for Reaching Community

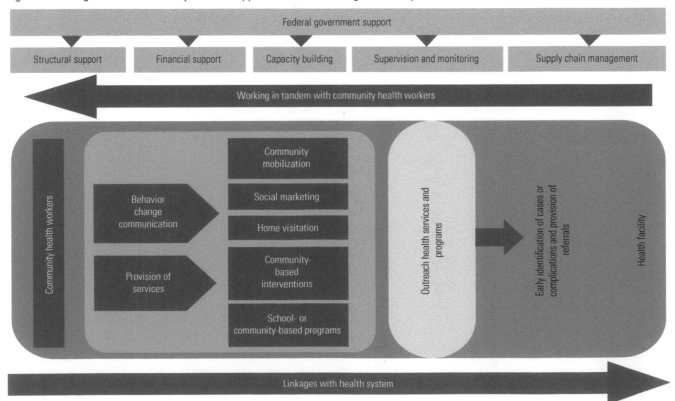

care around childbirth, and emergency perinatal and postnatal obstetric and neonatal care. Using a frequently cited threshold, interventions are considered to be cost-effective when the cost per disability-adjusted life year (DALY) averted is less than per capita gross domestic product (GDP) and very cost-effective when less than three times GDP per capita (WHO 2001).

Community-based strategies that deliver a package of child health interventions including vitamin A (Fiedler and Chuko 2008), ITN distribution (Ross and others 2011), home-based management of fever (Nonvignon and others 2012), treatment for severely malnourished children (Puett, Sadler, and others 2013; Puett, Salpéteur, and others 2013), and training TBAs to improve neonatal health (Sabin and others 2012) are cost-effective at less than US$100 per DALY averted (figure 14.4). Many of the studies rely on CHWs to deliver services, yet studies focused explicitly on the cost-effectiveness of CHWs are scarce. Lehmann and Sanders's (2007) review of the cost-effectiveness of CHW programs notes the dearth of data on the cost-effectiveness of CHW programs, despite assumptions that services provided by CHWs are expected to be less expensive and reach larger numbers of underserved people compared with clinic-based services. A similar finding is noted in a review of the cost-effectiveness

of lay health workers delivering vaccines (Corluka and others 2009). Methodologically, cost-effectiveness analyses may also miss key elements of CHW programs that enhance equity, increase communities' self-reliance, and contribute to other social benefits and community norms (Lehmann and Sanders 2007).

RCTs have also been used to generate cost-effectiveness results for community-based interventions. In a multicountry study conducted in Bangladesh (Fottrell and others 2013), India (Tripathy and others 2010), Malawi (Lewycka and others 2013), and Nepal (Manandhar and others 2004), community mobilization through women's groups was effective in preventing neonatal deaths. Using a systematic review and meta-analysis from these RCTs, Prost and others (2013) model the cost-effectiveness of women's groups for newborn care and find that the cost per averted neonatal year of life lost was US$91 in India and US$753 in Nepal, and was considered cost-effective when compared with GDP per capita. In Zambia, an RCT evaluating the Lufwanyama Neonatal Survival Project shows that training TBAs to manage birth asphyxia, hypothermia, and neonatal sepsis reduced all-cause neonatal mortality by 45 percent (Gill and others 2011) and was cost-effective for all scenarios. Scaling up the intervention from 2011 to 2020 was considered cost-effective at

Figure 14.4 Cost per DALY Averted in Community-Based Programs for Reproductive, Maternal, Newborn, and Child Health

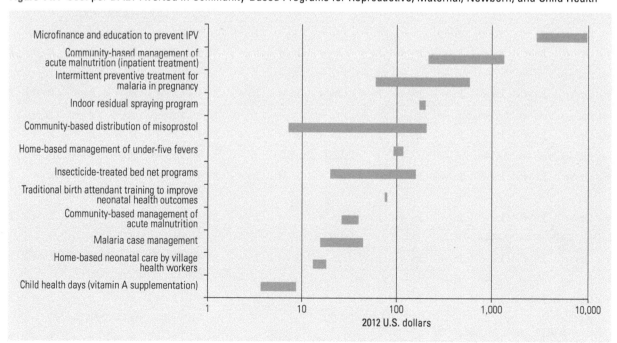

Sources: Based on Bachmann 2009; Bang, Bang, and Reddy 2005; Fiedler and Chuko 2008; Jan and others 2011; Nonvignon and others 2012; Puett and others 2013; Ross and others 2011; Sabin and others 2012; Sutherland and others 2010; Wilford, Golden, and Walker 2012; Yukich and others 2008; Yukich and others 2009.
Note: IPV = intimate partner violence.

US$74 per DALY averted at the baseline and improved to US$24 per DALY averted for an optimistic scale-up scenario. A strategy of using trained TBAs to reduce neonatal mortality can be highly cost-effective (Sabin and others 2012). Other community-based programs, such as social marketing or employer-based schemes for ITN distribution, are also cost effective at US$72 per DALY averted (Hanson and others 2003) and US$40 per DALY averted (Bhatia, Fox-Rushby, and Mills 2004), respectively.

Table 14.7 Average Intervention Costs for Community-Based RMNCH Services, 2012 U.S. Dollars

Community-based RMNCH services	Mean cost per beneficiary (range) (US$ 2012)	Sources of costs
Maternal and neonatal		
Volunteer peer counselling	$30.60 ($4.97–$68.04)	Nepal; Borghi and others (2005)
Traditional birth attendants and birth preparedness		Malawi; Lewycka and others (2013)
Home-based neonatal care		India; Bang, Bang, and others (2005)
Community health worker maternal care		Cambodia; Skinner and Rathavy (2009)
		Bangladesh; LeFevre and others (2013)
		Zambia; Sabin and others (2012)
Breastfeeding		
Peer counseling, education, and support	$166.50 ($162.55–$170.44)	Uganda; Chola and others (2011)
		South Africa; Nkonki and others (2014)
Child health		
Deworming campaigns	$3.47 ($0.34–9.69)	Lao PDR; Boselli and others (2011)
Child health days and weeks		Ethiopia; Fiedler and Chuko (2008)
		Honduras; Fiedler (2008)
		Zambia; Fiedler and others (2014)
		Somalia; Vijayaraghavan and others (2012)
		Vietnam; Casey and others (2011)
Immunization		
School-based and community-based vaccine programs	$26.75 ($3.50–$50)	South Asia; Jeuland and others (2009)
Mobile community health workers		Ecuador; San Sebastián and others (2001)
Malaria		
IPT with volunteer health workers	$5.02 ($1.350–$10.10)	Gambia, The; Bojang and others (2011)
Community health worker malaria treatment		Ghana; Nonvignon and others (2012)
		Ghana; Patouillard and others (2011)
Severe acute malnutrition		
Community-based therapeutic care	$153.85 ($116.11–$180.37)	Zambia; Bachmann (2009)
		Bangladesh; Puett, Sadler, and others (2013)
		Ethiopia; Tekeste and others (2012)
Gender-based violence		
Microfinance Gender/HIV training for prevention of GBV	$54.12	South Africa; Jan and others (2011)

Note: GBV = gender-based violence; HIV = human immunodeficiency virus; IPT = intermittent preventive treatment; RMNCH = reproductive, maternal, newborn, and child health; USD = U.S. dollars.

Costs of Community-Based Programs

On average, community-based interventions range from US$3 per beneficiary for child health days to US$166 for peer counseling, education, and support to promote breastfeeding. As seen in table 14.7, community strategies can cost as low as US$0.34 per beneficiary for a national deworming campaign in the Lao People's Democratic Republic (Boselli and others 2011) to a high of US$180.00 for community-based therapeutic care to treat severe acute malnutrition in Ethiopia (Tekeste and others 2012). The main cost drivers relate to the intensity of the intervention and the numbers covered. Even in cases in which intensive resources are required, the cost per capita can be quite low.

In Vietnam, weekly deworming and iron and folic acid supplementation delivered by CHWs to women of reproductive age required considerable resources to train caregivers and sustain the program over a year, yet the cost per woman treated was US$0.88 per year (Casey and others 2011).

A key factor in most of the studies described in table 14.7 is the reliance on CHWs to deliver services. McCord, Liu, and Singh (2013) estimate that it would cost US$2.6 billion a year to deploy CHWs to serve the entire Sub-Saharan African rural population, at a cost of US$6.86 per person for each CHW catchment area, and US$2.72 per person per year.

RESEARCH AGENDA

Since 2000, a substantial amount of research has been conducted on community based health interventions, particularly those carried out by CHWs. Yet numerous research gaps exist that, if studied, could have a significant impact on the delivery of health care. The studies available for review are mostly program evaluations without comprehensive and high-quality study designs. RCTs are limited to evaluation of interventions to improve newborn, child, and maternal outcomes.

The majority of community-based health programs are based in South Asian and Sub-Saharan African countries, and CHWs remain the core of the community-based care concept. Many program evaluations have been conducted to examine the effect of these programs on maternal and child health parameters, yet very few exist that study the quality of life and satisfaction among the CHWs themselves. There is also scarce evidence about whether the CHWs are over- or underutilized, and the impact of incentives, work hours, and job-related satisfaction on the performance of CHWs.

Evidence is also needed on the cost-effectiveness of small and large nutrition and other community-based

programs, the role of public and private partnerships, and the effect of political will and stability on health care delivery.

It is important to support routine implementation research while programs are being implemented and to identify hurdles and review and revise programs as necessary. More learning is also needed from community-based programs from HICs, with lessons adapted to LMICs.

CONCLUSIONS

As countries grow as a result of increased global economic development, existing health care systems are ill equipped to deal with the new population increments. Even with the expansion of health care systems, resources may be limited or facilities may be inaccessible to increasing segments of the population. Maternal, neonatal, and child mortality and morbidity continue to be persistent challenges, particularly in rural areas. Issues of cultural barriers, political instability, poverty, and poor educational systems contribute to ill health.

Improving reproductive, maternal, newborn, and child health requires successful community engagement. A combination of efforts is required to mobilize communities to take charge of their own needs, as well as to provide outreach activities to bring care to communities. Based on the evidence and examples mentioned in this chapter, we conclude that a bottom-up approach that actively involves communities, and that employs and recognizes CHWs as a formal cadre of the national health system, will bring about substantial changes to health care. The integration of community care subsystems into the primary care health system will have wide-ranging effects on the sustainability, effectiveness, and longevity of community health systems, bringing all closer to achieving the Millennium Development Goals.

ANNEX

The annex in this chapter is as follows. It is available at http://dcp-3.org/rmnch:

- Annex 14A. Additional Information on the Effect of Select Community-Based Interventions on Neonatal Health Indicators.

NOTES

1. The number of women who die annually during pregnancy and childbirth has fallen globally from 526,300 in 1980 to 303,000 in 2008 (Hogan and others 2010; WHO 2015). A number of countries in Sub-Saharan Africa have

halved the levels of maternal mortality since 1990 (*PLoS Medicine* Editors 2010).

2. See CCM Central (http://ccmcentral.com/about/iccm/). iCCM is typically delivered by community health workers at the community level and encompasses treatment for (1) childhood pneumonia with antibiotics, (2) diarrhea with zinc and oral rehydration solution, and (3) malaria with artemisinin combination therapy. The joint statement on iCCM also supports the identification (but not treatment) of severe acute malnutrition and home visits (but not treatment) for newborns (Bennett and others 2014; UNICEF 2012).

REFERENCES

Adam, T., S. S. Lim, S. Mehta, Z. A. Bhutta, H. Fogstad, and others. 2005. "Cost Effectiveness Analysis of Strategies for Maternal and Neonatal Health in Developing Countries." *British Medical Journal* 331 (7525): 1107.

Arifeen, S. E., D. M. Hoque, T. Akter, M. Rahman, M. E. Hoque, and others. 2009. "Effect of the Integrated Management of Childhood Illness Strategy on Childhood Mortality and Nutrition in a Rural Area in Bangladesh: A Cluster Randomised Trial." *The Lancet* 374 (9687): 393–403.

Arshad, A., R. A. Salam, Z. S. Lassi, J. K. Das, I. Naqvi, and others. 2014. "Community Based Interventions for the Prevention and Control of Tuberculosis." *Infectious Diseases of Poverty* 3: 27.

Azad, K., S. Barnett, B. Banerjee, S. Shaha, K. Khan, and others. 2010. "Effect of Scaling Up Women's Groups on Birth Outcomes in Three Rural Districts in Bangladesh: A Cluster-Randomised Controlled Trial." *The Lancet* 375 (9721): 1193–202.

Bachmann, M. O. 2009. "Cost Effectiveness of Community-Based Therapeutic Care for Children with Severe Acute Malnutrition in Zambia: Decision Tree Model." *Cost Effectiveness and Resource Allocation* 7: 2.

Balachander, J. 1993. "Tamil Nadu's Successful Nutrition Effort." In *Reaching Health for All*, edited by J. Rohde, M. Chatterjee, and D. Morley. Delhi, India: Oxford University Press.

Bang, A. T., R. A. Bang, S. B. Baitule, M. H. Reddy, and M. D. Deshmukh. 1999. "Effect of Home-Based Neonatal Care and Management of Sepsis on Neonatal Mortality: Field Trial in Rural India." *The Lancet* 354 (9194): 1955–61.

———. 2005. "Management of Birth Asphyxia in Home Deliveries in Rural Gadchiroli: The Effect of Two Types of Birth Attendants and of Resuscitating with Mouth-to-Mouth, Tube-Mask or Bag-Mask." *Journal of Perinatology* 25 (1): S82–91.

Bang, A. T., R. A. Bang, and H. M. Reddy. 2005. "Home-Based Neonatal Care: Summary and Applications of the Field Trial in Rural Gadchiroli, India (1993 to 2003)." *Journal of Perinatology* 25: S108–22.

Bang, A. T., H. M. Reddy, M. D. Deshmukh, S. B. Baitule, and R. A. Bang. 2005. "Neonatal and Infant Mortality in the Ten years (1993 to 2003) of the Gadchiroli Field Trial: Effect of Home-Based Neonatal Care." *Journal of Perinatology* 25: S92–107.

Baqui, A. H., S. El-Arifeen, G. L. Darmstadt, S. Ahmed, E. K. Williams, and others. 2008. "Effect of Community-Based Newborn-Care Intervention Package Implemented through Two Service-Delivery Strategies in Sylhet District, Bangladesh: A Cluster-Randomised Controlled Trial." *The Lancet* 371 (9628): 1936–44.

Bari, S., I. Mannan, M. A. Rahman, G. L. Darmstadt, M. H. R. Seraji, and others. 2006. "Trends in Use of Referral Hospital Services for Care of Sick Newborns in a Community-Based Intervention in Tangail District, Bangladesh." *Journal of Health, Population, and Nutrition* 24 (4): 519–29.

Bayer, A. 2001. *Executive Summary: Maternal Mortality and Morbidity*. Population Resource Center.

Bennett, S., A. George, D. Rodriguez, J. Shearer, B. Diallo, and others. 2014. "Policy Challenges Facing Integrated Community Case Management in Sub-Saharan Africa." *Tropical Medicine and International Health* 19 (7): 872–82.

Bhandari, N., R. Bahl, V. Bhatnagar, and M. K. Bhan. 1996. "Treating Sick Young Infants in Urban Slum Setting." *The Lancet* 347 (9017): 1774–75.

Bhatia, M. R., J. Fox-Rushby, and A. Mills. 2004. "Cost-Effectiveness of Malaria Control Interventions when Malaria Mortality Is Low: Insecticide-Treated Nets versus In-House Residual Spraying in India." *Social Science and Medicine* 59 (3): 525–39.

Bhutta, Z. A., J. K. Das, A. Rizvi, M. F. Gaffey, N. Walker, and others. 2013. "Evidence-Based Interventions for Improvement of Maternal and Child Nutrition: What Can Be Done and at What Cost?" *The Lancet* 382 (9890): 452–77.

Bhutta, Z. A., and Z. S. Lassi. 2010. "Empowering Communities for Maternal and Newborn Health." *The Lancet* 375 (9721): 1142–44.

Bhutta, Z. A., Z. S. Lassi, G. Pariyo, and L. Huicho. 2010. *Global Experience of Community Health Workers for Delivery of Health Related Millennium Development Goals: A Systematic Review, Country Case Studies, and Recommendations for Integration into National Health Systems*. Geneva: Global Health Workforce Alliance.

Bhutta, Z. A., Z. A. Memon, S. Soofi, M. S. Salat, S. Cousens, and others. 2008. "Implementing Community-Based Perinatal Care: Results from a Pilot Study in Rural Pakistan." *Bulletin of the World Health Organization* 86 (6): 452–59.

Black, R. E., C. G. Victora, S. P. Walker, Z. A. Bhutta, P. Christian, and others. 2013. "Maternal and Child Undernutrition and Overweight in Low-Income and Middle-Income Countries." *The Lancet* 382 (9890): 427–51.

Bojang, K. A., F. Akor, L. Conteh, E. Webb, O. Bittaye, and others. 2011. "Two Strategies for the Delivery of IPTc in an Area of Seasonal Malaria Transmission in The Gambia: A Randomised Controlled Trial." *PLoS Medicine* 8 (2): e1000409.

Borghi, J., B. Thapa, D. Osrin, S. Jan, J. Morrison, and others. 2005. "Economic Assessment of a Women's Group Intervention to Improve Birth Outcomes in Rural Nepal." *The Lancet* 366 (500): 1882–84.

Boselli, G., A. Yajima, P. E. Aratchige, K. E. Feldon, A. Xeuatvongsa, and others. 2011. "Integration of Deworming into an Existing Immunisation and Vitamin A Supplementation Campaign Is a Highly Effective Approach to Maximise Health Benefits with Minimal Cost in Lao PDR." *International Health* 3 (4): 240–45.

Bundy, D., N. de Silva, S. Horton, D. T. Jamison, and G. Patton, editors. Forthcoming. *Disease Control Priorities* (third edition): Volume 8, *Child and Adolescent Development.* Washington, DC: World Bank.

Casey, G. J., D. Sartori, S. E. Horton, T. Q. Phuc, L. B. Phu, and others. 2011. "Weekly Iron-Folic Acid Supplementation with Regular Deworming Is Cost-Effective in Preventing Anaemia in Women of Reproductive Age in Vietnam." *PLoS One* 6 (9): e23723.

Central Bureau of Statistics. 2001. *Statistical Year Book of Nepal 2001.* Kathmandu: Government of Nepal, National Planning Commission Secretariat.

Chola, L., L. Nkonki, C. Kankasa, J. Nankunda, J. Tumwine, and others. 2011. "Cost of Individual Peer Counselling for the Promotion of Exclusive Breastfeeding in Uganda." *Cost Effectiveness and Resource Allocation* 9 (1): 11.

Coe, A. 2001. "Health, Rights and Realities: An Analysis of the ReproSalud Project in Peru." Center for Health and Gender Equity Working Paper, Takoma Park, MD. http://www.popline.org/node/253834.

CORE Group. 2005. "'Scale' and Scaling Up: A CORE Group Background Paper on 'Scaling Up' Maternal, Newborn and Child Health Services." http://www.coregroup.org/resources/meetings/april05/Scaling_Up_Background_Paper_7-13.pdf.

Corluka, A., D. G. Walker, S. Lewin, C. Glenton, and I. B. Scheel. 2009. "Are Vaccination Programmes Delivered by Lay Health Workers Cost-Effective? A Systematic Review." *Human Resources for Health* 7 (1): 81.

Das, J., Z. Lassi, R. Salam, and Z. Bhutta. 2013. "Effect of Community Based Interventions on Childhood Diarrhea and Pneumonia: Uptake of Treatment Modalities and Impact on Mortality." *BMC Public Health* 13 (Suppl. 3): S29.

Dean, S. V., A. M. Imam, Z. S. Lassi, and Z. A. Bhutta. 2011. *Systematic Review of Preconception Risks and Interventions.* Karachi, Pakistan: Aga Khan University. http://globalresearchnurses.tghn.org/site_media/media/articles/Preconception_Report.pdf.

Department of Reproductive Health and Research, WHO (World Health Organization). 2012. *WHO Recommendations for the Prevention and Treatment of Postpartum Haemorrhage.* Geneva: WHO. http://www.who.int/iris/bitstream/10665/75411/1/9789241548502_eng.pdf.

do Monte, C. M., A. Ashworth, M. L. Sa, and R. L. Diniz. 1998. "Effectiveness of Nutrition Centers in Ceara State, Northeastern Brazil." *Revista Panamericana de Salud Pública* 4 (6): 375–82.

Fiedler, J. L., and T. Chuko. 2008. "The Cost of Child Health Days: A Case Study of Ethiopia's Enhanced Outreach Strategy (EOS)." *Health Policy and Planning* 23 (4): 222–33.

Fiedler, J. L., F. Mubanga, W. Siamusantu, M. Musonda, K. F. Kabwe, and others. 2014. "Child Health Week in Zambia: Costs, Efficiency, Coverage and a Reassessment of Need." *Health Policy and Planning* 29 (1): 12–29.

Flandermeyer, D., C. Stanton, and D. Armbruster. 2010. "Uterotonic Use at Home Births in Low-Income Countries: A Literature Review." *International Journal of Gynaecology and Obstetrics* 108 (3): 269–75.

Fottrell, E., K. Azad, A. Kuddus, L. Younes, S. Shaha, and others. 2013. "The Effect of Increased Coverage of Participatory Women's Groups on Neonatal Mortality in Bangladesh: A Cluster Randomized Trial." *JAMA Pediatrics* 167 (9): 816–25.

Freifeld, C. C., R. Chunara, S. R. Mekaru, E. H. Chan, T. Kass-Hout, and others. 2010. "Participatory Epidemiology: Use of Mobile Phones for Community-Based Health Reporting." *PLoS Medicine* 7 (12): e1000376.

Getachew, I. 2011. "Community-Based Nutrition Programme Targets Children at Risk in Ethiopia." United Nations Children's Fund, New York. http://www.unicef.org/infobycountry/ethiopia_59657.html.

Gill, C. J., G. Phiri-Mazala, N. G. Guerina, J. Kasimba, C. Mulenga, and others. 2011. "Effect of Training Traditional Birth Attendants on Neonatal Mortality (Lufwanyama Neonatal Survival Project): Randomised Controlled Study." *British Medical Journal* 342: d346.

Gogia, S., and H. S. Sachdev. 2010. "Home Visits by Community Health Workers to Prevent Neonatal Deaths in Developing Countries: A Systematic Review." *Bulletin of the World Health Organization* 88 (9): 658–66B.

Gupta, A., S. K. Gupta, and N. Baridalyne. 2013. "Integrated Child Development Services (ICDS) Schemes: A Journey of 37 Years." *Indian Journal of Community Health* 25 (1): 77–81.

Guy, R., J. Hocking, H. Wand, S. Stott, H. Ali, and others. 2012. "How Effective Are Short Message Service Reminders at Increasing Clinic Attendance? A Meta-Analysis and Systematic Review." *Health Service Research* 47 (2): 614–32.

Hanson, K., N. Kikumbih, J. Armstrong Schellenberg, H. Mponda, R. Nathan, and others. 2003. "Cost-Effectiveness of Social Marketing of Insecticide-Treated Nets for Malaria Control in the United Republic of Tanzania." *Bulletin of the World Health Organization* 81 (4): 269–76.

Hogan, M. C., K. J. Foreman, M. Naghavi, S. Y. Ahn, M. Wang, and others. 2010. "Maternal Mortality for 181 Countries, 1980–2008: A Systematic Analysis of Progress towards Millennium Development Goal 5." *The Lancet* 375 (9726): 1609–23.

Holmes, K. K., S. Bertozzi, B. Bloom, P. Jha, and R. Nugent, editors. Forthcoming. *Disease Control Priorities* (third edition): Volume 6, *HIV/AIDS, STIs, Tuberculosis, and Malaria.* Washington, DC: World Bank.

Howard-Grabman, L., G. Seoane, and C. Davenport. 1994. *The Warmi Project: A Participatory Approach to Improve Maternal and Neonatal Health: An Implementor's Manual.* Arlington, VA: John Snow, Mother Care.

Jan, S., G. Ferrari, C. H. Watts, J. R. Hargreaves, J. C. Kim, and others. 2011. "Economic Evaluation of a Combined Microfinance and Gender Training Intervention for the Prevention of Intimate Partner Violence in Rural South Africa." *Health Policy and Planning* 26 (5): 366–72.

Jeuland, M., J. Cook, C. Poulos, J. Clemens, and D. Whittington. 2009. "Cost-Effectivenes of New-Generation Oral Cholera Vaccines: A Multistate Analysis." *Value in Health* 12 (6): 899–908.

Jha, A. K., C. M. DesRoches, E. G. Campbell, K. Donelan, S. R. Rao, and others. 2009. "Use of Electronic Health Records in U.S. Hospitals." *New England Journal of Medicine* 360 (16): 1628–38.

Kerber, K. J., J. E. de Graft-Johnson, Z. A. Bhutta, P. Okong, A. Starrs, and others. 2007. "Continuum of Care for Maternal, Newborn, and Child Health: From Slogan to Service Delivery." *The Lancet* 370 (9595): 1358–69.

Kidane, G., and R. H. Morrow. 2000. "Teaching Mothers to Provide Home Treatment of Malaria in Tigray, Ethiopia: A Randomised Trial." *The Lancet* 356 (9229): 550–55.

Kidney, E., H. R. Winter, K. S. Khan, A. M. Gülmezoglu, C. A. Meads, and others. 2009. "Systematic Review of Effect of Community-Level Interventions to Reduce Maternal Mortality." *BMC Pregnancy and Childbirth* 9: 2.

Kumar, V., S. Mohanty, A. Kumar, R. P. Misra, M. Santosham, and others. 2008. "Effect of Community-Based Behaviour Change Management on Neonatal Mortality in Shivgarh, Uttar Pradesh, India: A Cluster-Randomised Controlled Trial." *The Lancet* 372 (9644): 1151–62.

Lassi, Z. S., B. A. Haider, and Z. A. Bhutta. 2010. "Community-Based Intervention Packages for Reducing Maternal and Neonatal Morbidity and Mortality and Improving Neonatal Outcomes." *Cochrane Database of Systematic Reviews* 10 (11): CD007754.

Lassi, Z. S., A. Majeed, S. Rashid, M. Y. Yakoob, and Z. A. Bhutta. 2013. "The Interconnections between Maternal and Newborn Health—Evidence and Implications for Policy." *Journal of Maternal-Fetal and Neonatal Medicine* 26 (Suppl. 1): 3–53.

Lee, S., A. Chib, and J. N. Kim. 2011. "Midwives' Cell Phone Use and Health Knowledge in Rural Communities." *Journal of Health Communication* 16 (9): 1006–23.

LeFevre, A. E., S. D. Shillcutt, H. R. Waters, S. Haider, S. El Arifeen, and others. 2013. "Economic Evaluation of Neonatal Care Packages in a Cluster-Randomized Controlled Trial in Sylhet, Bangladesh." *Bulletin of the World Health Organization* 91 (10): 736–45.

Lehmann, U., and D. Sanders. 2007. "Community Health Workers: What Do We Know about Them? The State of the Evidence on Programmes, Activities, Costs and Impact on Health Outcomes of Using Community Health Workers." School of Public Health, University of the Western Cape.

Lemay, N. V., T. Sullivan, B. Jumbe, and C. P. Perry. 2012. "Reaching Remote Health Workers in Malawi: Baseline Assessment of a Pilot mHealth Intervention." *Journal of Health Communications* 17 (Suppl. 1): 105–17.

Lewin, S., S. Munabi-Babigumira, C. Glenton, K. Daniels, X. Bosch-Capblanch, and others. 2010. "Lay Health Workers in Primary and Community Health Care for Maternal and Child Health and the Management of Infectious Diseases." *Cochrane Database of Systematic Reviews* 3 (3): CD004015.

Lewycka, S., C. Mwansambo, M. Rosato, P. Kazembe, T. Phiri, and others. 2013. "Effect of Women's Groups and Volunteer Peer Counselling on Rates of Mortality, Morbidity, and Health Behaviours in Mothers and Children in Rural Malawi (MaiMwana): A Factorial, Cluster-Randomised Controlled Trial." *The Lancet* 381 (9879): 1721–35.

Liu, L., K. Hill, S. Oza, D. Hogan, S. Cousens, and others. 2016. "Levels and Causes of Mortality under Age Five." In *Disease Control Priorities* (third edition): Volume 2, *Reproductive, Maternal, Newborn, and Child Health*, edited by R. E. Black, R. Laxminarayan, N. Walker, and M. Temmerman. Washington, DC: World Bank.

Lozano, R., H. Wang, K. J. Foreman, J. K. Rajaratnam, M. Naghavi, and others. 2011. "Progress towards Millennium Development Goals 4 and 5 on Maternal and Child Mortality: An Updated Systematic Analysis." *The Lancet* 378 (9797): 1139–65.

Manandhar, D. S., D. Osrin, B. P. Shrestha, N. Mesko, J. Morrison, and others. 2004. "Effect of a Participatory Intervention with Women's Groups on Birth Outcomes in Nepal: Cluster-Randomised Controlled Trial." *The Lancet* 364 (9438): 970–79.

Mason, J. B., D. Sanders, P. Musgrove, Soekirman, and R. Galloway. 2006. "Community Health and Nutrition Programs." In *Disease Control Priorities in Developing Countries*, 2nd ed., edited by D. T. Jamison, J. G. Breman, A. R. Measham, G. Alleyne, M. Claeson, D. B. Evans, P. Jha, A. Mills, and P. Musgrove, 1053–74. Washington, DC: World Bank and Oxford University Press.

McCord, G. C., A. Liu, and P. Singh. 2013. "Deployment of Community Health Workers across Rural Sub-Saharan Africa: Financial Considerations and Operational Assumptions." *Bulletin of the World Health Organization* 91 (4): 244–53b.

Medhanyie, A., M. Spigt, Y. Kifle, N. Schaay, D. Sanders, and others. 2012. "The Role of Health Extension Workers in Improving Utilization of Maternal Health Services in Rural Areas in Ethiopia: A Cross-Sectional Study." *BMC Health Services Research* 12 (1): 352.

Mukund, B. K. C., and P. J. Murray. 2010. "Cell Phone Short Messaging Service (SMS) for HIV/AIDS in South Africa: A Literature Review." *Studies in Health, Technology and Information* 160 (Pt 1): 530–34.

Newton, O., and M. English. 2006. "Newborn Resuscitation: Defining Best Practice for Low-Income Settings." *Transactions of the Royal Society of Tropical Medicine and Hygiene* 100 (10): 899–908.

Nguyen, D. T., K. K. Leung, L. McIntyre, W. A. Ghali, and R. Sauve. 2013. "Does Integrated Management of Childhood Illness (IMCI) Training Improve the Skills of Health Workers? A Systematic Review and Meta-Analysis." *PLoS One* 8 (6): e66030.

Nkonki, L. L., E. Daviaud, D. Jackson, L. Chola, T. Doherty, and others. 2014. "Costs of Promoting Exclusive Breastfeeding at Community Level in Three Sites in South Africa." *PLoS One* 9 (1): e79784.

Nonvignon, J., M. A. Chinbuah, M. Gyapong, M. Abbey, E. Awini, and others. 2012. "Is Home Management of Fevers a Cost-Effective Way of Reducing Under-Five Mortality in Africa? The Case of a Rural Ghanaian District." *Tropical Medicine and International Health* 17 (8): 951–57.

Olds, D. L., J. Robinson, L. Pettitt, D. W. Luckey, J. Holmberg, and others. 2004. "Effect of Home Visits by Paraprofessionals and by Nurses: Age 4 Follow-Up Results of a Randomized Trial." *Pediatrics* 114 (6): 1560–68.

PAIMAN (Pakistan Initiative for Mothers and Newborns). 2006. "Assessment of District Health Supervisory System." Report. Islamabad, Pakistan. http://paiman.jsi.com/Resources/Docs/assessment-of-district-health-supervisory-system.pdf.

Patouillard, E., L. Conteh, J. Webster, M. Kweku, D. Chandramohan, and others. 2011. "Coverage, Adherence and Costs of Intermittent Preventive Treatment of Malaria in Children Employing Different Delivery Strategies in Jasikan, Ghana." *PLoS One* 6 (11): e24871.

PLoS Medicine Editors. 2010. "Maternal Health: Time to Deliver." *PLoS Medicine* 7 (6): e1000300.

Pradhan, A., and E. R. A. New. 1997. *Nepal Family Health Survey, 1996.* Family Health Division, Department of Health Services, Ministry of Health, Government of Nepal.

Prost, A., T. Colbourn, N. Seward, K. Azad, A. Coomarasamy, and others. 2013. "Women's Groups Practising Participatory Learning and Action to Improve Maternal and Newborn Health in Low-Resource Settings: A Systematic Review and Meta-Analysis." *The Lancet* 381 (9879): 1736–46.

Puett, C., K. Sadler, H. Alderman, J. Coates, J. L. Fiedler, and others. 2013. "Cost-Effectiveness of the Community-Based Management of Severe Acute Malnutrition by Community Health Workers in Southern Bangladesh." *Health Policy and Planning* 28 (4): 386–99.

Puett, C., C. Salpéteur, E. Lacroix, F. Houngbé, M. Aït-Aïssa, and others. 2013. "Protecting Child Health and Nutrition Status with Ready-to-Use Food in Addition to Food Assistance in Urban Chad: A Cost-Effectiveness Analysis." *Cost Effectiveness and Resource Allocation* 11 (1): 27.

Ricca, J., N. Kureshy, K. Leban, D. Prosnitz, and L. Ryan. 2013. "Community-Based Intervention Packages Facilitated by NGOs Demonstrate Plausible Evidence for Child Mortality Impact." *Health Policy and Planning* 29 (2): 204–16.

Ronsmans, C., M. E. Chowdhury, S. K. Dasgupta, A. Ahmed, and M. Koblinsky. 2010. "Effect of Parent's Death on Child Survival in Rural Bangladesh: A Cohort Study." *The Lancet* 375 (9730): 2024–31.

Rosato, M., G. Laverack, L. H. Grabman, P. Tripathy, N. Nair, and others. 2008. "Community Participation: Lessons for Maternal, Newborn, and Child Health." *The Lancet* 372 (9642): 962–71.

Ross, A., N. Maire, E. Sicuri, T. Smith, and L. Conteh. 2011. "Determinants of the Cost-Effectiveness of Intermittent Preventive Treatment for Malaria in Infants and Children." *PLoS One* 6 (4): e18391.

Sabin, L. L., A. B. Knapp, W. B. MacLeod, G. Phiri-Mazala, J. Kasimba, and others. 2012. "Costs and Cost-Effectiveness of Training Traditional Birth Attendants to Reduce Neonatal Mortality in the Lufwanyama Neonatal Survival Study (LUNESP)." *PLoS One* 7 (4): e35560.

Salam, R. A., J. K. Das, Z. S. Lassi, and Z. A. Bhutta. 2014. "Impact of Community-Based Interventions for the Prevention and Control of Malaria on Intervention Coverage and Health Outcomes for the Prevention and Control of Malaria." *Infectious Diseases of Poverty* 3: 25.

Salam, R. A., S. D. Haroon, H. H. Ahmed, J. K. Das, and Z. A. Bhutta. 2014. "Impact of Community-Based Interventions on HIV Knowledge, Attitudes, and Transmission." *Infections Disease of Poverty* 3:36. doi:10.1186/2049-9957-3-26.

Salam, R. A., H. Maredia, J. K. Das, Z. S. Lassi, and Z. A. Bhutta. 2014. "Community-Based Interventions for the Prevention and Control of Helmintic Neglected Tropical Diseases." *Infectious Diseases of Poverty* 3: 23.

San Sebastián, M., I. Goicolea, J. Avilés, and M. Narváez. 2001. "Improving Immunization Coverage in Rural Areas of Ecuador: A Cost-Effectiveness Analysis." *Tropical Doctor* 31 (1): 21–24.

Sanghvi, H., N. Ansari, N. J. Prata, H. Gibson, A. T. Ehsan, and others. 2010. "Prevention of Postpartum Hemorrhage at Home Birth in Afghanistan." *International Journal of Gynaecology and Obstetrics* 108 (3): 276–81.

Sazawal, S., and R. E. Black. 2003. "Effect of Pneumonia Case Management on Mortality in Neonates, Infants, and Preschool Children: A Meta-Analysis of Community-Based Trials." *Lancet Infectious Disease* 3 (9): 547–56.

Schiffman, J., G. L. Darmstadt, S. Agarwal, and A. H. Baqui. 2010. "Community-Based Intervention Packages for Improving Perinatal Health in Developing Countries: A Review of the Evidence." *Seminars in Perinatology* 34 (6): 462–76.

Sines, E., A. Tinker, and J. Ruben. 2006. "The Maternal–Newborn–Child Health Continuum of Care: A Collective Effort to Save Lives." Washington, DC: Save the Children and Population Reference Bureau. www.prb.org/pdf06/snl-contofcare_eng.pdf.

Singh, P., and J. D. Sachs. 2013. "1 million Community Health Workers in Sub-Saharan Africa by 2015." *The Lancet* 382 (9889): 363–65.

Skinner, J., and T. Rathavy. 2009. "Design and Evaluation of a Community Participatory, Birth Preparedness Project in Cambodia." *Midwifery* 25 (6): 738–43.

Smith, J. M., R. Gubin, M. Holston, J. Fullerton, and N. Prata. 2013. "Misoprostol for Postpartum Hemorrhage Prevention at Home Birth: An Integrative Review of Global Implementation Experience to Date." *BMC Pregnancy and Childbirth* 13 (1): 44.

Stanton, C. K., S. Newton, L. C. Mullany, P. Cofie, C. Tawiah Agyemang, and others. 2013. "Effect on Postpartum Hemorrhage of Prophylactic Oxytocin (10 IU) by Injection by Community Health Officers in Ghana: A Community-Based, Cluster-Randomized Trial." *PLoS Medicine* 10 (10): e1001524.

Sutherland, T., C. Meyer, D. M. Bishai, S. Geller, and S. Miller. 2010. "Community-Based Distribution of Misoprostol for Treatment or Prevention of Postpartum Hemorrhage: Cost-Effectiveness, Mortality, and Morbidity Reduction

Analysis." *International Journal of Gynecology and Obstetrics* 108 (3): 289–94.

Svoronos, T., D. Mjungu, P. Dhadialla, R. Luk, and C. Zue. 2010. "Automated Quality Improvement to Strengthen Community-Based Health: The Need for Quality Improvement for CHWs." Program for Health Systems, Development and Research, Center for Global Health and Economic Development, The Earth Institute, Columbia University, New York, NY.

Tekeste, A., M. Wondafrash, G. Azene, and K. Deribe. 2012. "Cost Effectiveness of Community-Based and In-Patient Therapeutic Feeding Programs to Treat Severe Acute Malnutrition in Ethiopia." *Cost-Effectiveness and Resource Allocation* 10 (4): 1–10.

Theodoratou, E., S. Al-Jilaihawi, F. Woodward, J. Ferguson, A. Jhass, and others. 2010. "The Effect of Case Management on Childhood Pneumonia Mortality in Developing Countries." *International Journal of Epidemiology* 39 (Suppl. 1): i155–71.

Tripathy, P., N. Nair, S. Barnett, R. Mahapatra, J. Borghi, and others. 2010. "Effect of a Participatory Intervention with Women's Groups on Birth Outcomes and Maternal Depression in Jharkhand and Orissa, India: A Cluster-Randomised Controlled Trial." *The Lancet* 375 (9721): 1182–92.

UNFPA (United Nations Population Fund) and Guttmacher Institute. 2010. *Adding It Up: The Benefits of Investing in Sexual and Reproductive Health Care.* New York: Guttmacher Institute.

UNICEF (United Nations Children's Fund). 2012. *Levels and Trends in Child Mortality 2012: Estimates Developed by the UN Inter-agency Group for Child Mortality Estimation.* New York: UNICEF.

Vijayaraghavan, M., A. Wallace, I. R. Mirza, R. Kamadjeu, R. Nandy, and others. 2012. "Economic Evaluation of a Child Health Days Strategy to Deliver Multiple Maternal and Child Health Interventions in Somalia." *Journal of Infectious Diseases* 205 (Suppl. 1): S134–40.

Wall, S. N., A. C. Lee, S. Niermeyer, M. English, W. J. Keenan, and others. 2009. "Neonatal Resuscitation in Low-Resource Settings: What, Who, and How to Overcome Challenges to Scale Up?" *International Journal of Gynaecology and Obstetrics* 107 (Suppl. 1): S47–62.

WHO (World Health Organization). 1979. *Alma-Ata 1978: Primary Health Care.* Report of the International Conference on Primary Health Care, Alma-Ata, USSR. Geneva: WHO.

———. 1986. *Ottawa Charter for Health Promotion.* Geneva: WHO. http://www.who.int/healthpromotion/conferences /previous/ottawa/en/.

———. 2001. *Macroeconomics and Health: Investing in Health for Economic Development.* Geneva: WHO. http://www.who.int/macrohealth/infocentre/advocacy/en /investinginhealth02052003.pdf.

———. 2006. "Improving Health Worker Performance: In Search of Promising Practices." Report. WHO, Geneva. http://www.who.int/hrh/resources/improving _hw_performance.pdf.

———. 2008. *The World Health Report 2008: Primary Health Care Now More Than Ever.* Geneva: WHO.

———. 2011. *Rio Political Declaration on Social Determinants of Health.* Rio de Janeiro: WHO.

———. 2012. "WHO Recommendations: Optimizing Health Worker Roles to Improve Access to Key Maternal and Newborn Health Interventions through Task Shifting." WHO, Geneva.

———. 2015. *Trends in Maternal Mortality: 1990 to 2015— Estimates by WHO, UNFPA, The World Bank, and the United Nations Population Division.* Geneva: WHO.

Wilford, R., K. Golden, and D. G. Walker. 2012. "Cost-Effectiveness of Community-Based Management of Acute Malnutrition in Malawi." *Health Policy and Planning* 27 (2): 127–37.

World Bank. 2005. "Persistent Child Undernutrition and India's ICDS Program." South Asia Human Development Sector. World Bank, Washington, DC.

———. 2012. "Ethiopia Community-Based Nutrition Program Helps Reduce Child Malnutrition." World Bank, Washington, DC. http://www.worldbank.org/en/news /feature/2012/10/16/ethiopia-community-based-nutrition -program-helps-reduce-child-malnutrition.

Yambi, O., and R. Mlolwa. 1992. "Improving Nutrition in Tanzania in the 1980s: The Iringa Experience." UNICEF, International Child Development Centre.

Yeboah-Antwi, K., P. Pilingana, W. B. Macleod, K. Semrau, K. Siazeele, and others. 2010. "Community Case Management of Fever Due to Malaria and Pneumonia in Children under Five in Zambia: A Cluster Randomized Controlled Trial." *PLoS Medicine* 7 (9): e1000340

Yukich, J. O., C. Lengeler, F. Tediosi, N. Brown, J. A. Mulligan, and others. 2008. "Costs and Consequences of Large-Scale Vector Control for Malaria." *Malaria Journal* 7 (1): 1.

Yukich, J. O., M. Zerom, T. Ghebremeskel, F. Tediosi, and C. Lengeler. 2009. "Costs and Cost-Effectiveness of Vector Control in Eritrea Using Insecticide-Treated Bed Nets." *Malaria Journal* 8 (1): 1–14.

Zurovac, D., R. K. Sudoi, W. S. Akhwale, M. Ndiritu, D. H. Hamer, and others. 2011. "The Effect of Mobile Phone Text-Message Reminders on Kenyan Health Workers' Adherence to Malaria Treatment Guidelines: A Cluster Randomised Trial." *The Lancet* 378 (9793): 795–803.

15

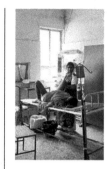

Innovations to Expand Access and Improve Quality of Health Services

Lori A. Bollinger and Margaret E. Kruk

INTRODUCTION

The first two editions of *Disease Control Priorities* contained extensive discussions of which health care services should be delivered to reduce the global burden of disease for a wide variety of diseases. These editions also provided justification, including by calculating cost-effectiveness ratios, for prioritizing the particular interventions (Jamison and others 1993; Jamison and others 2006). There was, however, little discussion of which service delivery platforms could be used to deliver the prioritized health care services.

To facilitate this discussion, we describe the existing health care service delivery mechanisms for reproductive, maternal, newborn, and child health (RMNCH) that are not community based. (The availability of community-based RMNCH service delivery is discussed in chapter 14 of this volume, Lassi, Kumar, and Bhutta 2016). We discuss different ways of organizing service delivery, including innovative approaches and their impacts on the quality of services delivered.

We begin with a landscape analysis of RMNCH indicators, organized by the conceptual framework used throughout this volume and described in detail in chapter 1: structure, including human resources; process; and outcomes. We next discuss different ways of organizing service delivery for RMNCH, including task-shifting, as well as examples unrelated to personnel. We examine coverage gaps and efforts to boost coverage, and we describe innovations to improve quality. Although evidence exists regarding the benefits of increasing coverage with innovative methods, little support is available on the effects of this increased coverage on quality. This paucity of data is due partly to a lack of an agreed-upon methodological framework, as well as to the poor quality of studies that do attempt to evaluate the innovative interventions.

LANDSCAPE ANALYSIS OF INDICATORS

To ensure the most consistent and comparable results, we present data from the World Bank World Development Indicators database, retrieving the most recent data for each country and averaging across available countries for each indicator to calculate regional averages for low- and middle-income countries (LMICs) in six regions: East Asia and Pacific, Europe and Central Asia, Latin America and the Caribbean, the Middle East and North Africa, South Asia, and Sub-Saharan Africa.

- First, we discuss indicators that represent the structure of the service delivery platforms, measured by the number of nurses and midwives per 1,000 people, the number of physicians per 1,000 people, and the number of hospital beds per 1,000 people.
- Second, we present indicators measuring the process of health care service delivery. For children, these are the

Corresponding author: Lori A. Bollinger, Avenir Health, Glastonbury, Connecticut, United States, LBollinger@avenirhealth.org.

percentage of children under age five years being taken to health providers for treatment of acute respiratory infection, the percentage under age five years with a fever receiving antimalarial drugs, and the percentage under age five years receiving a packet of oral rehydration solution for the treatment of diarrhea. For women, these indicators are the percentage of births being attended by skilled health staff and the percentage of pregnant women receiving antenatal care.

- Finally, we examine indicators for outcome measures. For children, these are the percentage ages 12–23 months being immunized against diphtheria, pertussis, and tetanus (DPT); the percentage ages 12–23 months being immunized against measles; the percentage of newborns being immunized against tetanus; the percentage under age five years using insecticide-treated bednets; and the percentage ages 6–59 months receiving vitamin A supplementation. For women, this is the percentage of married or in-union women ages 15–49 years having an unmet need for contraception.

Structure of Service Delivery Platforms

Dramatic differences in absolute numbers of structural resources can be seen across regions. Europe and Central Asia contain the highest average number of resources, while South Asia and Sub-Saharan Africa contain the lowest.

Of the 49 countries that the World Bank has categorized as low income, only five meet the minimum standard established by the World Health Organization (WHO) of 23 nurses, midwives, and physicians per 10,000 population (Global Health Workforce Statistics, http://www.who.int/hrh/workforce).

A number of structural resources is associated with each region (table 15.1, panel A).

Number of Nurses and Midwives per 1,000 People

Europe and Central Asia has 5.36 nurses and midwives per 1,000 people, almost twice as many as the next three best-served regions: Latin America and the Caribbean (2.76), East Asia and Pacific (2.52), and the Middle East and North Africa (2.40). After these four regions, the number of nurses and midwives per 1,000 people drops dramatically to about 1 in Sub-Saharan Africa; South Asia has only about 0.5 nurses and midwives, less than 10 percent of the value observed in Europe and Central Asia.

Number of Physicians per 1,000 People

At 2.78, Europe and Central Asia also has the highest number of physicians per 1,000 people. This is almost twice as high as the values for the next regions; Latin America and the Caribbean and the Middle East and North Africa each have 1.5 physicians per 1,000 people. East Asia and Pacific drops significantly below that figure, with only 0.9. This value drops again by half in South Asia, which has 0.4. Sub-Saharan Africa has only 0.16 physicians per 1,000 people, which is not quite 5 percent of the value observed in Europe and Central Asia, an even greater differential than that between the highest-covered and lowest-covered regions for nurses and midwives.

Number of Hospital Beds per 1,000 People

The number of hospital beds per 1,000 people varies from a high of 5.34 in Europe and Central Asia to a low of 1.41 in Sub-Saharan Africa. Europe and Central Asia has more than double the number of hospital beds as in the next region, 2.56 in East Asia and Pacific. Latin America and the Caribbean and the Middle East and North Africa have similar values, at approximately 1.9 hospital beds; South Asia and Sub-Saharan Africa have the fewest number of hospital beds, at 1.50 and 1.41 per 1,000 people, respectively. This value is approximately 25 percent of Europe and Central Asia, indicating a relatively lower level of inequality in the distribution of resources.

Process of Health Care Service Delivery

Indicators Related to Children

The indicators measuring the health care delivery process, which contribute to the final set of indicators—health outcomes—are displayed in table 15.1, panel B. The values for the two process indicators related to children are much more similar across regions than are the values for the structural indicators. The values for the first indicator, the percentage of children with acute respiratory infection taken to health providers, range from a high of 70 percent in Europe and Central Asia; to East Asia and Pacific and the Middle East and North Africa, with values of 69 percent and 68 percent, respectively; to a low of 50 percent in Sub-Saharan Africa. Latin America and the Caribbean and South Asia fall in between, at 64.5 percent and 56.7 percent, respectively. The lowest value is fully 70 percent of the highest value, which is significantly better than the differential that exists for structural indicators.

The same is true for the second process indicator related to children, the percentage of children under age five years receiving oral rehydration solution for diarrhea. East Asia and Pacific displays the highest percentage at 50.7 percent, followed by South Asia at 47.4 percent, Latin America and the Caribbean at 44.5 percent, the Middle East and North Africa at 38.8 percent, Europe and Central Asia at 38.7 percent, and Sub-Saharan Africa at 34.2 percent. The difference between the highest and

Table 15.1 Structure, Process, and Outcomes Indicators for RMNCH, by Region

Indicators	Region					
	Europe and Central Asia	East Asia and Pacific	Latin America and the Caribbean	Middle East and North Africa	South Asia	Sub-Saharan Africa
A. Structure (including human resources)						
Nurses and midwives (per 1,000 people)	5.36	2.52	2.76	2.40	0.46	0.99
Physicians (per 1,000 people)	2.78	0.86	1.49	1.47	0.44	0.16
Hospital beds (per 1,000 people)	5.34	2.56	1.95	1.86	1.50	1.41
B. Process						
ARI treatment (percent of children under age five years taken to health providers)	70.3	69.0	64.5	68.0	56.7	50.3
Diarrhea treatment (percent of children under age five years who received ORS packet)	38.7	50.7	44.5	38.8	47.4	34.2
Births attended by skilled health staff (percent of total)	98.0	81.2	86.7	84.8	40.3	57.8
Pregnant women receiving prenatal care at least once (percent)	95.3	91.6	94.4	87.5	59.4	81.9
C. Outcomes						
Immunization, DPT (percent of children ages 12–23 months completing three doses)	91.7	90.1	89.9	89.3	81.2	78.0
Immunization, measles (percent of children ages 12–23 months)	93.2	88.9	91.1	88.9	80.0	76.1
Newborns protected against tetanus (percent)	83.9	82.1	83.2	86.0	79.6	80.7
Unmet need for contraception (percent of married women ages 15–49)	15.2	21.4	16.1	13.8	20.5	25.1
Vitamin A supplementation coverage rate (percent of children ages 6–59 months)	95.0	75.9	31.0	42.2	88.2	70.9

Source: Calculations based on World Bank World Development Indicators database.

Note: ARI = acute respiratory infection; DPT = diphtheria, pertussis, and tetanus; ORS = oral rehydration solution; RMNCH = reproductive, maternal, newborn, and child health.

lowest observations is about the same as for the previous indicator, with the lower statistic approximately 67 percent the level of the higher statistic.

Indicators Related to Women

The percentage of births attended by skilled health staff reaches 98 percent in Europe and Central Asia. The next three regions follow closely: Latin America and the Caribbean at 86.7 percent, the Middle East and North Africa at 84.8 percent, and East Asia and Pacific at 81.2 percent. The value for the next region, Sub-Saharan Africa, drops to 57.8 percent. The lowest level is in South Asia; skilled health personnel attend only 40.3 percent of births; this rate is only 40 percent of the value in Europe and Central Asia.

The percentage of women receiving some antenatal care (ANC) shows a slightly more compressed distribution of values across regions. The highest value is observed again in Europe and Central Asia, followed even more closely by Latin America and the Caribbean (94.4 percent), East Asia and Pacific (91.6 percent), and the Middle East and North Africa (87.5 percent); Sub-Saharan Africa is only slightly lower at 81.9 percent. South Asia lags, with only 59.4 percent of women receiving some prenatal care; this lowest value is still about 60 percent of the value observed in Europe and Central Asia.

Health Outcomes

The indicators representing health outcomes as a result of the performance of the RMNCH health care service delivery system are displayed in table 15.1, panel C.

Immunizations

The recent push to increase coverage in immunizations is reflected in the relatively high rates shown in table 15.1, with only one region's immunization coverage rate dropping below 80 percent for each of the first three indicators. The first four regions show rates of about 90 percent for fully immunizing children against DPT and measles; South Asia and Sub-Saharan Africa report child immunization rates of about 80 percent. The lowest percentages for these two immunization rates are about 85 percent of the value of the highest percentages, indicating a fairly even distribution of immunization rates across all LMICs. The percentage of newborns protected against tetanus is slightly lower overall; the highest value is 86 percent in the Middle East and North Africa. However, the lowest value is 79.6 percent in South Asia, fully 93 percent of the highest value.

Unmet Need for Contraception

The unmet need for contraception varies from 25.1 percent in Sub-Saharan Africa to 13.8 percent in the Middle East and North Africa. Both Latin America and the Caribbean and Europe and Central Asia have values similar to those of the Middle East and North Africa, 15.2 percent and 16.1 percent, respectively. South Asia and East Asia and Pacific have similar levels of unmet need at 20.5 percent and 21.4 percent, respectively.

Vitamin A Supplementation

The percentage of children receiving vitamin A supplementation varies widely from 95 percent in Europe and Central Asia to 31 percent in Latin America and the Caribbean.

ORGANIZING SERVICE DELIVERY

Task-Shifting Related to Personnel

Given the significant financial requirements for health systems in LMICs, which are confronted by personnel costs that account for a large proportion of budgets and shortages of health personnel, one innovative approach to delivering more services is by reassigning part or all of certain tasks to lower cadres of workers. Because the quality of services may be affected through task-shifting, the WHO undertook an extensive review of the literature to determine which interventions could be delivered safely and effectively by different cadres, and in a sustainable fashion (WHO 2012).

Based on the evidence, the following classification can be used to determine whether task-shifting is appropriate for specific interventions:

- Recommend
- Recommend with targeted monitoring and evaluation
- Recommend only in the context of rigorous research
- Recommend against the practice.

Based on the literature review referred to above, and documented in the 2012 recommendations, the Guidance Panel made 119 recommendations for tasks that could be potentially shifted: 36 for lay health workers, 23 for auxiliary nurses, 17 for auxiliary nurse midwives, 13 for nurses, 13 for midwives, 8 for associate clinicians, 8 for advanced-level associate clinicians, and 1 for nonspecialist doctors.

In addition, the Guidance Panel refers to several factors that might create difficulties when task-shifting is implemented:

- *Management of programs:* If sufficient and trained management personnel are not available to supervise the lower cadre of workers, quality and efficiency may suffer. However, local implementation of programs might improve with local knowledge.
- *Financial issues:* Financial management capacity may not be available at more decentralized levels, which would impede the success of task-shifting. In addition, if higher cadres are compensated on a fee-for-service basis, shifting tasks may affect their income and hence encounter resistance.
- *Supply issues:* Shifting to more decentralized service delivery may result in stock-outs if logistical systems are overwhelmed.
- *Effects of task-shifting on personnel:* Task-shifting will affect providers from whom and to whom tasks are shifted, along with their interactions. Ensuring their inclusion in the design process could help smooth the transition.
- *Health workforce impacts:* The demand for both pre-service and in-service training is likely to increase. In addition, lower cadres will likely need higher levels of supervision and support, which should be included in any analysis of the financial implications of task-shifting.

Task-Shifting Related to Other Approaches

Several innovative approaches unrelated to personnel have been reported.

- Two studies evaluate the safety and efficacy of using sublingual misoprostol for incomplete abortions instead of surgical techniques, basically shifting the task from expensive personnel to a medication, although some personnel were involved in the implementation of the interventions (Ngoc and others 2013; Shochet and others 2012).
- An example of innovative task-shifting was reported in Ethiopia in measuring maternal mortality. A community-based approach in a rural area was tested at three health posts and one health center. Instead of tasking physicians with attributing cause of death, this approach trained priests, traditional birth attendants, and community-based reproductive health agents in reporting all births and deaths to the community health post (Prata, Gerdts, and Gessessew 2012).
- A review article of the use of ultrasound to diagnose obstetrical conditions in LMICs finds that it was highly effective, resulting in different clinical management in more than 30 percent of cases. The authors recommend expanding its use for tropical and noncommunicable diseases (Groen and others 2011).

EXPANDING COVERAGE AND IMPROVING QUALITY OF CARE

Achieving health improvements for women and children requires high coverage of essential interventions. It also requires that those interventions be effective in combating disease and promoting health. The success of the RMNCH agenda hinges on achieving both coverage and quality. In this section, we review selected current approaches to improving the coverage of priority RMNCH health care services, as well as efforts to improve their effectiveness. The list is not comprehensive; rather, it focuses on initiatives that have been (1) implemented in multiple LMIC settings in the past decade and (2) evaluated. We focus on strategies that receive substantial support from global funders, such as the World Bank, the WHO, and private foundations. The selection draws on several recent reviews, including Mangham-Jefferies and others (2014) and Dettrick, Firth, and Jimenez Soto (2013). A forthcoming overview of systematic reviews from the Cochrane Effective Practice and Organisation of Care Group (http://epoc.cochrane.org/) will provide more extensive guidance on what works to improve utilization and quality. An extensive review of strategies to improve provider performance is also near completion at the Centers

for Disease Control and Prevention (Rowe and others 2015). Although for child health in particular, many essential interventions are in the home and community, we focus here on improving access to and quality of care in clinical settings—clinics, health centers, or hospitals.

Expanding Coverage

The Millennium Development Goals proposed ambitious maternal and child health targets: two-thirds reduction in under-five mortality and three-quarters reduction in maternal mortality between 1990 and 2015. These goals were based on expert estimates that if existing health interventions could be distributed to all women and children in need in LMICs, it would be possible to reduce mortality dramatically without the need for further technical breakthroughs. This remarkable assertion shone the light on gaps in coverage of RMNCH services.

Bhutta and others (2010) review the progress on provision of 26 key maternal and child health intervention in 68 countries that accounted for more than 90 percent of maternal and child health deaths globally in 2010. As table 15.1 shows, they find substantial underprovision of a range of health services. Coverage tended to be highest for interventions that can be delivered vertically through specialized programs or campaigns and can be scheduled in advance. In contrast, coverage of curative interventions, and those that were more complex or required treatment on demand, was lower. An excellent example of this divergence is the high coverage of ANC versus the low coverage of deliveries by skilled birth attendants. The coverage gaps for curative and complex interventions result from weak health systems in which health workers are few and often unmotivated; facilities are deteriorating; and supplies, equipment, and medicines are lacking. Perhaps most important, accountability for results is weak: only one in three of the countries reviewed had policies for maternal death notification, and fewer than one in two had robust vital registration systems (Bhutta and others 2010). Accountability is even weaker at the facility level, where poor outcomes rarely lead to needed changes (Pattinson and others 2009).

Equity analyses show major variations in coverage levels within low-income, high-burden countries, with the rich utilizing maternal and child health services more than the poor. The differences are largest for health system interventions, such as skilled birth attendance, and for ANC visits, where the ratio of coverage between the richest and poorest wealth quintile ranges from 3:1 to 5:1 (Barros and others 2012).

Efforts to increase coverage of RMNCH services have largely centered on users. These demand-side interventions are intended to raise awareness of the need for health care and reduce the direct and opportunity costs of care seeking.

Community Mobilization and Community Health Workers

The formation of women's groups to promote effective parenting, feeding, and recognition of signs of illness has been tested in several settings. Fottrell and others (2013) find that introduction of women's groups that participated in a learning and action cycle to improve the health of mothers and children in a cluster randomized trial in Bangladesh was associated with a 38 percent reduction in neonatal mortality and was cost-effective. A study in Malawi reports reductions in both maternal mortality and infant mortality in areas with women's groups, compared with groups with peer counselors (Lewycka and others 2013). A meta-analysis including these and other rigorous studies suggests that women's participatory learning and action groups could potentially reduce maternal mortality by 37 percent and newborn mortality by 23 percent (Prost and others 2013).

Community health workers, most of whom are community members with modest health training, have been effective in increasing the uptake of some interventions, including immunization, as well as in promoting breastfeeding. There is less evidence on their ability to increase care seeking for childhood illness or improve effectiveness of tuberculosis treatment (Lewin and others 2010).

User Fee Removal

User fees, or payments for services at the point of care, have been extensively studied for their role in suppressing health care seeking. In the wake of the Millennium Development Goals, many LMICs in Sub-Saharan Africa removed user fees for maternal and newborn care in the mid-2000s to enhance ANC and skilled delivery coverage. User fee removals have typically resulted in increased utilization of the targeted service, sometimes by a large margin (Lagarde and Palmer 2008; Ponsar and others 2011). The effect is particularly pronounced for curative services, with the poor showing the largest increases in utilization (Nabyonga and others 2005). However, effects on quality of care and long-term health outcomes have not been systematically examined. Adequate preparation for user fee removal is required if facilities are not to be overwhelmed with new patients (Meessen and others 2011). At the national level, greater reliance on government health financing (versus out-of-pocket and private insurance) is associated with higher coverage of skilled delivery attendants and cesarean sections (Kruk, Galea, and others 2007).

It is increasingly evident that user fee removal, while promoting utilization, does not protect women and families from financial hardship (Kruk and others 2008; Xu and others 2006). This is particularly the case with complex services, such as emergency obstetric care, and for poor families. This hardship is driven by costs of travel, purchase of supplies and medicines out of stock in government clinics, informal payments, and the continued use of private providers where available (Nabyonga and others 2011). In short, removal of user fees is an important but partial solution to expanding coverage and providing financial protection.

Conditional Cash Transfers

Conditional cash transfers (CCTs) are negative user fees in the sense that they pay households for using services rather than charging them for services. Whereas LMICs have experimented with removing fees, many countries in Latin America and the Caribbean have introduced financial incentives for using care, with the aim of improving home health practices and health care utilization, as well as a wide range of other desired social behaviors, such as education and employment. A 2007 Cochrane review finds that conditional transfers were associated with higher utilization and may be an effective approach to promoting preventive interventions, such as immunization (Lagarde, Haines, and Palmer 2007).

Recent experiences with CCTs have been positive. Brazil's Bolsa Familia program, which provided households with cash transfers of US$18 to US$175 per month conditional on fulfilling the requirements on health and education, were associated with reduced under-five mortality. Effects increased with Bolsa Familia coverage and were greatest for mortality due to malnutrition (Rasella and others 2013). The Mexican program Oportunidades, which paid women for ANC visits, increased ANC attendance but also increased delivery by physicians or nurses by 40 percent to 90 percent in rural Mexico (Sosa-Rubi and others 2011). The same program raised cesarean section rates among underserved poor women in rural areas by 7.5 percent (Barber 2010).

A current debate is whether unconditional cash transfers (UCTs)—cash transfers to the poor not linked to specific desired behaviors—can accomplish similar outcomes while reducing administrative and logistical hurdles. A study in Zimbabwe shows that CCTs and UCTs achieved similar improvements in school attendance, and that CCTs but not UCTs increased the proportion of children with birth certificates (Robertson and others 2013). Another study finds that UCTs and CCTs reduced human immunodeficiency virus (HIV) and herpes simplex virus 2 infections in adolescent girls (Baird and others 2012). In addition to the debate about the effectiveness of UCTs and CCTs, very little evidence is available on the cost-effectiveness of these strategies (chapter 17 in this volume, Horton and Levin 2016). More research is needed to achieve efficient and effective policies.

Vouchers

Vouchers are another type of demand-side incentive. Vouchers are distributed or sold at a discount to target populations who can exchange them for health services by contracted providers or facilities. Vouchers often include private sector services, thereby enlarging the set of health service options for women and children. Because provider participation in voucher schemes is generally conditional on accreditation, voucher programs offer an opportunity to improve the quality of care in enrolled facilities. Vouchers have been extensively used to promote the uptake of family planning, facility birth delivery, and child preventive care. Although rigorous evaluations are few, vouchers have been linked to increases in utilization of facility delivery and family planning services (Bellows and others 2013; Bellows, Bellows, and Warren 2011). Vouchers appear to be less effective in areas with high levels of poverty, where contracted facilities are fewer, and where roads are poor (Kanya and others 2013). Transport vouchers are a promising intervention in these areas (Ekirapa-Kiracho and others 2011).

However, a quasi-random evaluation of a very large voucher-type scheme, India's Chiranjeevi Yojana, finds no differences in facility delivery rates or newborn complications, compared with nonprogram areas. This study is notable for contradicting earlier findings of large improvements in facility deliveries and reductions in maternal and child deaths, which the authors of the evaluation attribute to poor study design in earlier research. The Chiranjeevi Yojana program, which covered 800,000 deliveries between 2005 and 2012, paid contracted private sector hospitals a fixed fee (US$37) per vaginal or cesarean delivery per poor woman. The authors note that poor quality in contracted hospitals and high transport costs may have constrained demand for services (Mohanan and others 2013).

Performance-Based Financing

Performance-based financing (PBF), or paying for performance, is a supply-side financing method that rewards providers or health care organizations for achieving coverage or quality targets. These rewards typically are in the form of bonus payments in addition to regular salaries. A frequently cited study from Rwanda shows a 23 percent increase in facility delivery and larger increases in preventive care visits by young children in facilities enrolled in pay-for-performance schemes, as compared with randomly selected controls (Basinga and others 2011). These increases did not favor the rich or the poor, so additional measures would be required to close the equity gap in utilization (Priedeman Skiles and others 2012).

However, a Cochrane review suggests that the quality of evidence is too poor to draw general conclusions about the effectiveness of PBF, noting that several studies arrived at contradictory results (Witter and others 2012). Fretheim and others (2012) argue that PBF is a donor fad and unproven; others counter that whatever its direct effects, PBF may trigger constructive reforms in public health systems to make care at public facilities more efficient and responsive (Meessen, Soucat, and Sekabaraga 2011).

Improving Quality

Poor quality of care is a double obstacle to improved survival for mothers and children; it deters utilization and hinders achievement of good health outcomes. To improve health, health care has to effective and safe. Good-quality care is also respectful and considers the needs and preferences of patients. Interventions that are efficacious in clinical trials or in highly skilled settings in high-income countries have frequently been shown to be less effective when implemented in resource-constrained health systems in LMICs (Das and Gertler 2007; Das and others 2012; Leonard and Masatu 2007).

Quality of care for complex services is particularly problematic. Souza and others (2013) assess the use of evidence-based interventions in maternal health care and the frequency of poor maternal outcomes (near miss or maternal death) in large hospitals in 29 LMICs. The investigators find that mortality ratios were two to three times higher than expected on the basis of illness severity in high and very high maternal mortality ratio countries, which were the poorest countries in the sample; most were in Sub-Saharan Africa. These excess deaths occurred despite the high use of key interventions, such as magnesium sulfate for treating preeclampsia and eclampsia. Delays in the detection or treatment of complications, poor-quality critical supportive care (such as airway and fluid management), and weak infection control explained the poor outcomes (Souza and others 2013).

In addition to affecting health outcomes, quality of care can influence coverage. Good quality promotes trust in the health system and encourages utilization; poor quality can dissuade people from using health care.

One indicator of population preferences for care is bypassing—going to a more-distant facility when a nearby health facility is available. Bypassing is considered a strong sign of revealed preference, given that attending distant facilities takes longer and is more costly. Leonard, Mliga, and Mariam (2002) show that Tanzanian patients travel farther if they can access providers with greater medical knowledge and facilities that are better stocked. In examining the utilization of facilities for delivery, our research finds that 4 in 10 women bypassed local facilities to deliver in hospitals in western Tanzania, despite wide availability of nearby dispensaries that could provide the service (Kruk, Mbaruku, and others 2009). Bypassing was highest among first-time mothers, who were likely motivated by perceived higher risk of first delivery; it was also higher among women who perceived the local clinic to provide low-quality care.

In a separate paper, Kruk, Paczkowski, and others (2009) find strong preference for quality-of-care attributes in shaping women's decisions on where to seek care. We conclude that these data are consistent with high home delivery rates, given that few facilities can provide the quality that women expect. A range of qualitative studies supports the notion that women avoid low-quality facilities and may forgo care altogether if better options are not accessible (Abelson, Miller, and Giacomini 2009; Gilson 2003; Russell 2005).

Quality improvement in RMNCH is a vast enterprise with a long history. The initiatives here are not a comprehensive list; we focus on the strategies that have been recently applied in LMICs at scale, that have received donor support, and that have been evaluated.

Measurement and Accreditation

Accreditation of health facilities, common in high-income countries, is increasingly used as a quality-of-care intervention in LMICs. Accreditation is a formal process of assessing whether a health facility meets agreed-upon quality standards; it is typically conducted by an independent body. Published data suggest that accreditation is more common in middle-income countries than in low-income countries. Quimbo and others (2008) find that clinical performance in pediatric care was better in providers who worked in accredited hospitals in the Philippines. An even more influential factor was receipt of insurance payments, which were disbursed, at least in part, on the basis of compliance with clinical practice guidelines—and so could be seen as a payment for performance.

In Sub-Saharan Africa, accreditation is still rare, and evidence of its effects is rarer still. The Zambian Ministry of Health implemented a comprehensive accreditation program for its hospitals with support from the United States Agency for International Development (USAID). The program succeeded in raising compliance with standards, but the complex logistics and high costs (US$10,000 per hospital) of the accreditation process resulted in its cancellation (Bukonda and others 2002). Liberia, which is rebuilding its health system after 14 years of civil war, introduced more streamlined tablet-based data collection for accreditation in all 437 facilities in the country as a requirement for receiving funding. Facilities were rated using a star system. Although the baseline data were successfully collected, the follow-up assessment to demonstrate quality improvements has not been completed. However, the initial data showing large deficiencies in laboratory functions spurred national purchase of laboratory equipment (Cleveland and others 2011).

Performance-Based Financing

One of the potential reasons for poor-quality care may be a mismatch between provider knowledge and the effort providers make when treating patients. This might occur if providers are unmotivated or underpaid. PBF has been applied to improving the quality as well as the quantity of services.

A randomized trial in the Philippines tested the effect of a 5 percent salary bonus paid to physicians upon improvement on clinical vignettes—tests of clinical competence (Peabody and others 2014). The study finds improvements in self-reported health and wasting in children under age five years who attended intervention facilities. The authors note that the measurement and feedback to providers about their performance on the clinical vignettes was an essential element of the intervention.

Rusa and others (2009) find that PBF payments representing 40 percent to 80 percent of nurses' salaries that were paid in part on improved quality metrics were temporally associated with improved quality of maternal and child health services in health centers in Rwanda. The metrics included completed partograms, growth curves, follow-up for missed visits, and mother and child alive on discharge. Overall, the centers involved in PBF reached quality metrics between 80 percent and 95 percent of total possible scores within 18 months. However, the study design makes it impossible to disentangle the effects of PBF from overall salary increases, monthly supervision visits introduced as part of PBF, and other health system reforms at the same time in the country.

A lively discussion about the role of PBF in global health has ensued on the basis of these and other experiences. Some argue that PBF can catalyze essential health system reforms (Meessen, Soucat, and Sekabaraga 2011). Others believe that it is at best a partial solution and may create important distractions from more fundamental health system reform, such as expanding the heath workforce and raising the salary floor (Ireland, Paul, and Dujardin 2011). Most agree that the jury is still out about the extent to which paying for performance—apart from raising salaries and increasing oversight—is transformative in improving quality (Basinga, Mayaka, and Condo 2011). The lack of evidence has not stopped adoption: 22 countries in Sub-Saharan Africa have introduced PBF in the past several years (Soeters and Vroeg 2011; Spector and others 2012).

Training and Supportive Supervision

Supportive supervision is managerial support for front-line health workers, typically through periodic visits from first-level hospitals to peripheral facilities. It is intended to support quality of care and improve provider motivation and retention through nonpunitive review of practices and mentoring. It is popular in many countries where health services are decentralized and where structures to perform supportive supervision exist, at least in theory (Rowe and others 2005).

A Cochrane review of the evidence on supportive supervision in general primary care, not solely maternal and child health, is conducted by Bosch-Capblanch, Liaqat, and Garner (2011). They assess nine studies and find generally small benefits for provider practice and knowledge. They note that the quality of the assessments was weak.

A few country studies since 2011 show more positive results. Hoque and others (2013) find that monthly supportive supervision, combined with Integrated Management of Childhood Illness training, allowed health workers with 18 months of training to provide similar care to providers with four years of training in Tanzania. McAuliffe and others (2013) report that formal systems of supportive supervision were associated with high levels of job satisfaction and low intention to leave among clinical officers in Malawi, Mozambique, and Tanzania.

Continuous Quality Improvement and Quality Collaboratives

Continuous quality improvement (CQI) strategies rely on engaging facility and health system leaders in reflection on and measurement of performance in health care settings. This process involves identifying poor outcomes (for example, postpartum infections) and brainstorming about root and proximal causes. The quality improvement team then identifies causes that are both important and amenable to change and proposes strategies for addressing the cause. CQI initiatives have shown good results in selected hospitals in the United States, but they have been not been widely used in LMICs. One study from Colombia finds that CQI methods used in two nonprofit hospitals in Bogota led to reduction in surgical site infections immediately after the improvements (Weinberg and others 2001).

A related initiative is known as quality collaboratives. First advanced by the Institute for Healthcare Improvement, these consist of multiple facility-based teams working in parallel to apply improvement in a single area of care then sharing results and best practices in learning sessions (Øvretveit and others 2002). Although these initiatives have mostly been implemented in the United States, the USAID has funded quality collaboratives in 14 LMICs. A 2011 review of 27 collaboratives in 12 countries finds generally positive results with 87.4 percent of time-series charts reaching at least 80 percent performance levels on practices such as oxytocin administration within one minute of delivery and retaining HIV-infected patients in care, with gains sustained on average for 13 consecutive months (Franco and Marquez 2011). These data are encouraging but require a substantial health system effort to succeed (Wilson, Berwick, and Cleary 2003). The potential for scale up and the long-term sustainability of these results in the context of weak systems require further study.

Use of Checklists

Surgical safety checklists have been promoted as a means of reducing human errors in health care by ensuring a systematic approach to each patient and procedure. Similar checklists have been introduced for intrapartum care. A pilot study of a 29-point checklist consisting of items such as hand hygiene, administration of uterotonics, and management of complications was piloted at a large hospital in Karnataka, India. The researchers find that the proportion of indicated practices increased from 10 of 29 to an average of 25 (Spector and others 2012). This approach has to be tested to ensure the result can be obtained with a proper counterfactual and, if so, if it can be sustained.

COST-EFFECTIVENESS OF INTERVENTIONS TO EXPAND COVERAGE AND IMPROVE QUALITY OF CARE

Although limited in number, economic evaluations demonstrate that health center and community-based approaches to improving access to care and quality of services are cost-effective as measured by

Table 15.2 Cost-Effectiveness of Interventions to Improve Quality of Care
(Compared with no intervention)

Source	Country	Unit	Cost-effectiveness as presented ($/DALY averted)	Currency (year)	Cost-effectiveness (2012 U.S. dollars)
Bishai and others (2015)	Myanmar	Adding ORS-Z to an additional product line in existing social franchise program (platform)	339.00	US$ (2010)	3.42
Broughton and others (2011)	Nicaragua	Quality improvement intervention (improved compliance with clinical standards)	Cost saving	US$ (2010)	0.50
Broughton and others (2013)	Niger	Increasing compliance with high-impact, evidence-based care standards in maternal health care facilities	147.00	US$ (2008)	150.48
Colbourn and others (2015)	Malawi	Community intervention: Participatory women's groups mobilizing communities around maternal and neonatal health using volunteer facilitators supported by program staff for monthly meetings	79.00	$Int (2013)	1.30
Colbourn and others (2015)	Malawi	Facility intervention: Quality improvement to train staff, change packages, death reviews, leadership training, protocol-based trainings	281.00	$Int (2013)	4.63
Colbourn and others (2015)	Malawi	Both community and facility-based interventions	146.00	$Int (2013)	2.40
Grimes and others (2014)	Malawi	To relieve physician workload, trained orthopedic clinical officers for six months to treat patients needing a manipulation or operation	138.75	US$ (2012)	168.26

Note: DALY = disability-adjusted life year; $Int = International dollar; ORS-Z = oral rehydration solution plus zinc.

cost per disability-adjusted life year (DALY) averted (table 15.2). In Nicaragua, learning approaches used through quality improvement collaboration in a hospital setting reduced the length of stay for children with pneumonia and diarrhea and was also cost saving. In Niger, a similar quality improvement collaborative for obstetric and newborn care was both less costly and cost-effective. In Malawi, a community approach using both women's groups and health facility quality improvement that reduced maternal and neonatal deaths was cost-effective. Task-shifting through use of community health workers and lower-level health care providers can be both cost saving and cost-effective (Babigumira and others 2009; Grimes and others 2014; Kruk, Pereira, and others 2007). It is challenging to measure costs and cost-effectiveness associated with programs and policies designed to increase uptake, access, and quality. Part of the challenge lies in the absence of standard metrics for measuring quality; moreover, the health impacts of policies and programs established and implemented at multiple levels of health systems are harder to evaluate.

CONCLUSIONS

Good maternal and child health care is critical to improving survival and quality of life. Both expansion of access and improvements to quality are crucial elements of good care. Despite growing awareness of serious quality deficits, research on interventions to improve quality has not produced clear guidance on what works and which models improve quality at scale. This void in guidance is due in part to the lack of coherent conceptual frameworks that would direct the testing of promising quality interventions in different settings. Where interventions are tried, the evaluation is often of poor quality.

The situation is better for interventions aimed at increasing coverage of services where good evidence exists for demand-side interventions to motivate service uptake. Particularly effective interventions to expand access include task-shifting, community groups, and CCTs. However, as the epidemiology of maternal and child death shifts to more complex causes, insufficient quality of care will be an increasing barrier to reducing mortality and morbidity and to achieving global health goals. Indeed, expanding coverage will yield diminishing returns unless quality deficits are also tackled.

NOTE

World Bank Income Classifications as of July 2014 are as follows, based on estimates of gross national income (GNI) per capita for 2013:

- Low-income countries (LICs) = US$1,045 or less
- Middle-income countries (MICs) are subdivided:
  a) lower-middle-income = US$1,046–US$4,125
  b) upper-middle-income (UMICs) = US$4,126–US$12,745
- High-Income countries (HICs) = US$12,746 or more.

REFERENCES

Abelson, J., F. A. Miller, and M. Giacomini. 2009. "What Does It Mean to Trust a Health System? A Qualitative Study of Canadian Health Care Values." *Health Policy* 91 (1): 63–70.

Aboud, F. E., and A. K. Yousafzai. 2016. "Very Early Childhood Development." In *Disease Control Priorities* (third edition): Volume 2, *Reproductive, Maternal, Newborn, and Child Health*, edited by R. Black, R. Laxminarayan, M. Temmerman, and N. Walker. Washington, DC: World Bank.

Babigumira, J. B., B. Castelnuovo, M. Lamorde, A. Kambugu, A. Stergachis, and others. 2009. "Potential Impact of Task-Shifting on Costs of Antiretroviral Therapy and Physician Supply in Uganda." *BMC Health Services Research* 9 (1): 192.

Baird, S. J., R. S. Garfein, C. T. McIntosh, and B. Ozler. 2012. "Effect of a Cash Transfer Programme for Schooling on Prevalence of HIV and Herpes Simplex Type 2 in Malawi: A Cluster Randomised Trial." *The Lancet* 379 (9823): 1320–29.

Barber, S. L. 2010. "Mexico's Conditional Cash Transfer Programme Increases Cesarean Section Rates among the Rural Poor." *European Journal of Public Health* 20 (4): 383–88.

Barros, A. J., C. Ronsmans, H. Axelson, E. Loaiza, A. D. Bertoldi, and others. 2012. "Equity in Maternal, Newborn, and Child Health Interventions in Countdown to 2015: A Retrospective Review of Survey Data from 54 Countries." *The Lancet* 379 (9822): 1225–33.

Basinga, P., P. J. Gertler, A. Binagwaho, A. L. Soucat, J. Sturdy, and others. 2011. "Effect on Maternal and Child Health Services in Rwanda of Payment to Primary Health-Care Providers for Performance: An Impact Evaluation." *The Lancet* 377 (9775): 1421–28.

Basinga, P., S. Mayaka, and J. Condo. 2011. "Performance-Based Financing: The Need for More Research." *Bulletin of the World Health Organization* 89 (9): 698–99.

Bellows, N. M., B. W. Bellows, and C. Warren. 2011. "Systematic Review: The Use of Vouchers for Reproductive Health Services in Developing Countries." *Tropical Medicine and International Health* 16 (1): 84–96.

Bellows, B., C. Kyobutungi, M. K. Mutua, C. Warren, and A. Ezeh. 2013. "Increase in Facility-Based Deliveries Associated with a Maternal Health Voucher Programme in Informal Settlements in Nairobi, Kenya." *Health Policy and Planning* 28 (2): 134–42.

Bhutta, Z. A., M. Chopra, H. Axelson, P. Berman, T. Boerma, and others. 2010. "Countdown to 2015 Decade Report (2000–10): Taking Stock of Maternal, Newborn, and Child Survival." *The Lancet* 375 (9730): 2032–44.

Bishai, D., K. Sachathep, A. LeFevre, H. N. Nwe Thant, M. Zaw, and others. 2015. "Cost-Effectiveness of Using a Social Franchise Network to Increase Uptake of Oral Rehydration Salts and Zinc for Childhood Diarrhea in Rural Myanmar." *Cost Effectiveness and Resource Allocation* 13 (1): 3.

Bosch-Capblanch, X., S. Liaqat, and P. Garner. 2011. "Managerial Supervision to Improve Primary Health Care in Low- and Middle-Income Countries." *Cochrane Database of Systematic Reviews* (9): CD006413.

Broughton, E., I. Gomez, O. Nuñez, and Y. Wong. 2011. "Cost-Effectiveness of Improving Pediatric Hospital Care in Nicaragua." *Revista Panamericana de Salud Pública* 30 (5): 453–60.

Broughton, E., Z. Saley, M. Boucar, D. Alagane, K. Hill, and others. 2013. "Cost-Effectiveness of a Quality Improvement Collaborative for Obstetric and Newborn Care in Niger." *International Journal of Health Care Quality Assurance* 26 (3): 250–61.

Bukonda, N., P. Tavrow, H. Abdallah, K. Hoffner, and J. Tembo. 2002. "Implementing a National Hospital Accreditation Program: The Zambian Experience." *International Journal for Quality in Health Care* 14 (Suppl. 1): 7–16.

Cleveland, E. C., B. T. Dahn, T. M. Lincoln, M. Safer, M. Podesta, and others. 2011. "Introducing Health Facility Accreditation in Liberia." *Global Public Health* 6 (3): 271–82.

Colbourn, T., A.-M. Pulkki-Brännström, B. Nambiar, S. Kim, A. Bondo, and others. 2015. "Cost-Effectiveness and Affordability of Community Mobilisation through Women's Groups and Quality Improvement in Health Facilities (Maikhanda Trial) in Malawi." *Cost Effectiveness and Resource Allocation* 13 (1): 1.

Das, J., and P. J. Gertler. 2007. "Variations in Practice Quality in Five Low-Income Countries: A Conceptual Overview." *Health Affairs* 26 (3): w296–309.

Das, J., A. Holla, V. Das, M. Mohanan, D. Tabak, and B. Chan. 2012. "In Urban and Rural India, a Standardized Patient Study Showed Low Levels of Provider Training and Huge Quality Gaps." *Health Affairs (Millwood)* 31 (12): 2774–84.

Dettrick, Z., S. Firth, and E. Jimenez Soto. 2013. "Do Strategies to Improve Quality of Maternal and Child Health Care in Lower and Middle Income Countries Lead to Improved Outcomes? A Review of the Evidence." *PLoS One* 8 (12): e83070.

Ekirapa-Kiracho, E., P. Waiswa, M. H. Rahman, F. Makumbi, N. Kiwanuka, and others. 2011. "Increasing Access to Institutional Deliveries Using Demand and Supply Side Incentives: Early Results from a Quasi-Experimental Study." *BMC International Health and Human Rights* 11 (Suppl. 1): S11.

Fottrell, E., K. Azad, A. Kuddus, L. Younes, S. Shaha, and others. 2013. "The Effect of Increased Coverage of Participatory

Women's Groups on Neonatal Mortality in Bangladesh: A Cluster Randomized Trial." *Journal of the American Medical Association Pediatrics* 167 (9): 816–25.

Franco, L. M., and L. Marquez. 2011. "Effectiveness of Collaborative Improvement: Evidence from 27 Applications in 12 Less-Developed and Middle-Income Countries." *BMJ Quality and Safety* 20 (8): 658–65.

Fretheim, A., S. Witter, A. K. Lindahl, and I. T. Olsen. 2012. "Performance-Based Financing in Low- and Middle-Income Countries: Still More Questions Than Answers." *Bulletin of the World Health Organization* 90 (8): 559–59A.

Gilson, L. 2003. "Trust and the Development of Health Care as a Social Institution." *Social Science and Medicine* 56 (7): 1453–68.

Grimes, C. E., N. C. Mkandawire, M. L. Billingsley, C. Ngulube, and J. C. Cobey. 2014. "The Cost-Effectiveness of Orthopaedic Clinical Officers in Malawi." *Tropical Doctor* 44 (3): 128–34.

Groen, R. S., J. J. Leow, V. Sadasivam, and A. L. Kushner. 2011. "Review: Indications for Ultrasound Use in Low- and Middle-Income Countries." *Tropical Medicine and International Health* 16 (12): 1525–35. doi:10.1111/j.1365 -3156.2011.02868.x.

Hoque, D. E., S. E. Arifeen, M. Rahman, E. K. Chowdhury, T. M. Haque, and others. 2013. "Improving and Sustaining Quality of Child Health Care through IMCI Training and Supervision: Experience from Rural Bangladesh." *Health Policy and Planning* 29 (6): 753–62.

Horton, S., and C. Levin. 2016. "Cost-Effectiveness of Interventions for Reproductive, Maternal, Neonatal, and Child Health." In *Disease Control Priorities* (third edition): Volume 2, *Reproductive, Maternal, Newborn, and Child Health*, edited by R. Black, R. Laxminarayan, M. Temmerman, and N. Walker. Washington, DC: World Bank.

Ireland, M., E. Paul, and B. Dujardin. 2011. "Can Performance-Based Financing Be Used to Reform Health Systems in Developing Countries?" *Bulletin of the World Health Organization* 89 (9): 695–98.

Jamison, D. T., J. G. Breman, A. R. Measham, G. Alleyne, M. Claeson, D. B. Evans, P. Jha, A. Mills, and P. Musgrove, eds. 2006. *Disease Control Priorities in Developing Countries.* 2nd edition. Washington, DC: World Bank and Oxford University Press.

Jamison, D. T., W. Mosley, A. R. Measham, and J. Bobadilla. 1993. *Disease Control Priorities in Developing Countries.* New York: Oxford University Press.

Kanya, L., F. Obare, C. Warren, T. Abuya, I. Askew, and others. 2013. "Safe Motherhood Voucher Programme Coverage of Health Facility Deliveries among Poor Women in South-Western Uganda." *Health Policy and Planning* 29 (Suppl. 1): i4–11.

Kruk, M. E., S. Galea, M. Prescott, and L. P. Freedman. 2007. "Health Care Financing and Utilization of Maternal Health Services in Developing Countries." *Health Policy and Planning* 22 (5): 303–10.

Kruk, M. E., G. Mbaruku, C. W. McCord, M. Moran, P. C. Rockers, and others. 2009. "Bypassing Primary Care

Facilities for Childbirth: A Population-Based Study in Rural Tanzania." *Health Policy and Planning* 24 (4): 279–88.

Kruk, M. E., G. Mbaruku, P. C. Rockers, and S. Galea. 2008. "User Fee Exemptions Are Not Enough: Out-of-Pocket Payments for 'Free' Delivery Services in Rural Tanzania." *Tropical Medicine and International Health* 13 (12): 1442–51.

Kruk, M. E., M. Paczkowski, G. Mbaruku, H. de Pinho, and S. Galea. 2009. "Women's Preferences for Place of Delivery in Rural Tanzania: A Population-Based Discrete Choice Experiment." *American Journal of Public Health* 99 (9): 1666–72.

Kruk, M. E., C. Pereira, F. Vaz, S. Bergström, and S. Galea. 2007. "Economic Evaluation of Surgically Trained Assistant Medical Officers in Performing Major Obstetric Surgery in Mozambique." *BJOG* 114 (10): 1253–60.

Lagarde, M., A. Haines, and N. Palmer. 2007. "Conditional Cash Transfers for Improving Uptake of Health Interventions in Low- and Middle-Income Countries: A Systematic Review." *Journal of the American Medical Association* 298 (16): 1900–10.

Lagarde, M., and N. Palmer. 2008. "The Impact of User Fees on Health Service Utilization in Low- and Middle-Income Countries: How Strong Is the Evidence?" *Bulletin of the World Health Organization* 86 (11): 839–48.

Leonard, K. L., and M. C. Masatu. 2007. "Variations in the Quality of Care Accessible to Rural Communities in Tanzania." *Health Affairs* 26 (3): w380–92.

Leonard, K. L., G. R. Mliga, and D. H. Mariam. 2002. "Bypassing Health Centres in Tanzania: Revealed Preferences for Quality." *Journal of African Economics* (11): 441–71.

Lewin, S., S. Munabi-Babigumira, C. Glenton, K. Daniels, X. Bosch-Capblanch, and others. 2010. "Lay Health Workers in Primary and Community Health Care for Maternal and Child Health and the Management of Infectious Diseases." *Cochrane Database of Systematic Reviews* 20 (3): CD004015.

Lewycka, S., C. Mwansambo, M. Rosato, P. Kazembe, T. Phiri, and others. 2013. "Effect of Women's Groups and Volunteer Peer Counselling on Rates of Mortality, Morbidity, and Health Behaviours in Mothers and Children in Rural Malawi (Maimwana): A Factorial, Cluster-Randomised Controlled Trial." *The Lancet* 381 (9879): 1721–35.

Mangham-Jefferies, L., C. Pitt, S. Cousens, A. Mills, and J. Schellenberg. 2014. "Cost-Effectiveness of Strategies to Improve the Utilization and Provision of Maternal and Newborn Health Care in Low-Income and Lower-Middle-Income Countries: A Systematic Review." *BMC Pregnancy and Childbirth* 14: 243.

McAuliffe, E., M. Daly, F. Kamwendo, H. Masanja, M. Sidat, and H. de Pinho. 2013. "The Critical Role of Supervision in Retaining Staff in Obstetric Services: A Three Country Study." *PLoS One* 8 (3): e58415.

Meessen, B., D. Hercot, M. Noirhomme, V. Ridde, A. Tibouti, and others. 2011. "Removing User Fees in the Health Sector: A Review of Policy Processes in Six Sub-Saharan African Countries." *Health Policy and Planning* 26 (Suppl. 2): ii16–29.

Meessen, B., A. Soucat, and C. Sekabaraga. 2011. "Performance-Based Financing: Just a Donor Fad or a Catalyst towards

Comprehensive Health-Care Reform?" *Bulletin of the World Health Organization* 89 (2): 153–56.

Mohanan, M., S. Bauhoff, G. La Forgia, K. Singer, and G. Miller. 2013. "Effect of Chiranjeevi Yojana on Institutional Deliveries and Neonatal and Maternal Outcomes in Gujarat, India: A Difference-in-Differences Analysis." *Bulletin of the World Health Organization* 92 (3): 187–94.

Nabyonga, J., M. Desmet, H. Karamagi, P. Y. Kadama, F. G. Omaswa, and others. 2005. "Abolition of Cost-Sharing Is Pro-Poor: Evidence from Uganda." *Health Policy and Planning* 20 (2): 100–08.

Nabyonga Orem, J., F. Mugisha, C. Kirunga, J. Macq, and B. Criel. 2011. "Abolition of User Fees: The Uganda Paradox." *Health Policy and Planning* 26 (Suppl. 2): ii41–51.

Ngoc, N. T., T. Shochet, J. Blum, P. T. Hai, D. L. Dung, and others. 2013. "Results from a Study Using Misoprostol for Management of Incomplete Abortion in Vietnamese Hospitals: Implications for Task Shifting." *BMC Pregnancy and Childbirth* 13: 118. doi:10.1186/1471-2393-13-118.

Øvretveit, J., P. Bate, P. Cleary, S. Cretin, D. Gustafson, and others. 2002. "Quality Collaboratives: Lessons from Research." *Quality and Safety in Health Care* 11 (4): 345–51.

Pattinson, R., K. Kerber, P. Waiswa, L. T. Day, F. Mussell, and others. 2009. "Perinatal Mortality Audit: Counting, Accountability, and Overcoming Challenges in Scaling Up in Low- and Middle-Income Countries." *International Journal of Gynaecology and Obstetrics* 107 (Suppl. 1): S113–21, S21–22.

Peabody, J. W., R. Shimkhada, S. Quimbo, O. Solon, X. Javier, and others. 2014. "The Impact of Performance Incentives on Child Health Outcomes: Results from a Cluster Randomized Controlled Trial in the Philippines." *Health Policy and Planning* 29 (5): 615–21.

Ponsar, F., M. Van Herp, R. Zachariah, S. Gerard, M. Philips, and others. 2011. "Abolishing User Fees for Children and Pregnant Women Trebled Uptake of Malaria-Related Interventions in Kangaba, Mali." *Health Policy and Planning* 26 (Suppl. 2): ii72–83.

Prata, N., C. Gerdts, and A. Gessessew. 2012. "An Innovative Approach to Measuring Maternal Mortality at the Community Level in Low-Resource Settings Using Mid-Level Providers: A Feasibility Study in Tigray, Ethiopia." *Reproductive Health Matters* 20 (39): 196–204. doi:10.1016/S0968-8080(12)39606-7.

Priedeman Skiles, M., S. L. Curtis, P. Basinga, and G. Angeles. 2012. "An Equity Analysis of Performance-Based Financing in Rwanda: Are Services Reaching the Poorest Women?" *Health Policy and Planning* 28 (8): 825–37.

Prost, A., T. Colbourn, N. Seward, K. Azad, A. Coomarasamy, and others. 2013. "Women's Groups Practising Participatory Learning and Action to Improve Maternal and Newborn Health in Low-Resource Settings: A Systematic Review and Meta-Analysis." *The Lancet* 381 (9879): 1736–46.

Quimbo, S. A., J. W. Peabody, R. Shimkhada, K. Woo, and O. Solon. 2008. "Should We Have Confidence If a Physician Is Accredited? A Study of the Relative Impacts of Accreditation and Insurance Payments on Quality of Care in the Philippines." *Social Science and Medicine* 67 (4): 505–10.

Rasella, D., R. Aquino, C. A. Santos, R. Paes-Sousa, and M. L. Barreto. 2013. "Effect of a Conditional Cash Transfer Programme on Childhood Mortality: A Nationwide Analysis of Brazilian Municipalities." *The Lancet* 382 (9886): 57–64.

Robertson, L., P. Mushati, J. W. Eaton, L. Dumba, G. Mavise, and others. 2013. "Effects of Unconditional and Conditional Cash Transfers on Child Health and Development in Zimbabwe: A Cluster-Randomised Trial." *The Lancet* 381 (9874): 1283–92.

Rowe, A. K., D. de Savigny, C. F. Lanata, and C. G. Victora. 2005. "How Can We Achieve and Maintain High-Quality Performance of Health Workers in Low-Resource Settings?" *The Lancet* 366 (9490): 1026–35.

Rowe, A. K., S. Y. Rowe, D. H. Peters, K. A. Holloway, J. Chalker, and D. Ross-Degnan. 2015. "The Health Care Provider Performance Review: A Systematic Review of the Effectiveness of Strategies to Improve Health Care Provider Performance in Low- and Middle-Income Countries. Presentation of Preliminary Results." March 23.

Rusa, L., D. Ngirabega Jde, W. Janssen, S. Van Bastelaere, D. Porignon, and others. 2009. "Performance-Based Financing for Better Quality of Services in Rwandan Health Centres: 3-Year Experience." *Tropical Medicine and International Health* 14 (7): 830–37.

Russell, Steven. 2005. "Treatment-Seeking Behaviour in Urban Sri Lanka: Trusting the State, Trusting Private Providers." *Social Science and Medicine* 61 (7): 1396.

Shochet, T., A. Diop, A. Gaye, M. Nayama, A. B. Sall, and others. 2012. "Sublingual Misoprostol versus Standard Surgical Care for Treatment of Incomplete Abortion in Five Sub-Saharan African Countries." *BMC Pregnancy and Childbirth* 12: 127. doi:10.1186/1471-2393-12-127.

Soeters, R., and P. Vroeg. 2011. "Why There Is So Much Enthusiasm for Performance-Based Financing, Particularly in Developing Countries." *Bulletin of the World Health Organization* 89 (9): 700.

Sosa-Rubi, S. G., D. Walker, E. Servan, and S. Bautista-Arredondo. 2011. "Learning Effect of a Conditional Cash Transfer Programme on Poor Rural Women's Selection of Delivery Care in Mexico." *Health Policy and Planning* 26 (6): 496–507.

Souza, J. P., A. M. Gülmezoglu, J. Vogel, G. Carroli, P. Lumbiganon, and others. 2013. "Moving beyond Essential Interventions for Reduction of Maternal Mortality (WHO Multicountry Survey on Maternal and Newborn Health): A Cross-Sectional Study." *The Lancet* 381 (9879): 1747–55.

Spector, J. M., P. Agrawal, B. Kodkany, S. Lipsitz, A. Lashoher, and others. 2012. "Improving Quality of Care for Maternal and Newborn Health: Prospective Pilot Study of the WHO Safe Childbirth Checklist Program." *PLoS One* 7 (5): e35151.

Weinberg, M., J. M. Fuentes, A. I. Ruiz, F. W. Lozano, E. Angel, and others. 2001. "Reducing Infections among Women

Undergoing Cesarean Section in Colombia by Means of Continuous Quality Improvement Methods." *Archives of Internal Medicine* 161 (19): 2357–65.

WHO (World Health Organization). 2012. *WHO Recommendations: Optimizing Health Worker Roles to Improve Access to Key Maternal and Newborn Health Interventions through Task Shifting.* Geneva: WHO.

Wilson, T., D. M. Berwick, and P. D. Cleary. 2003. "What Do Collaborative Improvement Projects Do? Experience from Seven Countries." *Joint Commission Journal on Quality and Safety* 29 (2): 85–93.

Witter, S., A. Fretheim, F. L. Kessy, and A. K. Lindahl. 2012. "Paying for Performance to Improve the Delivery of Health Interventions in Low- and Middle-Income Countries." *Cochrane Database of Systematic Reviews* 2: CD007899.

World Bank. 2013. World Development Indicators Database. http://www.databank.worldbank.org.

Xu, K., D. B. Evans, P. Kadama, J. Nabyonga, P. O. Ogwal, and others. 2006. "Understanding the Impact of Eliminating User Fees: Utilization and Catastrophic Health Expenditures in Uganda." *Social Science and Medicine* 62 (4): 866–76.

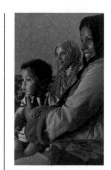

Chapter 16

Returns on Investment in the Continuum of Care for Reproductive, Maternal, Newborn, and Child Health

Karin Stenberg, Kim Sweeny, Henrik Axelson,
Marleen Temmerman, and Peter Sheehan

INTRODUCTION

The continuum of care for reproductive, maternal, newborn, and child health (RMNCH) addresses three key dimensions of service delivery across time, space, and type of care (Kerber and others 2007):

- Access to needed services throughout the lifecycle, including adolescence, pregnancy, childbirth, the postnatal period, and childhood
- Access to interventions with functional linkages among levels of care in the health system provided by families and communities, outpatient and outreach services, and health facilities
- Access to different types of health services and activities, including prevention, promotion, and curative and palliative care (World Health Assembly 2009).

Assessing the returns on investments in the continuum of care for RMNCH requires specification of a package of interventions and an estimate of the full costs incurred in the health system to deliver those interventions. On the benefits side, the outcome of the continuum of care is evidenced in the many dimensions of the health benefits arising from an integrated care program. These benefits are not only lives saved; they also include

the improved health and welfare of mothers and children, and the benefits that arise from expanding the ability of women to plan their pregnancies. These diverse health gains will have a wide range of economic and social benefits. Thus, assessing the returns on investment in the continuum of care for RMNCH also requires a comprehensive attempt to measure the various benefits that accrue to communities, at different stages of the lifecycle, as a result of the interventions. The overall analysis compares costs and benefits, taking into consideration their varying patterns over time, to generate benefit-cost ratios and rates of return on investment.

This chapter assesses the costs and benefits of delivering a set of integrated RMNCH interventions across the continuum of care in countries with high child and maternal mortality. The purpose is twofold:

- To demonstrate that very high returns can be achieved by strengthening investments in the delivery of a suite of high-impact interventions
- To underscore the importance of an accurate assessment of those returns, including the full range of costs involved in delivering integrated care across the continuum and the full range of benefits that flow from the interventions.

Corresponding author: Karin Stenberg, Department of Health Systems Governance and Financing, World Health Organization, Geneva, Switzerland, stenbergk@who.int.

This chapter is based on the first attempt, to our knowledge, to undertake such a comprehensive analysis of the returns on investment in the continuum of care for RMNCH (Stenberg and others 2014).

CONTEXT OF THE ANALYSIS

The benefits of improving the health of mothers and children are indisputable, and considerable progress has been made in reducing maternal and child deaths since the publication of *Disease Control Priorities in Developing Countries*, second edition (Jamison and others 2006). The global maternal mortality ratio decreased 25 percent, from 288 per 100,000 live births in 2005 to 216 in 2015 (Alkema and others 2015; WHO, UNICEF, UNFPA, and World Bank 2015). The global mortality rate for children under age five years decreased 32 percent, from 63 per 1,000 live births in 2005 to 42.5 in 2015 (UNICEF, WHO, World Bank, UN 2013; You and others 2015). Although several factors have contributed to these reductions, including general socioeconomic development, the increased coverage of essential RMNCH interventions has played an important role (WHO and UNICEF 2013).

Notwithstanding this progress, 5.9 million children died before their fifth birthdays in 2015, and 303,000 pregnant women died in 2015 from preventable complications related to pregnancy and birth. Moreover, progress has been uneven—both among countries and within countries (Barros and others 2012); a number of countries did not reach Millennium Development Goal (MDG) 4, to reduce child mortality, and MDG 5, to improve maternal health, by 2015 (Alkema and others 2015; You and others 2015).

The remaining challenges in reducing maternal and child mortality are, to a large extent, the effects of uneven attention to the full continuum of care. For example, in the 75 low- and middle-income countries (LMICs) that account for more than 95 percent of global maternal and child deaths, coverage of routine diphtheria-tetanus-pertussis immunization has reached a median level of more than 80 percent; however, coverage of other life-saving interventions is much lower, especially those delivered in the immediate postnatal period (median coverage of less than 45 percent) such as postnatal care for mothers and babies (WHO and UNICEF 2013). Similarly, adolescence remains a neglected period, as highlighted by a series in *The Lancet* on adolescent health (Cappa and others 2012). The continuum of care, including referral chain, is often less than fully functional in these countries (Bossyns and Van Lerberghe 2004; Font and others 2002).

Additional investments are required to sustain gains achieved and to accelerate efforts to address the remaining gaps. With LMICs facing the double burden of communicable and noncommunicable diseases, priorities need to be set to allocate resources to the most effective outcomes.

INVESTMENT "WINS"

This chapter demonstrates the considerable social and economic returns realized through the effect of investments in RMNCH interventions, building on and adding more specificity to earlier results. For example, it has previously been estimated that 30 percent to 50 percent of East Asia's dramatic economic growth during 1965–90 can be attributed to reduced child mortality and subsequent lower fertility rates (Bloom and Williamson 1997), and that gross domestic product (GDP) per capita is increasing by 1.0 percent per year in China and 0.7 percent per year in India as a result of the effect of lower fertility on age structures (Bloom and others 2010).

There are additional reasons why investing in women's and children's health is not only the right thing to do; it is also the smart thing to do.

Improved and Equitable Access

Well-targeted investments along the continuum of care can respond to a fundamental human right: the right to health. Increasing equitable access to RMNCH services is a key strategy for moving closer to universal health coverage, defined by the WHO as when all people obtain the health services they need without suffering financial hardship when paying for them (WHO 2010, ix).

Health System Benefits

Investments in women's and children's health strengthen the entire health system. For example, the capacity to provide 24-hour emergency obstetric care requires that health system components, such as qualified health workers, medications, facilities, and a functioning referral system, be in place across geographic areas.

Extended Lifecycle Benefits

Investments in RMNCH bring benefits across age groups. For example, investments in nutrition have long-lasting effects beyond the immediate improvement in nutritional status, such as improvements in cognitive development, school performance, and future earnings (Ruger and others 2012).

Cost-Effective Interventions

A considerable body of research, including *Disease Control Priorities in Developing Countries*, second edition, has established that RMNCH interventions are among the most effective and cost-effective available (Jamison and others 2006). Recent evidence confirms these findings. A study of diarrhea and pneumonia interventions finds that 15 highly cost-effective interventions exist that, if implemented at scale, would prevent 95 percent of deaths from diarrhea and 67 percent of deaths from pneumonia in children under age five years by 2025 (Bhutta and others 2013). Evidence from Afghanistan suggests that an approach combining improved family planning with incremental improvements in skilled birth attendance, transport, referral, and appropriate intrapartum care in high-quality facilities could prevent 75 percent of maternal deaths at a cost of less than US$200 per year of life saved (Carvalho, Salehi, and Goldie 2012).

Improved Integration of Services

Opportunities exist to deliver packages of interventions when women and children present at health facilities,

for example, to prevent sexually transmitted infections in conjunction with family planning programs (Church and Mayhew 2009). Findings of the Multi-Country Evaluation of the Integrated Management of Childhood Illness (IMCI) suggest that integrated care can lead to cost savings: the annual cost of providing health care to children was considerably lower in districts with IMCI compared with districts without it (Adam and others 2005).

ANALYTICAL FRAMEWORK FOR ASSESSING INVESTMENTS IN THE CONTINUUM OF CARE

The conceptual and methodological framework used is summarized in figure 16.1. This framework has three main elements:

- Identification of a suite of essential, cost-effective interventions

Figure 16.1 Conceptual and Methodological Framework

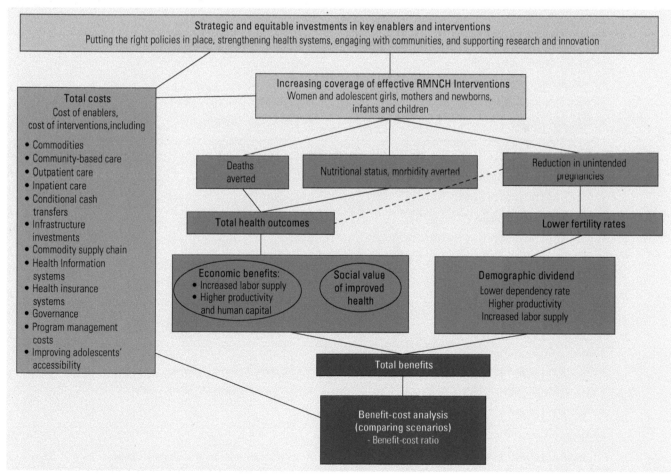

Source: Adapted from Stenberg and others 2014.
Note: RMNCH = Reproductive, maternal, newborn, and child health.

- Estimation of the health and fertility impacts and the total cost of specific levels of additional investment in these interventions
- Assessment of the economic and social benefits arising from these health and fertility impacts.

Selecting the Interventions

National policy makers must choose which services to provide, taking into account budgetary constraints and financial ceilings allocated by the ministry of finance and other financing partners. Evidence on cost-effectiveness, current health system capacity, feasibility, and acceptability will inform investment strategies. The framework outlined in this chapter includes interventions that were identified in a 2011 review as essential and cost-effective RMNCH interventions (PMNCH, WHO, and Aga Khan University 2011). Table 16.1 lists the 50 selected interventions grouped into six broad packages that follow program structures in many national health systems: family planning, maternal and newborn health, malaria, HIV/AIDS, immunization, and child health, with nutrition included in several packages.

The effective delivery of high-quality interventions depends on key enablers, including national policies, functional health systems, community engagement, and innovation. Strategies modeled include those supporting both the supply side (for example, expanding health

Table 16.1 Preventive and Treatment Interventions Modeled[a]

Promotive and preventive interventions	Treatment interventions
Family planning	
Modern family planning methods, including pill, condom, injectable, IUD, implant, female sterilization, male sterilization, LAM, vaginal barrier method, and vaginal tablets	
Maternal and newborn health	
• Multiple micronutrient supplementation[b]	• Safe abortion[c]
• Balanced energy supplementation[b]	• Postabortion case management
• Preventive postnatal care	• Ectopic case management
• Periconceptional folic acid supplementation	• Syphilis detection and treatment in pregnant women
• Calcium supplementation for prevention and treatment of preeclampsia and eclampsia	• Management of preeclampsia with magnesium sulphate
• Induction of labor (beyond 41 weeks)	• Detection and management of diabetes in pregnancy[b]
• Labor and delivery management	• Detection and management of fetal growth restriction[b]
• Clean practices and immediate essential newborn care	• Basic and emergency obstetric care
• Active management of the third stage of labor	• Management of eclampsia with magnesium sulphate
• Kangaroo mother care	• Neonatal resuscitation in institutions
	• Antenatal corticosteroids for preterm labor
	• Antibiotics for preterm premature rupture of membranes
	• Full supportive care for neonatal infections
Malaria	
• Insecticide treated materials	• Treatment of malaria in children
• Pregnant women sleeping under ITNs	• Treatment of malaria in pregnant women
• Intermittent preventive treatment for pregnant women	
HIV/AIDS	
• Prevention of mother-to-child transmission	• ART (first-line treatment) for pregnant women
• Cotrimoxazole for children	• Pediatric ART

table continues next page

Table 16.1 Preventive and Treatment Interventions Modeled (continued)

Promotive and preventive interventions	Treatment interventions
Immunization	
• Tetanus toxoid vaccine	
• Rotavirus vaccine	
• Measles vaccine	
• DPT vaccination	
• Hib vaccine	
• Polio vaccine	
• BCG vaccine	
• Pneumococcal vaccine	
• Meningitis vaccine[b]	
Child health	
• Breastfeeding counseling and support; complementary feeding counseling and support	• Oral rehydration therapy
	• Zinc for diarrhea treatment
• Vitamin A supplementation in infants and children ages 6–59 months	• Antibiotics for treatment of dysentery
	• Pneumonia treatment in children
	• Management of severe malnutrition in children
	• Management of moderate acute malnutrition[b]
	• Vitamin A for measles treatment in children

Source: Based on Stenberg and others 2014.
Note: ART = antiretroviral therapy; BCG = bacille Calmette-Guérin; DPT = diphtheria, pertussis, and tetanus; Hib = *Haemophilus influenzae* type B; ITN = insecticide-treated bednet; IUD = intrauterine device; LAM = lactational amenorrhea method.
a. Some interventions may have both preventive and curative elements.
b. Current analysis includes impact only, not cost.
c. In countries where abortion is legal.

Estimating the Costs

system access by constructing new hospitals and facilities) and the demand side (for example, mass media campaigns to encourage breastfeeding and care seeking for childhood illnesses).

The second stage of the analysis is to use modeling tools to estimate the health and fertility impacts of the interventions and the investment costs required.

With respect to costs, attempts have been made to estimate the resources required to scale up the provision of essential RMNCH services in LMICs. Most of these are disease- or program-specific cost studies that determine costs more or less specific to the disease or age group (Bhutta and others 2013; Singh and Darroch 2012; Stenberg and others 2007). Such studies tend to include patient-level costs for intervention-specific commodities, such as vaccines, bednets, and nutritional supplements,

as well as some estimates of the time and related cost of health workers involved in providing the health services. Ideally, these studies would also include program support costs, for example, for training in disease-specific management, epidemiological surveillance, and provision of vehicles specific to the program activities. However, the studies may not always do so, or the specific methods used to estimate such costs are not always well described. Finally, program- or disease-specific estimates may miss resources needed for broader health-system-strengthening activities, thereby underestimating the true resource needs for the provision of services. Health-system-strengthening activities to consider include preservice training and deployment of clinical staff, development of a functioning referral system, strengthening the health information system, and upgrading facility infrastructure. Figure 16.1 shows the 12 components of the full cost of scaling up the interventions that are estimated in the analysis presented in this chapter.

Estimating Health and Fertility Impacts

The scale up of a comprehensive package of care will have interactions across diseases and age groups. The interlinkages built into the OneHealth Tool and accompanying impact modules (box 16.1) eliminate double counting of lives saved, and they take into account the reduction in need for treatment as preventive care is scaled up. Increases in coverage are translated into reductions in maternal, newborn, and child mortality, along with declines in some aspects of morbidity such as prevalence of wasting and stunting. Fertility rates are modeled to decrease with increasing targets for contraceptive prevalence rates, in turn affecting population growth projections over time.

Assessing the Economic and Social Benefits of Achieved Outcomes

Once the improved health outcomes arising from the interventions—lives saved, morbidity averted, and unwanted pregnancies avoided—are determined, the task is to measure the benefits arising from these better outcomes. Some of these benefits will be strictly economic, reflected in higher GDP from increased workforce participation and from higher productivity. However, other benefits, although equally real and certainly economic in a broader welfare sense, will not be reflected in conventional GDP measures. A mother's life saved so that she is able to look after her children and support her community has great social value even if she does not enter the paid workforce. Equally, the value of a child's life saved does not depend only on his or her participation in the labor force when an adult. We refer to the benefits not captured in existing GDP measures as *social benefits.*

A strong consensus exists among economists that measurements of economic and social change need to move beyond production or conventional GDP to sustainable well-being (Stiglitz and others 2009) and that these more inclusive measures are especially important in relation to health (Arrow and others 2013; Suhrcke and others 2012). These more inclusive methods can be referred to as *full income methods.* They include additional benefits from improved health outcomes and more inclusive gauges of income than those included in GDP as it is currently measured.

The Lancet Commission on Investing in Health (Jamison and others 2013) argues strongly for a full income approach to measuring the benefits of investment in health, defined as measured increases in conventional GDP plus the value of additional life years gained. The approach presented in this chapter goes further, because it does not limit the analysis to the benefits arising from lives saved. We attempt to include in an explicit manner estimates of economic and social benefits from morbidity averted, and to estimate the economic benefits

---

Box 16.1

Translating Coverage Increases into Cost and Health Impacts: The OneHealth Tool

The OneHealth Tool (OHT) is a software program that aims to support integrated planning processes in low- and middle-income countries by bringing together disease-specific program planning and health systems planning. The tool was born out of a review of tools for strategic planning and costing that found that existing tools did not adequately allow for sector-wide scenario analysis (PMNCH 2008). The OHT aims to facilitate planning that incorporates health promotion, prevention, treatment, and disease management. Version 4 includes detailed modules for programs such as nutrition, child health, malaria, and noncommunicable diseases, as well as modules for health systems planning, for example, human resources, logistics, and infrastructure. It is prepopulated with demographic and epidemiological data by country, as well as input assumptions for prevention and treatment interventions based on World Health Organization–recommended treatment protocols. The tool estimates the likely health impact (mortality and morbidity) of scaling up coverage. The OHT incorporates preexisting models used by various United Nations' epidemiological reference groups such as the Lives Saved Tool (Winfrey, McKinnon, and Stover 2011); the AIDS Impact Model for HIV/AIDS interventions (USAID 2007; Stover and others 2010); and the FamPlan model, which computes the relationship between family planning and the total fertility rate (Bongaarts 1978; USAID 2004).

derived from control of fertility and hence from the reduction in unwanted pregnancies—the *demographic dividend*. Accordingly, the approach in this chapter allows for a more comprehensive approximation of the estimated benefits than that used in Jamison and others (2013) and other studies.

MEASURING THE HEALTH IMPACTS AND FULL COSTS OF INVESTMENTS IN THE CONTINUUM OF CARE

Estimates were derived for 74 high-burden countries in which more than 95 percent of the world's child and maternal mortality occurs (WHO and UNICEF 2013).[1] The list includes 35 low-income countries (LICs), 27 LMICs, 11 upper-middle-income countries (UMICs), and one high-income country (HIC). The investment occurs during 2013–35, and only health and fertility outcomes brought about by investment up to 2035 are considered. The economic and social benefits of those outcomes, such as lives saved or morbidity averted, continue to accrue for some decades to come and can be taken account of in the investment appraisal.

Modeling an Increase in Coverage Level

An investment case may take into account different scenarios of specific packages of services (content), levels of investment (level of ambition), and strategies (for example, community-based versus facility-based delivery) to achieve the set goals. At the country level, the various different scenarios should be assessed to inform national policy discussions regarding the most-effective resource allocations. Here, for illustrative purposes and in the interest of assessing the benefits of investing in a set of high-mortality countries, we scale up the same package of interventions across all countries. A scenario that maintains current baseline (2012) coverage is defined as *Low*, while an ambitious scenario with coverage increasing for all 50 interventions until 2035 is defined as *High* (table 16.2).[2]

The relative level of coverage across the scenarios drives the differences in intervention costs and impact so that the incremental effect of an investment strategy (that is, the High scenario) compared with maintaining current coverage without strengthening the health system (the Low scenario) can be assessed and valued. The analysis is centered on the comparison between

Table 16.2 Parameters of the Investment Analysis

Overall parameters	Scope of the analysis
Years of investment cost	2013–35
Years for which benefits are estimated	2013–35 (health benefits)
	2013–70 (economic and social benefits)
Population considered	4.9 billion in 2013 (74 countries) (UN 2013)
Costs considered	
Service delivery costs[a]	• **Inpatient care**: Costs comprise the "hotel" component of hospital costs, that is, excluding the cost of drugs and diagnostic tests but including costs for personnel and infrastructure running costs.
	• **Outpatient care**: Personnel and infrastructure running costs.
	• **Community-based care**: A proxy value is applied, assuming that the running cost of community-based care would be one-third the cost of care provided at health centers.
Intervention-specific direct costs[b]	Drugs, vaccines, laboratory tests, and medical supplies based on treatment guidelines
Program administration costs[c]	• **General**: Resource needs are estimated using a bottom-up ingredients approach for each specific area (child health, maternal health, immunization) and comprise in-service training activities, development of preservice training materials, distribution of printed information materials, mass media campaigns, supervision of community health workers, routine program management, conditional cash transfers, and other activities considered essential for ensuring an expansion of quality services.
	• **Specific for improving adolescents' access to health services**: Costs for general program coordination at national and district level of adolescent-friendly health services (AFHS), development and distribution of national standards for AFHS, in-service training on AFHS, information and communication activities, and upgrade of infrastructure and equipment to adolescent-friendly standards

table continues next page

Table 16.2 Parameters of the Investment Analysis *(continued)*

Overall parameters	Scope of the analysis
Health systems costs[d]	• Capital investments in infrastructure, primarily related to construction of hospitals, facilities, and health posts. Capital investments are assumed to take place during the first 12 years only (2013–24) to accommodate expansion in service delivery and effective referral systems. • Operational costs for transporting additional RMNCH commodities throughout the supply chain.[e] • Investments in equipment and procedures for better health information management. • Administration of social health insurance in 13 countries classified as having or planning to set up insurance schemes. • Investments in procedures for improved governance and management of resources.

Scenarios considered	Health interventions	Family planning	Economic growth assumptions
LOW This scenario assumes that coverage is maintained at current levels.	• Coverage is maintained at predicted current levels (2012). • It is assumed that with constant coverage, mortality rates do not change over time.	• Coverage is maintained at predicted current levels (2012). • Population growth is as would occur with current contraceptive use and fertility and mortality profiles of the 74 countries. The total population will continue to increase over time, along with the cost of providing services; the total absolute number of deaths will increase.	GDP per capita converges from current estimates to an annual growth rate of 2 percent by 2070.
HIGH This ambitious scenario scales up coverage by accelerating current trends using a best-performer approach.	Projected coverage values are derived from historical trends using the fastest rate of change achieved by countries at specific coverage levels. • For newer vaccines (rotavirus, *Haemophilus influenzae* type b [Hib], and pneumococcal vaccines), predictions of rollouts by Gavi, the Vaccine Alliance were used. • For predictions of HIV incidence, PMTCT, ART for children and adults, and treatment with cotrimoxazole, we applied global targets of 80 percent by 2015, and 95 percent by 2035. • The average coverage level attained for the 50 interventions is 88 percent by 2035.	Family planning and contraceptive use increase based on best-performer trends, with TFR limited from going below 2.1 (unless currently below 2.1).	GDP per capita and year are calculated based on economic benefits and social benefits valued in monetary terms.

Source: Based on Stenberg and others 2014.
Note: ART = antiretroviral therapy; GDP = gross domestic product; PMTCT = prevention of mother-to-child transmission; RMNCH = reproductive, maternal, newborn, and child health; TFR = total fertility rate.
a. WHO-CHOICE estimates of service delivery costs by country.
b. Commodity, vaccine, test, and supply costs included as defaults within the OneHealth Tool, multiplied by quantities of services delivered based on intervention scale up.
c. Program administration and support activity costs calculated as part of previous analysis, notably WHO (2009) and Deogan, Ferguson, and Stenberg (2012).
d. Health-system-strengthening costs calculated as part of previous analysis (WHO 2009).
e. Supply chain costs calculated as a mark-up rate on the variable commodity costs associated with intervention scale up.

scenarios; it is important to note that the main counterfactual in our example is the Low scenario with constant coverage levels and a growing population. Accordingly, the results should not be interpreted as additional spending above current levels of health expenditure, but rather as the cost and impact of bending the curve and accelerating progress compared with a Low scenario in which coverage remains at the 2012 level while population increases.

We applied tools that have been developed by the international community, including the OneHealth Tool (box 16.1) to assess intervention-specific costs and health and fertility impacts. Intervention-specific costs are driven by increases in coverage, with costs distributed to different levels of care (community, outreach, facility, and hospital). Program- and systems-related costs draw upon estimates made by the Taskforce on Innovative International Financing for Health Systems (WHO 2009) and are described in detail in Stenberg and others (2014). Costs are generally estimated using an ingredients approach (quantity times price), with the exception of supply chain costs, for which a mark-up ratio is applied.

ESTIMATING THE FULL BENEFITS OF INVESTMENT IN THE CONTINUUM OF CARE

Key Methodological Assumptions

The costs and the benefits are defined as the incremental costs and benefits between two scenarios. However, when fertility management tools are an important part of the suite of interventions, the populations in the two scenarios diverge substantially. The approach we adopt is to assess only those benefits that apply to those alive in the High scenario, and we compare their situation to what it would have been in the Low scenario.

Three broad types of benefit are identified:

- Some have the benefit of life because their lives were saved through the interventions.
- Others are in much better health because of the morbidity averted.
- The whole community has the benefit of higher per capita incomes arising from the reduction in unintended pregnancies and from the processes that the fall in fertility rates sets in motion.

The difference in deaths and in morbidity for children between the Low and High scenarios will reflect two different factors: the impact of the health interventions for a given level of births, and the reduction in the number of births (due to expanding family planning) for a given level of health. We partition the reduction in child deaths and in morbidity between the Low and High scenarios into these two components. We use only the former, which we refer to as *lives saved*, in calculating benefits.[3] The reduction in child mortality from scaling up contraceptives is thus counted in the health impact results but not in the cost-benefit analysis. All maternal deaths prevented are considered to be lives saved; that is, the full reduction in maternal mortality is translated into economic benefits.

GDP per capita paths were derived from World Bank data and were combined with population estimates from the OneHealth Tool projections; these were extended to 2070 on the basis of convergence to zero population growth in each country by that year. Per capita GDP estimates and assumptions about productivity are combined with data on labor force participation of those affected by the intervention[4] (ILO 2013).

Economic and Social Benefits of Years of Life Saved

A vast literature discusses the value of a statistical life[5] and, by implication, the value of life years saved (VLY). Most studies use a willingness-to-pay approach, either in the form of analyses of revealed preferences evident in wage and risk data or analyses of stated preferences. Viscusi and Aldy (2003) review the revealed preference literature and suggest, albeit with a wide uncertainty margin, an implied value for a life year of about 4.0 times GDP per capita, with an income elasticity of about 0.6. These two facts, in turn, imply a value of a life year for LICs of 1.5 to 2.0 times GDP per capita.

Jamison and others (2012) estimate the VLY as 2.3 times GDP per capita in LMICs at a 3 percent discount rate, with estimates by World Bank region ranging from 1.4 for Latin America and the Caribbean and for the Middle East and North Africa to 4.2 for Sub-Saharan Africa. Cropper, Hammitt, and Robinson (2011) note the recent expansion of the stated preference literature, in which individuals are asked about how they would act in hypothetical situations, and that the value of a statistical life emerging from these studies is much lower than for revealed preference studies.

The revealed preference studies refer to both the economic and social value of a life year; by economic value we mean the value that would be captured in conventional GDP measures, primarily through labor force effects; the social value refers to all other benefits of an additional year of life to an individual or a community not captured in GDP. We regard it as useful to distinguish between the social and economic components of the VLY because they may have different roles in some investment analyses.

We have constrained the total value of a life year across these two components to 1.5 times GDP per capita for the sample as a whole, which we regard as being at the lower end of the range used in the literature. The calculated economic benefits of increased labor force participation amount to about 1.0 times GDP per capita, calculated as the sum of GDP for all 74 countries divided by the population for all 74 countries. A social VLY equal to 0.5 times the GDP per capita of the full set of sample countries is then applied as a common value across countries. Although the strictly economic value of an additional year of life will vary with local economic parameters, there is no reason to think that the social value is lower in poorer countries than in richer ones. Although we do not use any age adjustment for the social value of a life, our procedure results in some discounting of the overall value of a life year for age, and the economic benefits of children's lives saved only begin to accrue when they enter the labor force.

Benefits of Morbidity Averted

Many women and children who survive adverse RMNCH events suffer serious and sustained disabilities (Ashford 2002; Blencowe and others 2013; Mwaniki and others 2012; Souza and others 2013) that undoubtedly have substantial human, social, and economic costs. The interventions studied here should be expected to generate important benefits through lower morbidity. In spite of its acknowledged importance, few attempts have been made to quantify the burden of maternal and child morbidity or to estimate its economic and social cost; we attempt to begin the process in this study.

Although the OneHealth Tool estimates the lives saved as a result of scaling up the interventions, it does not measure the morbidity averted (other than for wasting and stunting) or the impact on mortality in subsequent years from averting morbidity in the initial year. We estimate morbidity averted for four causes for children (preterm birth complications, birth injury, congenital abnormalities, and malnutrition) and two for mothers (obstructed labor and other maternal disorders), and calculate economic and social benefits.[6] Moreover, we derive parameters relating improved nutritional outcomes—prevention of low stature and low birth weight—to lifetime earnings and apply these to estimates of reduced wasting and stunting by country.

Benefits of Reduced Fertility Rates

The third benefit is the economic impact of the reduction in fertility rates, which is well documented in the literature.[7] Ashraf, Weil, and Wilde (2013) identify a range of channels through which a reduction in the total fertility rate (TFR), that is, the number of children born to the average woman during her lifetime, affects growth in GDP per capita; these channels can be grouped into three types of effect, each affecting GDP:

- A dependency effect because a reduction in births reduces the dependent population. Given that the nondependent population produces the GDP, the fall in the dependent population for a given level of GDP increases the level of GDP per capita.

- A labor supply effect because adults are able to devote more time to working. (With fewer births, women and other caregivers will have an increased propensity to enter the labor force, leading to increased labor supply per capita and hence to increased GDP per head.)

- A productivity effect covering a range of factors influencing long-term productivity, such as higher saving by households and higher investment in schooling. More generally, with lower birth rates, more of a society's resources can be devoted to capital deepening, thereby increasing productivity, rather than to capital widening to meet the needs of the expanding population.

The estimates of the demographic dividend draw on and adjust the methods of Ashraf, Weil, and Wilde (2013), who developed estimates of key parameters based on a review of relevant literature. We derive from their model an aggregate relationship between the reduction in the TFR and the change in GDP per capita over time, out to 2070, and apply this to the change in the TFR in each country to estimate the impact on per capita GDP and hence on overall GDP.[8]

In summary, we present economic benefits, valued in GDP terms, derived from the following:

- Lives saved
- Morbidity averted
- Demographic dividend.

Social benefits, also valued in GDP terms, are derived from the following:

- Lives saved
- Morbidity averted.

In the Low scenario, GDP per capita paths converge to an annual growth rate of 2 percent by 2070. The economic benefits here refer to the difference in GDP growth between the High and Low scenarios.

Two Country Case Studies

To illustrate how the investment framework could be applied at the country level, we present two case studies of LICs. One is a country in Asia that has seen increased coverage of RMNCH interventions and reductions in the fertility rate to about 2.5. The other is a country in Sub-Saharan Africa with low coverage of many RMNCH interventions and continued high fertility rates (table 16.3).

Table 16.3 Parameters of Country Case Studies

	Asia case study country	Sub-Saharan Africa case study country
Description	High coverage of maternal and child health interventions; fertility rates of less than 2.5	Low coverage of most RMNCH interventions; high child and maternal mortality and high fertility rates
U5MR per 1,000 live births	Low (< 60)	High (> 100)
Maternal Mortality Ratio per 100,000 live births	Low (< 100)	Medium (between 100 and 300)
TFR	Low (< 2.5)	High (> 4)
Current health expenditure per capita (2011 U.S. dollars)	Low (< 50)	Low (< 50)
Women's labor participation rate	Low (50–70 percent)	Medium (70–80 percent)
GDP per capita	US$700–US$1,000	US$500–US$800
Coverage increase, High scenario	• Use of modern contraceptives increases to 53 percent from 50 percent	• Use of modern contraceptives scaled up to 49 percent from 13 percent
	• Interventions surrounding child birth are scaled to 95–99 percent from ≈ 30 percent	• Interventions surrounding child birth are scaled up to 95–99 percent from around 50 percent
	• Management of childhood illness and other child interventions reach levels of universal coverage approaching 95 percent	• Management of childhood illness and other child interventions reach levels of universal coverage approaching 95–100 percent
	• Exclusive breastfeeding rates (1–5 months) increase to 75 percent from 41 percent	• Exclusive breastfeeding rates (1–5 months) increase to 99 percent from 22 percent
	• HIV interventions reach 67–100 percent coverage by 2035	• HIV interventions reach 73–100 percent coverage by 2035
Additional estimated costs (2011 U.S. dollars) and deaths prevented for High scenario compared with Low scenario	• Cumulative additional costs 2013–35 of US$17.9 million	• Cumulative additional costs 2013–35 of US$2.4 million
	• Per capita costs in 2035 = US$2.65	• Per capita costs in 2035 = US$6.88
	• 3.1 million deaths prevented 2013–35	• 3.4 million deaths prevented 2013–35

Source: Based on Stenberg and others 2014.
Note: GDP = gross domestic product; HIV = human immunodeficiency virus; RMNCH = reproductive, maternal, newborn, and child health; TFR = total fertility rate; U5MR – under-five mortality rate.

RESULTS: INVESTMENT METRICS AND COMPONENTS OF COSTS AND BENEFITS

We present benefit-cost ratios of investing in RMNCH. For details on costs (in 2011 U.S. dollars) and health benefits, see Stenberg and others (2014). In brief, the High scenario would require an extra US$4.48 per capita in 2035, with country estimates ranging from US$1.2 to US$112.7, although the per capita numbers will be higher in earlier years because of frontloading in infrastructure costs and the increase in population over time. Total costs reach US$30 billion in the third year and remain at that level until 2035.[9]

Table 16.4 shows estimates of total deaths prevented, apportioned between deaths averted (the reduction in births due to enhanced access to contraceptives) and lives saved (the impact of the health interventions on those who are born). The distribution of deaths across these two categories varies across countries and regions, largely reflecting the importance of fertility reduction in individual countries. In UMICs, for example, where fertility rates are in general already fairly low, 75.6 percent of deaths prevented are lives saved.

Benefit-Cost Ratios for Investments

Applying a discount rate enables benefits and costs to be expressed as a net present value (NPV). The benefit-cost ratio for a given discount rate is the ratio of the NPV of benefits and costs at that discount rate.

Table 16.5 reports for all countries considered as a whole, and for groups of countries, the benefit-cost

Table 16.4 Costs and Deaths Prevented, High versus Low Scenarios, 2013–35

Country grouping (number of countries in parentheses)	Cost (billion 2011 US$)	Deaths prevented (millions)	Stillbirths Lives saved (percent)	Stillbirths Deaths averted (percent)	Maternal deaths Lives saved (percent)	Child deaths Lives saved (percent)	Child deaths Deaths averted (percent)	Total lives saved (millions)
Low-income countries (35)	173.6	78.9	30	70	100	46	54	40.4
Lower-middle-income countries (27)	316.3	98.1	40	60	100	58	42	59.9
Upper-middle- and high-income countries (12)	188.8	7.8	43	57	100	67	33	5.9
Total (74)	678.1	184.9	36	64	100	53	47	106.3
Sub-Saharan Africa (43)	232.9	109.3	27	73	100	45	55	54.5
Latin America and the Caribbean (6)	46.8	2.9	42	58	100	64	36	1.9
Middle East and North Africa (5)	24.1	4.7	22	78	100	48	52	2.2
Europe and Central Asia (5)	10.0	0.2	55	45	100	71	29	0.6
South Asia (5)	165.3	60.4	47	53	100	64	36	40.7
East Asia and Pacific (10)	199.0	7.4	61	39	100	86	14	6.5

Source: Based on Stenberg and others 2014.
Note: Numbers may not sum precisely because of rounding.

Table 16.5 Benefit-Cost Ratios for High Compared with Low Scenarios, Selected Periods and Discount Rates

Country grouping	Number of countries	To 2035 (3 percent discount rate)	To 2050 (5 percent discount rate)	To 2070 (7 percent discount rate)
All 74 countries	74	8.7	27.6	34.2
Low-income countries	35	7.2	16.9	18.5
Lower-middle-income countries	27	11.3	34.0	41.0
Upper-middle-income countries, excluding China	10	6.1	22.5	30.1
China	1	0.7	2.7	3.8
India	1	15.0	42.8	52.6
Sub-Saharan Africa	43	11.0	32.3	37.9
South Asia	5	12.7	36.2	43.4
High fertility impact countries[a]	27	13.7	40.6	47.4
Asia case study country	1	4.0	9.4	10.5
Sub-Saharan Africa case study country	1	9.9	24.6	27.4

Source: Based on Stenberg and others 2014.
a. The 27 high fertility impact countries are those in which the estimated demographic dividend by 2035 (comparing the High and Low scenarios) is 8 percent of gross domestic product or greater. These are Afghanistan, Angola, Benin, Burkina Faso, Cameroon, Chad, Comoros, the Democratic Republic of Congo, the Republic of Congo, Equatorial Guinea, The Gambia, Guinea, Guinea-Bissau, Iraq, Kenya, Liberia, Malawi, Mali, Mozambique, Niger, Nigeria, Rwanda, Senegal, Sierra Leone, Somalia, Tanzania, Uganda, and Zambia.

ratios calculated using rising discount rates over the period: 3 percent for 2013–35, 5 percent for 2013–50, and 7 percent for 2013–70. We present results individually for China and India given the significant size of these countries. China is also a particular case in that there is limited additional demographic dividend to gain (table 16.6). Although the 3 percent rate is commonly used in this type of analysis (appendix 3 in Jamison and others 2013), the use of rising discount rates for longer periods is one way of taking account of higher uncertainty over the longer term as well as myopic time preferences and likely increases in consumption over time.

The benefit-cost ratios shown in table 16.5 indicate high returns on increased investment in RMNCH in most countries, especially when benefits beyond the intervention period are included. For all countries considered as a group, the benefit-cost ratio is 8.7 for the intervention period to 2035 at a 3 percent discount rate, 27.6 at 5 percent for the period to 2050, and 34.2 at 7 percent for the period to 2070. The benefit-cost ratio is generally higher for lower-middle-income countries and UMICs than for LICs, especially post 2035, as well as for those 43 countries in Sub-Saharan Africa and 5 in South Asia where maternal and child mortality are highest.

Analysis of Benefits and Benefit-Cost Ratios by Type of Benefit

Tables 16.6 and 16.7 show the contribution from the three sources of benefits to 2050 comparing the High and Low scenarios (using a 5 percent discount rate) expressed in two ways: as a contribution to the overall benefit-cost ratio and as a percentage share of all benefits in NPV terms. These tables illustrate four points about the distribution of benefits.

Uneven Distribution of Demographic Dividend

First, the demographic dividend is unevenly distributed across countries, depending on each country's projected fertility rate reduction. Overall, the reduced fertility generates a benefit-cost ratio of 13.3 by 2050 (the demographic dividend in table 16.6), but the estimated impact of reduced fertility rates in the High scenario is particularly high in 27 countries, where it could lead

Table 16.6 Analysis of Contribution to Benefit-Cost Ratio, High versus Low Scenarios, 5 percent Discount Rate for Net Present Value, 2013–50

Country grouping	Benefit-cost ratio	Direct workforce-related benefits			Demographic dividend	Economic benefits	Social benefits			All benefits
		Lives saved	Morbidity averted	Increase in GDP			Lives saved	Morbidity averted	Total	
		(a)	(b)	(c) = (a) + (b)	(d)	(e) = (c) + (d)	(f)	(g)	(h) = (f) + (g)	(t) = (e) + (h)
All 74 countries	27.6	5.7	1.4	7.1	13.3	20.4	6.7	0.5	7.2	27.6
Low-income countries	16.9	1.4	0.3	1.7	5.5	7.1	9.2	0.6	9.8	16.9
Lower-middle-income countries	34.0	4.2	1.2	5.4	20.0	25.4	8.0	0.6	8.6	34.0
Upper-middle-income countries, excluding China	22.5	6.7	1.8	8.5	11.0	19.5	2.8	0.2	3.0	22.5
China	2.7	1.3	0.3	1.5	0.0	1.5	1.1	0.0	1.2	2.7
India	42.8	5.1	1.5	6.6	21.3	27.9	13.9	1.0	14.9	42.8
Sub-Saharan Africa	32.3	4.1	0.8	4.9	17.4	22.3	9.4	0.6	10.0	32.3
South Asia	36.2	4.4	1.3	5.7	18.1	23.8	11.5	0.9	12.4	36.2
High fertility impact countries	40.6	4.7	0.9	5.6	22.0	27.6	12.2	0.7	13.0	40.6
Asia case study country	9.4	1.0	0.4	1.4	1.8	3.2	5.5	0.7	6.1	9.4
Sub-Saharan Africa case study country	24.6	2.0	0.3	2.3	9.6	11.9	12.2	0.5	12.7	24.6

Source: Based on Stenberg and others 2014.
Note: Total direct health benefits = increase in gross domestic product (GDP) from work-related benefits (c) + total social benefits (h). Numbers may not sum precisely because of rounding.

Table 16.7 Analysis of Contribution to Benefits, High versus Low Scenarios, by percentage Shares, 5 percent Discount Rate for Net Present Value, 2013–50

Country grouping	Direct workforce-related benefits			Demographic dividend	Economic benefits	Social benefits			All benefits
	Lives saved	Morbidity averted	Total			Lives saved	Morbidity averted	Total	
	(a)	(b)	(c) = (a) + (b)	(d)	(e) = (c) + (d)	(f)	(g)	(h) = (f) + (g)	(t) = (e) + (h)
All 74 countries	20.6	5.1	25.7	48.3	74.0	24.2	1.7	26.0	100
Low-income countries	8.2	1.8	10.0	32.2	42.1	54.4	3.4	57.9	100
Lower-middle-income countries	12.4	3.4	15.8	58.9	74.7	23.4	1.9	25.3	100
Upper-middle-income countries, excluding China	29.7	7.8	37.5	49.0	86.6	12.6	0.7	13.4	100
China	46.4	10.6	57.0	0.0	57.0	41.9	1.1	43.0	100
India	11.9	3.5	15.5	49.7	65.2	32.4	2.4	34.9	100
Sub-Saharan Africa	12.6	2.5	15.1	54.0	69.1	29.1	1.8	30.9	100
South Asia	12.2	3.5	15.6	50.1	65.8	31.7	2.6	34.2	100
High fertility impact countries	11.5	2.3	13.8	54.3	68.1	30.1	1.8	31.9	100
Asia case study country	10.5	4.8	15.2	20.0	34.3	58.1	7.6	65.7	100
Sub-Saharan Africa case study country	7.8	1.3	9.1	39.0	48.1	49.4	2.6	51.9	100

Source: Based on Stenberg and others 2014.

Note: Total direct health benefits = increase in gross domestic product (GDP) from work-related benefits (c) + total social benefits (h).

to an increase in GDP per capita of 8 percent or more by 2035. In these countries, which are mainly lower-middle-income countries, the demographic dividend on total investment generates a benefit-cost ratio of 22.

High Direct Health Benefits

Second, the direct health benefits, excluding the demographic dividend, are very high at 14.3 for the sample as a whole. These direct benefits are much more evenly distributed across countries, 11.4 for LICs and 11.5 for UMICs, excluding China.

Total Economic and Social Benefits Are Fairly Equal

Third, the workforce-related economic benefits (excluding the demographic dividend) and the social benefits are about equal for the sample as a whole. The benefit-cost ratio generated by the direct workforce benefits alone is 7.1, and that generated by the social benefits alone is 7.2 for the 74 countries. The contribution of direct workforce benefits versus social benefits varies significantly across country income groups; social benefits are much greater than workforce-related benefits in LICs, but the reverse is true in UMICs. This finding presumably reflects the lower economic value of lives saved and morbidity averted in poorer countries, whereas the social benefits are valued using a sample-wide metric.

Significant Morbidity Benefits

Finally, in spite of the very preliminary nature of the morbidity analysis, the morbidity benefits are significant, representing 6.8 percent of the total benefits (table 16.7). These results suggest that further detailed work on maternal and child morbidity is both appropriate and necessary.

Results from Two Case Studies

The Asian country is considerably larger in both population and GDP than the Sub-Saharan African country and has a somewhat higher level of GDP per capita. The Sub-Saharan African country has higher mortality rates for both children and mothers in addition to a higher fertility rate and a higher level of labor force participation by women (table 16.3).

Although the total cost of the intervention for the Asian country is larger than that for the Sub-Saharan African country, reflecting the disparity in population size, the additional cost per person for the High versus the Low scenario is considerably lower at US$2.65 (versus US$6.88). This result is due to the higher fertility and maternal and child death rates in the Sub-Saharan African country, which require a higher level of intervention and a greater cost per capita. Despite the differences in population size, the numbers of maternal, child, and stillbirth deaths prevented by the interventions are similar in the two countries, with a proportionally greater impact in the Sub-Saharan African country.

Table 16.5 shows a high benefit-cost ratio for the Sub-Saharan African country, with results similar to those for the average of all 74 countries and for the group of LICs. Although positive, the benefit-cost ratio for the Asian country is more modest, again reflecting the differences in initial fertility and death rates.

A more detailed description of the sources of the benefits that arise from the intervention for the two country case studies is provided in tables 16.6 and 16.7. For the Asian country, the biggest contributors to the benefit-cost ratio are those benefits arising from the social value of lives saved and morbidity averted (65.7 percent). The contributions from the increase in GDP from workforce-related benefits (15.2 percent) and from the demographic dividend (20.0 percent) are more modest but still significant. Considered solely as a function of either the increase in GDP from workforce-related benefits or from the demographic dividend, the benefit-cost ratio still shows benefits outweighing costs (ratios of 1.4 and 1.8, respectively).

For the Sub-Saharan African country, in contrast, the contributions from the economic and social benefits are virtually equal (48.1 percent and 51.9 percent, respectively). The demographic dividend is about twice as important as for the Asian country (39.0 percent), while the contribution from additional GDP is lower (9.1 percent). Again as a function of either the increase in GDP from workforce-related benefits or from the demographic dividend, the benefit-cost ratio shows benefits outweighing costs (ratios of 2.3 and 9.6, respectively) and the ratios are higher than for the Asian country.

IMPLICATIONS OF THE ANALYSIS

The analysis presented refers to 74 countries that account for more than 95 percent of global maternal and child deaths. This approach goes beyond the standard full income approach to allow for a more comprehensive picture of the returns on investment by explicitly including estimates of economic and social benefits from morbidity averted, and by estimating the effect of the demographic dividend. The analysis points to six main findings.

Large Economic and Social Returns

First, investments in high-impact interventions across the continuum of care in RMNCH have large economic and social returns in addition to the impact on health outcomes. The benefit-cost ratio of investments in the High scenario for the full country sample is 8.7 in 2035. Findings are robust to variations in the methods of analysis, such as discount rates.

Affordable Investments

Second, the required investments are affordable for most countries. On average for the 74 countries, an additional US$4.48 per capita would be needed in 2035 to finance the High scenario. However, affordability needs to be examined in the context of fiscal sustainability as issues related to universal coverage, financial protection, quality, responsiveness, and efficiency will affect the policy dialogue around public investment in health, and macroeconomic conditions will set the overall boundaries for what can be achieved. The Global Financing Facility to Advance Women's and Children's Health, created in 2014, will support countries in overcoming fiscal constraints in the short term and in setting up mechanisms to achieve long-term sustainable domestic financing.[10]

Variable Returns on Investment

Third, the magnitude of returns on investment varies across country groupings. By income, the highest returns are realized in lower-middle-income countries. This finding might be explained by two factors: First, economies of lower-middle-income countries with higher GDP have higher returns operating through workforce benefits and the demographic dividend compared with LICs. Second, returns in UMICs might be lower than in LMICs, given their already lower mortality rates and more strongly diminishing returns.

The findings vary by individual countries, reflecting the epidemiological and demographic situation in each, current health systems performance, and country-specific economic factors. The substantially different findings of the two country case studies confirms that individual countries will find considerable value in undertaking their own investment analyses, to give results specific to their circumstances. For example, the returns on investment in the Sub-Saharan African case study country, with low coverage of most RMNCH interventions, and therefore still facing high child and maternal mortality rates and high fertility rates, are more than twice as large as the case study country in Asia, which has managed to increase coverage of RMNCH interventions and reduce fertility rates to less than 2.5. The country case studies confirm the importance of investing in family planning; the effect of the demographic dividend is substantial even when the investment reduces the TFR by a small amount.

Similarly, we present results for China and India separately, given the size of their populations and economies. Given current low birth rates in China, no significant economic benefits are to be derived from increasing the availability of family planning. This is not to argue that significant benefits could not be bought by increasing the quality of current programs and ensuring their responsiveness to population needs (Kane and Choi 1999). In India, our model estimates high economic benefits from increasing the contraceptive prevalence rate to respond to the unmet need.

High Rates of Return for a Comprehensive Approach, Including Family Planning

Fourth, investment in each of the elements in the continuum of care matters. The analysis finds that family planning programs generate particularly high returns, especially in countries with current high fertility rates, primarily through its effect on the demographic dividend. We have not separated out the rate of return on investment in maternal versus child health because the analysis deals with investing across the full spectrum of RMNCH; however, we note that there may be specifically high returns on investment in maternal care for adolescents, given that adolescent pregnancies pose a much higher risk for both mother and newborn compared with pregnancies among women of older age groups (Patton and others 2009; WHO 2008, 2011).

Returns on Investment Vary over Time

Fifth, the different types of interventions often generate benefits in different time frames, so that the rate of return varies over time. Returns increase substantially over time, particularly beyond the investment period of 2013–35. For example, at a discount rate of 3 percent, the benefit-cost ratio for the full sample of 74 countries is about four times larger in 2070 (34.2) as in 2035 (8.7). Although policy makers often make decisions in much shorter time horizons, it is nevertheless important to note that returns are realized well beyond the investment period.

An Extended Modeling Approach

Finally, on a methodological note, the overall economic and social benefits are driven by the demographic dividend generated by the investment. For example, in 2050 the demographic dividend accounts for 48.3 percent of the benefit-cost ratio (for the 74 countries). Workforce-related benefits and social benefits account for about 25 percent each. The relative share of morbidity-averted benefits compared with lives saved benefits is low because only a few sources of morbidity are included in the model, and the gains in morbidity are adjusted for the degree of disability averted. For LICs, the social benefits predominate because these are valued using the average GDP per capita of all countries; the workforce-related benefits are valued using country GDP per person in the workforce.

CONCLUSIONS

The analysis extends the full income approach to include estimates of economic and social benefits from morbidity averted and estimates of the effect of the demographic dividend, thereby providing a more comprehensive picture of the returns on investment in RMNCH interventions.

The analysis is limited to the health sector and does not include all sexual and reproductive health interventions; notably, surgical care is omitted because of a lack of data to enable us to model related costs and impacts. Estimates do not take into account costs and returns of some interventions that contribute to improving RMNCH outcomes, such as water supply, sanitation and hygiene, girls' education, empowerment of women and girls, and food fortification. Moreover, it should be acknowledged that the high returns calculated here are dependent on those investments being made, for example, in the education sector, to empower women with greater decision-making authority in relation to planning family size. To realize high returns, countries need to consider effective multisectoral policies to deliver public goods associated with family planning and maternal and reproductive health, including for adolescents.

Despite these limitations, the results underscore the value of addressing remaining gaps. RMNCH concerns should feature prominently in the post-2015 landscape, for example, in the Sustainable Development Goals that are to supersede the MDGs. The development of models focused more strongly on the morbidity elements of maternal and child health, and the evolution of that morbidity over time, is an important topic for future research. Further work should also consider nonhealth interventions, including activities that affect social determinants of health.

NOTES

World Bank Income Classifications as of July 2014 are as follows, based on estimates of gross national income (GNI) per capita for 2013:

- Low-income countries (LICs) = US$1,045 or less
- Middle-income countries (MICs) are subdivided:
  a) lower-middle-income (LMICs) = US$1,046 to US$4,125
  b) upper-middle-income (UMICs) = US$4,126 to US$12,745
- High-income countries (HICs) = US$12,746 or more.

1. Of the 75 countries accounting for more than 95 percent of global maternal and child mortality, data limitations prevented inclusion of South Sudan in the analysis.
2. The original analysis also includes an intermediate *Medium* scenario.
3. The methods by which this is done are discussed in Stenberg and others (2014).
4. For assumptions on participation rates and labor market productivity of women and children upon entering the labor force, see Stenberg and others (2014).
5. For reviews see Viscusi and Aldy (2003); Jamison and others (2012); and Cropper and others (2011).
6. For more details, see Stenberg and others (2014).
7. For a recent review, see Canning and Schultz (2012).
8. In subsequent work it would be appropriate to take account of the specific characteristics, especially of the population structure, of each country.
9. Per capita costs in 2035 for *High versus Low*, refer to the difference between the estimated costs in the High and in the Low scenarios in 2035, divided by the population in the High scenario in 2035.
10. http://www.worldbank.org/en/news/press-release /2014/09/25/development-partners-support-creation -global-financing-facility-women-children-health (accessed October 24, 2014).

REFERENCES

Adam, T., F. Manzi, J. R. M. Armstrong Schellenberg, L. Mgalula, D. de Savigny, and others. 2005. "Does the Integrated Management of Childhood Illness Cost More than Routine Care? Results from Tanzania." *Bulletin of the World Health Organization* 83 (5): 369–77.

Alkema, L. D. Chou, D. Hogan, S. Zhang, A.-B. Moller, and others. 2015. "Global, Regional, and National Levels and Trends in Maternal Mortality between 1990 and 2015, with Scenario-Based Projections to 2030: A Systematic Analysis by the UN Maternal Mortality Estimation Inter-Agency Group." *The Lancet*. Epub November 13, 2015. doi:10.1016/ S0140-6736(15)00838-7.

Arrow, K. J., P. Dasgupta, L. H. Goulder, K. J. Mumford, and K. Oleson. 2013 "Sustainability and the Measurement of Wealth: Further Reflections." *Environment and Development Economics* 18 (4): 504–16.

Ashford, L. 2002. *Hidden Suffering: Disabilities from Pregnancy and Childbirth in Less Developed Countries.* Washington, DC: Population Reference Bureau. http://www.prb.org/pdf /HiddenSufferingEng.pdf.

Ashraf, Q., D. Weil, and J. Wilde. 2013. "The Effect of Fertility Reduction on Economic Growth." *Population and Development Review* 39 (1): 97–130.

Barros, A. J. D., C. Ronsmans, H. Axelson, E. Loaiza, A. D. Bertoldi, and others. 2012. "Equity in Maternal, Newborn, and Child Health Interventions in Countdown to 2015: A Retrospective Review of Survey Data from 54 Countries." *The Lancet* 379 (9822): 1225–33.

Bhutta, Z. A., J. K. Das, A. Rizvi, M. F. Gaffey, N. Walker, and others. 2013. "Evidence-Based Interventions for Improvement of Maternal and Child Nutrition: What Can Be Done and at What Cost?" *The Lancet* 382 (9890): 452–77.

Blencowe, H., A. C. Lee, S. Cousens, A. Bahalim, R. Narwal, and others. 2013. "Preterm Birth-Associated Neuro-developmental Impairment Estimates at Regional and Global Levels for 2010." *Pediatric Research* 74 (Suppl 1): 35–49.

Bloom, D. E., D. Canning, L. Hu, Y. Liu, A. Mahal, and others. 2010. "The Contribution of Population Health and Demographic Change to Economic Growth in China and India." *Journal of Comparative Economics* 38 (1): 17–33.

Bloom, D. E., and J. G. Williamson. 1997. "Demographic Transitions and Economic Miracles in Emerging Asia." Working Paper 6268, National Bureau of Economic Research, Cambridge, MA.

Bongaarts, J. 1978. "A Framework for Analyzing the Proximate Determinants of Fertility." *Population and Development Review* 4 (1): 105–32.

Bossyns, P., and W. Van Lerberghe. 2004. "The Weakest Link: Competence and Prestige as Constraints to Referral by Isolated Nurses in Rural Niger." *Human Resources for Health* 2 (1): 1.

Canning, D., and T. Schultz. 2012. "The Economic Consequences of Reproductive Health and Family Planning." *The Lancet* 380 (9837): 165–71.

Cappa, C., T. Wardlaw, C. Lengevin-Falcon, and J. Diers. 2012. "Progress for Children: A Report Card on Adolescents." *The Lancet* 379 (9834): 2323–25.

Carvalho, N., A. S. Salehi, and S. J. Goldie. 2012. "National and Sub-National Analysis of the Health Benefits and Cost-Effectiveness of Strategies to Reduce Maternal Mortality in Afghanistan." *Health Policy and Planning* 28 (1): 62–74.

Church, K., and S. H. Mayhew. 2009. "Integration of STI and HIV Prevention, Care, and Treatment into Family Planning

Services: A Review of the Literature." *Studies in Family Planning* 40 (3): 171–86.

Cropper, M., J. Hammitt, and L. Robinson. 2011. "Valuing Mortality Risk Reductions: Progress and Challenges." *Annual Review of Resource Economics* 3 (1): 313–36.

Deogan, C., J. Ferguson, and K. Stenberg. 2012. "Resource Needs for Adolescent Friendly Health Services: Estimates for 74 Low- and Middle-Income Countries." *PLoS One* 7: e51420.

Font, F., L. Quinto, H. Masanja, R. Nathan, C. Ascaso, and others. 2002. "Paediatric Referrals in Rural Tanzania: The Kilombero District Study: A Case Series." *BMC International Health and Human Rights* 2 (1): 4.

ILO (International Labour Organization). 2013. LABORSTA Database. *Economically Active Population, Estimates and Projections.* 6th edition. Geneva: ILO Department of Statistics. http://laborsta.ilo.org/applv8/data/EAPEP /eapep_E.html.

Jamison, D. T., J. G. Breman, A. R. Measham, G. Alleyne, M. Claeson, D. B. Evans, P. Jha, A. Mills, and P. Musgrove, eds. 2006. *Disease Control Priorities in Developing Countries.* 2nd edition. Washington, DC: World Bank and Oxford University Press.

Jamison, D. T., P. Jha, R. Laxminarayan, and T. Ord. 2012. "Infectious Disease, Injury, and Reproductive Health." In *Global Problems, Smart Solutions: Costs and Benefits*, edited by B. Lomborg, 390–426. Cambridge, UK: Cambridge University Press. http://www.cambridge.org/us/academic /subjects/economics/public-economics-and-public-policy /global-problems-smart-solutions-costs-and-benefits #contentsTabAnchor.

Jamison, D. T., L. H. Summers, G. Alleyne, K. J. Arrow, S. Berkley, and others. 2013. "Global Health 2035: A World Converging within a Generation." *The Lancet* 382 (9908): 1898–955.

Kane, P., and C. Y. Choi. 1999. "China's One Child Family Policy." *BMJ* 319 (7215): 992–94.

Kerber, K., J. E. de Graft-Johnson, Z. A. Bhutta, P. Okong, A. Starrs, and others. 2007. "Continuum of Care for Maternal, Newborn, and Child Health: From Slogan to Service Delivery." *The Lancet* 370 (9595): 1358–69.

Mwaniki, M. K., M. Atieno, J. E. Lawn, and C. R. Newton. 2012. "Long-Term Neurodevelopmental Outcomes after Intrauterine and Neonatal Insults: A Systematic Review." *The Lancet* 379 (9814): 445–52.

Patton, G. C., C. Coffey, S. M. Sawyer, R. M. Viner, D. M. Haller, and others. 2009. "Global Patterns of Mortality in Young People: A Systematic Analysis of Population Health Data." *The Lancet* 374 (9693): 881–92.

PMNCH (The Partnership for Maternal Health, Newborn and Child Health). 2008. *Review of Costing Tools Relevant to the Health MDGs.* Meeting Report, Technical Consultation. Saly Portudal, Senegal, January 8–10. Geneva: World Health Organization. http://www.who.int/pmnch/topics /economics/ctoolssenegalconsultation.pdf.

PMNCH, WHO, and Aga Khan University. 2011. *Essential Interventions, Commodities and Guidelines: A Global Review of Key Interventions Related to Reproductive, Maternal,* *Newborn and Child Health.* Geneva: PMNCH. http:// www.who.int/pmnch/knowledge/publications/201112 _essential_interventions/en/index.html.

Ruger, J. P., D. T. Jamison, D. E. Bloom, and D. Canning. 2012. "Health and the Economy." In *Global Health: Diseases, Programs, Systems and Policies*, 3rd edition, edited by M. Merson, R. E. Black, and A. Mills, 757–813. Burlington, MA: Jones & Bartlett Learning.

Singh, S., and J. E. Darroch. 2012. *Adding It Up: Costs and Benefits of Contraceptive Services—Estimates for 2012.* New York: Guttmacher Institute and United Nations Population Fund. http://www.guttmacher.org/pubs/AIU -2012-estimates.pdf.

Stenberg, K., H. Axelson, P. Sheehan, I. Anderson, A. M. Gülmezoglu, and others. 2014. "Advancing Social and Economic Development by Investing in Women's and Children's Health: A New Global Investment Framework." *The Lancet* 383 (9925): 1333–54. doi: 10.1016 /S0140-6736(13)62231-X.

Stenberg, K., B. Johns, R. W. Scherpbier, and T. T. Edejer. 2007. "A Financial Road Map to Scaling Up Essential Child Health Interventions in 75 Countries." *Bulletin of the World Health Organization* 85 (4): 305–14.

Stiglitz, J. E., A. Sen, and J.-P. Fitoussi. 2009. "The Measurement of Economic Performance and Social Progress Revisited." Working Paper 2009-33, Centre de recherche en économie de SciencesPo, Paris. http://www.ofce.sciences-po.fr/pdf /dtravail/WP2009-33.pdf.

Stover, J., P. Johnson, T. Hallett, M. Marston, R. Becquet, and others. 2010. "The Spectrum Projection Package: Improvements in Estimating Incidence by Age and Sex, Mother-to-Child Transmission, HIV Progression in Children and Double Orphans." *Sexually Transmitted Infections* 86 (Suppl 2): ii16–21. doi:10.1136/sti.2010 .044222.

Souza, J. P., A. M. Gülmezoglu, J. P. Vogel, G. Carroli, P. Lumbiganon, and others. 2013. "Moving beyond essential interventions for reduction of maternal mortality (the WHO Multicountry Survey on Maternal and Newborn Health): a cross-sectional study." *The Lancet* 381 (9879): 1747–55.

Suhrcke, M., R. S. Arce, M. McKee, and L. Rocco. 2012. "Economic Costs of Ill Health in the European Region," in *Health Systems, Health, Wealth and Societal Well-Being: Assessing the Case for Investing in Health Systems*, edited by M. McKee and J. Figueras. European Observatory on Health Systems and Policies Series. Maidenhead, Berkshire, U.K.: Open University Press.

UN (United Nations). 2013. *World Population Prospects: The 2012 Revision, Key Findings and Advance Tables.* Department of Economic and Social Affairs, Population Division, United Nations, New York. http://esa.un.org/wpp/Documentation /pdf/WPP2012_%20KEY%20FINDINGS.pdf.

UNICEF, WHO, World Bank, and UN (United Nations Children's Fund, World Health Organization, World Bank, and United Nations). 2013. *Levels and Trends in Child Mortality—Report 2013.* New York, New York: United Nations Children's Fund. http://www.childinfo.org/files /Child_Mortality_Report_2013.pdf.

USAID (United States Agency for International Development). 2004. *FamPlan: A Computer Program for Projecting Family Planning Requirements.* Washington, DC: USAID.

———. 2007. *AIM: A Computer Program for Making HIV/ AIDS Projections and Examining the Demographic and Social Impacts of AIDS.* Washington, DC: USAID.

Viscusi, W., and J. Aldy. 2003. "The Value of a Statistical Life: A Critical Review of Market Estimates throughout the World." *Journal of Risk and Uncertainty* 27 (1): 5–76.

WHO (World Health Organization). 2008. "10 Facts on Adolescent Health." WHO, Geneva. http://www.who .int/features/factfiles/adolescent_health/facts/en/index2 .html.

———. 2009. *Constraints to Scaling Up and Costs.* Taskforce on Innovative International Financing for Health Systems, Working Group 1 Report. Geneva: WHO. http://www.who .int/pmnch/media/membernews/2009/htltf_wg1_report _EN.pdf.

———. 2010. *World Health Report 2010. Health Systems Financing: The Path to Universal Coverage.* Geneva: WHO.

———. 2011. *Mortality Estimates by Cause, Age, and Sex for the Year 2008.* Geneva: WHO. http://www.who.int/healthinfo /global_burden_disease/en/.

WHO and UNICEF (World Health Organization and United Nations Children's Fund). 2013. *Accountability for Maternal, Newborn, and Child Survival: The 2013 Update.* Geneva: WHO; New York: UNICEF. http:// www.countdown2015mnch.org/documents/2013Report /Countdown_2013-Update_withprofiles.pdf.

WHO, UNICEF, UNFPA, and World Bank (World Health Organization, United Nations Children's Fund, United Nations Population Fund, and World Bank). 2014. *Trends in Maternal Mortality: 1990 to 2013.* Geneva: WHO.

———. 2015. *Trends in Maternal Mortality: 1990 to 2015. Estimates by WHO, UNICEF, UNFPA, the World Bank and the United Nations Population Division.* Geneva: WHO.

Winfrey, W., R. McKinnon, and J. Stover. 2011. "Methods Used in the Lives Saved Tool (LiST)." *BMC Public Health* 11 (Suppl 3): S32.

World Health Assembly. 2009. Resolution 62/82.

You, D., L. Hug, S. Ejdemyr, P. Idele, D. Hogan, and others. 2015. 'Global, Regional, and National levels and Trends in Under-5 Mortality between 1990 and 2015, with Scenario-Based Projections to 2030: A Systematic Analysis by the UN Inter-Agency Group for Child Mortality Estimation. *The Lancet* 386: 2275–86.

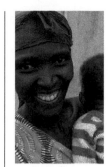

Chapter **17**

Cost-Effectiveness of Interventions for Reproductive, Maternal, Neonatal, and Child Health

Susan Horton and Carol Levin

INTRODUCTION

Substantial efforts and investment have been made in global reproductive, maternal, newborn, and child health (RMNCH) since 2000. The Millennium Development Goals (MDGs) have been one focus for efforts. The establishment of international funds—such as the Global Alliance for Vaccines and Immunization (Gavi, founded in 2000); and smaller foundations, such as the Clinton Health Access Initiative founded in 2007; the Children's Investment Fund Foundation, which made its first significant investments in 2009; and the Bill & Melinda Gates Foundation, founded in 1997—has brought new resources as well as an emphasis on value for money.

The amount of funding has been significant. In 1990, the members of the Development Assistance Committee of the Organisation for Economic Co-operation and Development provided an estimated US$5.6 billion for international health assistance (Ravishankar and others 2009). In 2011, this amount had grown to US$27.7 billion (Leach-Kemon and others 2012). Part of the increase was due to spending for human immunodeficiency virus/acquired immunodeficiency syndrome human immunodeficiency virus/acquired immunodeficiency syndrome (HIV/AIDS) (US$7.7 billion), but the increase in other areas was also substantial: RMNCH was the second largest component (US$6.1 billion) (IHME 2014).

The increase in resources and the growing interest in results combined to greatly increase the number of economic analyses of maternal and child health interventions. This chapter summarizes the findings of a systematic search of the cost-effectiveness literature on RMNCH, which builds on previous work, including several chapters in *Disease Control Priorities in Developing Countries*, second edition (Jamison and others 2006), as well as other systematic surveys and reviews on specific topics. The chapter's focus is on the cost-effectiveness of interventions; one section summarizes the findings on cost, building on a longer systematic search on unit cost (Levin and Brouwer 2014).

The studies identified in this chapter do not cover all of the interventions that affect maternal and child health. Some are covered in other volumes in this series (see table 17.1). The literature also has biases. Studies tend to concentrate on areas of current policy interest; for example, the literature on vaccines concentrates disproportionately on new vaccines—particularly those for pneumococcus and rotavirus, but also hepatitis B and *Haemophilus influenzae* B (HiB)—and not on older interventions known to be cost-effective, such as the original Expanded Program of Immunization (EPI) vaccines. Ideally, when resources are allocated across interventions, the full range would be considered. Funding could potentially be reallocated

Corresponding author: Susan Horton, Centre for International Governance Innovation Chair in Global Health Economics, University of Waterloo, sehorton@uwaterloo.ca.

Table 17.1 Interventions Covered in This Chapter: Topics Covered in Other Volumes

Topics covered in this volume	Topics covered in other volumes
Reproductive health: Family planning, safe abortion, intimate partner violence	Adult male circumcision in volume 6 (*HIV/AIDS, STIs, Tuberculosis, and Malaria*)
Maternal and child mortality: Antenatal, intrapartum, and postpartum care; care of newborns	Intrapartum care also covered in volume 1 (*Essential Surgery*)
Febrile child: Diagnosis and treatment of malaria and pneumonia	Prevention of malaria covered in volume 6 (*HIV/AIDS, STIs, Tuberculosis, and Malaria*)
Diarrheal diseases: Treatment of diarrhea; brief review of interventions to prevent diarrhea, including water and sanitation	Water and sanitation also covered in volume 7 (*Injury Prevention and Environmental Health*)
Vaccines: 16 conditions (BCG, DPT, polio, measles, hepatitis B, *Haemophilus influenzae* B [HiB], Japanese encephalitis, meningitis A, yellow fever, pneumococcus, rubella, rotavirus, typhoid, and cholera)	HPV covered in volume 3 (*Cancer*)
Nutrition: Management of severe acute malnutrition, and infant and child growth	
Platforms for health care and public health interventions	

Note: BCG = Bacillus Calmette–Guérin; DPT = diphtheria, pertussis, and tetanus; HIV/AIDS = human immunodeficiency virus/acquired immunodeficiency syndrome (HIV/AIDS); HPV = human papillomavirus; STIs = sexually transmitted infections.

from old but cost-ineffective interventions to promising new ones, or coverage of older and very cost-effective interventions could be completed before new ones that are less cost-effective are incorporated.

The next section discusses the methods used for the search and analysis of the literature. The findings are then organized according to the sequence of chapters in this volume:

- Reproductive health (chapter 6)
- Maternal and newborn child morbidity and mortality (chapter 7)
- Febrile conditions (chapter 8)
- Diarrheal disease (chapter 9)
- Vaccines (chapter 10)
- Treatment of severe acute malnutrition (chapter 11)
- Infant and young child growth (chapter 12)
- Platforms for the delivery of interventions (chapters 14 and 15).

Following a discussion of the literature on the cost and affordability of interventions, we provide conclusions. Throughout the chapter, unless otherwise specified, costs and cost-effectiveness are converted to 2012 U.S. dollars.

METHODS

We undertook a systematic survey of the literature beginning in 2000 on the cost-effectiveness of interventions for RMNCH, detailed in Horton and others (2015). The studies discussed here are primarily those measured as cost per discounted disability-adjusted life year (DALY) averted,[1] the most commonly considered outcome, but we also provide figures showing results for deaths averted. Studies using cost per quality-adjusted life year (QALY) saved and life-year saved (LYS) are included in the working paper (Horton and others 2015), as are studies using other outcomes, for example, per patient correctly treated. For studies that express outcomes in life-years or deaths, we have in some cases made an approximate conversion to DALYs, where one life-year is approximately 0.5 DALY for a newborn in low-income countries (LICs). Similarly the conversion from deaths to DALYs assumes that a newborn life is approximately 32 DALYs (a life expectancy of about 60 years, discounted at 3 percent). The flow charts for the searches on cost-effectiveness and cost are presented in Horton and others (2015).

In all, 222 articles were identified; of these, 21 covered reproductive care, 26 maternal and newborn morbidity, 10 febrile conditions, 10 diarrheal diseases, 131 vaccines, 3 community management of severe acute malnutrition (SAM), and 28 growth of infants and young children. Seven articles covered more than one category, and 104 included DALYs as one of the outcome measures. We benefited from several recent systematic reviews, including Gyles and others (2012); Mangham-Jefferies and others (2014); Ozawa and others (2012); and White and others (2011). All studies were read by two reviewers to extract the cost-effectiveness data; one reviewer graded the article quality using the Drummond Checklist (Drummond and others 2005); grades are presented in Horton and others (2015). In some cases we augmented systematic reviews with additional searches. For vaccines (Ozawa and others 2012), we added literature from 2010 onward for HiB, meningitis, pneumococcal, rotavirus, and syncytial virus. Small, focused searches in PubMed only were undertaken to find additional studies on meningitis, yellow fever, and rubella, which are not covered in Ozawa's review; however, no studies for these conditions report results in DALYs.

Cost-effectiveness data were converted to 2012 U.S. dollars using the original study country currency and consumer price index (World Bank 2013). Several studies provided multiple cost-effectiveness estimates for different interventions. This chapter discusses those that provided an incremental cost-effectiveness ratio compared with a clear alternative. Cost-effectiveness data from more complex interventions, for example, switching from fortification to supplementation combined with another package of interventions, are not summarized here but are listed in Horton and others (2015).

The cost-effectiveness results measured in DALYs are summarized in figure 17.1; figure 17.2 provides similar results for deaths averted. The studies used to generate the figures are cited in tables 3 and 4, respectively, in Horton and others (2015). To interpret the results, a useful yardstick comes from the WHO (2001), which suggests that interventions costing less than per capita gross national income (GNI) per DALY averted can be termed "very cost-effective," and those costing less than three times per capita GNI can be termed "cost-effective." In 2012, according to the World Bank's World Development Indicators (World Bank 2013), only one country had a GNI per capita of less than US$320, and LICs' GNI per capita was up to and including US$1,035. Thus, all interventions costing less than US$320 per DALY averted are "very cost-effective" in all countries but one, and those costing less than about US$1,000 per DALY averted are cost-effective in LICs, and very cost-effective in middle-income countries.

REPRODUCTIVE HEALTH

Economic studies of family planning preceded those of health, just as international assistance and lending for family planning preceded that for health; the cost-effectiveness of modern contraceptives is well established. Only two surveys were identified on the cost-effectiveness of modern contraception using DALYs (Babigumira and others 2012; Seamans and Harner-Jay 2007); both indicate that contraceptives are very cost-effective in all countries as measured by the benefits to mothers' and children's health. Other studies were identified in which the outcome (couple-year of protection) is specific to contraception; these are discussed in chapter 6 of this volume (Stover and others 2016).

Safe abortion is cost saving compared with unsafe abortion, which leads to adverse health outcomes for mothers as demonstrated by Hu and others (2010) for Ghana and Nigeria; other studies with outcomes such as maternal lives saved are summarized in Horton and others (2015). Safe abortion remains an issue for policy; safe abortion methods are not available in all low- and middle-income countries (LMICs), and the availability of new methods, such as medical abortion, increases the options.

Only one economic study was found on intimate partner violence (Jan and others 2010); this study examines a microfinance initiative combined with gender training in South Africa. Although the cost-effectiveness was less than the per capita GNI for South Africa and thereby "very cost-effective" for that country, the cost of US$2,908 per DALY averted is at the higher end compared with other interventions in this chapter.

MATERNAL AND NEWBORN MORBIDITY AND MORTALITY

Expanding access to existing essential and cost-effective interventions for maternal and newborn care, while also focusing on impact, costs, and affordability, has been a priority for reaching MDG 4 (reduce child mortality) and MDG 5 (improve maternal health) (Bhutta and others 2014). Several new interventions have also become available, and efforts to deliver interventions more inexpensively and to encourage uptake have been undertaken. Goldie and others (2010) model an "expansion path" of interventions, suggesting that starting with family planning and safe abortion is the most cost-effective first step, followed by increasing the availability of skilled birth attendants, then improving antenatal and postpartum care. Shifting births to facilities comes next, and finally increasing referral for complicated cases and providing transport. The study by Goldie and others (2010) was restricted to India, but the findings are confirmed by the studies identified for this chapter.

A few innovations studied used new modest-cost health inputs and have costs per DALY averted in the range of US$20 to US$100, for example, skin emollients to help keep small newborns warm (Lefevre and others 2010), single-use injection devices for oxytocin delivery during labor (Tsu and others 2009), and clean delivery kits for in-home births (Sabin and others 2012). However, the total amount of DALYs averted by these methods are modest. Several studies (Borghi and others 2005; Fottrell and others 2013; Lewycka and others 2013; Tripathy and others 2010) look at the cost-effectiveness of participatory women's groups on health outcomes; cost per DALY averted ranges from US$150 to US$1,000. Training initiatives for village health workers and midwives have a similar range of costs per DALY averted (Lefevre and others 2013).

Safe motherhood initiatives (a package combining antenatal and postpartum care with trained birth attendants, potentially in a health facility) in various countries fall in the same range of US$150 to US$1,000 per DALY averted (Carvalho, Salehi, and Goldie 2013 for Afghanistan; Erim, Resch, and Goldie 2012 for Nigeria; Goldie and others 2010 for India; Hu and others 2007 for Mexico). Cesarean sections for obstructed labor have a wider range, from US$200 to US$4,000 per DALY averted, depending on the country, with a median of US$400 (Alkire and others 2012).

Figure 17.1 Cost-Effectiveness of Interventions for RMNCH, in 2012 U.S. Dollars per DALY Averted

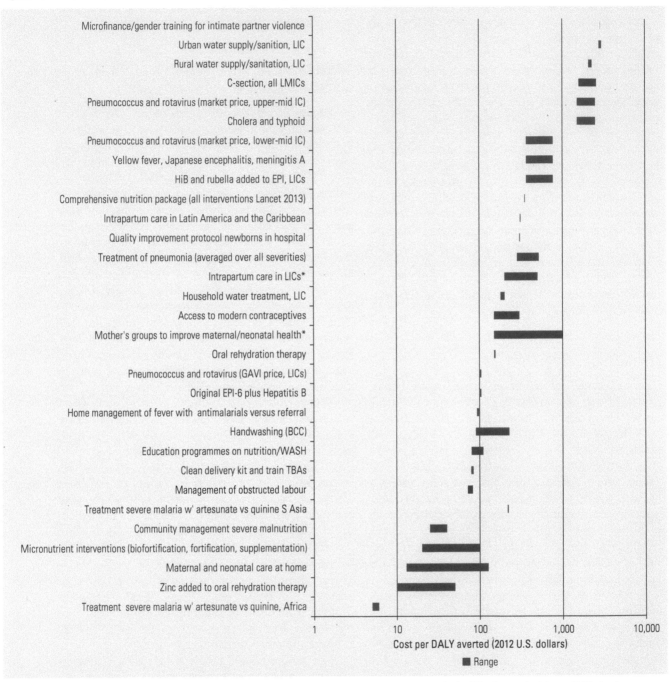

Note: DALY = disability-adjusted life year; EPI = Expanded Program of Immunization; Gavi = Global Alliance for Vaccines and Immunization; HiB = *Haemophilus influenzae* B; LIC = low-income country; RMNCH = reproductive, maternal, newborn, and child health; WASH = water, sanitation, and hygiene.
a. Converted from life-years, assuming that a newborn life is equivalent to 32 DALYs or 60 life-years.

Bhutta and others (2014) undertake a more ambitious estimate of the cost-effectiveness of a package involving scaling up effective interventions in the 75 high-burden Countdown countries; the annual cost of the package would be US$5.65 billion. This investment would reduce maternal and neonatal deaths and prevent stillbirths at a cost of US$1,928 per life saved or US$60 per DALY averted. Bhutta and others (2014) estimate that 82 percent of the effect in lives saved would be from facility-based care.

Figure 17.2 Cost-Effectiveness of Interventions for RMNCH, 2012 U.S. Dollars per Death Averted

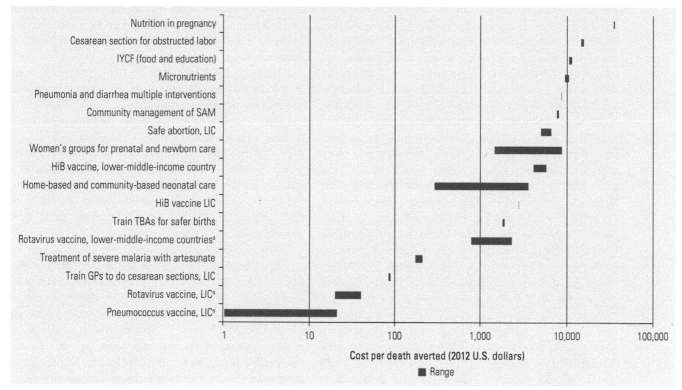

Note: If country group is not specified, results refer to low- and lower-middle-income countries combined. GP = general practitioner; HiB= *Haemophilus influenzae* B; IYCF = infant and young child feeding interventions (combine education with food distribution to poorest); LIC = low-income country; RMNCH = reproductive, maternal, newborn, and child health; SAM = severe acute malnutrition; TBA = traditional birth attendants.

a. Cost-effectiveness of vaccines is sensitive to vaccine price. Rotavirus and pneumococcus vaccine costs to LICs are a fraction (for example, 5 percent) of the price paid by Gavi, the Vaccine Alliance, to procure the vaccines; and Gavi in turn receives prices that are more favorable than in upper-middle income countries because of volume discounts and the like.

UNDER-FIVE ILLNESS

Febrile Conditions

The most recent cost-effectiveness estimates for the treatment of pneumonia are from the second edition of *Disease Control Priorities in Developing Countries* (Simoes and others 2006), and suggest that cost-effectiveness is US$516 per DALY averted in LMICs overall (US$342 per DALY averted in South Asia and US$282 per DALY averted in Sub-Saharan Africa). These costs are averaged across nonsevere cases treated in communities or local facilities along with severe and very severe cases treated in hospitals.

A significant amount of work has been done on malaria in the past decade, alongside policy efforts such as the Roll Back Malaria Partnership. Recent studies suggest that treatment of severe malaria with artesunate is very cost-effective, even in LICs. White and others (2011) identify four studies of treatment of severe malaria using artesunate. Lubell and others (2009) estimate the cost-effectiveness of artesunate compared with quinine as US$14 per DALY averted, pooling

results for four countries in Sub-Saharan Africa; in pooled results for four countries in the WHO regions of South Asia and Southeast Asia, the cost-effectiveness is US$152 per DALY averted. Buchanan and others (2010) and Tozan and others (2010) examine the cost-effectiveness of presumptive treatment in the community with rectal artesunate for severe malaria in Sub-Saharan Africa. Cost-effectiveness is US$20 per DALY averted compared with no treatment (Buchanan and others 2010), and US$122 to US$1,855 per DALY averted compared with parenteral treatment (Tozan and others 2010). Nonvignon and others (2012) examine the cost-effectiveness of presumptive community-based treatment of malaria, using an artemisin combination therapy compared to standard care; standard care is a combination of treatment at health facilities, purchase of antimalarials at a pharmacy, and other types of treatment. They estimate the cost per DALY averted compared to standard care to be US$93.

In contrast, the literature suggests that rapid diagnostic tests (RDTs) for malaria are not generally very cost-effective in program settings. However, where microscopy is poorly done, RDTs become more cost-effective. Microscopy has been considered the gold standard for the diagnosis of malaria, but it is not always feasible in low-resource environments. If not well done, it can lead to a relatively high rate of misdiagnosis, and can entail long waits for treatment, depending on the capacity for reading slides. In areas without microscopy, presumptive diagnosis has been used. Clinicians use their expert knowledge to determine whether a patient presenting with fever has malaria or another infection and treat accordingly. Thus, RDTs are potentially more cost-effective where *P. falciparum* predominates and the more effective but more costly artemisinin combination drugs are being used. RDTs are also cost-effective where transmission rates are low because presumptive treatment involves overuse of antimalarials and, possibly, delays antibiotic treatment if the underlying infection is bacterial rather than malarial (Ansah and others 2013; Babigumira and Gelband, forthcoming; Lemma and others 2011; Rolland and others 2006). RDTs and microscopy both perform more favorably if clinicians are more likely to use the results of the diagnosis in their prescription behavior, that is, if they only prescribe antimalarials if the test indicates malaria is the likely diagnosis, and only prescribe antibiotics if malaria is not the likely diagnosis (Yukich and others 2010). Two studies with outcomes measured in cost per deaths averted (Chanda, Castillo-Riquelme, and Masiye 2009; Uzochukwu and others 2009) suggest that RDTs do not rank as particularly cost-effective in program settings because clinicians apparently do not always prescribe according to test results. Chapter 8 in this volume (Hamer and others 2016) discusses some of these issues in more detail and cites other studies that did not fit the inclusion criteria here.

Diarrheal Disease

New developments for diarrheal disease since 2000 include the use of zinc as adjunct therapy in combination with oral rehydration solution (ORS), a substantial decrease in the cost of rotavirus vaccine, and additional research separating the cost-effectiveness of water supply from that of sanitation.

The most cost-effective interventions for diarrhea, based on cost per DALY averted, are prophylactic zinc supplementation as an adjunct to ORS (US$10 to US$50 per DALY averted), ORS (US$150 per DALY averted), rotavirus vaccine (US$100 per DALY averted at the Gavi price in LICs), and household-level water treatment in rural areas using chlorination or solar disinfection (US$180 to US$200 per DALY averted) (figure 17.1). The next most cost-effective

group includes rural sanitation; piped water; and in selected countries, cholera vaccine (US$2,000 per DALY averted). Urban sanitation and cholera vaccine in lower mortality countries can cost US$3,000 or more per DALY averted.

The systematic search identified only one recent study of behavior change. Behavior change interventions tend to have heterogeneous results, and some are not effective (let alone cost-effective), but the one identified—a hand-washing education intervention in Burkina Faso (Borghi and others 2002)—falls into the very cost-effective group (US$88 per DALY averted). It is quite possible that well-designed behavior change interventions to increase the use of clean water, of latrines where available, of ORS, of prophylactic zinc, and of vaccines could all be cost-effective.

Most studies estimate the cost-effectiveness of adding a single intervention to "usual care." If interventions are added in combination, the incremental cost-effectiveness of each additional individual intervention can decline. Fischer Walker and others (2011) estimate the combined effect of 10 interventions designed to reduce diarrhea in 68 countries with high child mortality, using the Lives Saved Tool (LiST). Two scenarios are modeled: an ambitious strategy designed to reach MDG 4 goals; and a universal strategy designed to bring coverage of many interventions to 90 percent or more, and water, sanitation, and handwashing interventions to 55 percent or more. Both strategies are scaled up from current coverage to the target over five years.

The ambitious strategy saves 3.8 million lives during a five-year period, at a cost of US$49.2 billion, which is US$12,847 per death averted or approximately US$405 per DALY averted in 2008 U.S. dollars. The universal strategy saves 5 million lives at a cost of US$19,460 per death averted, approximately US$608 per DALY averted in 2008 U.S. dollars. Although $608 per DALY averted certainly falls in the cost-effective or very cost-effective range for most countries, affordability remains problematic. The water and sanitation component is the main issue, accounting for 84 percent of the cost of the ambitious package and 87 percent of the universal one.

Vaccines

Vaccines rank among the most cost-effective health interventions because of their life-saving potential. The original EPI-6 vaccines (against tuberculosis, diphtheria, tetanus, pertussis, measles, and polio) are very cost-effective (less than $100 per DALY averted), although no studies on the basic six antigens that typically comprise a national EPI were identified by the systematic search.

One study published after our search examines Vietnam's national EPI, and estimates that 26,000 deaths were prevented by EPI since 1980, with a cost-effectiveness of about US$1,000 to US$27,000 (in 2010 U.S. dollars) per death averted (based on financial data for that same period) (Jit and others 2015). Since 2000, the focus has been on the introduction of new and underutilized vaccines and those in the pipeline. Of the 57 studies since 2000 using DALYs as an outcome, more than half focus on pneumococcus and rotavirus vaccines. Whether, and how, to adopt these vaccines has been the major LMIC childhood vaccine policy preoccupation of the past decade. Vaccine cost-effectiveness studies are frequently undertaken before governments or donors decide to fund the intervention.

The cost-effectiveness of new childhood vaccines is very much dependent on the price of the vaccine. For well-established vaccines with long-expired patent protection, a clear world market price may exist based on the cost of production. For new vaccines, the price is less clear. The companies that develop new vaccines retain patents but have increasingly been willing to offer differentiated prices to different markets. To take advantage of economies of scale, international organizations (particularly Gavi, but also the United Nations Children's Fund) have entered into agreements for bulk purchase or have made advance market commitments. Hence, cost-effectiveness studies are often undertaken at a variety of price points to gauge ability to develop a market for different groups of countries. Our summary is undertaken using current prices, which vary between Gavi-eligible countries, recent Gavi graduates, countries covered by the Pan-American Health Organization's revolving fund, and upper-middle-income countries facing the world market.

Table 10.1 (chapter 10 in this volume [Feikin and others 2016]) summarizes the cost-effectiveness findings in DALYs at current key price points and adds information for meningitis A (Miller and Shahab 2005), and yellow fever (Monath and Nasidi 1993).

Among the new and underutilized vaccines, cost-effectiveness ranges from about US$24 to US$2,500 per DALY averted in low-income settings, depending on the vaccine, geographic setting, income level, and associated price point. Rotavirus and Japanese encephalitis are the most cost-effective at less than US$50 per DALY averted in high-burden, LICs in Asia and Sub-Saharan Africa, followed by pneumococcal vaccines. Some vaccines in LICs have not yet been incorporated into EPI programs because their cost-effectiveness is less favorable, at more than US$1,000 per DALY averted. These vaccines include cholera and typhoid, which may meet the WHO's cost-effective criterion, but only in countries of high endemicity. However, these vaccines are planned for rollout by Gavi and its partners before 2020, assuming prices come down or effectiveness goes up (or both).

Cost-effectiveness ratios increase with country income per capita, but the general ranking of what is considered cost-effective stays the same. In lower-middle-income countries, hepatitis B, HiB, and rotavirus vaccines range between US$60 and US$350 per DALY averted and are among the most cost-effective. Rubella, pneumococcal, and polio vaccines are between US$1,000 and US$3,000 per DALY averted.

The estimates of cost per DALY averted for yellow fever and meningitis fall between US$100 and US$1,040 (converting from deaths prevented in children). For the rubella vaccine, the only study from LMICs (from the English-speaking Caribbean) reports that the vaccination is cost saving (Irons and others 2000). Other vaccines, such as meningitis A and yellow fever in selected countries that are being considered for EPI expansion, are typically between US$100 and US$200 per DALY averted or at least below US$500 in LICs (Miller and Shahab 2005). Cost-effectiveness of even newer vaccines, for example, malaria and respiratory syncytial virus, is more speculative, given that the effectiveness is still being investigated and price points are unknown.

Eradication through immunization—although costly in the short and medium terms—may be cost saving in the long term by eliminating the need for vaccination; smallpox is the best example. Polio eradication is potentially cost saving in the long term, but it requires a switch from oral polio vaccine (OPV) to the inactivated polio vaccine to prevent outbreaks from vaccine-derived polioviruses. However, the inactivated polio vaccine is 20 or more times more costly than OPV (Duintjer Tebbens and others 2010) and correspondingly less cost-effective and less affordable in the short term. Measles eradication is also potentially cost saving (Bishai and others 2010), but the second measles immunization needed to approach eradication has to be given outside of the traditional EPI schedule and hence incurs additional delivery cost. This delivery schedule also affects rubella because measles and rubella vaccines are typically delivered together.

A systematic review of studies of interventions to affect the demand side of vaccine uptake (Shea, Andersson, and Henry 2009) finds that the literature was of variable quality, with only two randomized controlled trials. Some of the interventions, such as mass media campaigns, do not lend themselves to randomized controlled trials. The review concludes that mass media campaigns might be effective, but their effectiveness depends on the context.

Incentives to households might help. Other interventions have been tried, such as conditional cash transfers and use of text message reminders, but no results on cost-effectiveness of these methods were found.

NUTRITION

Interventions for Severe Acute Malnutrition

Community management of SAM is attractive from a cost-effectiveness perspective, ranging from US$26 to US$39 per DALY averted across three studies. This finding is driven in part by the high probability, as high as 20 percent, that children will die if not treated. Initially, programs cost as much as US$200 per child for a four-month course of treatment; however, during the past decade or so the cost has declined by at least a third, with greater program efficiency. Experience suggests that substituting cheaper ready-to-use therapeutic food for proprietary ones does not lead to outcomes that are quite as good, although it may lower costs. All three studies examined in this section used Plumpy'Nut, a popular ready-to-use therapeutic food.

Interventions for Infant and Young Child Growth

The majority (14) of the studies of nutrition for the general population focus on micronutrient interventions, 1 on nutrition education, 1 on the effects of scaling up a comprehensive package of nutrition intervention, and 1 on outcomes other than nutrition. No new studies of cost-effectiveness were identified for breastfeeding.

Nutrition interventions are associated with impacts on multiple outcomes of importance. Some nutrition interventions reduce morbidity and save lives in the more malnourished populations. In these cases, the outcomes can be measured using cost-effectiveness methods, such as deaths averted, LYS, QALYs saved, or DALYs averted. In other cases, nutrition is associated with impacts on cognitive improvements, and these benefits are better measured using benefit-cost ratios because benefits can be measured in financial units (higher wages).

From the literature search, five studies for folic acid, iron, and iodine interventions all had very favorable benefit-cost ratios (Horton, Alderman, and Rivera 2008; Horton and Ross 2003, 2006; Sayed and others 2008; Sharieff, Horton, and Zlotkin 2006; Sharieff and others 2008). Hoddinott and others (2013) undertake a benefit-cost analysis for a comprehensive set of nutrition interventions. These studies cannot be compared with those using DALY outcomes without assigning a dollar value to DALYs, a task that involves judgments about the value of human life.

As in previous studies (Hoddinott, Rosegrant, and Torero 2012; Horton, Alderman, and Rivera 2008), micronutrient interventions remain very cost-effective (typically less than US$100 per DALY averted, and often less than US$50 per DALY averted), with some variation. Interventions are often more cost-effective in LICs with more widespread deficiencies; for example, the cost per DALY averted is lower in South Asia and Sub-Saharan Africa than in China. Fortification is more cost-effective than supplementation for micronutrients where deficiencies are widely spread throughout the population and the micronutrient is relatively cheap, for example, iron; the opposite is true for micronutrients that are relatively more expensive, and where the benefits are concentrated particularly in vulnerable groups, for example, vitamin A. Biofortification appears to be very cost-effective, with some estimates in the US$0 to US$20 range. However, the biofortification estimates for staple food crops, such as rice, were early stage projections, and it remains to be proven whether these optimistic projections can be realized. There has been more success to date for more minor crops (orange-flesh sweet potato, beans, and vitamin A–rich cassava), although iron-rich rice and wheat seeds are now beginning to be disseminated to farmers (Harvest Plus 2013).

The only intervention identified for nutrition education (Waters and others 2006) costs slightly more than US$100 per DALY averted; this was a modest-cost intervention (US$6 per child in 2001 U.S. dollars). Estimated costs per DALY averted for earlier, more elaborate interventions were at least two to three times higher than the single case here.

Another innovation since 2000 has been the evaluation of packages of nutritional interventions. When interventions are combined, the cost-effectiveness of each individual component tends to become less attractive. Either vitamin A supplements or measles immunization can save lives, but the combined effect of both vitamin A supplements and measles immunization saves fewer lives than the sum of the two individually. Bhutta, Das, Rizvi, and others (2013) estimate that the cost per DALY averted of three components of a comprehensive nutrition intervention—micronutrients, nutrition education with selected supplements regarding infant and young child feeding, and SAM management—ranges from US$240 to US$340 per DALY averted; this cost per DALY averted is three to five times higher than the cost per DALY averted of the components introduced individually. Hoddinott and others (2013) use the same intervention package and estimate that the median benefit-cost ratio is 35 to 1 for a group of 17 LMICs for interventions provided to children.

The cost per DALY averted for nutrition interventions provided to mothers is higher still—more than US$1,100, but still in the cost-effective range for middle-income countries (Bhutta, Das, Rivzi, and others 2013).

PLATFORMS FOR DELIVERY OF INTERVENTIONS

Maternal and child health services can be delivered from a variety of platforms, including the following:

- The household level or through mobile outreach
- The community level
- At health facilities, which range from health posts and community clinics to higher-level facilities such as first-level hospitals.

Service delivery can be combined on any of the platforms if doing so increases cost-effectiveness.

In part, the type of health activity determines the appropriate platform: surgical interventions related to delivery need to be provided at the facility level, whereas immunizations have achieved better coverage in some countries through mobile outreach or community-level delivery. Outreach and community-based strategies that deliver a package of child health interventions, including vitamin A (Fiedler and Chuko 2008); distribute insecticide-treated bednets (Ross and others 2011); provide home-based management of fevers (Nonvignon and others 2012); treat severely acute malnourished children (Puett and others 2013); and train traditional birth attendants to improve neonatal health (Sabin and others 2012) are cost-effective at less than US$100 per DALY averted (chapter 14 in this volume [Bhutta and Lassi 2016]).

Community health workers (CHWs) have become essential facilitators in delivering outreach and community-based services. They are also critical for linking beneficiaries to health facilities for preventive care and treatment, when essential. Depending on the country, condition, and setting, CHWs play different roles that change with the level of coverage of fixed health facilities and urbanization. For example, outreach workers, by going to households to provide family planning and maternal and child health services in Bangladesh, played an important role in reducing birth rates; but Routh and Khuda (2000) show that in urban Dhaka, the delivery of family planning and maternal and child health services at clinics now become more cost-effective. However, the delivery of vaccinations by community-based workers cost less and achieved greater coverage than outreach by health workers in communities reached by river in the Amazon (San Sebastian and others 2001).

Despite the growing evidence on effectiveness of CHW programs, data on the cost-effectiveness of such programs are still lacking. Cost-effectiveness analyses of CHW programs may pose methodological challenges because they do not capture the full benefits of enhanced equity, increased self-reliance by communities, and contributions to other social benefits and community norms (Lehmann and Sanders 2007).

Task-shifting through the use of lay workers sheds some light on the potential cost reductions and improved cost-effectiveness. Lewin and others (2010) undertake a Cochrane review on effectiveness of lay health workers for selected maternal and child health care interventions (not restricted to LMICs), and conclude that the use of lay health workers could increase vaccine uptake. A systematic review of the cost-effectiveness of vaccination programs delivered by lay health workers in LMICs (Corluka and others 2009) finds insufficient data to allow conclusions to be drawn. Sabin and others (2012) find that training traditional birth attendants in treating birth asphyxia, hypothermia, and sepsis was very cost-effective in situations in which access to facility care was not readily available; but this intervention would not be effective in addressing obstructed labor and deliveries requiring cesarean section. The cost-effectiveness of task-shifting is underresearched for LMICs, and additional studies are needed to strengthen policy guidance.

An emerging area of interest is the integration of services to improve impact and reduce costs. The cost-effectiveness of integrating services while maintaining the effectiveness of individual interventions is a high priority research area, given the investments in individual interventions. Some of the considerable interest in the cost-effectiveness of different delivery platforms has been driven by the literature on vertical services for HIV/AIDS, tuberculosis, and malaria that have been successful but where sustainability requires integration of services. Kahn and others (2012), for example, conclude that an integrated service in Kenya that provided HIV testing and early treatment, insecticide-treated nets for malaria prevention, and water filters for diarrhea prevention saved lives and was cost-effective. For some preventive services, there may be trade-offs between cost-effectiveness and coverage. However, campaigns and mobile delivery may be essential to achieve high and equitable levels of coverage in countries with poorer availability of facilities or greater population dispersion. Verguet and others (2013) find that child health campaigns that integrated supplementary immunization activity for measles with vitamin A supplements, deworming medications, and OPVs were more cost-effective than measles supplementary immunization activity alone.

Bartlett and others (2014) use the LiST to model the effect of scaling up an integrated midwifery, obstetrics, and family planning intervention in 58 LMICs. They conclude that scaling up any of the three individually is attractive in cost per death averted, but that scaling up midwifery combined with family planning costs half as much per death averted as scaling up obstetrics combined with family planning; the lowest cost per death averted occurs when all three are scaled up together. Midwifery saves lives across the continuum of prepregnancy, prenatal, delivery, and neonatal care; obstetrical care has a strong effect on mortality during delivery.

The only cost-effectiveness study undertaken for Integrated Management of Childhood Illness finds that mortality was lower in the intervention district than in the control, and the costs were no higher and possibly lower (Armstrong-Schellenberg and others 2004). However, experience was not uniformly positive in other effectiveness trials, and there have been some difficulties scaling up this intervention. No cost-effectiveness studies were identified on the Integrated Management of Neonatal and Child Illness (IMNCI) or integrated community case management. Prinja and others (2013) note that even though overall health expenditures per case did not increase as IMNCI was implemented, there was an increase from the perspective of the government, which they estimate to be 1 percent to 1.5 percent of the government's health budget (US$0.61 to US$2.60 per child covered), depending on which field workers implement the program. The additional costs arose because the program was effective, which led to increased utilization as households switched from using private health providers.

COSTS

The country setting, type and level of the facility, severity of the event, and specific treatment offered influence costs. Service delivery platforms that reach large numbers of beneficiaries close to their homes increase the coverage and lower the cost of services. Child health days in Ethiopia, Somalia, and Zambia offer a package of preventive services that cost US$1 to US$2 per child reached; facility-based integrated care offering similar services is closer to US$10 per child treated and may be as high as US$20, as in Brazil (Adam and others 2005; Adam and others 2009; Bryce and others 2005; Fiedler and Chuko 2008; Vijayaraghavan and others 2012). For many interventions, effective and cost-effective interventions exist but suffer from low uptake or coverage. Many of the studies that present specific costs of facility-based programs do not capture the shared health system costs or costs of demand creation to increase access to and use of services.

Information on RMNCH unit costs comes from a large selection of literature published primarily after 2007. The review assessed the quality of cost data found in 146 articles and chose to liberally include unit costs if the data sources and methods were clearly explained (Levin and Brouwer 2014). Unit costs vary substantially across country settings for similar interventions. In addition, a variety of methodological approaches confound the expected variation in costs due to country context and different choices of interventions evaluated. Identifying sources of heterogeneity is challenging because many studies lack detailed information on resource use and how costs were estimated (Crowell and others 2013; Pegurri, Fox-Rushby, and Walker 2004; Shearer, Walker, and Vlassoff 2010; Walker and others 2004).

In some areas in which cost or cost-effectiveness studies have been conducted and published dating back to the 1990s, representative and standardized data on long-running interventions, such as vitamin A or iron capsule supplementation or food-based strategies, is surprisingly lacking despite consistent calls for improved information on the costs and cost-effectiveness of nutrition interventions (Fiedler and Puett 2015; Gyles and others 2012; Morris, Gogill, and Uauy 2008; Ruel 2001; Ruel, Alderman, and the Maternal and Child Nutrition Study Group 2013). Similarly, in the area of family planning, for which effective coverage of modern contraceptive use still lags, little new information is available on country-level costs of scaling up interventions to increase the supply of and demand for services (Singh, Darroch, and Ashford 2014).

In general, average unit costs are relatively low for family planning interventions, antenatal care visits for pregnant women, and normal deliveries at home or at health centers with trained birth attendants. Unit costs tend to increase with the complexity of the service. For example, clinic-based breastfeeding support and prevention of micronutrient deficiencies are inexpensive, compared with home visits and peer counseling to support breastfeeding and optimal child feeding or community-based treatment of SAM. Treatment of febrile illness and diarrheal disease are less expensive per child (US$20 to US$100) than treatment of pneumonia and meningitis, which typically require inpatient admission (US$150 per visit, or US$800 per child treated for pneumonia; US$300 to US$500 for inpatient care). Although the treatment of diarrhea is typically between US$2 and US$20 per visit for outpatient visits, treatment costs can be much higher and more variable when inpatient hospital care is required.

Other interventions for which affordability is an issue, and has likely slowed the rate of scale up, include community management of SAM (US$120 per child), and facility-based delivery. Safe motherhood interventions including facility-based delivery are estimated to cost US$1.15 per person in the population, not including the initial investment in new facilities (Bhutta and others 2014). The year for the costing is not specified, so these amounts are assumed to be in 2014 U.S. dollars. Although US$1.15 per person sounds modest, with a crude birth rate of 25–30 per 1,000 population, it amounts to an increased cost per birth of US$33 to US$40, not a small sum in resource-constrained settings.

Similarly, the relatively high cost for water and sanitation has likely hindered scale up. In 2007 the initial investment costs per household for standard urban requirements, namely, water piped to the house and a sewer connection, were estimated to be US$102 and US$120, respectively. For the lowest-cost interventions in a rural area, these costs were still substantial: the lowest-cost clean water supply was US$21 per household for a dug well and US$23 for a borehole. The lowest cost sanitation, a pit latrine, was US$39 per household (all costs from Haller, Hutton, and Bartram [2007] in 2000 U.S. dollars).

An enormous international effort has gone into universalizing coverage of children with the EPI. According to Brenzel (2015), the cost per fully immunized child was US$25 in LICs (higher in higher-income regions) in 2008–11. She estimates that HiB, pneumococcus, and rotavirus will increase this amount to US$45 or more per fully immunized child. This cost may lead to affordability issues, even though these immunizations are cost-effective.

CONCLUSIONS

The large literature surveyed in this chapter suggests that many very cost-effective interventions could be used to address maternal, neonatal, and child health conditions. Simple solutions for newborn health, treatment of febrile illness, immunization against preventable childhood diseases, and micronutrient interventions are among the most cost-effective interventions and are affordable in many settings. Other studies explore how to provide existing interventions using new platforms to increase outreach or decrease cost per person covered, or both. Interventions provided in the community— for example, community management of SAM—may achieve both purposes to differing extent. Task-shifting, such as training lay health workers to provide vaccines, may decrease costs. Training traditional birth attendants in skills for safer deliveries may increase coverage.

The main challenge is to increase coverage of interventions known to be effective and cost-effective.

These include many old interventions for which no new cost-effectiveness findings were identified past 2000, as well as new innovations whose cost-effectiveness is assessed in this chapter, such as vaccines for rotavirus and pneumococcus; biofortification of staple crops; RDTs for malaria; new protocols for community management of nutrition and of malaria or severe malaria; and prophylactic zinc for diarrhea. A few studies have focused on how to increase demand for services in settings in which supply is less the issue. Changing people's behavior can be more difficult than identifying ways to supply effective interventions. Some promising findings emerge for women's groups surveyed in the section on maternal and neonatal conditions. No cost-effectiveness studies were found for mHealth (that is, utilizing mobile phones to improve health), a growth area. Studies on cost-effectiveness of conditional cash transfers designed to enhance uptake of health interventions were not covered in the survey, and few studies provide such information, even though some conditional cash transfer programs have been found to be effective.

Despite the very large number of studies, research gaps persist. More information on cost-effective approaches to integration, task-sharing, and the use of CHWs to deliver community-based services is needed, along with new studies on costs and impacts for demand creation to increase coverage. The volume of studies in this area is so large that a single repository for cost-effectiveness studies for health in LMICs would be useful, along the lines of similar registries for high-income countries, for example, the Tufts Cost-Effectiveness Analysis Registry (https://research.tufts -nemc.org/cear4/Default.aspx) or that maintained at the University of York. Although published systematic reviews and the rise of common standards for grading studies are extremely helpful, the reviews are undertaken in different years and costs are not standardized to a single year. There are plans for a single registry for unit costs for health for LMICs, and a parallel registry of cost-effectiveness studies for health interventions in LMICs would be valuable.

Methodological gaps exist as well. The method for standardizing costs is not uniform, whether done in the currency of the original study or in U.S. dollars. In vaccine studies, the vaccine prices are not adjusted for inflation when cost-effectiveness is adjusted to a different year. Studies done in international dollars for a region (as is the case for a number of WHO-CHOICE studies from the Choosing Interventions that are Cost-Effective project, http://www.who/int/choice/en) could not be updated to dollars of a common year, at the time of writing this chapter, because the WHO has not provided a time series for this price index. The resulting limitation is that none of those studies could be included here because they could not be updated to 2012 U.S. dollars. For some interventions, particularly the nutrition ones, benefits include improved quality of life rather than lives saved, and a benefit-cost analysis is a more appropriate methodology than cost-effectiveness. These and other methodological issues are addressed at more length in volume 9 of this series.

A larger unresolved issue is that of the DALY measure itself. More studies surveyed here used the discounted DALY measure than the other main measures—QALY, life-years, or deaths. The recent suggestion by the Institute for Health Metrics and Evaluation (Murray and others 2012) not to discount DALYs is likely to lead to confusion in the literature, with practitioners unsure about whether a particular study uses discounted or undiscounted DALYs. It will also drive a wedge between studies of HICs, where QALYs are discounted on a standard basis, and those of LMICs. Already, the lack of a single outcome measure makes comparisons of interventions more difficult, and this recent methodological advice will exacerbate the difficulties.

An innovation in modeling the cost-effectiveness of integrated interventions has been the use of LiST to estimate the impact and costs of packages of RMNCH interventions (Bartlett and others 2014; Bhutta, Das, Rivzi, and others 2013; Bhutta, Das, Walker, and others 2013; Bhutta and others 2014). The LiST model accounts for the synergies in effects such that lives saved are not double counted. However, the extent to which services can remain effective when management of them becomes more complicated, and when demands increase on the time of community-level personnel, remains to be verified in practice.

Analysis of cost and cost-effectiveness data has been an important tool in progress toward the MDGs and seems likely to continue to be useful with the transition to the Sustainable Development Goals.

NOTES

Susan Horton acknowledges support from the Grand Challenges Grant 0072-03 to the Grantee, the Trustees of the University of Pennsylvania.

World Bank Income Classifications as of July 2014 are as follows, based on estimates of gross national income (GNI) per capita for 2013:

- Low-income countries (LICs) = US$1,045 or less
- Middle-income countries (MICs) are subdivided:
  a) lower-middle-income (LMICs) = US$1,046 to US$4,125
  b) upper-middle-income (UMICs) = US$4,126 to US$12,745
- High-income countries (HICs) = US$12,746 or more.

1. Note that the WHO uses the term DALY to mean the loss of a healthy year of life; hence, deaths and DALYs are bad things that health interventions try to avert, whereas life-years and Quality-Adjusted Life Years are good things that health interventions try to save ("Health Statistics and Information Systems: Metrics: Disability-Adjusted Life Year [DALY])." http://www.who.int/healthinfo/global_burden_disease/metrics_daly/en/).

REFERENCES

Aboud, F. E., and A. K. Yousafzai. 2016. "Very Early Childhood Development." In *Disease Control Priorities* (third edition): Volume 2, *Reproductive, Maternal, Newborn, and Child Health*, edited by R. Black, R. Laxminarayan, M. Temmerman, and N. Walker. Washington, DC: World Bank.

Adam, T., S. J. Edwards, D. G. Amorim, J. Amaral, C. G. Victora, and others. 2009. "Cost Implications of Improving the Quality of Child Care Using Integrated Clinical Algorithms: Evidence from Northeast Brazil." *Health Policy* 89 (1): 97–106.

Adam, T., S. S. Lim, S. Mehta, Z. A. Bhutta, H. Fogstad, and others. 2005. "Cost Effectiveness Analysis of Strategies for Maternal and Neonatal Health in Developing Countries." *British Medical Journal* 331 (7525):1107–12.

Alkire, B. C., J. R. Vincent, C. T. Burns, I. S. Metzler, P. E. Farmer, and others. 2012. "Obstructed Labor and Caesarean Delivery: The Cost and Benefit of Surgical Intervention." *PLoS One* 7: E34595.

Ansah, E. K., M. Epokor, C. J. M. Whitty, S. Yeung, and K. S. Hansen. 2013. "Cost-Effectiveness Analysis of Introducing RDTs for Malaria Diagnosis as Compared to Microscopy and Presumptive Diagnosis in Central and Peripheral Public Health Facilities in Ghana." *American Journal of Tropical Medicine and Hygiene* 89 (4): 724–36.

Armstrong-Schellenberg, J. R., T. Adam, H. Mshinda, H. Masanja, G. Kabadi, and others. 2004. "Effectiveness and Cost of Facility-Based Integrated Management of Childhood Illness (IMCI) in Tanzania." *The Lancet* 364 (9445): 1583–94.

Babigumira, J. B., I. Morgan and A. Levin. 2013. "Health Economics of Rubella: A Systematic Review to Assess the Value of Rubella Vaccination." *BMC Public Health* 13: 406–17.

Babigumira, J. B., A. Stergachis, D. L. Veenstra, J. S. Gardner, J. Ngonzi, and others. 2012. "Potential Cost-Effectiveness of Universal Access to Modern Contraceptives in Uganda." *PLoS One* 7 (2): e30735.

Babigumira, J. B., and H. Gelband. Forthcoming. "Cost-Effectiveness of Strategies for Diagnosis and Treatment of Febrile Illness in Children." In *Disease Control Priorities* (third edition): Volume 6, *HIV/AIDS, STIs, Tuberculosis, and Malaria*, edited by K. Holmes, S. Bertozzi, P. Jha, B. Bloom, and R. Nugent. Washington, DC: World Bank.

Bartlett, L., E. Weissman, R. Gubin, R. Patton-Molitors, and I. K. Friberg. 2014. "The Impact and Cost of Scaling Up Midwifery and Obstetrics in 58 Low- and Middle-Income Countries." *PLoS One* 9: e98550.

Bhutta, Z. A., J. K. Das, R. Bahl, J. E. Lawn, R. A. Salam, and others. 2014. "Can Available Interventions End Preventable Deaths in Mothers, Newborn Babies, and Stillbirths, and at What Cost?" *The Lancet* 384 (9940): 347–70.

Bhutta, Z. A., J. K. Das, A. Rizvi, M. F. Gaffey, N. Walker, and others. 2013. "Evidence-Based Interventions for Improvement of Maternal and Child Nutrition: What Can Be Done and at What Cost?" *The Lancet* 382 (9890): 452–77.

Bhutta, Z. A., J. K. Das, N. Walker, A. Rizvi, H. Campbell, and others. 2013. "Interventions to Address Deaths from Childhood Pneumonia and Diarrhoea Equitably: What Works and at What Cost?" *The Lancet* 381 (9875): 1417–29.

Bhutta, Z., and Z. Lassi. 2016. "Community-Based Care." In *Disease Control Priorities* (third edition): Volume 2, *Reproductive, Maternal, Newborn, and Child Health*, edited by R. Black, R. Laxminarayan, M. Temmerman, and N. Walker. Washington, DC: World Bank.

Bishai, D., B. Johns, A. Lefevre, and D. Nair. 2010. *Cost Effectiveness of Measles Eradication*. Baltimore, MD: Johns Hopkins Bloomberg School of Public Health.

Borghi, J., L. Guinness, J. Ouedraogo, and V. Curtis. 2002. "Is Hygiene Promotion Cost-Effective? A Case Study in Burkina Faso." *Tropical Medicine and International Health* 7 (11): 960–69.

Borghi, J., B. Thapa, D. Osrin, S. Jan, J. Morrison, and others. 2005. "Economic Assessment of a Women's Group Intervention to Improve Birth Outcomes in Rural Nepal." *The Lancet* 366 (9500): 1882–84.

Brenzel, L. 2015. "What Have We Learned on Costs and Financing of Routine Immunization from the Comprehensive Multi-Year Plans in GAVI Eligible Countries?" *Vaccine* 33 (Suppl. 1): A93–98.

Bryce, J., E. Gouws, T. Adam, R. E. Black, J. A. Schellenberg, and others. 2005. "Improving Quality and Efficiency of Facility-Based Child Health Care through Integrated Management of Childhood Illness in Tanzania." *Health Policy and Planning* 20 (S1): I69–76.

Buchanan, J., B. Mihaylova, A. Gray, and N. White. 2010. "Cost-Effectiveness of Pre-Referral Antimalarial, Antibacterial, and Combined Rectal Formulations for Severe Febrile Illness." *PLoS One* 5: e14446.

Carvalho, N., A. S. Salehi, and S. J. Goldie. 2013. "National and Sub-National Analysis of the Health Benefits and Cost-Effectiveness of Strategies to Reduce Maternal Mortality in Afghanistan." *Health Policy and Planning* 28: 62–74.

Chanda, P., M. Castillo-Riquelme, and F. Masiye. 2009. "Cost-Effectiveness Analysis of the Available Strategies for Diagnosing Malaria in Outpatient Clinics in Zambia." *Cost-Effectiveness and Resource Allocation* 7: 5. doi: 10.1186 /1478-7547-7-5.

Corluka, A., D. G. Walker, S. Lewin, C. Glenton, and I. B. Scheel. 2009. "Are Vaccination Programmes Delivered by Lay Health Workers Cost-Effective? A Systematic Review." *Human Resources for Health* 7: 81.

Crowell, V., A. Levin, K. Galactionova, and F. Tediosi. 2013. *Costing and Budgeting for Malaria Service Delivery*. Basel: Swiss Tropical and Public Health Institute.

Drummond, M. F., M. J. Schulpher, G. W. Torrance, D. J. O'Brien, and G. L. Stoddart. 2005. *Methods for the Economic Evaluation of Health Care Programmes*. 3rd ed. New York: Oxford University Press.

Duintjer Tebbens, R. J., M. A. Pallansch, S. L. Cochi, S. G. F. Wassilak, J. Linkins, and others. 2010. "Economic Analysis of the Global Polio Eradication Initiative." *Vaccine* 29 (2): 334–43.

Erim, D. O., S. C. Resch, and S. J. Goldie. 2012. "Assessing Health and Economic Outcomes of Interventions to Reduce Pregnancy-Related Mortality in Nigeria." *BMC Public Health* 12: 786.

Feikin, D. R., B. Flannery, M. J. Hamel, M. Stack, and P. Hansen. "Vaccines for Children in Low- and Middle-Income Countries." 2006. In *Disease Control Priorities* (third edition): Volume 2, Reproductive, Maternal, Newborn, and Child Health, edited by R. Black, R. Laxminarayan, M. Temmerman, and N. Walker. Washington, DC: World Bank.

Fiedler, J. L., and T. Chuko. 2008. "The Cost of Child Health Days: A Case Study of Ethiopia's Enhanced Outreach Strategy (EOS)." *Health Policy and Planning* 23 (4): 222–33.

Fiedler, J. L., and C. Puett. 2015. "Micronutrient Program Costs: Sources of Variations and Noncomparabilities." *Food and Nutrition Bulletin* 36 (1): 43–56.

Fischer Walker, C. L., I. K. Friberg, N. Binkin, M. Young, N. Walker, and others. 2011. "Scaling Up Diarrhea Prevention and Treatment Interventions: A Lives Saved Tool Analysis." *PLoS Medicine* 8: E1000428.

Fottrell, E., K. Azad, A. Kuddus, L. Younes, S. Shaha, and others. 2013. "The Effect of Increased Coverage of Participatory Women's Groups on Neonatal Mortality in Bangladesh: A Cluster Randomized Trial." *JAMA Pediatrics* 167 (9): 816–25.

Goldie, S. J., S. Sweet, N. Carvalho, U. C. M. Natchu, and D. Hu. 2010. "Alternative Strategies to Reduce Maternal Mortality in India: A Cost-Effectiveness Analysis." *PLoS Medicine* 7 (4): e1000264.

Gyles, C. L., I. Lenoir-Wijnkoop, J. G. Carlbert, V. Senanayake, I. Gutierrez-Ibarluzea, and others. 2012. "Health Economics and Nutrition: A Review of Published Evidence." *Nutrition Reviews* 70 (12): 693–708.

Haller, L., G. Hutton, and J. Bartram. 2007. "Estimating the Costs and Health Benefits of Water and Sanitation Improvements at Global Level." *Journal of Water and Health* 5 (4): 467–80.

Hamer, D., J. Herlihy, V. D'Acremont, and D. Burgess. 2016. "Diagnosis and Treatment of a Febrile Child." In *Disease Control Priorities* (third edition): Volume 2, *Reproductive, Maternal, Newborn, and Child Health*, edited by R. Black, R. Laxminarayan, M. Temmerman, and N. Walker. Washington, DC: World Bank.

Harvest Plus. 2013. *Diving into Delivery: 2013 Annual Report*. Washington, DC: International Food Policy Research Institute.

Hoddinott, J., H. Alderman, J. R. Behrman, L. Haddad, and S. Horton. 2013. "The Economic Rationale for Investing in Stunting." *Maternal and Child Nutrition* 9 (S2): 69–82.

Hoddinott, J., M. Rosegrant, and M. Torero. 2012. *Copenhagen Consensus 2012 Challenge Paper: Hunger and Malnutrition*. Washington: International Food Policy Research Institute.

Horton, S., H. Alderman, and J. Rivera. 2008. *Copenhagen Consensus 2008 Challenge Paper: Hunger and Malnutrition.* Copenhagen Consensus Center.

Horton, S., and J. Ross. 2003. "The Economics of Iron Deficiency." *Food Policy* 28 (1): 51–75.

———. 2006. "Corrigendum to the Economics of Iron Deficiency [Food Policy 28 (2003) 51–75]." *Food Policy* 32 (1): 141–43.

Horton, S., D. C. N. Wu, E. Brouwer, and C. Levin. 2015. "Methodology and Results for Systematic Search, Cost and Cost-Effectiveness Analysis: RMNCH." Working Paper, *Disease Control Priorities,* third edition. http://www.dcp-3 .org/resources/working-papers.

Hu, D., S. M. Bertozzi, E. Gakidou, S. Sweet, and S. J. Goldie. 2007. "The Costs, Benefits, and Cost-Effectiveness of Interventions to Reduce Maternal Morbidity and Mortality in Mexico." *PLoS One* 2 (8): e750.

Hu, D., D. Grossman, C. Levin, K. Blanchard, R. Adanu, and others. 2010. "Cost-Effectiveness Analysis of Unsafe Abortion and Alternative First-Trimester Pregnancy Termination Strategies in Nigeria and Ghana." *African Journal of Reproductive Health* 14 (2): 85–103.

IHME (Institute for Health Metrics and Evaluation). 2014. *Financing Global Health 2013: Transition in an Age of Austerity.* Seattle, WA: IHME.

Irons, B., M. J. Lewis, M. Dahl-Regis, C. Castillo-Solorzano, P. A. Carrasco, and C. A. de Quadros. 2000. "Strategies to Eradicate Rubella in the English-Speaking Caribbean." *American Journal of Public Health* 90 (10): 1545–49.

Jamison, D. T., J. Bremen, A. R. Measham, G. Alleyne, M. Claeson, D. B. Evans, P. Jha, A. Mills, and P. Musgrove. 2006. *Disease Control Priorities in Developing Countries,* second edition. Washington, DC: Oxford University Press and World Bank.

Jan, S., G. Ferrari, C. H. Watts, J. R. Hargreaves, J. C. Kim, and others. 2010. "Economic Evaluation of a Combined Microfinance and Gender Training Intervention for the Prevention of Intimate Partner Violence in Rural South Africa." *Health Policy and Planning* 26 (5): 366–72.

Jit, M., T. T. Dong, I. Friberg, V. M. Hoang, T. K. Pham Huy, and others. 2015. "Thirty Years of Vaccination in Vietnam: Impact and Cost-Effectiveness of the National Expanded Programme on Immunization." *Vaccine* 335 (Supp. 1): A233–39.

Kahn, J. G., N. Munguri, B. Harris, E. Mugada, T. Clasen, and others. 2012. "Integrated HIV Testing, Diarrhea and Malaria Prevention Campaign in Kenya: Modeled Health Impact and Cost-Effectiveness." *PLoS One* 7 (2): e31316.

Leach-Kemon, K., D. P. Chou, M. T. Schneider, A. Tardif, J. L. Dieleman, and others. 2012. "The Global Financial Crisis Has Led to a Slowdown in Growth of Funding to Improve Health in Many Developing Countries." *Health Affairs* 31 (1): 228–35.

Lefevre, A. E., S. D. Shillcut, S. K. Saha, A. S. Ahmed, S. Ahmed, and others. 2010. "Cost-Effectiveness of Skin-Barrier-Enhancing Emollients among Pre-Term Infants in Bangladesh." *Bulletin of the World Health Organization* 88: 104–12.

Lefevre, A. E., S. D. Shillcut, H. R. Waters, S. Haider, S. El Arifeen, and others. 2013. "Economic Evaluation of Neonatal Care Packages in a Cluster-Randomized Controlled Trial in Sylhet, Bangladesh." *Bulletin of the World Health Organization* 91: 736–45.

Lehmann, U., and D. Sanders. 2007. "Community Health Workers: What Do We Know about Them? The State of the Evidence on Programmes, Activities, Costs and Impact on Health Outcomes of Using Community Health Workers." *World Health Organization Policy Brief* 2: 1–42.

Lemma, H., M. San Sebastian, C. Lofgren, and G. Barnabas. 2011. "Cost-Effectiveness of Three Malaria Treatment Strategies in Rural Tigray, Ethiopia, Where Both Plasmodium Falciparum and Plasmodium Vivax Co-Dominate." *Cost Effectiveness and Resource Allocation* 9: 2.

Levin, C., and E. Brouwer. 2014. "Saving Brains: Literature Review of Reproductive, Neonatal, Child and Maternal Health and Nutrition Interventions to Mitigate Basic Risk Factors to Promote Child Development." Grand Challenges Canada Working Paper Series 14-08. http://repository .upenn.edu/gcc_economic_returns/17.

Lewin, S., S. Munabi-Babigumira, C. Glenton, K. Daniels, X. Bosch-Capblanch, and others. 2010. "The Effect of Lay Health Workers on Mother and Child Health and Infectious Diseases." http://summaries.cochrane.org/cd004015/epoc _the-effect-of-lay-health-workers-on-mother-and-child -health-and-infectious-diseases.

Lewycka, S., C. Mwansambo, M. Rosato, P. Kazembe, T. Phiri, and others. 2013. "Effect of Women's Groups and Volunteer Peer Counselling on Rates of Mortality, Morbidity, and Health Behaviours in Mothers and Children in Rural Malawi (Maimwana): A Factorial, Cluster-Randomised Controlled Trial." *The Lancet* 381 (9879): 1721–35.

Lubell, Y., S. Yeung, A. M. Dondorp, N. P. Day, F. Nosten, and others. 2009. "Cost-Effectiveness of Artesunate for the Treatment of Severe Malaria." *Tropical Medicine and International Health* 14 (3): 332–37.

Mangham-Jefferies, L., C. Pitt, S. Cousens, A. Mills, and J. Schellenberg. 2014. "Cost-Effectiveness of Strategies to Improve the Utilization and Provision of Maternal and Newborn Health Care in Low-Income and Lower-Middle-Income Countries: A Systematic Review." *BMC Pregnancy and Childbirth* 14: 243. doi: 10.1186/1471-2393-14-243.

Miller, M. A., and C. K. Shahab. 2005. "Review of the Cost-Effectiveness of Immunisation Strategies for the Control of Epidemic Meningococcal Meningitis." *Pharmacoeconomics* 23 (4): 333–43.

Monath, T. P., and A. Nasidi. 1993. "Should Yellow Fever Vaccine Be Included in the Expanded Program of Immunization in Africa? A Cost-Effectiveness Analysis for Nigeria." *American Journal of Tropical Medicine and Hygiene* 48 (2): 274–99.

Morris, S. S., B. Gogill, and R. Uauy. 2008. "Effective International Action against Undernutrition: Why Has It Proven So Difficult and What Can Be Done to Accelerate Progress?" *The Lancet* 371 (9612): 608–21.

Murray, C., T. Vos, R. Lozano, M. Naghavi, A. D. Flaxman, and others. 2012. "Disability-Adjusted Life Years (DALYs) for 291 Diseases and Injuries in 21 Regions, 1990–2010: A Systematic Analysis for the Global Burden of Disease Study 2010." *The Lancet* 380 (9859): 2197–223.

Nonvignon, J., M. A. Chinbuah, M. Gyapong, M. Abbey, E. Awini, and others. 2012. "Is Home Management of Fevers a Cost-Effective Way of Reducing Under-Five Mortality in Africa? The Case of a Rural Ghanaian District." *Tropical Medicine and International Health* 17 (8): 951–57.

Ozawa, S., A. Mirelman, M. L. Stack, D. G. Walker, and O. S. Levine. 2012. "Cost-Effectiveness and Economic Benefits of Vaccines in Low- and Middle-Income Countries: A Systematic Review." *Vaccine* 31 (1): 96–108.

Pegurri, E., J. Fox-Rushby, and D. Walker. 2004. "The Effects and Costs of Expanding Coverage of Immunization Services in Developing Countries: A Systematic Literature Review." *Vaccine* 23 (13): 1624–35.

Prinja, S., N. Manchanda, P. Mohan, G. Gupta, G. Sethy, and others. 2013. "Cost of Neonatal Intensive Care Delivered through District Level Public Hospitals in India." *Indian Pediatrics* 50 (9): 839–46.

Puett, C., K. Sadler, H. Alderman, J. Coates, J. L. Fiedler, and M. Myatt. 2013. "Cost-Effectiveness of the Community-Based Management of Severe Acute Malnutrition by Community Health Workers in Southern Bangladesh." *Health Policy and Planning* 28 (4): 386–99.

Ravishankar, N., P. Gubbins, R. J. Cooley, K. Leach-Kemon, C. M. Michaud, and others. 2009. "Financing of Global Health: Tracking Development Assistance for Health from 1990 to 2007." *The Lancet* 373 (9681): 2113–24.

Rolland, E., F. Checchi, L. Pinoges, S. Balkan, J. P. Guthmann, and others. 2006. "Operational Response to Malaria Epidemics: Are Rapid Diagnostic Tests Cost-Effective?" *Tropical Medicine and International Health* 11 (4): 398–408.

Ross, A., N. Maire, E. Sicuri, T. Smith, and L. Conteh. 2011. "Determinants of the Cost-Effectiveness of Intermittent Preventive Treatment for Malaria in Infants and Children." *PLoS One* 6 (4): e18391.

Routh, S., and Barkat-e-Khuda. 2000. "An Economic Appraisal of Alternative Strategies for the Delivery of MCH-FP Services in Urban Dhaka, Bangladesh." *International Journal of Health Planning and Management* 15 (2): 115–32.

Ruel, M. T. 2001. *Can Food Based Strategies Help Reduce Vitamin A and Iron Deficiencies? A Review of Recent Evidence.* Washington DC: International Food Policy Research Institute.

———. H. Alderman, and the Maternal and Child Nutrition Study Group. 2013. "Nutrition-Sensitive Interventions and Programmes: How Can They Help to Accelerate Progress in Improving Maternal and Child Nutrition?" *The Lancet* 382 (9891): 536–51.

Sabin, L. L., A. B. Knapp, W. B. Macleod, G. Phiri-Mazala, J. Kasimba, and others. 2012. "Costs and Cost-Effectiveness of Training Traditional Birth Attendants to Reduce Neonatal Mortality in the Lufwanyama Neonatal Survival Study (LUNESP)." *PLoS One* 7: E35560.

San Sebastian, M., I. Goicolea, J. Aviles, and M. Narvaez. 2001. "Improving Immunization Coverage in Rural Areas of Ecuador: A Cost-Effectiveness Analysis." *Tropical Doctor* 31 (1): 21–24.

Sayed, A. R., D. Bourne, R. Pattinson, J. Nixon, and B. Henderson. 2008. "Decline in the Prevalence of Neural Tube Defects Following Folic Acid Fortification and Its Cost-Benefit in South Africa." *Birth Defects Research Part A: Clinical and Molecular Teratology* 82 (4): 211–16.

Seamans, Y., and C. M. Harner-Jay. 2007. "Modelling Cost-Effectiveness of Different Vasectomy Methods in India, Kenya, and Mexico." *Cost Effectiveness and Resource Allocation* 5: 8.

Sharieff, W., S. E. Horton, and S. Zlotkin. 2006. "Economic Gains of a Home Fortification Program: Evaluation of 'Sprinkles' from the Provider's Perspective." *Canadian Journal of Public Health* 97 (1): 20–23.

Sharieff, W., S. H. Zlotkin, W. J. Ungar, B. Feldman, M. D. Krahn, and others. 2008. "Economics of Preventing Premature Mortality and Impaired Cognitive Development in Children through Home-Fortification: A Health Policy Perspective." *International Journal of Technology Assessment in Health Care* 24 (3): 303–11.

Shea, B., N. Andersson, and D. Henry. 2009. "Increasing the Demand for Childhood Vaccination in Developing Countries: A Systematic Review." *BMC International Health and Human Rights* 9 (Suppl. 1): S5. doi: 10.1186/1472-698X-9-S1-S5.

Shearer, J. C., D. G. Walker, and M. Vlassoff. 2010. "Costs of Post-Abortion Care in Low- and Middle-Income Countries." *International Journal of Gynaecology and Obstetrics* 108 (2): 165–69.

Simoes, E. A. F., T. Cherian, J. Chow, S. Shahid-Salles, R. Laxminarayan, and T. J. John. 2006. "Acute Respiratory Infections in Children." In *Disease Control Priorities in Developing Countries*, second edition edited by D. T. Jamison, J. G. Breman, A. R. Measham, G. Alleyene, M. Claeson, D. B. Evans, P. Jha, A. Mills, and P. Musgrove. Washington, DC: World Bank and Oxford University Press.

Singh, S., J. E. Darroch, and L. S. Ashford. 2014. *Adding It Up: The Costs and Benefits of Investing in Sexual and Reproductive Health 2014.* New York: Guttmacher Institute. ISBN: 978-1-934387-18-4.

Stover, J., K. Hardee, B. Ganatra, C. García Moreno, and S. E. Horton. 2016. "Interventions to Improve Reproductive Health." In *Disease Control Priorities* (third edition): Volume 2, *Reproductive, Maternal, Newborn, and Child Health*, edited by R. Black, R. Laxminarayan, M. Temmerman, and N. Walker. Washington, DC: World Bank.

Tozan, Y., E. Y. Klein, S. Darley, R. Panicker, R. Laxminarayan, and others. 2010. "Prereferral Rectal Artesunate for Treatment of Severe Childhood Malaria: A Cost-Effectiveness Analysis." *The Lancet* 376 (9756): 1910–15.

Tripathy, P., N. Nair, S. Barnett, R. Mahapatra, J. Borghi, and others. 2010. "Effect of a Participatory Intervention with Women's Groups on Birth Outcomes and Maternal Depression in Jharkhand and Orissa, India: A Cluster-Randomized Controlled Trial." *The Lancet* 375 (9721): 1182–92.

Tsu, V. D., C. Levin, M. P. T. Tran, M. V. Hoang, and H. T. T. Luu. 2009. "Cost-Effectiveness Analysis of Active Management of Third-Stage Labour in Vietnam." *Health Policy and Planning* 24 (6): 438–44.

Tu, H. A., J. J. Woerdenbag, S. Kane, A. Riewaiboon, M. Van Hulst, and others. 2009. "Economic Evaluations of Hepatitis B Vaccination for Developing Countries." *Expert Review of Vaccines* 8 (7): 907–20.

Uzochukwu, B. S., E. N. Obikeze, O. E. Onwujekwe, C. A. Onoka, and U. K. Griffiths. 2009. "Cost-Effectiveness Analysis of Rapid Diagnostic Test, Microscopy and Syndromic Approach in the Diagnosis of Malaria in Nigeria: Implications for Scaling-Up Deployment of ACT." *Malaria Journal* 8: 265.

Verguet, S., W. Jassat, M. Y. Bertram, S. M. Tollman, C. J. Murray, and others. 2013. "Supplementary Immunization Activities (SIAs) in South Africa: Comprehensive Economic Evaluation of an Integrated Child Health Delivery Platform." *Global Health Action* 6: 1–9.

Vijayaraghavan, M., A. Wallace, I. R. Mirza, R. Kamadjeu, R. Nandy, and others. 2012. "Economic Evaluation of a Child Health Days Strategy to Deliver Multiple Maternal and Child Health Interventions in Somalia." *Journal of Infectious Diseases* 205 (Supp. 1): S134–40.

Walker, D., N. R. Mosqueira, M. E. Penny, C. F. Lanata, A. D. Clark, and others. 2004. "Variation in the Costs of Delivering Routine Immunization Services in Peru." *Bulletin of the World Health Organization* 82 (9): 676–82.

Waters, H. R., M. E. Penny, H. M. Creed-Kanashiro, R. C. Roberts, R. Narro, and others. 2006. "The Cost-Effectiveness of a Child Nutrition Education Programme in Peru." *Health Policy and Planning* 21 (4): 257–64.

White, M. T., L. Conteh, R. Cibulskis, and A. C. Ghani. 2011. "Costs and Cost-Effectiveness of Malaria Control Interventions: A Systematic Review." *Malaria Journal* 10: 337. doi: 10.1186/1475-2875-10-337.

World Bank. 2013. "World Bank World Development Indicators." http://data.worldbank.org/indicator/ny.gnp.pcap.cd/countries/sg--xr?page=1&display=default.

WHO (World Health Organization). 2001. *Macroeconomics and Health: Investing in Health for Economic Development.* Geneva: WHO.

———. "Choosing Interventions That are Cost-Effective (CHOICE)." http://www.who/int/choice/en. Accessed October 2, 2015.

Yukich, J., V. D'Acremont, J. Kahama, N. Swai, and C. Lengeler. 2010. "Cost Savings with Rapid Diagnostic Tests for Malaria in Low-Transmission Areas: Evidence from Dar es Salaam, Tanzania." *American Journal of Tropical Medicine and Hygiene* 83 (1): 61–68.

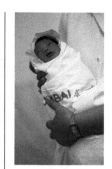

Chapter **18**

The Benefits of a Universal Home-Based Neonatal Care Package in Rural India: An Extended Cost-Effectiveness Analysis

Ashvin Ashok, Arindam Nandi, and Ramanan Laxminarayan

INTRODUCTION

Each year, 27 percent of the world's newborn deaths—about 748,000—occur in India according to 2013 estimates (UN IGME 2014). India's newborn mortality rate (NMR) has declined by nearly 43 percent since 1990. However, this decline has been much slower than the decline in the mortality rate for children under age five years, which has dropped by 58 percent during the same period. Consequently, the share of newborn deaths among all under-five deaths in India has risen from 41 percent in 1990 to 56 percent in 2013, highlighting the relative lack of progress made in newborn survival. Conditions associated with neonates—such as preterm birth complications and sepsis—rank among the top 10 causes of all premature mortality in India (CDC 2015). A study in 2005 found that prematurity and low birth weight, infections, birth asphyxia, and birth trauma caused nearly 80 percent of newborn deaths (Bassani and others 2010).

India's NMR of 29 per 1,000 live births continues to be among the highest in the world,[1] underscoring the need for a policy response (UN IGME 2014) (figure 18.1).[2] Although antenatal care and other preventive interventions such as encouraging institutional delivery and improving maternal health care access have been implemented, their impact on newborn survival has been minimal (Hollowell and others 2009; Lim and others 2010; Singh and others 2013). Good quality postnatal care may prevent about 67 percent of all newborn deaths (WHO 2012) in India. However, availability of and access to postnatal care remain low. Data from the District Level Household Survey conducted between 2007 and 2008 suggest that only 45 percent of newborns in India underwent a health examination within the first 24 hours (IIPS 2010).

In addition to low levels of access to newborn care in general, large regional and socioeconomic differences in access lead to significant variations in outcomes. The mortality among newborns in India's rural areas is twice that in urban areas—34 and 17 per 1,000 live births, respectively—with mortality rates substantially exceeding the national average in the poorer and larger states of Madhya Pradesh, Uttar Pradesh, Odisha, Rajasthan, Jammu and Kashmir, and Chhattisgarh (Chand and others 2013).

In this chapter, we examine the health and economic benefits and the cost to the government associated with scaling up a publicly financed home-based neonatal care (HBNC) package in rural India. We consider two intervention scenarios against a baseline of no HBNC:

- In the first scenario, we examine the scaling up of access to HBNC through the current network of

Corresponding author: Ramanan Laxminarayan, Center for Disease Dynamics, Economics & Policy, Washington, DC, ramanan@cddep.org.

Figure 18.1 Newborn, Infant, and Child Mortality in India, 1990–2015

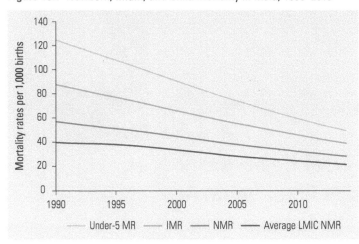

Source: UN IGME 2015.

Note: Newborn mortality rate (NMR) is defined as the ratio of the number of deaths in the first 28 days of life to the number of live births occurring in the same population during the same period. Infant mortality rate (IMR) is defined as the ratio of the number of deaths in one year, of children less than age one year to the number of live births in that year. Average LMIC NMR refers to the average neonatal mortality rate among low- and middle-income countries (excluding India) during the same period.

accredited social health activists (ASHA)—a group of community health workers (CHWs) that covers 60.1 percent of India's villages (or roughly 54 percent of the rural population)—to those not presently receiving care. Of rural newborns, 39.8 percent receive some form of home- or facility-based newborn care during the first 10 days of life (IIPS 2010). By extending HBNC within the current network of ASHA workers, 72 percent of the rural newborn population would have access to care either through the HBNC package or their existing home- or facility-based care.

- In the second scenario, we analyze a near-universal setting in which access to HBNC—through expansion of the network of CHWs—is extended to 83.4 percent of those not presently receiving care. With this extension, 90 percent of the rural neonate population would have access to the HBNC package or their existing home- or facility-based care.

Box 18.1 provides information on the types of CHWs and the primary health systems in which they operate.

HOME- AND COMMUNITY-BASED NEONATAL CARE IN INDIA

In 2011, the government of India introduced an HBNC package—to be delivered by ASHAs—that includes five or six home visits during the first month after birth for children born at health facilities or at home, respectively

(Ministry of Health and Family Welfare 2011). The ASHAs provide essential newborn care, particularly for preterm and low-birth-weight infants; identify illnesses; refer sick infants to health facilities; and provide information to mothers on care practices, such as thermal care and breastfeeding.

In their joint statement, the World Health Organization and the United Nations Children's Fund recognized the role of home-based care in providing postnatal care to mothers who are unable to access it otherwise because of financial, social, physical, or other barriers (WHO/UNICEF Joint Statement 2009). In a widely cited field trial in the Indian state of Maharashtra, Bang and others (1999) find that an HBNC package—the key components of which included a method of screening high-risk neonates; management of sepsis, low birth weight, and birth asphyxia; and education and training of mothers on newborn care—reduced mortality by more than 60 percent. Kumar and others (2008) also conducted an efficacy trial of a similar community-based prevention package of essential newborn care in Uttar Pradesh. This package comprised birth preparedness, clean delivery and cord care, thermal care including skin-to-skin care, breastfeeding promotion, danger sign recognition, and liquid crystal hypothermia indicators. The authors find mortality reductions of about 54 percent. Similar results in Bangladesh and Pakistan have contributed to the growing body of evidence demonstrating the effectiveness of home-based and community-based care in improving access to postnatal care and curbing newborn deaths in countries with high barriers to institutional care (Baqui and others 2008; Bhutta and others 2008).

Although the home-based care packages in these studies share similarities, they also contain important differences in the number of home visits, kind of training provided to community workers, extent of community mobilization, and quality of the local health infrastructure (community-worker-to-population ratio). These are important considerations that might affect the efficacy of the intervention as it is scaled up to the national level (Gogia and others 2011). We note these differences but still use parameters from various studies (with sensitivity analyses) to assess the potential magnitude of the benefits that can be derived from implementing a home-based package.

PRIORITY-SETTING METHODOLOGIES

Resource allocations are guided by evidence. Cost-effectiveness analysis (CEA) is an extremely useful and widely applied method that identifies interventions that provide the most value for money on the basis of

Community Health Workers in India

Structure of India's health system

India's primary care network consists of two types of institutions: primary health subcenters and primary health centers. As of March 2014, India had 152,326 primary health subcenters and 25,020 primary health centers (Health Management Information System 2014). Subcenters are established at the rate of one per 5,000 people in most areas, and one per 3,000 people in hilly, tribal, or remote areas.

Types of Community Health Workers

India has three main types of female community health workers (CHWs) supporting child health: accredited social health activists (ASHAs), auxiliary nurse midwives (ANMs), and nutrition workers known as *Anganwadi* workers.

ASHAs were introduced in 2005 as part of the National Rural Health Mission, to serve a population of 700 in tribal areas and 1,000 in rural villages. An ASHA is typically a woman residing in the village, reporting to the local ANM. Her primary responsibilities are to improve health awareness in the local communities while facilitating the use of health care services (including antenatal and postnatal care and ushering pregnant women to nearby health facilities at the time of delivery). She is also expected to track pregnant women and newborn children from the village. ASHAs are not paid a salary but receive allowances based on tasks performed. The 800,000 ASHAs constitute the largest group of CHWs in the world (Perry and Zulliger 2012) and presently cover about 60 percent of villages in rural India (IIPS 2010).

ANMs are posted at health subcenters and earn monthly salaries as employees of local health departments. They are responsible for providing treatment for basic ailments; antenatal, postnatal, and delivery care; family planning services; and immunization of children (Mavalankar and Vora 2008). Each ANM is typically supported by three to five ASHAs in carrying out these tasks (Sharma, Webster, and Bhattacharyya 2014).

Anganwadi workers were introduced under the Integrated Child Development Scheme of 1975, a large-scale supplementary nutrition program for pregnant women and young children. The Department of Women and Child Development employs them, and their primary focus is on providing supplementary nutrition under the scheme. However, they also provide health education services, immunizations, and health check-ups (Shashidhar 2012).

Although there is considerable overlap in the functions of these three groups of CHWs, this study evaluates the rollout of home-based neonatal care through the ASHA network because they are closest to the communities and most suited to providing home-based care.

cost per disability-adjusted life year (DALY) averted (Brouwer and Koopmanschap 2000; Garber and Phelps 1997; Jamison and others 2006; WHO 2003).

CEAs are relatively simple in application, but do not include the nonhealth benefits of interventions. Adverse health events in low- and middle-income countries (LMICs) are often associated with economic hardship (O'Donnell and others 2008; van Doorslaer and others 2006, 2007; Wagstaff 2008). Households experiencing health shocks may need to finance health care costs through out-of-pocket (OOP) expenditures, which may lead to borrowing or selling of assets, thereby causing impoverishment (Gertler and Gruber 2002; Kruk, Goldmann, and Galea 2009; Wagstaff 2007).

Such economic shocks may have a lasting intergenerational effect if they reduce resources available to children (Dillon 2012; Sun and Yao 2010). Free or subsidized health interventions can potentially prevent such economic shocks.

Although the literature on economic impacts of newborn morbidity is limited, several studies have shown that the financial burden of care is significant (Asian Development Bank 2012). Bonu and others (2009) find that 16 percent of households incur catastrophic expenditures of more than 10 percent of annual household consumption for antenatal and postnatal care in India. Complications caused by hemorrhage, sepsis, and dystocia were associated with 15 percent to 34 percent of total household expenditures in Benin and 5 percent to 8 percent in Ghana (Borghi and others 2003).

Therefore, the impoverishing effects of newborn morbidity should not be ignored; the economic benefits of an intervention need to be incorporated into priority-setting methodologies. Other methodologies, such as cost-consequence analysis and benefit-cost analysis, attempt to incorporate the nonhealth benefits of health interventions; but these approaches are computationally intensive and do not explicitly capture the financial risk protection that interventions provide.

In this study, we apply the method of extended cost-effectiveness analysis (ECEA) to estimate the economic benefits, in addition to health gains, of health interventions (Verguet, Laxminarayan, and Jamison 2014). ECEA has been used to examine the impacts of publicly financed interventions—for example, tuberculosis treatments in India (Verguet, Laxminarayan, and Jamison 2014) and rotavirus vaccinations in India and Ethiopia (Verguet and others 2013)—and thus to measure the distributional consequences of interventions on the health and financial outcomes for a population. Similarly, we measure the health benefits of scaling up the HBNC package in India by the resulting reductions in newborn morbidity and mortality. The economic benefits are measured from the perspective of health systems accounting, that is, the amount of OOP private medical expenditures and associated financial risk that could be averted by the HBNC.

Data and Methods

We extract information on disease epidemiology from existing studies; table 18.1 presents these input parameters and the interventions in our analysis. The lack of recent disease data presents a significant challenge in generating health and economic estimates that we overcome in two ways.

First, some of the parameters have been revised based on current conditions. For example, a newborn's risk of suffering from high-risk morbidity, such as sepsis, congenital anomaly, or birth asphyxia, was observed to be 48.2 percent by Bang and others (2001). This risk is likely to have changed significantly since the 1990s; therefore we assume that the baseline probability that a neonate suffers from high-risk morbidity equals 28.3 percent, based on the most recently available neonatal mortality rate of 29.2 per 1,000 live births in India (UN IGME 2014). We continue to use the case fatality rate of 10.3 percent from severe morbidity (Bang and others 1999) on the assumption that the underlying mortality risk after contracting the disease is unlikely to have changed significantly, even with progress in access or improved economic conditions. Furthermore, because of the lack of disease data disaggregated by population subgroups, we make the simplifying assumption that the incidence and mortality rates are the same across all income quintiles.

Second, recognizing the uncertainty surrounding the true morbidity and mortality risks of newborns, we

Table 18.1 Disease, Treatment, and Newborn Care Package Intervention Parameters for Community Health Worker Analysis

Parameter type	Value	Sensitivity analysis	Source
Disease parameters	*Disease: Newborn morbidity*		
Incidence	0.283	0.198–0.369	Based on NMR (UN IGME 2014)
Case fatality rate	0.103	0.072–0.134	Bang and others 1999
Treatment parameters	*Treatment: Intensive care treatment*		
Demand for treatment (%)	75.00	52.50–97.50	Assumed
Cost of treatment (US$)	108.97	76.28–141.66	Prinja, Manchanda, and others 2013
Intervention parameters	*Intervention: Home-based newborn care as defined in Bang and others (2005)*		
Baseline coverage of intervention (%)	0	n.a.	Assumed
Baseline coverage of ASHA workers (%)	54	n.a.	IIPS 2010
Cost at 54% coverage (US$)	5.89 per neonate	4.12–7.66	Prinja, Mazumder, and others 2013
Cost at 83% coverage (US$)	6.54 per neonate	4.58–8.50	Prinja, Mazumder, and others 2013
Risk reduction in incidence	0.5035	0.3520–0.6550	Bang and others 2005
Risk reduction in mortality	0.540	0.378–0.702	Kumar and others 2008

Note: ASHA = accredited social health activist; DLHS = District Level Household Survey; NMR = newborn mortality rate. n.a. = not applicable.

conducted a 100-simulation Latin hypercube sampling sensitivity analysis on these risks and other intervention and cost parameters (table 18.1). Results from the sensitivity analysis are used to produce 95 percent uncertainty ranges for our mean estimates. These ranges are reported in the results in the next section.

Intervention and Treatment Data

Parameters with respect to the efficacy of interventions on prevention of newborn morbidity and mortality were obtained from published studies and secondary household survey data in India. According to the District Level Household Survey–3, 39.8 percent of rural newborns receive some form of home- or facility-based newborn care during the first 10 days of life (IIPS 2010). We assumed that the HBNC package in our analysis would be administered to the remaining 60.2 percent of the neonate population without access to care (that is, baseline coverage rate of 0). We scaled up the HBNC package in our model in two scenarios. First, responsibilities of the existing ASHAs (who were available to 54 percent of the neonate population) were extended to include the HBNC. In the second scenario, access to HBNC was extended to 83.4 percent of newborns without care by assuming that more ASHAs would be used. In this scenario, a total of 90 percent of newborns born in rural India would access care either directly through the intervention or through the home- or facility-based care provided in the baseline.

Studies have shown that care packages in Gadchiroli, Maharashtra, and in Shivgarh, Uttar Pradesh, reduced the incidence of severe newborn morbidity and mortality by 50.4 percent and 54.0 percent, respectively (Bang and others 2005; Kumar and others 2008). We assumed these efficacy rates on incidence and mortality for our study, but performed a sensitivity analysis on the parameters to estimate the impact of a wide range of possible levels of intervention effectiveness. Baqui and others (2007) observe a lower efficacy on mortality reduction (34 percent) in Bangladesh of a community-led intervention, which is significant given that the intervention was conducted in India's geographic neighborhood. Because this effect size falls below the lower limit (37.8 percent) of the efficacy on mortality reduction parameter in our sensitivity analysis, we conducted a separate analysis using an effectiveness rate of 34 percent to report the corresponding reduction in deaths.

Under our intervention scenario, the government bears the full cost of administering or expanding the HBNC program. The cost of this program is derived from the costs of administering the Integrated Management of Childhood Illnesses (IMCI) program through CHWs in Faridabad district, examined by Prinja, Mazumder, and others (2013).

Within the current ASHA network, we assumed that the cost of implementing the intervention would approximate the annual per child cost under the IMCI program of US$1.52, in addition to the US$4.37 per neonate incentive provided to each ASHA worker for delivering care, which totals US$5.89.[3] Prinja, Mazumder and others (2013) also estimate the incremental costs (including increased time commitments of ASHA workers and additional monitoring time) of expanding coverage of the IMCI program. We assumed that similar costs would be incurred to expand the intervention beyond the current network of ASHA workers. These additional costs of US$0.65 per newborn (including the cost of enlarging the ASHA network), result in a total cost of US$6.54 (2013 dollars) per neonate under this scenario.

Finally, we assumed the demand for newborn intensive treatment to be 75 percent, which means that the parents or guardians of 75 percent of neonates suffering from severe morbidity seek intensive care, if available, with an OOP treatment expenditure of US$108.97 (Prinja, Manchanda, and others 2013). As with other parameters, we considered a wide range of additional demand and cost scenarios in our sensitivity analysis.

Methods

Our analysis was conducted on an annual cohort of 10.48 million Indian newborns as of 2013. This cohort size was estimated in two steps. First, based on India's birth rate of 20.438 per 1,000 and the total rural population of 852 million (World Bank, World Development Indicators),[4] we estimated 17.40 million new births in rural India per year. We subtracted the 39.8 percent of rural newborns receiving some form of home- or facility-based care during the first 10 days of life (IIPS 2010) from this birth cohort to obtain the resultant cohort of 10.48 million neonates who do not receive any care each year.

We estimated the incident cases and deaths averted from severe newborn morbidity by the HBNC package under each of the two intervention scenarios, compared with the baseline. Our analysis is similar to the well-known Lives Saved Tool (LiST)—a powerful tool developed to model the impact on children of scaling up health interventions (Steinglass and others 2011). However, our estimates differ from its projections because the LiST is based on the effectiveness of interventions gathered from scientific evidence that is not restricted to a specific country. The ECEA method enables us to estimate the impacts of interventions based on the efficacy literature available for the target country. In addition to health outcomes, we estimated economic benefits of the HBNC including incremental OOP expenditures averted and the money-metric value of insurance provided. For simplicity, we only considered OOP expenditures related to treatment expenditure for newborn morbidity. Higher levels of access to HBNC are likely to lower the incidence of morbidity, reducing the need for treatment and associated expenditure.

The money-metric value of insurance is a metric that measures the financial protection provided by the HBNC package. It estimates the risk premium, that is, the amount of money an individual is willing to pay to avoid an ailment. To calculate the value of insurance, we started with a mean per capita gross domestic product (GDP) in India of US$1,489 (in 2013 U.S. dollars) (World Bank World Development Indicators).

We used a constant relative risk aversion utility function of the form $u(y) = \dfrac{y^{1-\rho}}{1-\rho}$ with a coefficient of relative risk aversion of $\rho = 3$ (McClellan and Skinner 2006). The probability of receiving treatment for a disease is denoted by $r(y)$, a function of income. Therefore, the expected value of income will be as follows:

$$E(y) = (1 - r)y + r(y - c), \qquad (18.1)$$

in which c denotes the OOP cost of treatment. The certainty equivalent of this expected income, denoted by y^* is as follows:

$$y^* = u^{-1}[(1-r)u(y) + ru(y-c)] \qquad (18.2)$$
$$= [(1-r)y^{1-\rho} + r(y-c)^{1-\rho}]^{\frac{1}{1-\rho}}.$$

The money-metric value of insurance denoted by v is as follows:

$$v = E(y) - y^*$$
$$= [(1-r)y + r(y-c) - [(1-r)y^{1-\rho} + r(y-c)^{1-\rho}]^{\frac{1}{1-\rho}}.$$
$$(18.3)$$

RESULTS

Table 18.2 reports the health and financial consequences of the HBNC package based on the disease and intervention parameters listed in table 18.1. For our study cohort of neonates, we found that if the current

network of ASHA workers were utilized with a coverage rate of 54 percent of the population, the corresponding reduction in incidence of morbidity and deaths would be 805,000 (95 percent uncertainty range 477,000 to 1,218,000) and 89,000 (95 percent uncertainty range 44,200 to 149,100), respectively, compared with the baseline. Extending the coverage of the care package in scenario 2 could avert a total of 1.25 million cases (95 percent uncertainty range 750,000 to 1,950,000) of newborn morbidity and 138,000 deaths (95 percent uncertainty range 76,400 to 244,100) compared with the baseline (figure 18.2). Even at a more conservative efficacy rate of 34 percent on mortality based on Baqui and others (2008), we found that the package averts 55,900 deaths (95 percent uncertainty range 34,700 to 85,100) when scaled up to the present ASHA coverage level, and 86,800 deaths (95 percent uncertainty range 49,000 to 130,000) when scaled up in scenario 2.

The financial benefits of the estimated health reductions are significantly large as well. At US$108.97 for newborn intensive care (Prinja, Manchanda, and others 2013), the OOP expenditures averted by the care package amount to US$66 million (95 percent uncertainty range $35 million to $106 million) at the existing ASHA coverage, and US$102 million (95 percent uncertainty range $51 million to $182 million) under intervention scenario 2. At a relative risk averseness coefficient of 3 and income per capita of US$1,489, we estimate that the financial risk protection (value of insurance) afforded by the HBNC package amounts to US$474 (95 percent uncertainty range $222 to $885) per 1,000 births in the cohort within existing ASHA coverage levels, and US$826 (95 percent uncertainty range $351 to $1,626) per 1,000 births when scaled up further in the second intervention scenario.

The financial burden of the newborn care package on the government would amount to US$33 million (95 percent uncertainty range $24 million to $42 million) when the package is rolled out within the present ASHA network, and US$53 million (95 percent uncertainty range $41 million to $66 million) when extended to 83 percent of the population in scenario 2. To put this figure in context, the government allocated US$386.1 million (23.2 billion Indian rupees, assuming US$1 = 60 Indian rupees) for *all* child health-related programs in fiscal year 2013/14 (CBGA 2013).

The value of this package measured by costs per death averted indicates that it is cost saving under both scenarios (if we include the OOP expenditure averted). Otherwise, if we only consider programmatic costs and ignore OOP costs averted, the first intervention scenario extending the package to current ASHA worker levels costs US$373 per death averted from the baseline; the second scenario costs US$387 per death averted from

Table 18.2 Estimates of the Impact of Home-Based Neonatal Care through Community Health Workers

	Intervention 1		Intervention 2	
	At 54 percent coverage	95 percent uncertainty range	At 83 percent coverage	95 percent uncertainty range
Incidence averted	804,718	476,612–1,217,799	1,246,812	751,155–1,950,785
Deaths averted	89,022	44,199–149,050	138,162	76,358–244,072
OOP expenses averted (US$ millions)	66	35–106	102	51–182
Cost to government (US$ millions)	33	24–42	53	41–66
Value of insurance per 1,000 newborn (US$ millions)	474	222–885	826	351–1,626

Note: OOP = out-of-pocket.

Figure 18.2 Estimated Impact of Home-Based Neonatal Care Package on the Incidence of Morbidity and Mortality

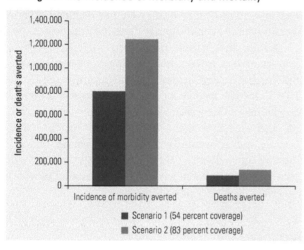

■ Scenario 1 (54 percent coverage)
■ Scenario 2 (83 percent coverage)

the baseline. These costs suggest that these interventions are "very cost-effective" by the cost-effectiveness threshold of the WHO (WHO 2003).

DISCUSSION AND CONCLUSION

We assessed the health and financial benefits of expanding access to an HBNC package. Although the health benefits may be of primary importance, the direct and indirect costs of newborn care are also significant (Asian Development Bank 2012). Newborn morbidity poses a significant economic risk for households, and evaluating the financial risk protection benefits of the HBNC package is important.

Incorporating this aspect of financial risk protection and OOP expenditures averted favorably differentiates the ECEA method from other priority-setting tools.[5]

For the purpose of this analysis, we assumed that the government bears the full cost of the intervention and expands coverage to either 54 percent or 83 percent of the population that does not have access to care. The total cost to the government under these two intervention scenarios would be $33 million (up to $42 million) and $53 million (up to $66 million), respectively. The HBNC is a new program and the details of its budget allocations are not yet publicly available. However, we can compare the estimated financial requirements of the HBNC with other large-scale maternal and child health programs in India. The Janani Suraksha Yojana[6] (Safe Motherhood Scheme) is one such program. It provides cash incentives to pregnant women for delivering their babies at health facilities (instead of home births). Implemented across the country beginning in 2005, it has led to some modest improvements in newborn and perinatal death rates (Lim and others 2010). However, in comparison with the estimated cost of HBNC, Janani Suraksha Yojana has a much larger budget of more than $300 million per year (Ministry of Health and Family Welfare 2012).

The two intervention scenarios in our analysis reflect some of the options available to the government. The policies can be adapted as needed, for example, by setting a lower threshold for coverage or by paying a percentage of the cost of the intervention. At the given rates of intervention efficacy, this adaptability would help strike a balance between the potential benefits and financial viability for the government.

The health and financial outcome estimates in this analysis illustrate the potential benefits under an ideal policy implementation scenario. The effectiveness of policy depends on more than access to ASHAs. On the demand side, it is essential to change the care-seeking practices and behaviors of mothers. Only 17 percent of pregnant women in rural Uttar Pradesh received at least one antenatal checkup during their entire period of pregnancy (Baqui and others 2007). Furthermore, only 5 percent of women were informed about thermal care and breastfeeding. These alarming statistics highlight the need to improve health education for mothers and increase incentives to seek proper care through programs like Janani Suraksha Yojana.

In addition to improving the demand for care and changing the practices of mothers, it is important to focus on improving health care delivery channels. The quality of training provided to ASHAs, motivation levels, and remuneration of workers are factors that contribute to the effectiveness of the intervention and influence its uptake among the population (Bang and others 1999). The challenges of delivery were highlighted by a recent situational analysis of the new HBNC program in Uttar Pradesh. The assessment found that ASHAs failed to identify critical signs and did not follow program guidelines. Furthermore, they were misclassifying sickness categories of a staggering 80 percent of newborn children (Das and others 2014).

Based on available evidence on the efficacy of the interventions, our results indicate that expanding the HBNC package within the current network of ASHA workers to 54 percent and further expanding it to 83 percent would significantly prevent newborn morbidity, extend the lives of neonates, and yield significant financial risk protection. Considering that newborn mortality constitutes 71 percent of infant mortality and 56 percent of mortality under age five years in India (UN IGME 2014), the HBNC has tremendous potential to lower NMR in India. Recognizing this potential and its ability to overcome the demand-side barriers to accessing postnatal care at health facilities, HBNC was recommended as the primary strategy for combating NMR by the Eleventh Five-Year Plan of India (2007–12) (Planning Commission of India 2008).

Furthermore, expanding coverage of the HBNC is in complete alignment with the objectives of continuum of care as outlined in India's Newborn Action Plan (2014)—which aims to reduce preventable newborn deaths and stillbirths. It is also in harmony with the future goals of universal health coverage in India. The 2010 World Health Report (WHO 2010) outlines the need for public financing of health interventions in the developing world to reduce OOP private medical expenditure and protect vulnerable populations from catastrophic health shocks in an equitable way. The report also highlights the need to ensure that interventions are prepaid (through some form of progressive taxation), to enable the poor and the sick to benefit from the implicit subsidy provided to them by rich and healthy population groups through such a mechanism. The Indian Planning Commission's report on universal health coverage has also emphasized such public financing (High Level Expert Group on Universal Health Coverage 2011).

The following factors circumscribe the conclusions of our study. Because data on HBNC are limited, we have relied on a research study conducted in 1996 for newborn morbidity and efficacy of interventions in a district of India. Although this study is dated and localized, we overcame the uncertainty in these estimates by conducting a rigorous sensitivity analysis. The estimates of this model would be enriched by the availability of geographic or economic segmentation in the data on incidence and mortality to provide an understanding of the distributional consequences of the intervention. As a result of the absence of such data, we were unable to estimate the equity impacts of the HBNC intervention and account for any spatial or economic heterogeneity, such as costs or income, in our results. Furthermore, differences in quality of interventions or factors that could affect behavioral responses to the intervention were not included. A more dynamic model could capture these heterogeneities.

Despite these limitations, our analysis takes an important step toward highlighting the overall magnitude of health and economic benefits provided by the HBNC for the welfare of India's newborn population. Further research on the role of community worker training and supervision, the health system in which they operate, and community mobilization would lead to a broader understanding about the impacts of home- and community-based interventions in improving newborn survival in a variety of conditions.

NOTES

World Bank Income Classifications as of July 2014 are as follows, based on estimates of gross national income (GNI) per capita for 2013:

- Low-income countries (LICs) = US$1,045 or less
- Middle-income countries (MICs) are subdivided:
  a) lower-middle-income = US$1,046–US$4,125
  b) upper-middle-income (UMICs) = US$4,126–US$12,745
- High-income countries (HICs) = US$12,746 or more.

1. By comparison, the average NMR among countries in the same economic category as India (lower-middle-income) is 20.7 per 1,000 live births.
2. In 1990, India's NMR was 51.1 per 1,000 live births, which declined to 29.2 in 2013 (UN IGME 2014).
3. Unless otherwise specified, all cost data in our analysis are in 2013 U.S. dollars.
4. In 2013, 68 percent of India's total population of 1.252 billion was rural.
5. In a traditional CEA framework, priority setting is based on the health benefits of an intervention, measured by

the cost per DALY averted. DALYs put greater emphasis on early life by discounting future life years. Therefore, a neonatal care package will avert a very large number of DALYs and be highly cost-effective. However, when the financial benefits of an intervention are considered (as in the ECEA) in a priority-setting analysis, they may shift the policy makers' focus away from early life to future life years. Although an HBNC will be very attractive on the basis of DALYs, other health interventions may significantly outweigh it based on economic benefits.

6. The Janani Suraksha Yojana is a conditional cash transfer scheme introduced in 2005 to encourage demand for institutional deliveries and provide mothers with incentives to give birth at health facilities.

REFERENCES

Asian Development Bank. 2012. *Impact of Maternal and Child Health Private Expenditure on Poverty and Inequity*. Manila: Asian Development Bank.

Bang, A. T., R. A. Bang, S. B. Baitule, M. H. Reddy, and M. D. Deshmukh. 1999. "Effect of Home-Based Neonatal Care and Management of Sepsis on Neonatal Mortality: Field Trial in Rural India." *The Lancet* 354 (9194): 1955–61.

Bang, A. T., R. A. Bang, S. Baitule, M. Deshmukh, and M. H. Reddy. 2001. "Burden of Morbidities and the Unmet Need for Health Care in Rural Neonates—A Prospective Observational Study in Gadchiroli, India." *Indian Pediatrics* 38: 952–65.

Bang, A. T., R. A. Bang, M. H. Reddy, M. Deshmukh, and S. Baitule. 2005. "Reduced Incidence of Neonatal Morbidities: Effect of Home-Based Neonatal Care in Rural Gadchiroli, India." *Journal of Perinatology* 25 (Suppl 1): S51–61.

Baqui, A. H., S. El-Arifeen, G. L. Darmstadt, S. Ahmed, E. K. Williams, and others. 2008. "Effect of Community-Based Newborn-Care Intervention Package Implemented through Two Service-Delivery Strategies in Sylhet District, Bangladesh: A Cluster-Randomised Controlled Trial." *The Lancet* 371 (9628): 1936–44.

Baqui, A. H., E. K. Williams, G. L. Darmstadt, V. Kumar, T. U. Kiran, and others. 2007. "Newborn Care in Rural Uttar Pradesh." *Indian Journal of Pediatrics* 74 (3): 241–47.

Bassani, D. G., R. Kumar, S. Awasthi, S. K. Morris, V. K. Paul, and others. 2010. "Causes of Neonatal and Child Mortality in India: A Nationally Representative Mortality Survey." *The Lancet* 376 (9755): 1853–60.

Bhutta, Z. A., Z. A. Memon, S. Soofi, M. S. Salat, S. Cousens, and J. Martines. 2008. "Implementing Community-Based Perinatal Care: Results from a Pilot Study in Rural Pakistan." *Bulletin of the World Health Organization* 86 (6): 452–59.

Bonu, S., I. Bhushan, M. Rani, and I. Anderson. 2009. "Incidence and Correlates of 'Catastrophic' Maternal Health Care Expenditure in India." *Health Policy and Planning* 24 (6): 445–56.

Borghi, J., K. Hanson, C. A. Acquah, G. Ekanmian, V. Filippi, and others. 2003. "Costs of Near-Miss Obstetric Complications for Women and Their Families in Benin and Ghana." *Health Policy and Planning* 18 (4): 383–90.

Brouwer, W. B., and M. A. Koopmanschap. 2000. "On the Economic Foundations of CEA. Ladies and Gentlemen, Take Your Positions!" *Journal of Health Economics* 19 (4): 439–59.

CBGA (Centre for Budget and Governance Accountability). 2013. *How Has the Dice Rolled? Response to Union Budget 2013–14*. New Delhi: Centre for Budget and Governance Accountability.

CDC (Centers for Disease Control and Prevention). 2015. "CDC in India." Center for Global Health, Atlanta, Georgia, United States. July. http://www.cdc.gov/globalhealth/countries/india/pdf/india.pdf.

Chand, R., B. Das, D. P. Awasthi, and R. Bisht. 2013. *Heath and Family Welfare Statistics in India 2013*. New Delhi: Ministry of Health and Family Welfare, Government of India.

Das, E., D. S. Panwar, E. A. Fischer, G. Bora, and M. C. Carlough. 2014. "Performance of Accredited Social Health Activists to Provide Home-Based Newborn Care: A Situational Analysis." *Indian Pediatrics* 51 (November 2012): 142–44.

Dillon, A. 2012. "Child Labour and Schooling Responses to Production and Health Shocks in Northern Mali." *Journal of African Economies* 22 (2): 276–99.

Garber, A. M., and C. E. Phelps. 1997. "Economic Foundations of Cost-Effectiveness Analysis." *Journal of Health Economics* 16 (1): 1–31.

Gertler, P., and J. Gruber. 2002. "Insuring Consumption against Illness." *American Economic Review* 92 (1): 51–76.

Gogia, S., S. Ramji, P. Gupta, T. Gera, D. Shah, and others. 2011. "Community Based Newborn Care: A Systematic Review and Meta-Analysis of Evidence: UNICEF-PHFI Series on Newborn and Child Health, India." *Indian Pediatrics* 48 (7): 537–46.

Health Management Information System. 2014. "Rural Health Statistics 2013–14." Ministry of Health and Family Welfare, New Delhi. https://nrhm-mis.nic.in/RURAL HEALTH STATISTICS/(A) RHS - 2014/Rural Health Care System in India.pdf.

High Level Expert Group on Universal Health Coverage. 2011. *High Level Expert Group Report on Universal Health Coverage for India*. New Delhi: Public Health Foundation of India.

Hollowell, J., J. J. Kurinczuk, L. Oakley, P. Brocklehurst, and R. Gray. 2009. *A Systematic Review of the Effectiveness of Antenatal Care Programmes to Reduce Infant Mortality and Its Major Causes in Socially Disadvantaged and Vulnerable Women, Final Report*. Oxford: National Perinatal Epidemiology Unit.

IIPS (International Institute of Population Sciences). 2010. *DLHS-3 District Level Household and Facility Survey, 2007–2008*. IIPS, Mumbai, India: IIPS.

Jamison, D. T., J. G. Breman, A. R. Measham, G. Alleyne, M. Claeson, and others, eds. 2006. *Disease Control Priorities in Developing Countries*. 2nd ed. Washington, DC: Oxford University Press and World Bank.

Kruk, M. E., E. Goldmann, and S. Galea. 2009. "Borrowing and Selling to Pay for Health Care in Low- and Middle-Income Countries." *Health Affairs* 28 (4): 1056–66.

Kumar, V., S. Mohanty, A. Kumar, R. P. Misra, M. Santosham, and others. 2008. "Effect of Community-Based Behaviour Change Management on Neonatal Mortality in Shivgarh, Uttar Pradesh, India: A Cluster-Randomised Controlled Trial." *Lancet* 372 (9644): 1151–62.

Lim, S. S., L. Dandona, J. A. Hoisington, S. L. James, M. C. Hogan, and others. 2010. "India's Janani Suraksha Yojana, a Conditional Cash Transfer Programme to Increase Births in Health Facilities: An Impact Evaluation." *The Lancet* 375 (9730): 2009–23.

Mavalankar, D. V., and K. S. Vora. 2008. "The Changing Role of Auxiliary Nurse Midwife (ANM) in India: Implications for Maternal and Child Health (MCH)." Working Papers, Indian Institute of Management Ahmedabad, Ahmedabad, India.

McClellan, M., and J. Skinner. 2006. "The Incidence of Medicare." *Journal of Public Economics* 90 (1–2): 257–76.

Ministry of Health and Family Welfare. 2011. *Home-Based Newborn Care Operational Guidelines.* New Delhi: Ministry of Health and Family Welfare.

———. 2012. *Annual Report 2011–12: Ministry of Health and Family Welfare.* New Delhi: Ministry of Health and Family Welfare.

O'Donnell, O., E. R. van Doorslaer, R. P. Rannan-Eliya, A. Somanathan, S. R. Adhikari, and others. 2008. "Who Pays for Health Care in Asia?" *Journal of Health Economics* 27 (2): 460–75.

Perry, H., and R. Zulliger. 2012. *How Effective Are Community Health Workers?* Baltimore, MD: Johns Hopkins Bloomberg School of Public Health.

Planning Commission of India. 2008. *Eleventh Five Year Plan (2007–2012).* New Delhi: Oxford University Press. planningcommission.nic.in/plans/planrel/fiveyr/11th/11_v2/11th_vol2.pdf?

Prinja, S., N. Manchanda, P. Mohan, G. Gupta, G. Sethy, and others. 2013. "Cost of Neonatal Intensive Care Delivered through District Level Public Hospitals in India." *Indian Pediatrics* 50 (9): 839–46.

Prinja, S., S. Mazumder, S. Taneja, P. Bahuguna, N. Bhandari, and others. 2013. "Cost of Delivering Child Health Care through Community Level Health Workers: How Much Extra Does IMNCI Program Cost?" *Journal of Tropical Pediatrics* 59 (6): 489–95.

Sharma, R., P. Webster, and S. Bhattacharyya. 2014. "Factors Affecting the Performance of Community Health Workers in India: A Multi-Stakeholder Perspective." *Global Health Action* 7: 1–8.

Shashidhar, R. 2012. "India's Integrated Child Development Scheme and Its Implementation: Performance of Anganwadis and Analysis." *OIDA International Journal of Sustainable Development* 5 (6): 29–38.

Singh, A., S. Pallikadavath, F. Ram, and M. Alagarajan. 2013. "Do Antenatal Care Interventions Improve Neonatal Survival in India?" *Health Policy and Planning* 29: 842–48.

Steinglass, R., T. Cherian, J. Vandelaer, R. D. Klemm, and J. Sequeira. 2011. "Development and Use of the Lives Saved Tool (LiST): A Model to Estimate the Impact of Scaling Up Proven Interventions on Maternal, Neonatal and Child Mortality." *International Journal of Epidemiology* 40 (2): 519–20.

Sun, A., and Y. Yao. 2010. "Health Shocks and Children's School Attainments in Rural China." *Economics of Education Review* 29 (3): 375–82.

UN IGME (UN Inter-Agency Group for Child Mortality Estimation). 2014. *Levels and Trends in Child Mortality: Report 2014: Estimates Developed by the UN Inter-Agency Group for Child Mortality Estimation (IGME).* New York: United Nations Children's Fund; World Health Organization; The World Bank; United Nations, Department of Economic and Social Affairs, Population Division; United Nations Economic Commission for Latin America and the Caribbean, Population Division.

———. 2015. *Levels and Trends in Child Mortality: Report 2015: Estimates Developed by the UN Inter-Agency Group for Child Mortality Estimation (IGME).* New York: United Nations Children's Fund; World Health Organization; The World Bank; United Nations, Department of Economic and Social Affairs, Population Division; United Nations Economic Commission for Latin America and the Caribbean, Population Division.

van Doorslaer, E., O. O'Donnell, R. P. Rannan-Eliya, A. Somanathan, S. R. Adhikari, and others. 2006. "Effect of Payments for Health Care on Poverty Estimates in 11 Countries in Asia: An Analysis of Household Survey Data." *The Lancet* 368 (9544): 1357–64.

———. 2007. "Catastrophic Payments for Health Care in Asia." *Health Economics* 16 (11): 1159–84.

Verguet, S., S. Murphy, B. Anderson, K. A. Johansson, R. Glass, and others. 2013. "Public Finance of Rotavirus Vaccination in India and Ethiopia: An Extended Cost-Effectiveness Analysis." *Vaccine* 31 (42): 4902–10.

Verguet, S., R. Laxminarayan, and D. T. Jamison. 2014. "Universal Public Finance of Tuberculosis Treatment in India: An Extended Cost-Effectiveness Analysis." *Health Economics* 24 (3): 318–32.

Wagstaff, A. 2007. "The Economic Consequences of Health Shocks: Evidence from Vietnam." *Journal of Health Economics* 26: 82–100.

———. 2008. "Measuring Financial Protection in Health." Policy Research Working Paper 4554, World Bank, Washington, DC.

WHO (World Health Organization). 2003. *Making Choices in Health: WHO Guide to Cost-Effectiveness Analysis.* Edited by T. Tan-Torres Edejer, R. Baltussen, T. Adam, R. Hutubessy, A. Acharya, and others. Geneva: World Health Organization.

———. 2010. *The World Health Report—Health Systems Financing: The Path to Universal Coverage.* Geneva: World Health Organization.

———. 2012. "Newborns: Reducing Mortality [Fact Sheet]." World Health Organization, Geneva.

WHO/UNICEF Joint Statement. 2009. *Home Visits for the Newborn Child: A Strategy to Improve Survival.* Geneva: World Health Organization.

World Bank, World Development Indicators. "Data: India." World Development Indicators. http://data.worldbank.org/country/india.

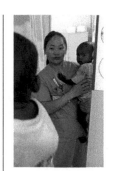

Chapter 19

Health Gains and Financial Risk Protection Afforded by Treatment and Prevention of Diarrhea and Pneumonia in Ethiopia: An Extended Cost-Effectiveness Analysis

By Stéphane Verguet, Clint Pecenka, Kjell Arne Johansson,
Solomon Tessema Memirie, Ingrid K. Friberg,
Julia R. Driessen, and Dean T. Jamison

INTRODUCTION

Universal health coverage (UHC) continues to receive considerable attention from the global health community. UHC was the main topic of the 2010 *World Health Report* (WHO 2010), the main topic in 2012 issues of *The Lancet* (2012) and *Health Policy and Planning* (McIntyre and Mills 2012), and the theme of the Second Global Symposium on Health Systems Research in Beijing in 2012. Margaret Chan, Director-General of the World Health Organization (WHO), stated that "universal health coverage [is] the single most powerful concept that public health has to offer" (Chan 2012). This continued attention led to the 2013 *World Health Report*, which discusses the role that research can play in answering important questions about UHC (WHO 2013).

Although substantial variation is a hallmark of UHC initiatives, UHC is generally viewed along three dimensions: who is covered, what services are covered, and the proportion of the costs that are covered (WHO 2010). One financing option, universal public finance (UPF), involves the government shouldering the entire cost of specific services, regardless of who receives them. The potential benefits of UPF include improved health outcomes and improved financial risk protection (FRP). However, the evidence available to policy makers is limited with respect to the magnitude and distribution of these benefits.

Extended cost-effectiveness analysis (ECEA) (Verguet, Gauvreau, and others 2015; Verguet and Jamison 2015; Verguet, Laxminarayan, and Jamison 2015; Verguet, Olson, and others 2015; Verguet and others 2013) provides a tool with which to gain a more complete understanding of the health and financial benefits associated with different health policies and interventions. ECEA combines the traditional health system perspective of cost-effectiveness analysis (CEA) with the patient perspective, notably through the quantification of the benefits associated with avoiding medical impoverishment and the assessment of the distributional consequences, that is equity, of policies (Verguet, Laxminarayan, and Jamison 2015). This tool helps policy makers make decisions based on the joint benefits and tradeoffs associated with different policies and interventions, specifically in health gains, FRP and equity benefits.

Corresponding author: Stéphane Verguet, Department of Global Health and Population, Harvard T.H. Chan School of Public Health, Boston, Massachusetts, United States, verguet@hsph.harvard.edu.

In 2013 in Ethiopia, about 60,000 children under age five years died as a result of pneumonia or diarrhea, the fifth-highest absolute level worldwide (IVAC 2013). Studies have associated the incidence of both conditions with socioeconomic status (Fekadu, Terefe, and Alemie 2014; Mihrete, Alemie, and Teferra 2014), suggesting that an evaluation of the impact of prevention and treatment services by income quintile would be suitable.

This chapter uses ECEA methods to examine UPF of the prevention and treatment of pneumonia and diarrhea in Ethiopia, with a focus on children under age five years. The combination of prevention and treatment options illustrates health and FRP benefits brought by the different intervention packages available to decision makers. This analysis also examines these benefits by income quintile so that policy makers can better understand how each package affects different segments of the population—a critical element of UHC. A 20 percentage point increase in coverage is modeled. Our purpose is to expose with simplicity the broad implications for policy makers rather than to provide them with definitive estimates, hence the presentation of limited rudimentary sensitivity analyses. After we summarize current child health services in Ethiopia, we outline the methods used in this chapter, which draw from the ECEA methodology (Verguet, Laxminarayan, and Jamison 2015). Then, we present results—both health and financial protection—for the following:

- Pneumonia treatment
- Combined pneumonia treatment and pneumococcal conjugate vaccination (PCV)
- Diarrhea treatment
- Combined diarrhea treatment and rotavirus vaccination.

Finally, we discuss the implications of the findings and conclude.

CHILD HEALTH AND HEALTH CARE SERVICES IN ETHIOPIA

Ethiopia has made substantial progress in reducing the mortality rate of children under age five years—from 205 deaths per 1,000 live births in 1990 to 68 in 2012 and to 59 in 2015 (You and others 2015)—achieving Millennium Development Goal 4 three years early (UNICEF 2013a, 2013b; UN IGME 2015). Despite this progress, substantial need remains for child health interventions. In 2012, approximately 205,000 Ethiopian children died from preventable causes and treatable diseases before reaching their fifth birthday. Apart from neonatal causes, the two major killers of children in Ethiopia were acute respiratory infections and diarrhea (Liu and others 2012).

The coverage of child health care services remains very low compared with other low- and middle-income countries (LMICs) (WHO 2015). According to Ethiopia's 2011 Demographic and Health Survey (DHS) (Central Statistical Agency and ICF International 2011), coverage of measles vaccine, pentavalent 3 (third dose of diphtheria, pertussis, tetanus, *Haemophilus influenzae* type b, and hepatitis B vaccines), care-seeking for acute respiratory infection, and care-seeking for diarrhea were 56 percent, 35 percent, 27 percent, and 32 percent, respectively. Inequities in child mortality and access to care between urban and rural dwellers and across wealth quintiles remain large. According to Ethiopia's 2011 DHS, infant mortality is 29 percent higher in rural areas than in urban areas. The urban-rural difference is even more pronounced for mortality in children under age five years, and up to 37 percent higher in rural areas than in urban areas. Furthermore, wide regional variations are observed in mortality rates in infants and children, with more than a twofold difference, for example, between Addis Ababa and Benishangul-Gumuz in the western part of the country. In addition to the increased risk of diarrheal illnesses and pneumonia among children from the lowest wealth quintile, children from the wealthiest quintiles were considerably more likely to receive care from health facilities or providers (Central Statistical Agency and ICF International 2011).

There are about 12 million children under age five years in Ethiopia (table 19.1) and strong demographic and mortality disparities exist between the different wealth strata of the Ethiopian population (table 19.2). More specifically, strong inequalities in pneumonia- and diarrhea-related deaths can be observed in the country. Using the Lives Saved Tool (LiST), a partial cohort model that projects mortality by age and cause of death using inputs on health status and intervention coverage

Table 19.1 Distribution of the Population of Children Younger than Age Five Years, by Gender, Ethiopia

Age group in years	Population	
	Male	Female
0–1	1,230,000	1,210,000
1–2	1,220,000	1,200,000
2–3	1,200,000	1,180,000
3–4	1,190,000	1,170,000
4–5	1,180,000	1,170,000
Total	6,020,000	5,930,000

Source: United Nations 2014.

Table 19.2 Demographic and Mortality Disparities between the Different Wealth Strata of the Population, Ethiopia

Wealth quintile	Total fertility rate	Under-five mortality rate (per 1,000 live births)
I (poorest)	6.0	137
II	5.7	121
III	5.3	96
IV	5.0	100
V (richest)	2.8	86

Source: Central Statistical Agency and ICF International 2011.

Figure 19.1 Estimated Mortality in Children Younger than Age Five Years Due to Pneumonia and Diarrhea across Income Groups in Ethiopia

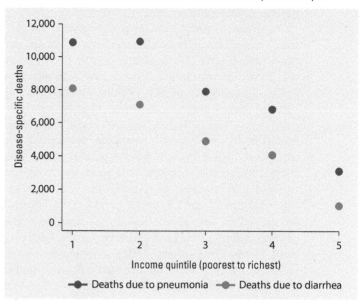

and effectiveness (Winfrey, McKinnon, and Stover 2011), and methods described elsewhere (Amouzou and others 2010), we estimate total under-five deaths due to pneumonia and diarrhea by income group (figure 19.1). Subsequently, we see that such disease-specific mortality rates are about four times higher in the poorest quintile than in the wealthiest quintile.

As in many low-income countries, government per capita spending on health in Ethiopia is very low at about US$15 (WHO 2015). The national health policy strongly emphasizes fulfilling the needs of the underserved rural population, which constitutes 84 percent of the total population. Ensuring health care accessibility for the whole population is one of the main strategic objectives of Ethiopia's health sector development program IV (2011–15) (Federal Democratic Republic of Ethiopia 2010). The Ministry of Health envisages the health extension program (HEP) as a primary vehicle for delivering critical and basic preventive and curative care to the community (Banteyerga 2011). The HEP is an innovative, community-based program that makes essential health services available at the grassroots level. It proposes a package of basic preventive and curative health services that targets rural households (Banteyerga 2011).

HEP comprises the following four health subprograms, which correspond to the elements of primary health care as defined in the Alma Ata Declaration (WHO 1978):

- Disease prevention
- Family health
- Environmental hygiene and sanitation
- Health education and communication.

Every village with at least 1,000 households—about 5,000 residents—builds a health post. Two female health extension workers (HEWs), who have completed tenth grade, are recruited from the same community and trained in HEP modules for one year; upon completion of their training, they return home as salaried frontline health care staff. The major goals of the HEWs are to provide communities and households with increased knowledge and skills regarding preventable diseases, accessible health services at health posts, and facilitated referrals to health centers and hospitals.

Ample evidence suggests that community health workers can identify, refer, or treat childhood illnesses outside of health facilities (Bang and others 1999; Baqui and others 2009; Bhutta and others 2005; Haines and others 2007). The HEWs have substantial potential to increase coverage of highly cost-effective child survival interventions at the community level. Starting in 2011, the government of Ethiopia took an additional step and allowed the HEWs to provide community case management of childhood pneumonia, malaria, and diarrheal illnesses. The HEP offers an opportunity to scale up child health services in Ethiopia and is expected to narrow the gap between different income quintiles and geographic locations.

Despite the government's current attempt to provide certain essential services free of charge—including those that relate to family health, communicable disease control, hygiene and environmental sanitation, and health education and communication—34 percent of health expenditure is privately financed as of 2012

(WHO 2012). This expenditure consists of households' direct outlays, including gratuities and in-kind payments, for health services.

To prevent deaths from pneumonia and diarrhea, the two biggest killers for those younger than age five years in Ethiopia (Liu and others 2012), preventive and curative interventions must be intensified to reach all segments of the population. Establishing healthy environments to protect children from pneumonia and diarrhea, and increasing access to cost-effective interventions for both prevention and treatment, will greatly reduce mortality rates from those conditions. Although little work has examined the cost-effectiveness of pneumonia and diarrhea interventions in an Ethiopian or other low-income setting (Kim and others 2010; Laxminarayan and others 2006; Rheingans, Atherly, and Anderson 2012; Sinha and others 2007), efficacious rotavirus and PCVs have been licensed (Fischer Walker and Black 2011; Theodoratou, Johnson, and others 2010). Treatment interventions for pneumonia (for example, community case management with antibiotics) and diarrhea (for example, oral rehydration salts) have proven to be effective (Munos, Fischer Walker, and Black 2010; Theodoratou, Al-Jilaihawi, and others 2010). Evidence-based information on the expected health, equity, and FRP outcomes for various diarrhea and pneumonia strategies is crucial for setting priorities. Verguet and others (2013) conducted a preliminary ECEA of public finance of rotavirus vaccination in Ethiopia that points to the substantial health benefits (such as deaths averted) and FRP benefits (such as prevention of medical impoverishment) that would accrue to the poorest socioeconomic groups.

Here we use ECEA methods to evaluate the consequences of UPF on health, equity, and impoverishment for a hypothetical program targeting children under age five years in Ethiopia. This program would consist of four interventions:

- Pneumonia treatment
- Combined pneumonia treatment and PCV
- Diarrhea treatment
- Combined diarrhea treatment and rotavirus vaccination.

We measure program impact along four dimensions: under-five deaths averted, household expenditures averted, FRP afforded, and distributional consequences across the wealth strata of the country population.

METHODS

Extended Cost-Effectiveness Analysis

ECEA (Verguet, Gauvreau, and others 2015; Verguet and Jamison 2015; Verguet, Laxminarayan, and Jamison 2015; Verguet, Olson, and others 2015; Verguet and others 2013) expands on the standard approach to economic evaluation proposed by CEA, by evaluating aspects of health policies that are important for policy makers. Specifically, in addition to health benefits, ECEA estimates the impact of policies along three dimensions: (1) household out-of-pocket (OOP) expenditures averted by the policy, (2) FRP benefits provided, and (3) distributional consequences (for example, according to socioeconomic status or geographical setting). Thus, this study examines provision of diarrhea and pneumonia interventions within the broader framework of UPF. The broader household financial consequences of publicly financed prevention and treatment interventions could then be analyzed, evaluating their impact on the reduction of household OOP expenditures and FRP. The distributional impact is also considered across income quintiles, highlighting the equity potential of UPF.

Interventions Analyzed

Pneumonia Treatment with Antibiotics

We assume that current coverage of pneumonia treatment (antibiotics) across all income groups is increased by 20 percentage points (table 19.3). The average baseline coverage of pneumonia treatment was 27 percent before UPF. After UPF, coverage increases, on average, to 47 percent. Health gains as measured by deaths averted are calculated for the increase. We chose a 20 percentage point increase, a rather small increase, to capture a realistic scenario that can be achieved by the Ethiopian health system. The effectiveness of pneumonia treatment also drew on a meta-analysis of studies used for populating LiST; community case management with antibiotics was found to reduce pneumonia-related deaths by 70 percent (Theodoratou, Al-Jilaihawi and others 2010).

Combined Pneumonia Treatment and Pneumococcal Conjugate Vaccination

As a complement to the scale-up of pneumonia treatment, we assume that UPF scales up coverage of PCV from 0 percent to 20 percent across income groups (table 19.3).

PCV-13 protects against the 13 serotypes (1, 3, 4, 5, 6A, 6B, 7F, 9V, 14, 18C, 19A, 19F, 23F) that are typically associated with invasive diseases like pneumonia, sepsis, and meningitis. These 13 serotypes have been estimated to cause 70 percent of all invasive pneumococcal diseases in Gavi-eligible countries (Johnson and

Table 19.3 Input Parameters Used for Analysis of Pneumonia Treatment and Combined Pneumonia Treatment and Pneumococcal Conjugate Vaccination

Parameter	Value	Sources
Epidemiology		
Under-five deaths due to pneumonia in 2011, from poorest to richest (income quintiles 1–5)	10,900; 11,000; 7,900; 6,800; 3,100	Authors' calculations using LiST based on Amouzou and others 2010; Fischer Walker and others 2013
Proportion of under-five pneumonia deaths attributed to pneumococcal disease	33 percent	Fischer Walker and others 2013
Interventions		
Antibiotic effectiveness	0.70	Theodoratou, Al-Jilaihawi, and others 2010
Vaccine (PCV-13) effectiveness (per three-dose course)		
• Pneumonia (all causes)	0.26	Theodoratou, Johnson, and others 2010
• Pneumonia (pneumococcal)	0.68	Cutts and others 2005
• Meningitis	0.64	Hsu and others 2009
• Nonpneumonia nonmeningitis	0.89	Black and others 2000
Coverage of antibiotics, from poorest to richest (income quintiles 1–5), before UPF	16%; 25%; 22%; 33%; 62%	Central Statistical Agency and ICF International 2011
Coverage of antibiotics, from poorest to richest (income quintiles 1–5), after UPF	36%; 45%; 42%; 53%; 82%	
Coverage of vaccine, from poorest to richest (income quintiles 1–5), before UPF	0%; 0%; 0%; 0%; 0%	Central Statistical Agency and ICF International 2011
Coverage of vaccine, from poorest to richest (income quintiles 1–5), after UPF	20%; 20%; 20%; 20%; 20%	
Costs (2011 US$)		
Hospitalization cost for disease[a]		Stack and others 2011;
Pneumonia	$84	WHO-CHOICE 2014
Meningitis or nonpneumonia nonmeningitis	$182	
Outpatient clinic visit cost for pneumonia	$45	Stack and others 2011; WHO-CHOICE 2014
Probability of hospitalization, from poorest to richest (income quintiles 1–5)	0.09 for pneumonia cases; 0.75 for meningitis and nonpneumonia nonmeningitis cases	Rudan and others 2004;
Probability of outpatient visit, from poorest to richest (income quintiles 1–5)	0.16; 0.25; 0.22; 0.33; 0.62	Central Statistical Agency and ICF International 2011
Pneumococcal conjugate vaccine price (per vial, 3 doses needed)		Gavi 2014
Base case	$3.5	
With Gavi subsidy	$0.2	
Vaccination system cost (per vial, 3 doses needed)	$0.5	Griffiths and others 2009

table continues next page

Table 19.3 Input Parameters Used for Analysis of Pneumonia Treatment and Combined Pneumonia Treatment and Pneumococcal Conjugate Vaccination (continued)

Parameter	Value	Sources
Ethiopia's gross domestic product per capita	$360	World Bank 2013
Ethiopia's Gini index	0.3	
Utility function as a function of individual income y	$\frac{y^{1-r}}{1-r}$ with $r = 3$	McClellan and Skinner 2006; Verguet, Laxminarayan, and Jamison 2015
	(r = coefficient of relative risk aversion)	

Note: LiST = Lives Saved Tool; PCV = pneumococcal conjugate vaccine; UPF = universal public finance.

a. Severe infections and hospitalizations were not included.

others 2010). We found no studies reporting serotype distribution in Ethiopia. Our estimates of the efficacy of PCV-13 come from clinical trials (Black and others 2000; Cutts and others 2005; Hsu and others 2009) and from a meta-analysis of PCV-9 and PCV-11 used for populating LiST, where all-valent PCV was found to reduce radiologically confirmed pneumonia by 26 percent (Theodoratou, Johnson and others 2010).

To estimate pneumococci deaths averted—33 percent of all pneumonia deaths are due to pneumococci (Fischer Walker and others 2013)—the model follows the current Ethiopian birth cohort. Depending on disease-specific mortality (pneumonia, meningitis, nonpneumonia nonmeningitis), we estimated intervention coverage, intervention effectiveness, and reductions in disease-specific deaths in each income group. This static approach does not capture epidemiological changes such as herd immunity and serotype replacement from vaccination, which could be captured more fully in, for example, a dynamic transmission model. However, the extent of such indirect effects on the nonvaccinated population is unclear, leading to their exclusion from this analysis (Weinberger, Malley, and Lipsitch 2011).

Diarrhea Treatment with Oral Rehydration Salts

Oral rehydration salts (ORS) are evaluated as a treatment for diarrhea in this analysis. To determine the number of deaths averted by UPF of ORS, we assume a 20 percentage point increase in treatment-seeking above the level reported for each income quintile in the DHS (Central Statistical Agency and ICF International 2011). We also assume ORS is 93 percent effective in preventing deaths from diarrhea, following estimates based on a systematic review from the Child Health Epidemiology Reference Group (Munos, Fischer Walker, and Black 2010). Deaths averted by income quintile are

the product of the baseline number of diarrhea deaths, the increase in treatment coverage, and the effectiveness of treatment.

Combined Diarrhea Treatment and Rotavirus Vaccination

As a complement to the scale up of diarrhea treatment, we assume that UPF scales up rotavirus vaccination from 0 percent to 20 percent coverage across income groups (table 19.4) to mimic coverage achievable by the Ethiopian health system.

After determining the baseline number of diarrhea deaths by income quintile, we attribute 27 percent of diarrhea deaths to rotavirus (Fischer Walker and others 2013). This yields the number of rotavirus-attributable deaths by income quintile (table 19.4). Although estimates of vaccine efficacy vary in Sub-Saharan Africa and by strain, we use an effectiveness of 50 percent taken from a meta-analysis (Fischer Walker and Black 2011) and assume it prevented visits to health facilities as well as mortality (Verguet and others 2013). Specifically, to estimate rotavirus deaths averted, the model follows the current Ethiopian birth cohort; rotavirus deaths averted are the product of baseline rotavirus deaths, vaccine coverage, and vaccine effectiveness (Verguet and others 2013). This static approach is unable to capture epidemiological changes such as herd immunity, which has only been documented in a few countries (Buttery and others 2011; Tate and others 2011; Yen and others 2011).

Treatment Expenditures Averted

Household private expenditures averted through UPF of vaccinations are calculated differently than for treatment. Vaccine intervention–related private

Table 19.4 Input Parameters Used for Analysis of Diarrhea Treatment and Combined Diarrhea Treatment and Rotavirus Vaccination

Parameter	Value	Sources
Epidemiology		
Under-five deaths due to diarrhea in 2011, from poorest to richest (income quintiles 1–5)	8,100; 7,100; 4,900; 4,100; 1,100	Authors' calculations using LiST based on Amouzou and others 2010; Fischer Walker and others 2013
Proportion of under-5 diarrhea deaths attributed to rotavirus	27%	Fischer Walker and others 2013
Interventions		
ORS effectiveness	0.93	Munos, Fischer Walker, and Black 2010
Rotavirus vaccine effectiveness (per two-dose course)	0.50	Fischer Walker and Black 2011
Coverage of ORS, from poorest to richest (income quintiles 1–5), before UPF	22%; 25%; 35%; 33%; 53%	Central Statistical Agency and ICF International 2011
Coverage of ORS, from poorest to richest (income quintiles 1–5), after UPF	42%; 45%; 55%; 53%; 73%	
Coverage of vaccine, from poorest to richest (income quintiles 1–5), before UPF	0%; 0%; 0%; 0%; 0%	Central Statistical Agency and ICF International 2011
Coverage of vaccine, from poorest to richest (income quintiles 1–5), after UPF	20%; 20%; 20%; 20%; 20%	
Costs (2011 US$)		
Hospitalization cost for diarrhea[a]	$49	Stack and others 2011; WHO-CHOICE 2014
Outpatient clinic visit cost for diarrhea	$9	Stack and others 2011; WHO-CHOICE 2014
Probability of hospitalization for diarrhea, from poorest to richest (income quintiles 1–5)	0.02; 0.02; 0.01; 0.02; 0.01	Authors' calculations based on Central Statistical Agency [Ethiopia] and ICF International 2011; and Lamberti, Fischer Walker, and Black 2012
Probability of outpatient visit for diarrhea, from poorest to richest (income quintiles 1–5)	0.22; 0.25; 0.35; 0.33; 0.53	Central Statistical Agency and ICF International 2011
Rotavirus vaccine price (per vial, two doses needed)		Gavi 2014
Base case	$2.5	
With Gavi subsidy	$0.2	
Vaccination system cost (per vial, two doses needed)	$0.5	Griffiths and others 2009
Ethiopia's gross domestic product per capita	$360	World Bank 2013
Ethiopia's Gini index	0.3	
Utility function as a function of individual income y	$\dfrac{y^{1-r}}{1-r}$ with $r = 3$ (r = coefficient of relative risk aversion)	McClellan and Skinner 2006; Verguet, Laxminarayan, and Jamison 2015

Note: LiST = Lives Saved Tool; ORS = oral rehydration salts; UPF = universal public finance.
a. Severe infections and hospitalizations were not included.

expenditures averted depend on the number of cases of a specific infection (a subset of total cases), vaccine coverage, vaccine effectiveness, probability of seeking either inpatient or outpatient care in the absence of the vaccine, and cost of inpatient and outpatient care. Details of the methods are given elsewhere (Verguet and others 2013). Before UPF is implemented, households pay at a 34 percent level for inpatient and outpatient care (the remaining 66 percent is covered by the government) (WHO 2012). After UPF is implemented, individuals would pay 0 percent for inpatient and outpatient care, and the government would pay 100 percent of the costs.

Government Costs

Government costs due to UPF of the vaccine also differ from those for treatment. Government costs for the vaccine are based on the size of the birth cohort, vaccine coverage, the costs of the vaccine itself, and the associated system costs of delivery. Because the vaccine also averts future government treatment costs, these averted costs are subtracted from the cost of delivering the vaccine to estimate the net costs of the combined treatment-vaccine interventions from the government's perspective.

Government costs for diarrhea and pneumonia treatment include 66 percent of the costs for inpatient and outpatient care for currently covered households, plus 100 percent of the costs for inpatient and outpatient care for the 20 percentage point increment in coverage.

Financial Risk Protection

UPF provides FRP benefits to households by shielding them from the OOP costs and impoverishment-related consequences of the covered health care services. UPF "insures" households against the OOP cost of diarrhea and pneumonia treatment, and in doing so can prevent households from related impoverishment.

Several metrics can be used to quantify the FRP benefits of health policies. One approach is to estimate the amount of households' OOP expenditures averted by the policy; another is to estimate the number of cases of poverty averted (that is, counting the number of individuals no longer falling under a poverty line or threshold because of substantial OOP medical expenditures). In this study, we use the money-metric value of insurance provided by UPF as the FRP metric (Verguet, Laxminarayan, and Jamison 2015). The money-metric value of insurance metric quantifies "insurance risk premiums"; it reflects risk aversion, in which individuals

would prefer the certainty of insurance to the uncertainty or risk of possible OOP expenditures, and hence they are willing to pay a certain amount of money to avoid that risk.

As explained in great detail in Verguet, Laxminarayan, and Jamison (2015), to estimate the FRP (for example, the money-metric value of insurance) to an individual who is provided UPF, we first estimate the individual's expected income before UPF, depending on treatment coverage and associated costs. We then estimate the individual's certainty equivalent by assigning individuals utility functions that specify their risk aversion (tables 19.3 and 19.4), which is equivalent to calculating their willingness to pay for insurance against risks of medical expenditures. This certainty equivalent reflects the final income that individuals are willing to accept to make the outcome certain. Finally, we derive a money-metric value of insurance provided (risk premium) as the difference between the expected value of income and the certainty equivalent (Brown and Finkelstein 2008; Finkelstein and McKnight 2008; McClellan and Skinner 2006; Verguet, Laxminarayan, and Jamison 2015). Aggregating the money-metric value of insurance provided using an income distribution in the population (with a proxy based on country gross domestic product per capita and Gini coefficient [Salem and Mount 1974]) yields a dollar value of FRP at the societal level.

All mathematical derivations used are presented in annex 19A. All calculations are estimated using the R statistical software (www.r-project.org).

RESULTS

Pneumonia Treatment and Combined Pneumonia Treatment and Pneumococcal Conjugate Vaccination

Deaths Averted

Annually, pneumonia treatment would avert about 5,600 deaths; the combined treatment-vaccine package would avert about 7,500 deaths (figure 19.2, panel a). Pneumonia treatment would save more lives among the poorest income group because of the higher disease burden in this population and would evenly increase coverage among all income groups.

Combined pneumonia treatment and PCV would save more lives among the bottom income quintiles because the higher burden of disease is concentrated in the poorest income groups. Yet, 32,000 pneumonia-related deaths would still occur; of these, 8,000 would occur in the poorest income quintile.

Figure 19.2 Benefits of Pneumonia Treatment and Combined Pneumonia Treatment and Pneumococcal Vaccination

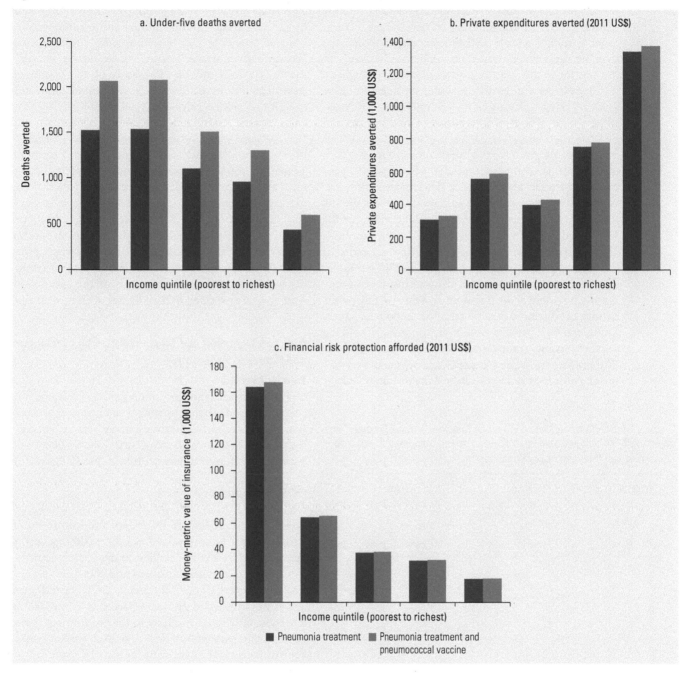

a. Under-five deaths averted

Income quintile (poorest to richest)

b. Private expenditures averted (2011 US$)

Income quintile (poorest to richest)

c. Financial risk protection afforded (2011 US$)

Income quintile (poorest to richest)

■ Pneumonia treatment ■ Pneumonia treatment and pneumococcal vaccine

OOP Expenditures Averted

The health benefits finding is the opposite of the distribution of OOP expenditures averted because of the variations in current coverage of pneumonia treatment, from 16 percent in the bottom income quintile to 62 percent in the top income quintile. Wealthier people have better access to care in both programs, which would lead to reductions in household private expenditures for those who have access (figure 19.2, panel b).

Financial Risk Protection

Both programs would offer the highest FRP for the poorest income quintile (figure 19.2, panel c). There would, however, be a shift in gradients between private expenditures averted and FRP. The poorest would have, in absolute terms, the lowest private expenditures averted but the highest FRP. This outcome occurs because the poorest quintile would have substantially lower disposable income than the richest in absolute terms; therefore the change in income due to the interventions would be much higher.

To illustrate the results per dollar of expenditure, an arbitrary budget constraint of US$1 million is introduced (figure 19.3). The two dimensions of health gains and FRP afforded (measured by a money-metric value of insurance) are given for the five income groups, for UPF of pneumonia treatment, and UPF of combined pneumonia treatment and PCV. Per dollar expenditure, the combined treatment-vaccine package would save slightly more lives compared with treatment alone. However, the FRP afforded would be slightly reduced in each quintile. This slight reduction in FRP, when vaccines are added, is due to the fact that vaccines provide less FRP per dollar spent than treatment. In particular, vaccines protect only against pneumococcal pneumonia, whereas full public finance of treatment is more targeted. In both instances, health and FRP benefits would disproportionally aid the poorest income groups given that both the health and FRP benefits would be substantially larger in the poorest income quintile than in the richest income quintile.

Figure 19.3 Health Benefits and Financial Risk Protection Afforded from Investing $1 Million in Pneumonia Treatment and Combined Pneumonia Treatment and Pneumococcal Vaccination

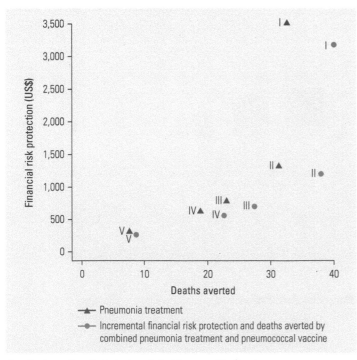

Note: Results are shown for five income quintiles (I is poorest; V is richest).

Program Costs

The total costs of scaling up pneumonia treatment by 20 percentage points across all income groups (and of providing UPF for those who currently have access to pneumonia treatment) would be approximately US$49.6 million. The costs of the combined treatment-vaccine package vary substantially, depending on the vaccine price and Gavi eligibility. The total costs of the combined pneumonia treatment and PCV package would be approximately US$56.1 million (88 percent of which is for pneumonia treatment, 12 percent of which is for pneumococcal vaccine) based on a vaccine price of US$3.50 per dose, which is the market price currently paid by Gavi. If the fully Gavi-subsidized cost of US$0.20 per dose were to be used, the total cost of the combined treatment-vaccine package would be US$50.6 million. Regardless of vaccine price, more of the combined treatment-vaccine program funding would go to the richest groups of the population, since they are expected to have higher utilization rates.

Diarrhea Treatment and Combined Diarrhea Treatment and Rotavirus Vaccination

Deaths Averted

UPF for diarrhea treatment would avert 4,700 deaths each year. Combined diarrhea treatment and rotavirus vaccination would avert 5,400 deaths each year. Yet, 20,000 diarrhea-related deaths would still occur; of these, 6,000 would occur in the poorest income quintile (figure 19.4, panel a).

OOP Expenditures Averted

On an annual basis, UPF for diarrhea treatment would avert US$43.8 million of OOP expenditures. It would also provide insurance valued at US$93,000 at a cost of approximately US$100.9 million to the government.

Combined diarrhea treatment and rotavirus vaccination would avert US$44.1 million in OOP expenditures, and it would provide insurance valued at US$96,000 at a net cost of US$103.3 million to the government (gross government expenditure for rotavirus vaccination is approximately US$3.2 million) (figure 19.4, panel b).

Financial Risk Protection

Diarrhea treatment would provide about US$1,000 in FRP benefits per US$1 million spent. Combined diarrhea treatment and rotavirus vaccination would provide approximately US$1,000 in FRP benefits per US$1 million spent. For both diarrhea treatment and combined diarrhea treatment and rotavirus vaccination, health and FRP benefits would be substantially larger among the poorer income quintiles than the richer income quintiles (figure 19.4, panel c; figure 19.5).

Figure 19.4 Benefits of Diarrhea Treatment and Combined Diarrhea Treatment and Rotavirus Vaccination

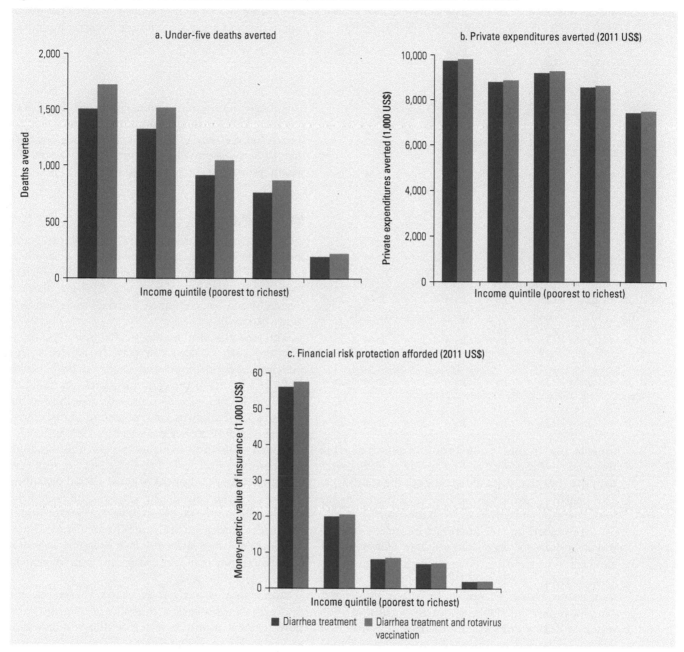

Program Costs

Diarrhea treatment would save lives at a cost of approximately US$21,000 per death averted; combined diarrhea treatment and rotavirus vaccination would save lives at an approximate cost of US$19,000 per death averted. If we view these results per US$1 million spent, diarrhea treatment would avert approximately 47 deaths and US$430,000 in private expenditures. Diarrhea treatment would provide about US$1,000 in FRP benefits per US$1 million spent (figure 19.5). Combined diarrhea treatment and rotavirus vaccination would avert 52 deaths and US$430,000 in private expenditures averted per US$1 million spent.

These results provide two outstanding messages. First, diarrhea treatment and combined diarrhea treatment and rotavirus vaccination provide similar FRP

Figure 19.5 Health Benefits (deaths averted) and Financial Risk Protection Afforded (Measured in 2011 US$) from Investing US$1 Million of Public Expenditures on Diarrhea Treatment and Combined Diarrhea Treatment and Rotavirus Vaccination

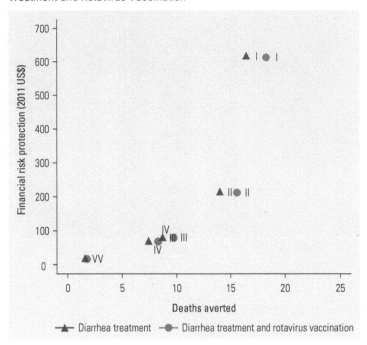

Note: Results are shown for five income quintiles (I is poorest; V is richest).

poorest tend to gain more FRP benefits because their incomes are lower, and the marginal value of the reduction of risk is of lower value for the wealthier quintiles.

DISCUSSION

This chapter illustrates the potential broader benefits of providing UPF for child health interventions for pneumonia and diarrhea in Ethiopia. It also demonstrates that UPF could provide different benefits across the wealth distribution, in addition to FRP and equity.

Main Findings

UPF for pneumonia treatment and for combined pneumonia treatment and PCV would provide substantially higher FRP for the poor and save more lives for the poor. Similar results are seen for UPF for diarrhea treatment and for combined diarrhea treatment and rotavirus vaccine.

This analysis also highlights the role that organizations such as Gavi can play. In particular, for rotavirus and pneumococcal vaccines, both health and FRP benefits of the combined packages could be enhanced if Gavi were to fully subsidize the vaccine prices to the Ethiopian government so that the government paid $0.20 per dose (tables 19.5 and 19.6). Although interesting in its own right, this situation may become a practical concern if Gavi support were to expire. Acknowledgment of these altered benefits is important when considering Gavi eligibility and the sustainability of the inclusion of vaccine interventions in benefits packages. This issue is particularly compelling when a strong rationale, such as equity, supports an intervention that a country may not implement under current incentives.

Although this analysis focuses on Ethiopia, the findings may also speak to the value of these interventions in other countries facing similar coverage gaps and mortality burdens related to diarrhea and pneumonia. Ethiopia is one of 15 countries that account for 75 percent of the worldwide child deaths from pneumonia and diarrhea (IVAC 2013; Liu and others 2012), all of which are characterized by inadequate coverage of ORS and antibiotic treatment. This coverage issue underscores the relevance of using ECEA to understand distributional impact. Furthermore, future applications of ECEA should examine the impact of UPF for all four interventions studied here combined, and more broadly for a package of highly cost-effective child health interventions.

benefits per income group, and combined diarrhea treatment and rotavirus vaccination averts more deaths than diarrhea treatment alone. Second, the scale of the FRP benefits provided by UPF is small relative to the health benefits and private expenditures averted.

The numbers provide important information on the overall impacts of these interventions. However, it is also critical to view the results through the equity lens to understand the effects of UPF. The figures show how an investment of US$1 million in UPF in these interventions is distributed throughout the population. With regard to deaths averted, both diarrhea treatment and combined diarrhea treatment and rotavirus vaccination generally provide greater benefits to the poor. A major reason that both packages benefit the poorest is the higher burden of diarrheal disease among the poorest. An examination of private expenditures averted demonstrates a different trend. For both diarrhea treatment and combined diarrhea treatment and rotavirus vaccination the wealthy tend to experience greater relative gains in private expenditures averted, since private expenditures averted by UPF are relatively flat across income quintiles. Finally, the FRP benefits provided by UPF again favor the poorest by a substantial margin. In general, the

Limitations of the Analysis

Our analysis has several limitations. First, consistent with much of the cost-effectiveness literature, our disease models are static rather than dynamic. Dynamic models can more accurately capture synergies but require greater reliance on additional data and assumptions about disease behavior that may not be readily available. The inclusion of secondary cases prevented would lead to increased deaths averted and FRP benefits. Longer-term benefits of vaccination at ages older than five years were not addressed, however, because the burden of disease is largely concentrated among children under age five years.

Second, a more comprehensive accounting of household medical payments could be included, and other costs associated with the short-term treatment and long-term impacts of disease could be considered. In particular, direct nonmedical costs, such as for transportation and housing, and indirect costs due to disease or condition, including loss of earnings and impact on labor productivity, can be substantial, although empirical data are sparse. The focus on child health interventions in this study magnifies the productivity impacts associated with disease, given the inevitability of lost work time for caregivers and the higher number of years of lost productivity associated with childhood disability or death. For example, an economic analysis of the benefits of an array of vaccines estimated caretaker productivity to be roughly 20 percent of averted treatment costs for both pneumonia and rotavirus (Stack and others 2011). Averted productivity losses due to death from rotavirus and pneumonia were, respectively, approximately 15 and 18 times greater than treatment costs (Stack and others 2011). An economic analysis of rotavirus vaccine in Brazil includes costs associated with transportation and missed work in the total cost of treating gastroenteritis, finding that these costs constituted approximately 20 percent of the total cost per inpatient and almost 75 percent of the total cost per outpatient (Constenla and others 2008). Given the magnitude of costs involved in treatment beyond those strictly due to medical care, inclusion of nonmedical and indirect costs would increase the FRP benefits reported here and would also bolster the argument for prevention over treatment.

Third, data on the existing mix of public and private provision and purchase of health care are limited. Fourth, we did not pursue an uncertainty analysis because the purpose of this chapter is to expose broad implications for policy makers with simplicity and not to provide definitive estimates. Nevertheless, many sources of uncertainty underlie this analysis, including the imputed mortality rates derived from estimation, the efficacy of rotavirus and pneumococcal vaccines, and more generally the leap from efficacy to effectiveness for the treatment and prevention interventions studied here. The pricing of vaccines can also affect the findings (tables 19.5 and 19.6), a difference that can be even more pronounced when vaccines are considered stand-alone interventions. In addition, our modeling choices embody inherent uncertainty. For example, we assumed a uniform increase of 20 percentage points across all income quintiles to facilitate the interpretation of the results, although richer quintiles currently have higher treatment coverage than do poorer quintiles (tables 19.3 and 19.4). Finally, we chose to represent FRP according to the money-metric value of insurance provided. Alternatives include number of cases of poverty averted and avoided cases of forced borrowing and forced sales (Kruk, Goldmann, and Galea 2009).

Table 19.5 Deaths Averted and Financial Risk Protection Afforded by Combined Pneumonia Treatment and Pneumococcal Conjugate Vaccines, under Different Gavi Subsidies for Vaccines

	Income quintile				
	I (poorest)	II	III	IV	V (richest)
Deaths averted (per US$ 1million spent)					
$0.20 per dose	33	37	31	26	17
$3.50 per dose	31	34	27	23	15
Financial risk protection afforded (2011 US$)					
$0.20 per dose	2,710	1,170	780	640	510
$3.50 per dose	2,490	1,060	700	580	440

Table 19.6 Deaths Averted and Financial Risk Protection Afforded by Combined Diarrhea Treatment and Rotavirus Vaccines, under Different Gavi Subsidies for Vaccines

	Income quintile				
	I (poorest)	II	III	IV	V (richest)
Deaths averted (per US$1 million spent)					
$0.20 per dose	22	15	11	15	5
$2.50 per dose	14	14	10	9	3
Financial risk protection afforded (2011 US$)					
$0.20 per dose	480	190	80	70	30
$2.50 per dose	470	190	80	70	30

CONCLUSIONS

Future research will expand on this analysis by incorporating other essential features that promote realism of the scenario. Financial barriers are not the only barriers preventing individuals from seeking care: lack of information, limited availability of services, and distance to facilities are also important. In countries with weak health infrastructures, such as Ethiopia, health services may not be available even after the removal of some financial barriers. In particular, expanding health services to rural areas may require additional investments, such as strengthening or upgrading health facilities through training and deployment of skilled health workers, providing essential equipment, and improving infrastructure for service delivery. Inability to make these investments will, in turn, limit the expansion of coverage that UPF is able to achieve. To account for this challenge, we chose a specified coverage increment of 20 percentage points for all interventions. In addition, marginal costs of health care provision may increase substantially with increases in coverage, and these marginal costs may vary substantially depending on the population subgroups targeted (Brenzel and Claquin 1994; Brenzel and others 2006). This analysis also points to the substantial data requirements for understanding household health-seeking behaviors, OOP expenditures, and time and wages associated with illness.

The case study presented in this chapter is tailored to specific selected child health interventions. The interventions chosen for an essential child health package will involve other considerations, such as the acceptability of an intervention from a public health or clinical standpoint, and the scope of the chosen intervention.

The scale and rate of intervention rollout should be evaluated in the context of a thorough understanding of the strengths and weaknesses of the host health systems.

Our approach permits the incorporation of FRP in the economic evaluation of health policies. This methodology enables packages of benefits to be selected based on the quantitative inclusion of information on how much FRP can be bought, in addition to how much health can be bought, per dollar expenditure on health care. Some interventions and packages will rank higher on one or both metrics relative to others. Although this methodology does not provide advice on what is to be selectively prioritized and included in a benefits package, it allows policy makers to take both health and FRP into account when making decisions and thereby to more effectively target scarce resources to specific policy objectives.

This analysis also provides policy makers with information on how they might sequence the development of health care packages as the health and financial needs of populations evolve and resource envelopes change. Here, we show that the interventions studied would largely benefit the poorest populations, which can help to both progressively and efficiently prioritize limited resources. In addition, we point to substantial FRP benefits, which can help demonstrate how worthwhile investments in health can be in comparison with investments in other sectors such as education or transport, which is critical from the viewpoints of ministries of finance and development. This is why, while most of the health economics literature has focused on determining the efficient purchase of health benefits, with ECEA we intend to directly estimate the efficient purchase of nonhealth benefits, starting with distributional consequences such as equity and FRP.

ANNEX

The annex to this chapter is as follows. It is available at http://www.dcp-3.org/RMNCH.

- Annex 19A. Health Gains and Financial Risk Protection Afforded by Treatment and Prevention of Diarrhea and Pneumonia in Ethiopia: An Extended Cost-Effectiveness Analysis.

NOTE

Portions of this chapter were previously published:

- K. A. Johansson, S. T. Memirie, C. Pecenka, D. T. Jamison, and S. Verguet. 2015. "Health Gains and Financial Protection from Pneumococcal Vaccination and Pneumonia Treatment in Ethiopia: Results from an Extended Cost-Effectiveness Analysis." *PLoSOne* 10 (12): e0142691. doi:10.1371/journal.pone.0142691. © COPYRIGHT OWNER Johansson and others. Licensed under Creative Commons Attribution (CC BY 4.0) available at: https://creativecommons.org/licenses/by/4.0/.
- C. Pecenka, K. A. Johansson, S. T. Memirie, D. T. Jamison, and S. Verguet. 2015. "Health Gains and Financial Risk Protection: An Extended Cost-Effectiveness Analysis of Treatment and Prevention of Diarrhoea in Ethiopia." *BMJ Open* 5:e006402. doi:10.1136/bmjopen-2014-006402. © COPYRIGHT OWNER Pecenka and others. Licensed under Creative Commons Attribution (CC BY 4.0) available at: https://creativecommons.org/licenses/by/4.0/.

World Bank Income Classifications as of July 2014 are as follows, based on estimates of gross national income (GNI) per capita for 2013:

- Low-income countries (LICs) = US$1,045 or less
- Middle-income countries (MICs) are subdivided:
  a) lower-middle-income = US$1,046 to US$4,125
  b) upper-middle-income (UMICs) = US$4,126 to US$12,745
- High-income countries (HICs) = US$12,746 or more.

ACKNOWLEDGMENTS

We thank the Bill & Melinda Gates Foundation for funding through the Disease Control Priorities Network grant to the University of Washington, Seattle. Kjell Arne Johansson and Solomon Tessema Memirie were funded through the project Priorities 2020 by a grant from NORAD/The Norwegian Research Council. An earlier version of this paper was presented at a meeting of the authors of this volume, in Ferney-Voltaire, France, in November 2013. We received valuable comments from participants, including Robert E. Black, Zulfiqar Bhutta, Jerry Keusch, and Carol Levin, as well as from Elizabeth Brouwer and Zachary Olson.

REFERENCES

Amouzou, A., S. A. Richard, I. K. Friberg, J. Bryce, A. H. Baqui, and others. 2010. "How Well Does LiST Capture Mortality by Wealth Quintile? A Comparison of Measured versus Modeled Mortality Rates among Children Under-Five in Bangladesh." *International Journal of Epidemiology* 39 (Suppl 1): i186–92.

Bang, A., R. Bang, S. Baitule, M. H. Reddy, and M. Deshmukh. 1999. "Effect of Home-Based Neonatal Care and Management of Sepsis on Neonatal Mortality: Field Trial in Rural India." *The Lancet* 354 (9194): 1955–61.

Banteyerga, H. 2011. "Ethiopia's Health Extension Program: Improving Health through Community Involvement." *MEDICC Review* 13 (3): 46–49.

Baqui, A. H., S. E. Arifeen, E. K. Williams, S. Ahmed, I. Mannan, and others. 2009. "Effectiveness of Home-Based Management of Newborn Infections by Community Health Workers in Rural Bangladesh." *Pediatric Infectious Disease Journal* 28 (4): 304–10.

Bhutta, Z. A., G. L. Darmstadt, B. S. Hasan, and R. A. Haws. 2005. "Community Based Interventions for Improving Perinatal and Neonatal Health Outcomes in Developing Countries: A Review of the Evidence." *Pediatrics* 115 (2 Suppl): 519–618.

Black, S., H. Shinefield, B. Fireman, E. Lewis, P. Ray, and others. 2000. "Efficacy, Safety and Immunogenicity of Heptavalent Pneumococcal Conjugate Vaccine in Children. Northern California Kaiser Permanente Vaccine Study Center Group." *Pediatric Infectious Disease Journal* 19 (3): 187–95.

Brenzel, L., and P. Claquin. 1994. "Immunization Programs and Their Costs." *Social Science and Medicine* 39: 527–36.

Brenzel, L., L. J. Wolfson, J. Fox-Rushby, M. Miller, and N. A. Halsey. 2006. "Vaccine-Preventable Diseases." In *Disease Control Priorities in Developing Countries*, 2nd ed., edited by D. T. Jamison, J. G. Bremen, A. R. Measham, G. Alleyne, M. Claeson D. B. Evans, P. Jha, A. Mills, and P. Musgrove, 39–411. Washington, DC: World Bank and Oxford University Press.

Brown, J. R., and A. Finkelstein. 2008. "The Interaction of Public and Private Insurance: Medicaid and the Long-Term Care Insurance Market." *American Economic Review* 98 (3): 1083–102.

Buttery, J. P., S. B. Lambert, K. Grimwood, M. D. Nissen, E. J. Field, and others. 2011. "Reduction in Rotavirus-Associated Acute Gastroenteritis Following Introduction of Rotavirus Vaccine into Australia's National Childhood Vaccine Schedule." *Pediatric Infectious Disease Journal* 30 (1): S25–29.

Central Statistical Agency [Ethiopia] and ICF International. 2011. *Ethiopia Demographic and Health Survey*. Addis Ababa, Ethiopia, and Calverton, MD: Central Statistical Agency and ICF International.

Chan, M. 2012. "Remarks to the 65th World Health Assembly." May 26. http://www.who.int/mediacentre/news/releases/2012/wha65_closes_20120526/en/.

Constenla, D. O., A. C. Linhares, R. D. Rheingans, L. R. Antil, E. A. Waldman, and others. 2008. "Economic Impact of a Rotavirus Vaccine in Brazil." *Journal of Health, Population, and Nutrition* 26 (4): 388–96.

Cutts, F. T., S. M. Zaman, G. Enwere, S. Jaffar, O. S. Levine, and others. 2005. "Efficacy of Nine-Valent Pneumococcal Conjugate Vaccine against Pneumonia and Invasive Pneumococcal Disease in The Gambia: Randomised, Double-Blind, Placebo-Controlled Trial." *The Lancet* 365 (9465): 1139–46.

Federal Democratic Republic of Ethiopia, Ministry of Health. 2010. "Health Sector Development Program IV 2010/11- 2014/15." Ministry of Health.

Fekadu, G. A., M. W. Terefe, and G. A. Alemie. 2014. "Prevalence of Pneumonia among Under-Five Children in Este Town and the Surrounding Rural Kebeles, Northwest Ethiopia: A Community Based Cross Sectional Study." *Science* 2 (3): 150–55.

Finkelstein, A., and R. McKnight. 2008. "What Did Medicare Do? The Initial Impact of Medicare on Mortality and Out-of-Pocket Medical Spending." *Journal of Public Economics* 92 (7): 1644–68.

Fischer Walker, C. L., and R. E. Black. 2011. "Rotavirus Vaccine and Diarrhea Mortality: Quantifying Regional Variation in Effect Size." *BMC Public Health* 11 (Suppl 3): S16.

Fischer Walker, C. L., I. Rudan, L. Liu, H. Nair, E. Theodoratou, and others. 2013. "Global Burden of Childhood Pneumonia and Diarrhoea." *The Lancet* 381 (9875): 1405–16.

Gavi, the Vaccine Alliance. 2014. "Pneumococcal Vaccine Support." http://www.gavialliance.org/support/nvs/pneumococcal/.

Griffiths, U. K., V. S. Korczak, D. Ayalew, and A. Yigzaw. 2009. "Incremental System Costs of Introducing Combined DTwP-Hepatitis B-Hib Vaccine into National Immunization Services in Ethiopia." *Vaccine* 27 (9): 1426–32.

Haines, A., D. Sanders, U. Lehmann, A. K. Rowe, J. E. Lawn, and others. 2007. "Achieving Child Survival Goals: Potential Contribution of Community Health Workers." *The Lancet* 369 (9579): 2121–31.

Hsu, H. E., K. A. Shutt, M. R. Moore, B. W. Beall, N. M. Bennett, and others. 2009. "Effect of Pneumococcal Conjugate Vaccine on Pneumococcal Meningitis." *New England Journal of Medicine* 360 (3): 244–56.

IVAC (International Vaccine Access Center). 2013. "Pneumonia and Diarrhea Progress Report 2013." http://www.jhsph .edu/research/centers-and-institutes/ivac/resources/IVAC -2013-Pneumonia-Diarrhea-Progress-Report.pdf.

Johnson, H. L., M. Deloria-Knoll, O. S. Levine, S. K. Stoszek, H. L. Freimanis, and others. 2010. "Systematic Evaluation of Serotypes Causing Invasive Pneumococcal Disease among Children under Five: The Pneumococcal Global Serotype Project." *PLoS Medicine* 7 (10): e1000348.

Kim, S.-Y., S. Sweet, D. Slichter, and S. J. Goldie. 2010. "Health and Economic Impact of Rotavirus Vaccination in GAVI-Eligible Countries." *BMC Public Health* 10: 253.

Kruk, M. E., E. Goldmann, and S. Galea. 2009. "Borrowing and Selling to Pay for Health Care in Low- and Middle-Income Countries." *Health Affairs* 28 (4): 1056–66.

Lamberti, L. M., C. L. Fischer Walker, and R. E. Black. 2012. "Systematic Review of Diarrhea Duration and Severity in Children and Adults in Low- and Middle-Income Countries." *BMC Public Health* 12: 276.

The Lancet. 2012. "Universal Health Coverage." *The Lancet.* Theme issue, 380 (9845): 859–948. http://www.thelancet .com/themed-universal-health-coverage.

Laxminarayan, R., A. J. Mills, J. G. Breman, A. R. Measham, G. Alleyne, and others. 2006. "Advancement of Global Health: Key Messages from the Disease Control Priorities Project." *The Lancet* 367 (9517): 1193–208.

Liu, L., H. L. Johnson, S. Cousens, J. Perin, S. Scott, and others. 2012. "Global, Regional, and National Causes of Child Mortality: An Updated Systematic Analysis for 2010 with Time Trends since 2000." *The Lancet* 379 (9832): 2151–61.

McClellan, M., and J. Skinner. 2006. "The Incidence of Medicare." *Journal of Public Economics* 90 (1–2): 257–76.

McIntyre, D., and A. Mills, eds. 2012. "Research to Support Universal Coverage Reforms in Africa: The SHIELD Project." *Health Policy and Planning* 27 (Suppl 1).

Mihrete, T. S., G. A. Alemie, and A. S. Teferra. 2014. "Determinants of Childhood Diarrhea among Under-Five Children in Benishangul Gumuz Regional State, North West Ethiopia." *BMC Pediatrics* 14 (1): 102.

Munos, M. K., C. L. Fischer Walker, and R. E. Black. 2010. "The Effect of Oral Rehydration Solution and Recommended Home Fluids on Diarrhea Mortality." *International Journal of Epidemiology* 39 (Suppl 1): i75–87.

Rheingans, R. D., D. Atherly, and J. Anderson. 2012. "Distributional Impact of Rotavirus Vaccination in 25 GAVI Countries: Estimating Disparities in Benefits and Cost-Effectiveness." *Vaccine* 30 (Suppl): A15–23.

Rudan, I., L. Tomaskovic, C. Boschi-Pinto, H. Campbell, and the WHO Child Health Epidemiology Reference Group. 2004. "Global Estimate of the Incidence of Clinical Pneumonia among Children under Five Years of Age." *Bulletin of the World Health Organization* 82 (12): 895–903.

Salem, A. B. Z., and T. D. Mount. 1974. "A Convenient Descriptive Model of Income Distribution: The Gamma Density." *Econometrica* 42 (6): 1115–27.

Sinha, A., O. Levine, M. D. Knoll, F. Muhib, and T. A. Lieu. 2007. "Cost-Effectiveness of Pneumococcal Conjugate Vaccination in the Prevention of Child Mortality: An International Economic Analysis." *The Lancet* 369 (9559): 389–96.

Stack, M. L., S. Ozawa, D. M. Bishai, A. Mirelman, Y. Tam, and others. 2011. "Estimated Economic Benefits during the 'Decade of Vaccines' Include Treatment Savings, Gains in Labor Productivity." *Health Affairs* 30 (6): 1021–28.

Tate, J. E., M. M. Cortese, D. C. Payne, A. T. Curns, C. Yen, and others. 2011. "Uptake, Impact, and Effectiveness of Rotavirus Vaccination in the United States." *Pediatric Infectious Disease Journal* 30 (1): S56–60.

Theodoratou, E., S. Al-Jilaihawi, F. Woodward, J. Ferguson, A. Jhass, and others. 2010. "The Effect of Case Management on Childhood Pneumonia Mortality in Developing

Countries." *International Journal of Epidemiology* 39 (Suppl 1): i155–71.

Theodoratou, E., S. Johnson, A. Jhass, S. A. Madhi, A. Clark, and others. 2010. "The Effect of Haemophilus Influenzae Type B and Pneumococcal Conjugate Vaccines on Childhood Pneumonia Incidence, Severe Morbidity and Mortality." *International Journal of Epidemiology* 39 (Suppl 1): i172–85.

UNICEF (United Nations Children's Fund). 2013a. *Committing to Child Survival: A Promise Renewed*. Progress Report 2013. New York: UNICEF.

———. 2013b. *Levels and Trends in Child Mortality*. Report, UN Inter-agency Group for Child Mortality Estimation. New York: UNICEF.

United Nations. 2014. *World Population Prospects, 2012 Revision*. New York: UN, Department of Economic and Social Affairs, Population Division.

UN IGME (UN Inter-agency Group for Child Mortality Estimation). 2015. "Levels and Trends in Child Mortality". United Nations Children's Fund, New York.

Verguet, S., and D. T. Jamison. 2015. "Seeking the Efficient Purchase of Non-Health Benefits Using the Extended Cost-Effectiveness Analysis (ECEA) Framework." Disease Control Priorities, 3rd edition, Working Paper 11. http:// dcp-3.org/resources/seeking-efficient-purchase-non-health -benefits-using-extended-cost-effectiveness-analysis.

Verguet, S., R. Laxminarayan, and D. T. Jamison. 2015. "Universal Public Finance of Tuberculosis Treatment in India: An Extended Cost-Effectiveness Analysis." *Health Economics* 24 (3): 318–32.

Verguet, S., S. Murphy, B. Anderson, K. A. Johansson, R. Glass, and R. Rheingans. 2013. "Public Finance of Rotavirus Vaccination in India and Ethiopia: An Extended Cost-Effectiveness Analysis." *Vaccine* 31 (42): 4902–10.

Verguet, S., C. L. Gauvreau, S. Mishra, M. MacLennan, S. M. Murphy, and others. 2015. "The Consequences of Tobacco Tax on Household Health and Finances in Rich and Poor Smokers in China: An Extended Cost-Effectiveness Analysis." *The Lancet Global Health* 3 (4): e206–16.

Verguet, S., Z. D. Olson, J. B. Babigumira, D. Desalegn, K. A. Johansson, and others. 2015. "Health Gains and Financial Risk Protection Afforded from Public Financing of Selected Interventions in Ethiopia: An Extended Cost-Effectiveness Analysis." *The Lancet Global Health* 3 (5): e288–96.

Weinberger, D. M., R. Malley, and M. Lipsitch. 2011. "Serotype Replacement in Disease after Pneumococcal Vaccination." *The Lancet* 378 (9807): 1962–73.

WHO (World Health Organization). 1978. "Declaration of Alma-Ata." International Conference on Primary Health Care, Alma-Ata, September 6–12. http://www.who.int /publications/almaata_declaration_en.pdf.

———. 2010. *World Health Report 2010: Health Systems Financing, the Path to Universal Coverage*. Geneva: WHO.

———. 2012. Global Health Expenditure Database. Geneva. http://www.who.int/nha/country/en/index.html.

———. 2013. *World Health Report 2013: Research for Universal Health Coverage*. Geneva: WHO.

———. 2014. WHO-CHOICE. http://www.who.int/choice /costs/en.

———. 2015. Global Health Observatory (GHO) data. http:// www.who.int/gho/en.

Winfrey, W., R. McKinnon, and J. Stover. 2011. "Methods Used in the Lives Saved Tool (LiST)." *BMC Public Health* 11 (Suppl 3): S32.

World Bank. 2013. "World Development Indicators." World Bank, Washington, DC. http://data.worldbank.org /data-catalog/world-development-indicators.

Yen, C., J. A. A. Guardado, P. Alberto, D. S. Rodriguez Araujo, C. Mena, and others. 2011. "Decline in Rotavirus Hospitalizations and Health Care Visits for Childhood Diarrhea Following Rotavirus Vaccination in El Salvador." *Pediatric Infectious Disease Journal* 30 (1): S6–10.

You, D., L. Hug, S. Ejdemyr, P. Idele, D. Hogan, and others. 2015. 'Global, Regional, and National levels and Trends in Under-5 Mortality between 1990 and 2015, with Scenario-Based Projections to 2030: A Systematic Analysis by the UN Inter-Agency Group for Child Mortality Estimation. *The Lancet* 386: 2275–86.

DCP3 Series Acknowledgments

Disease Control Priorities, third edition *(DCP3)* compiles the global health knowledge of institutions and experts from around the world, a task that required the efforts of over 500 individuals, including volume editors, chapter authors, peer reviewers, advisory committee members, and research and staff assistants. For each of these contributions we convey our acknowledgement and appreciation. First and fore- most, we would like to thank our 33 volume editors who provided the intellectual vision for their volumes based on years of professional work in their respective fields, and then dedicated long hours to reviewing each chapter, providing leadership and guidance to authors, and framing and writing the summary chapters. We also thank our chapter authors who collectively volunteered their time and expertise to writing over 160 comprehensive, evidence-based chapters.

We owe immense gratitude to the institutional sponsor of this effort: The Bill & Melinda Gates Foundation. The Foundation provided sole financial support of the Disease Control Priorities Network. Many thanks to Program Officers Kathy Cahill, Philip Setel, Carol Medlin, and (currently) Damian Walker for their thoughtful interactions, guidance, and encouragement over the life of the project. We also wish to thank Jaime Sepúlveda for his longstanding support, including chairing the Advisory Committee for the second edition and, more recently, demonstrating his vision for *DCP3* while he was a special advisor to the Gates Foundation. We are also grateful to the University of Washington's Department of Global Health and successive chairs King Holmes and Judy Wasserheit for providing a home base for the *DCP3* Secretariat, which included intellectual collaboration, logistical coordination, and administrative support.

We thank the many contractors and consultants who provided support to specific volumes in the form of economic analytical work, volume coordination, chapter drafting, and meeting organization: the Center for Disease Dynamics, Economics, & Policy; Center for Chronic Disease Control; Center for Global Health Research; Emory University; Evidence to Policy Initiative; Public Health Foundation of India; QURE Healthcare; University of California, San Francisco; University of Waterloo; University of Queensland; and the World Health Organization.

We are tremendously grateful for the wisdom and guidance provided by our advisory committee to the editors. Steered by Chair Anne Mills, the advisory committee assures quality and intellectual rigor of the highest order for *DCP3*.

The National Academies of Science, Engineering, and Medicine, in collaboration with the Interacademy Medical Panel, coordinated the peer-review process for all *DCP3* chapters. Patrick Kelley, Gillian Buckley, Megan Ginivan, and Rachel Pittluck managed this effort and provided critical and substantive input.

The World Bank External and Corporate Relations Publishing and Knowledge division provided exceptional guidance and support throughout the demanding production and design process. We would particularly like to thank Carlos Rossel, the publisher; Mary Fisk, Nancy Lammers, Rumit Pancholi, and Deborah Naylor for their diligence and expertise. Additionally, we thank Jose de Buerba, Mario Trubiano, Yulia Ivanova, and Chiamaka Osuagwu of the World Bank for providing professional counsel on communications and marketing strategies.

Several U.S. and international institutions contributed to the organization and execution of meetings that supported the preparation and dissemination of *DCP3*.

We would like to express our appreciation to the following institutions:

- University of Bergen, consultation on equity (June 2011)
- University of California, San Francisco, surgery volume consultations (April 2012, October 2013, February 2014)
- Institute of Medicine, first meeting of the Advisory Committee to the Editors ACE (March 2013)
- Harvard Global Health Institute, consultation on policy measures to reduce incidence of noncommunicable diseases (July 2013)
- Institute of Medicine, systems strengthening meeting (September 2013)
- Center for Disease Dynamics, Economics, and Policy (Quality and Uptake meeting Sept 2013, reproductive and maternal health volume consultation November 2013)
- National Cancer Institute cancer consultation (November 2013)
- Union for International Cancer Control cancer consultation (November 2013, December 2014)

Carol Levin provided outstanding governance for cost and cost-effectiveness analysis. Stéphane Verguet added invaluable guidance in applying and improving the extended cost-effectiveness analysis method. Shane Murphy, Zachary Olson, Elizabeth Brouwer, Kristen Danforth, David Watkins, Jennifer Nguyen, and Jennifer Grasso provided exceptional research assistance and analytic assistance. Brianne Adderley ably managed the budget and project processes. The efforts of these individuals were absolutely critical to producing this series, and we are thankful for their commitment.

Volume and Series Editors

VOLUME EDITORS

Robert E. Black

Robert E. Black, MD, MPH, has focused his research and professional activities on reducing the number of unnecessary child deaths in developing countries. He is conducting epidemiologic research on the interaction of infectious diseases and nutrition, clinical and community-based trials of new vaccines to prevent childhood infectious diseases, and trials of nutritional interventions to reduce infectious disease morbidity and mortality, as well as improve growth and development. He is also assisting with implementation of disease control and nutrition programs in developing countries and conducting evaluations of their effectiveness and mortality impact. He is currently a Professor of International Health at Johns Hopkins Bloomberg School of Public Health.

Ramanan Laxminarayan

Ramanan Laxminarayan is Vice President for Research and Policy at the Public Health Foundation of India, and he directs the Center for Disease Dynamics, Economics & Policy in Washington, D.C., and New Delhi. His research deals with the integration of epidemiological models of infectious diseases and drug resistance into the economic analysis of public health problems. He was one of the key architects of the Affordable Medicines Facility for malaria, a novel financing mechanism to improve access and delay resistance to antimalarial drugs. In 2012, he created the Immunization Technical Support Unit in India, which has been credited with improving immunization coverage in the country. He teaches at Princeton University.

Marleen Temmerman

Professor Marleen Temmerman is Chair, Department Obstetrics and Gynaecology, and Director, Women's Health and Research, Aga Khan University, East Africa, since 2015. She was previously Director, Reproductive Health and Research, World Health Organization. She is the Founding Director of the International Centre of Reproductive Health, Ghent University, Belgium, with sister organizations in Kenya and Mozambique. She has a strong academic background, with over 500 publications in the area of women's health, and she has mentored PhD students around the globe.

In 2007, she was elected Senator in the Belgian Parliament. She served as a member of the iERG (independent expert review group) of the United Nations Secretaries-Generals' Every Woman, Every Child platform to accelerate Millennium Development Goals (MDGs) 4 and 5. She is one of the penholders of the new Global Strategy for Women's, Children, and Adolescents' health, transitioning from the MDGs to the Sustainable Development Goals.

Neff Walker

Neff Walker is a Senior Scientist in the Institute for International Programs, Department of International Health, Bloomberg School of Public Health, Johns Hopkins University. Before coming to Johns Hopkins University, he spent four years at UNICEF as the Senior Advisor for estimation and modeling related to the impact of HIV/AIDS, as well as serving as UNICEF's focal point for the Child Health Epidemiology Reference Group (CHERG). From 1998 through 2003, Neff worked as the Senior Advisor for statistics and modeling at United Nations Program on HIV/AIDS. In both positions a primary focus of his work was the development and implementation of standard methods for estimation and modeling related to disease burden.

SERIES EDITORS

Dean T. Jamison

Dean T. Jamison is a Senior Fellow in Global Health Sciences at the University of California, San Francisco, and an Emeritus Professor of Global Health at the University of Washington. He previously held academic appointments at Harvard University and the University of California, Los Angeles; he was an economist on the staff of the World Bank, where he was lead author of the World Bank's *World Development Report 1993: Investing in Health*. He was lead editor of *DCP2*. He holds a PhD in economics from Harvard University and is an elected member of the Institute of Medicine of the U.S. National Academy of Sciences. He recently served as Co-Chair and Study Director of *The Lancet's* Commission on Investing in Health.

Rachel Nugent

Rachel Nugent is a Research Associate Professor in the Department of Global Health at the University of Washington. She was formerly Deputy Director of Global Health at the Center for Global Development, Director of Health and Economics at the Population Reference Bureau, Program Director of Health and Economics Programs at the Fogarty International Center of the National Institutes of Health, and senior economist at the Food and Agriculture Organization of the United Nations. From 1991–97, she was associate professor and department chair in economics at Pacific Lutheran University. She has advised the World Health Organization, the U.S. government, and nonprofit organizations on the economics and policy environment of noncommunicable diseases.

Hellen Gelband

Hellen Gelband is Associate Director for Policy at the Center for Disease Dynamics, Economics & Policy (CDDEP). Her work spans infectious disease, particularly malaria and antibiotic resistance, and noncommunicable disease policy, mainly in low- and middle-income countries. Before joining CDDEP, then Resources for the Future, she conducted policy studies at the (former) Congressional Office of Technology Assessment, the Institute of Medicine of the U.S. National Academies, and a number of international organizations.

Susan Horton

Susan Horton is Professor at the University of Waterloo and holds the Centre for International Governance Innovation (CIGI) Chair in Global Health Economics in the Balsillie School of International Affairs there. She has consulted for the World Bank, the Asian Development Bank, several United Nations agencies, and the International Development Research Centre, among others, in work carried out in over 20 low- and middle-income countries. She led the work on nutrition for the Copenhagen Consensus in 2008, when micronutrients were ranked as the top development priority. She has served as associate provost of graduate studies at the University of Waterloo, vice-president academic at Wilfrid Laurier University in Waterloo, and interim dean at the University of Toronto at Scarborough.

Prabhat Jha

Prabhat Jha is the founding director of the Centre for Global Health Research at St. Michael's Hospital and holds Endowed and Canada Research Chairs in Global Health in the Dalla Lana School of Public Health at the University of Toronto. He is lead investigator of the Million Death Study in India, which quantifies the causes of death and key risk factors in over two million homes over a 14-year period. He is also Scientific Director of the Statistical Alliance for Vital Events, which aims to expand reliable measurement of causes of death worldwide. His research includes the epidemiology and economics of tobacco control worldwide.

Ramanan Laxminarayan

See the list of Volume Editors.

Charles N. Mock

Charles N. Mock, MD, PhD, FACS, has training as both a trauma surgeon and an epidemiologist. He worked as a surgeon in Ghana for four years, including at a rural hospital (Berekum) and at the Kwame Nkrumah University of Science and Technology (Kumasi). In 2005–07, he served as Director of the University of Washington's Harborview Injury Prevention and Research Center. In 2007–10, he worked at the World Health Organization (WHO) headquarters in Geneva, where he was responsible for developing the WHO's trauma care activities. In 2010, he returned to his position as Professor of Surgery (with joint appointments as Professor of Epidemiology and Professor of Global Health) at the University of Washington. His main interests include the spectrum of injury control, especially as it pertains to low- and middle-income countries: surveillance, injury prevention, prehospital care, and hospital-based trauma care. He is President (2013–15) of the International Association for Trauma Surgery and Intensive Care.

Contributors

Frances E. Aboud
Department of Psychology, McGill University, Montreal, Canada

Fernando Althabe
Institute for Clinical Effectiveness and Health Policy, Buenos Aires, Argentina

Ashvin Ashok
Clinton Health Access Initiative, Boston, Massachusetts, United States

Henrik Axelson
Partnership for Maternal, Newborn and Child Health, World Health Organization, Phnom Penh, Cambodia

Rajiv Bahl
Department of Reproductive Health and Research, World Health Organization, Geneva, Switzerland

Akinrinola Bankole
Guttmacher Institute, New York, New York, United States

Zulfiqar A. Bhutta
Division of Women and Child Health, Aga Khan University Hospital, Karachi, Pakistan

Lori A. Bollinger
Avenir Health, Glastonbury, Connecticut, United States

Deborah C. Hay Burgess
Bill & Melinda Gates Foundation, Seattle, Washington, United States

Doris Chou
Department of Reproductive Health and Research, World Health Organization, Geneva, Switzerland

Yue Chu
Johns Hopkins Bloomberg School of Public Health, Baltimore, Maryland, United States

John Cleland
Department of Population Health, London School of Hygiene & Tropical Medicine, London, United Kingdom

Simon Cousens
MARCH Center, London School of Hygiene & Tropical Medicine, London, United Kingdom

Jai K. Das
Division of Women and Child Health, Aga Khan University, Karachi, Pakistan

Julia R. Driessen
Department of Health Policy and Management, University of Pittsburgh, Pittsburgh, Pennsylvania, United States

Valérie D'Acemont
Swiss Tropical and Public Health Institute, University of Basel, Basel, Switzerland

Alex Ezeh
African Population and Health Research Center, Nairobi, Kenya

Daniel R. Feikin
Centers for Disease Control and Prevention, Atlanta, Georgia, United States

Véronique Filippi
Department of Infectious Disease Epidemiology, London School of Hygiene & Tropical Medicine, London, United Kingdom

Mariel M. Finucane
Gladstone Institutes, University of California, San Francisco, San Francisco, California, United States

Christa Fischer Walker
Johns Hopkins Bloomberg School of Public Health, Baltimore, Maryland, United States

Brendan Flannery
Centers for Disease Control and Prevention, Atlanta, Georgia, United States

Ingrid K. Friberg
Johns Hopkins Bloomberg School of Public Health, Baltimore, Maryland, United States

Bela Ganatra
Department of Reproductive Health and Research, World Health Organization, Geneva, Switzerland

Marijke Gielen
Department of Paediatrics, University Hospitals Leuven, Leuven, Belgium

Wendy Graham
The Institute of Applied Health Sciences, University of Aberdeen, Aberdeen, United Kingdom

A. Metin Gülmezoglu
Department of Reproductive Health and Research, World Health Organization, Geneva, Switzerland

Demissie Habte
Board of Trustees, International Clinical Epidemiological Network, Addis Ababa, Ethiopia

Mary J. Hamel
Centers for Disease Control and Prevention, Atlanta, Georgia, United States

Davidson H. Hamer
Department of Global Health, Boston University School of Public Health, Boston, Massachusetts, United States

Peter M. Hansen
Gavi Alliance, Geneva, Switzerland

Karen Hardee
Population Council, New York, New York, United States

Julie M. Herlihy
Department of Global Health, Boston University School of Public Health, Boston, Massachusetts, United States

Natasha Hezelgrave
Division of Women's Health, King's College London School of Medicine, London, United Kingdom

Kenneth Hill
Harvard T. H. Chan School of Public Health, Boston, Massachusetts, United States

G. Justus Hofmeyr
Effective Care Research Unit, East London Hospital Complex, East London, South Africa

Dan Hogan
Department of Health Statistics and Informatics, World Health Organization, Geneva, Switzerland

Susan Horton
School of Public Health and Health Systems, University of Waterloo, Waterloo, Canada

Aamer Imdad
SUNY Upstate Medical University, Syracuse, New York, United States

Dean T. Jamison
Department of Global Health, University of Washington, Seattle, Washington, United States

Kjell Arne Johansson
Department of Public Health & Centre for International Health, University of Bergen, Bergen, Norway

Gerald T. Keusch
Boston University School of Medicine, Boston, Massachusetts, United States

Margaret E. Kruk
Harvard T.H. Chan School of Public Health, Boston, Massachusetts, United States

Rohail Kumar
Division of Women and Child Health, Aga Khan University, Karachi, Pakistan

Zohra S. Lassi
Division of Women and Child Health, Aga Khan University, Karachi, Pakistan

Joy E. Lawn
MARCH Center, London School of Hygiene & Tropical Medicine, London, United Kingdom

Theresa A. Lawrie
Department of Reproductive Health and Research, World Health Organization, Geneva, Switzerland

Lindsey Lenters
The Hospital for Sick Children, Toronto, Canada

Carol Levin
Department of Global Health, University of Washington, Seattle, Washington, United States

Li Liu
Johns Hopkins Bloomberg School of Public Health, Baltimore, Maryland, United States

Colin Mathers
Department of Health Statistics and Informatics, World Health Organization, Geneva, Switzerland

Agustina Mazzoni
Institute for Clinical Effectiveness and Health Policy, Buenos Aires, Argentina

Solomon Tessema Memirie
Department of Public Health & Centre for International Health, University of Bergen, Bergen, Norway

Claudia Garcia Moreno
Department of Reproductive Health and Research, World Health Organization, Geneva, Switzerland

Sheila Mwero
African Population and Health Research Center, Nairobi, Kenya

Arindam Nandi
Center for Disease Dynamics, Economics & Policy, Washington, DC, United States

Olufemi T. Oladapo
Department of Reproductive Health and Research, World Health Organization, Geneva, Switzerland

Shefali Oza
MARCH Center, London School of Hygiene & Tropical Medicine, London, United Kingdom

Christopher J. Paciorek
Department of Statistics, University of California, Berkeley, Berkeley, California, United States

Clint Pecenka
PATH, Seattle, Washington, United States

Carine Ronsmans
School of Public Health, Sichuan University, Chengdu, China

Rehana A. Salam
Division of Women and Child Health, Aga Khan University, Karachi, Pakistan

Lale Say
Department of Reproductive Health and Research, World Health Organization, Geneva, Switzerland

Peter Sheehan
Victoria Institute of Strategic Economic Studies, Melbourne, Victoria, Australia

João Paula Souza
Department of Social Medicine, Ribeirão Preto School of Medicine, University of São Paulo, São Paulo, Brazil

Meghan Stack
Johns Hopkins Bloomberg School of Public Health, Baltimore, Maryland, United States

Cynthia Stanton
Johns Hopkins Bloomberg School of Public Health, Baltimore, Maryland, United States

Karin Stenberg
Department of Health Systems Governance and Financing, World Health Organization, Geneva, Switzerland

Gretchen A. Stevens
Department of Health Statistics and Information Systems, World Health Organization, Geneva, Switzerland

John Stover
Avenir Health, Glastonbury, Connecticut, United States

Kim Sweeny
Victoria University, Melbourne, Victoria, Australia

Stéphane Verguet
Department of Global Health and Population, Harvard T. H. Chan School of Public Health, Boston, Massachusetts, United States

Kerri Wazny
The Hospital for Sick Children, Toronto, Canada

Aisha K. Yousafzai
Department of Paediatrics and Child Health, Aga Khan University, Karachi, Pakistan

Abdhalah Kasiira Ziraba
African Population and Health Research Center, Nairobi, Kenya

Advisory Committee to the Editors

Carol Medlin
Senior Health and Nutrition Specialist,
Health, Nutrition, and Population Global Practice,
World Bank, Washington, DC, United States

Alvaro Moncayo
Researcher, Universidad de los Andes, Bogotá,
Colombia

Jaime Montoya
Executive Director, Philippine Council for Health
Research and Development, Taguig City, the
Philippines

Ole Norheim
Professor, University of Bergen, Bergen, Norway

Folashade Omokhodion
Professor, University College Hospital, Ibadan,
Nigeria

Toby Ord
President, Giving What We Can, Oxford, United
Kingdom

K. Srinath Reddy
President, Public Health Foundation of India,
New Delhi, India

Sevkat Ruacan
Dean, Koç University School of Medicine, Istanbul,
Turkey

Jaime Sepúlveda
Executive Director, Global Health Sciences, University
of California, San Francisco, San Francisco, California,
United States

Richard Skolnik
Lecturer, Health Policy Department, Yale School
of Public Health, New Haven, Connecticut,
United States

Stephen Tollman
Professor, University of Witwatersrand, Johannesburg,
South Africa

Jürgen Unützer
Professor, Department of Psychiatry, University of
Washington, Seattle, Washington, United States

Damian Walker
Senior Program Officer, Bill & Melinda Gates
Foundation, Seattle, Washington, United States

Ngaire Woods
Director, Global Economic Governance Program,
Oxford University, Oxford, United Kingdom

Nopadol Wora-Urai
Professor, Department of Surgery, Phramongkutklao
Hospital, Bangkok, Thailand

Kun Zhao
Researcher, China National Health Development
Research Center, Beijing, China

Reviewers

Diego G. Bassani
University of Toronto Centre for Global Child Health, Toronto, Canada

Florencia Lopez Boo
Inter-American Development Bank, Washington, DC, United States

Lara Brearley

Edward I. Broughton
University Research Co., Washington, DC, United States

William Checkley
Johns Hopkins University School of Medicine, Baltimore, Maryland, United States

Jacqueline E. Darroch
Guttmacher Institute, Seattle, Washington, United States

Jai K. Das
Division of Women and Child Health, Aga Khan University, Karachi, Pakistan

Mercedes de Onis
Growth Assessment and Surveillance Unit, World Health Organization, Geneva, Switzerland

Shannon Doocy
Johns Hopkins Bloomberg School of Public Health, Baltimore, Maryland, United States

Karen Edmond
University of Western Australia School of Paediatrics and Child Health, Perth, Western Australia, Australia

Alex Ergo
Broad Band Associates, Yangon, Myanmar

Victoria Fan
Office of Public Health Studies, University of Hawaii, Honolulu, Hawaii, United States

Ingrid K. Friberg
Norwegian Institute of Public Health, Oslo, Norway

Anna Glasier
Society of Family Planning, University of Edinburgh, Edinburgh, Scotland

Joseph E. de Graft-Johnson
Save the Children, Accra, Ghana

Glenda Gray
Perinatal HIV Research Unit, Chris Hani Baragwanath Hospital, Johannesburg, South Africa

Richard L. Guerrant
University of Virginia School of Medicine, Charlottesville, Virginia, United States

Jane Hutchings
PATH, Seattle, Washington, United States

Claudio F. Lanata
Instituto de Investigación Nutricional, Lima, Peru

Karen Macours
Paris School of Economics, Paris, France

Matthews Mathai
Department of Maternal, Newborn, and Child and Adolescent Health, World Health Organization, Geneva, Switzerland

Jeff K. Mathe
Mbabane Government Hospital, Mbabane, Swaziland

William McGreevey
Department of International Health, Georgetown University, Washington, DC, United States

Regina Moench-Pfanner
Global Alliance for Improved Nutrition, Geneva, Switzerland

Luke C. Mullany
Johns Hopkins Bloomberg School of Public Health, Baltimore, Maryland, United States

Omotade Olayemi Olufemi-Julius
University of Ibadan Institute of Child Health, Ibadan, Nigeria

Walter A. Orenstein
Emory Vaccine Center, Emory University, Atlanta, Georgia, United States

Roman Prymula
University Hospital Hradec Králové, Hradec Králové, Czech Republic

Usha Ramakrishnan
Emory University Rollins School of Public Health, Atlanta, Georgia, United States

Helen Rees
Wits Reproductive Health and HIV Institute, Johannesburg, South Africa

Alexander K. Rowe
Center for Global Health, Centers for Disease Control and Prevention, Atlanta, Georgia, United States

Enrique Ruelas
Institute for Healthcare Improvement, Cambridge, Massachusetts, United States

Harhad Sanghvi
Jhpiego, Baltimore, Maryland, United States

Katherine Seib
Emory Vaccine Center, Emory University, Atlanta, Georgia, United States

Saba Shahid
Indus Hospital, Karachi, Pakistan

Karin Stenberg
Department of Health Systems Governance and Financing, World Health Organization, Geneva, Switzerland

Jorge E. Tolosa
Oregon Health & Science University, Portland, Oregon, United States

Nana A. Y. Twum-Danso
The Bill & Melinda Gates Foundation, Accra, Ghana

Index

Boxes, figures, maps, notes, and tables are indicated by b, f, m, n, and t following page numbers.

delivery platforms. *See also* community-based
   interventions; hospitals; primary health centers
   cost-effectiveness of interventions, 327–28
   cost of scaling up, 17–18
   interventions for maternal and child mortality and
      morbidity, 8, 11–13*t*
demand-side interventions, 19
Democratic Republic of Congo. *See* Congo, Democratic
   Republic of
Demographic and Health Surveys, 26, 51, 60, 85, 96,
   174, 176, 188*b*, 346
demographic dividend, 96, 305, 311–12
dengue fever, 147
depression, 5, 6, 39
   child development, effect of maternal
      depression on, 247
   postpartum depression, 60
Dettrick, Z., 289
Development Assistance Committee (Organisation for
   Economic Co-operation and Development), 319
diabetes, 6
   treatment, 125
diarrheal diseases, 1, 163–85
   antibiotics, use of, 170–71, 179
   behavioral interventions, 174–77
   burden of infection, 164
      by region, 164–65*f*
   child mortality (under five) and, 78, 79*t*, 163
   cholera, 172
   community-based interventions, 176, 266
   community-led total sanitation, 176–77
   cost-effectiveness of interventions, 177–78, 177*t*, 324
   cost of interventions, 177–78, 177*t*, 328
      scaling up, 18
   definitions and classification, 163–64
   early childhood development and, 246
   environmental enteric dysfunction, 167–69, 168*b*
   in Ethiopia, treatment and prevention, 345–61.
      See also Ethiopia
   etiologies, 164–65
   handwashing, 174–75
   health care seeking, 175–76
   incidence, 163, 164
   inflammatory diarrhea and dysentery, 166, 169
   interventions, 163, 164*b*, 169–77, 169*b*
   mortality due to, 78, 164
   natural history, 166
   nutrition, 173
   oral rehydration solutions (ORS). *See* oral
      rehydration solutions
   overview, 163
   persistent, 166–67
   preventive interventions, 169*b*

rotavirus, 165, 171–72, 350, 351*t*
subclinical infections, 167
therapeutic interventions, 169–71, 169*b*
transmission and epidemiology, 165–66
tropical enteropathy, 167
vaccines, 171
water, sanitation, and hygiene, 174
watery, 166
zinc supplementation, 173–74
diet. *See* nutrition; vitamin and mineral supplements
diphtheria, tetanus, and pertussis (DTP) vaccines, 188*b*,
   189, 190–91, 300, 324–25
disability-adjusted life years (DALYs)
   in CEA vs. ECEA framework, 343*n*5
   community-base care and, 277–78, 277*f*
   cost-effectiveness results using, 321, 330
   diarrheal diseases and, 177, 178
   malnutrition and, 217, 326
   maternal morbidity and, 61, 129–30
   pneumonia and, 323
   quality of services and, 293–94, 294*t*
   vaccination and, 187, 189, 197–98
   WHO metrics and, 330*n*1
*Disease Control Priorities in Developing
   Countries* (DCP)
   coverage of other volumes, 2, 320*t*
   evolution of series and third edition, xiii, 3*b*, 300,
      319
Djibouti, wasting in, 91*b*
Dolea, C., 58
domestic violence. *See* violence against women
Doppler ultrasound, use of, 125–26
dysentery, 166, 169

E
early childhood development, 8, 241–61
   cerebral malaria and, 246
   child nutrition and, 249–51, 254–55
   conditions affecting, 242–48, 249*f*
   cost-benefit of interventions, 254
   delayed mental development, 247
   diarrhea and, 246
   enteropathy and, 246
   environmental conditions and, 245–46
   Family Care Indicators, 243
   fatty acids and, 249–50
   Home Observation for Measurement of the
      Environment (HOME) Inventory, 243, 243*f*,
      248, 251*f*
   infections and, 246, 251–52, 255
   interventions to enhance, 248–54
   macronutrients and, 244, 244*f*
   maternal mental health and, 247, 255

height-for-age and. *See* stunting

iron supplementation, 231–32

maternal mortality and morbidity, 124–25, 124*t*

maternal nutrition, 234–35*t*, 246–47

interventions, 252–53

psychosocial stimulation integrated with child nutrition, 251

Nutrition Impact Model Study (NIMS), 85

O

obstetric fistula, 6, 60

obstetric hemorrhage. *See* postpartum hemorrhage

obstructed labor. *See* childbirth

official development assistance, 2

OneHealth Tool, 304, 304*b*, 307, 308

Onwujekwe, O., 103

open defecation, 176, 232

oral cholera vaccine, 188*b*, 197

oral rehydration salts, use of, 350

oral rehydration solutions (ORS), 169–70, 171, 173, 179, 286–87, 324, 350

Ouagadougou Declaration (West Africa, 2011), 100

overweight, 7, 8

oxytocin, 116, 117*t*, 118, 273

Ozawa, S., 320

P

Paciorek, C. J., 85

Paczkowski, M., 292

Pakistan

child mortality (under five) in, 78–79

community-based interventions in, 270

home visits and reduction in newborn deaths, 265

lady health worker program, 252*b*, 267*b*, 273

perinatal packages, 151

contraception in, 102

DTP vaccine in, 197

Early Child Development Scale-Up Trial, 252*b*

family planning in, 102

cost-effectiveness of, 103

handwashing in, 175

home visits and reduction in newborn deaths in, 336

Integrated Community Case Management (iCCM) in, 153, 154

maternal depression's effect on child development in, 248

pneumonia in, 153

stillbirth data from, 76

Thinking Healthy program, 253

vaccine costs in, 197

wasting in, 207

Palmer, N., 19

Pan-American Health Organization's revolving fund, 325

Papua New Guinea

Integrated Management of Neonatal and Childhood Illness (IMNCI) in, 151

wasting in, 91*b*

parasite infestations, 267–68

partograph, use of, 126

Peabody, J. W., 18

pelvic inflammatory disease (PID), 34–35

performance-based financing, 18, 102, 291, 292–93

perinatal morbidity and mortality

evidence-based policy making and interventions, 124*t*, 127*t*

levels and trends, 6

pertussis immunization. *See* diphtheria, tetanus, and pertussis vaccines

Peru

diarrheal diseases in, 167, 170

IMCI effectiveness in, 149

maternal depression's effect on child development in, 248

Philippines

accredited hospitals in, 292

Integrated Management of Neonatal and Childhood Illness (IMNCI) in, 151

payment-for-performance incentives in, 18, 292

physicians, 286. *See also* health workers/professionals

PID (pelvic inflammatory disease), 34–35

pneumococcal conjugate vaccines, 14, 15, 81, 188*b*, 193–94, 199, 325, 348–50, 349–50*t*

pneumonia, 1

antibiotics, use of, 348

child mortality (under five) and, 79*t*

in children under age of five, 6, 78

community-based care, 266

cost-effectiveness of interventions, 323, 353*f*

cost of scaling up treatment, 18

in Ethiopia, treatment and prevention, 345–61. *See also* Ethiopia

universal public finance for pneumonia treatment, 15

Pneumonia Etiology Research for Child Health project, 145

Polio Eradication and Endgame Strategic Plan 2013-2018, 191

polio vaccines, 188*b*, 191, 325

postnatal care, 128–29

postpartum depression, 60, 248

postpartum endometritis, 123

Child Health Epidemiology Reference Group (CHERG). *See* Child Health Epidemiology Reference Group
chlorhexidine application to umbilical cord, 129
cholera vaccines, approval of, 197
Choosing Interventions that are Cost-Effective project, 329
complementary feeding guidelines, 230
essential newborn care, 128
Expanded Program on Immunization, 178
female genital mutilation (FGM) study, 40
fever treatment guidelines, 140, 148, 149*f*
Gavi (Vaccine Alliance). *See* Gavi
Global Action Plan for Prevention and Control of Pneumonia, 145
Global Database on Child Growth and Malnutrition, 85
Global Health Estimates, 61, 96
Guidance Panel on Task Shifting, 18
health system building blocks, 64
hepatitis B vaccine recommendations, 193
infant and young child feeding (IYCF) guidelines, 225, 226*t*, 235–36
infertility, definition and measurement of, 35–36
Integrated Management of Childhood Illness (IMCI), 130, 137, 145, 146*t*, 148–50, 149*f*, 266
Japanese encephalitis (JE) vaccine recommendations, 195
Joint Malnutrition data set, 208
malaria vaccine recommendations, 147, 196
maternal morbidity study, 56
Maternal Morbidity Working Group, 56
maternal mortality study, 52
measle vaccine recommendations, 191
Multi-country Study on Women's Health and Domestic Violence against Women, 38, 119
nutrition guidelines, 216
oral rehydration solutions, recommendations for, 169
pneumonia guidelines, 145
polio vaccine recommendations, 191
preeclampsia and eclampsia prevention, 119
rotavirus recommendations, 194
safe abortion technologies, 106
SAFE (surgery, antibiotics, facial cleanliness, and environmental improvements) strategy for trachoma elimination, 251
Special Programme for Research and Training in Tropical Diseases, 152
Strategic Advisory Group of Experts on

Immunization and Malaria Policy Advisory Committee, 188*b*, 196
10-step malnutrition program, 214
universal health coverage and, 300, 345
unsafe abortion
    definition of, 28
    indirect approach to study of, 29, 31
uterine massage, 118
violence against women
    clinical and policy guidelines, 108
    estimates on, 38
WHO/CHOICE model, 276, 329
WHO/PRE-EMPT Calcium in Pre-eclampsia (CAP), 120
World Health Report (2010), 342
Young Infants Study Group and Young Infants Clinical Signs Study Group, 143
World Report on Disability (WHO & World Bank), 36
worm and parasite infestations, 267–68

Y
yellow fever vaccine, 188*b*, 195, 325
Yemen
    female genital mutilation (FGM) in, 39–40
    stunting and height-for-age in, 88
    teenage pregnancy in, 28
youth centers, 105

Z
Zaidi, A. K. M., 143
Zambia
    accredited hospitals in, 292
    child health services, costs of, 328
    community-based interventions in, 266
        Lufwanyama Neonatal Survival Project, 277
        nutrition, 217
    Integrated Community Case Management (iCCM) in, 153, 154
    malnutrition in, 215
    maternal mortality and morbidity in, 65
    pneumonia in, 145
    training of birth attendants to administer neonatal resuscitation in, 151
Zimbabwe
    adolescent-friendly contraceptive services in, 105
    cash transfers in, 290
    cholera in, 197
    contraceptive use in, 97, 100*f*
zinc deficiencies, 7, 8, 173, 227, 231
    diarrheal diseases and, 169, 173–74, 324
    supplementation, 13*t*, 125

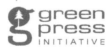